Oxford Medical Publications

Oxford Handbook of
Learning and Intellectual Disability Nursing

T0369596

Published and forthcoming Oxford Handbooks in Nursing

Oxford Handbook of Midwifery
Janet Medforth, Susan Battersby, Maggie Evans, Beverley Marsh, and Angela Walker

Oxford Handbook of Mental Health Nursing
Edited by Patrick Callaghan and Helen Waldock

Oxford Handbook of Children's and Young People's Nursing
Edited by Edward Alan Glasper, Gillian McEwing, and Jim Richardson

Oxford Handbook of Nurse Prescribing
Sue Beckwith and Penny Franklin

Oxford Handbook of Cancer Nursing
Edited by Mike Tadman and Dave Roberts

Oxford Handbook of Cardiac Nursing
Edited by Kate Johnson and Karen Rawlings-Anderson

Oxford Handbook of Primary Care Nursing
Edited by Vari Drennan and Claire Goodman

Oxford Handbook of Gastrointestinal Nursing
Edited by Christine Norton, Julia Williams, Claire Taylor, Annmarie Nunwa, and Kathy Whayman

Oxford Handbook of Respiratory Nursing
Terry Robinson and Jane Scullion

Oxford Handbook of Nursing Older People
Beverley Tabernacle, Marie Barnes, and Annette Jinks

Oxford Handbook of Clinical Skills in Adult Nursing
Jacqueline Randle, Frank Coffey, and Martyn Bradbury

Oxford Handbook of Emergency Nursing
Edited by Robert Crouch, Alan Charters, Mary Dawood, and Paula Bennett

Oxford Handbook of Dental Nursing
Kevin Seymour, Dayananda Samarawickrama, Elizabeth Boon and Rebecca Parr

Oxford Handbook of Diabetes Nursing
Lorraine Avery and Sue Beckwith

Oxford Handbook of Musculoskeletal Nursing
Edited by Susan Oliver

Oxford Handbook of Women's Health Nursing
Sunanda Gupta, Debra Holloway, and Ali Kubba

Oxford Handbook of Perioperative Practice
Suzanne Hughes and Andy Mardell

Oxford Handbook of Critical Care Nursing
Sheila Adam and Sue Osborne

Oxford Handbook of Neuroscience Nursing
Sue Woodward and Cath Waterhouse

Oxford Handbook of General and Adult Nursing
Ann Close and George Castledine

Oxford Handbook of
Learning and Intellectual Disability Nursing

Second Edition

Owen Barr
Professor of Nursing and Intellectual Disabilities,
Ulster University, Londonderry, UK,
Visiting Professor, Faculty of Health Sciences,
University of Maribor, Slovenia

Bob Gates
Professor of Learning Disabilities, University of
West London, UK, Emeritus Professor, University
of Hertfordshire, UK, Visiting Professor of Learning
Disabilities, University of Derby, and Editor in
Chief of the *British Journal of Learning Disabilities*

OXFORD
UNIVERSITY PRESS

OXFORD
UNIVERSITY PRESS

Great Clarendon Street, Oxford, OX2 6DP,
United Kingdom

Oxford University Press is a department of the University of Oxford.
It furthers the University's objective of excellence in research, scholarship,
and education by publishing worldwide. Oxford is a registered trade mark of
Oxford University Press in the UK and in certain other countries

First Edition published in 2009
Second Edition published in 2019

Impression: 3

Published in the United States of America by Oxford University Press
198 Madison Avenue, New York, NY 10016, United States of America

British Library Cataloguing in Publication Data
Data available

Library of Congress Control Number: 2018939874

ISBN 978-0-19-878287-2

Printed and bound in the UK by
Ashford Colour Press Ltd.

Preface

It is with considerable pride that the editors OB and BG of this text welcome you to the second edition of the *Oxford Handbook of Learning and Intellectual Disability Nursing*. This much revised textbook represents the culmination of a 2-year project that has sought, as in the previous edition, to involve leading practitioners and academics from the field of learning/intellectual disabilities from the UK, as well as the Republic of Ireland and much further beyond, in the production of an authoritative text able to offer essential facts and information on learning/intellectual disabilities. The editors set out on this renewed task, knowing that much of the landscape for the practice of learning/intellectual disability nursing has never been so complex, even more so that the last edition. Nurses for people with learning/intellectual disabilities can now be found working and supporting people in a variety of different care contexts such as community learning disability teams, treatment and assessment services, reach-out services, residential settings, day-care services, respite services, health facilitation, mental health and/or challenging behaviour services, special schools, and many other specialist services for people who are on the spectrum of autistic disorders. Additionally, they can be found working for many different agencies such as healthcare, social care, education, and the independent sector (this comprises the private, voluntary, and not-for-profit organizations), and also alongside numerous other professional disciplines such as clinical psychologists, social workers, occupational therapists, speech and language therapists, and consultant psychiatrists in intellectual disabilities, as well as a range of professionals within general healthcare, social services, and education. Given this complexity of context and practice, we believe that the *Oxford Handbook of Learning and Intellectual Disability Nursing* continues to offer students, and newly qualified practitioners alike, up-to-date and concise, practical, applied knowledge, as well as theoretical information, for use in the very many areas where nurses for people with learning/intellectual disabilities are located. Notwithstanding that nurses for people with learning/intellectual disabilities are the primary audience for this text, we continue to believe, and as evidenced by its use, the wider audience includes a range of other health and/or social care professionals, who often seek an authoritative text that provides essential facts and information on learning/intellectual disability.

In keeping with other handbooks in this series, the underlying philosophy of this text is to be both '*a guide and a friend*', adopting a '*person-centred*' approach that has incorporated space for the reader to record their own anecdotes, quotations, and notes. Therefore, as with other handbooks, the *Oxford Handbook of Learning and Intellectual Disability Nursing*'s content is organized, so that there is one topic per left-hand page, with the right-hand pages generally having some blank space for notes and local information, or for diagrams, flowcharts, tables, key point boxes, and other quick-reference information. The reader will also find a fully updated emergencies section at the back of the book that provides essential information for the management of, for example, status epilepticus, holding powers under mental health legislation, and dealing with abuse. We believe that unique to this Oxford Handbook is the continuing attention given to differences in legislation and social policy across the jurisdictions of the constituent countries of the UK, as well as the Republic of Ireland.

It is important for us to make a brief note on the terminology used in this text. Generally speaking, within the UK, the term 'learning disability' is used to describe that group of people who have significant developmental delay resulting in arrested or incomplete achievement of the 'normal' milestones of human development. The term learning disability is also used throughout the world, but where it may hold different meanings, paradoxically so too at times in the UK. It is this difference in meaning that might lead to confusion as to what we anticipate will be a continued international readership. Problematic has been determining as to what term we should adopt. Elsewhere in the world, alternative terms to 'learning disability' are used such as mental retardation and mental handicap, but these terms are felt by many to portray negative imagery concerning people with learning disabilities. Whereas we accept that 'naming is not a simple act' (Luckasson, 2003), the increasing internationalization of textbooks has led us to conclude that we needed to adopt a term to replace learning disability that would enable this book to be seen as relevant to as wide a readership as possible. That term which we believe seems most appropriate to this text, to the readership, and to those whom this book is principally about and that which seems to have the most universal consensus is that of 'intellectual disabilities'. Therefore, throughout the remainder of this text, we will not repeat the rather clumsy term used, that of learning/intellectual disability, and from hereon, in this book, we will use the term intellectual disability, save where certain Acts and/or other technical works require its use for accuracy. We have also made a purposeful decision to use the full words of 'intellectual disabilities', rather than the abbreviation 'ID' in order to highlight, rather than risk minimizing, the importance of intellectual disabilities in the lives of people who live with it. This is also important when considering your role as a nurse for people with intellectual disabilities, and we encourage you to refer to your role as a registered nurse for people with intellectual disabilities (or learning disabilities), rather than an intellectual or learning disability nurse.

We feel confident that the *Oxford Handbook of Learning and Intellectual Disability Nursing* has already become a highly regarded textbook—not only in the field of intellectual disabilities, but also more widely, and that it will be used just as widely by the many professionals and students from the range of different professional and academic backgrounds that have an interest in the lives of people with intellectual disabilities. Both editors also strongly believe that the excellent end-product that you have before you is due entirely to the excellent contributions that have been made by our many friends and colleagues from across the UK, the Republic of Ireland, and beyond, and we earnestly thank them for their trust in us by contributing to this textbook. We earnestly hope that all who read this book find it helpful and that its use will assist us all in helping people with intellectual disabilities enjoy health and well-being in their lives.

Owen Barr, Derry, Northern Ireland
Bob Gates, Taddington, Derbyshire, England
January 2018

References

Luckasson R (2003). Terminology and power. In: SS Her, LO Gostin, HH Koh, eds. *The Human Rights of Persons with Intellectual Disabilities: Different but Equal*. Oxford University Press: Oxford; pp. 49–58.

Foreword

There have been many developments in learning/intellectual disability nursing since I wrote the foreword to the 1st edition of this book in 2009. One such development was the publication of a new nursing strategy entitled 'Strengthening the Commitment' (Scottish Government, 2012). That report made a number of recommendations for modernizing the profession and aimed to ensure that nurses with the right skills and knowledge were available to meet the needs of people with learning/intellectual disabilities across their lifespan, in the right place, at the right time. Within that context, it highlighted new and developing roles that nurses for people with learning/intellectual disabilities were adopting, and this is certainly an area that has seen much development. As well as working within specialist learning disability community and residential services, nurses for people with learning/intellectual disabilities are increasingly working in a diverse and growing range of settings that include general hospital services, children's services, end-of-life care, schools, and prisons. For those of us that can remember the Cullen Report (1991), it would seem that the profession is truly demonstrating that its knowledge and skills are 'facility-independent'.

Recent years have also seen increased evidence that the health needs of people with learning/intellectual disabilities are not always appropriately identified and met, and that they experience an increased risk of premature and avoidable death (Heslop et al., 2013). One response to this growing awareness has been a call for all nurses to increase their awareness of the health needs of people with learning/intellectual disabilities and to develop their skills in identifying and meeting such needs. Indeed, at the time of writing this foreword, new standards for pre-registration nursing are being developed within the UK and the Republic of Ireland that will ensure a key element is the need for all nurses, at the point of registration, to be able to identify and address the health needs of people with learning/intellectual disabilities.

The need for nurses for people with learning/intellectual disabilities, along with nurses from other fields of practice, to have access to key knowledge to enable them to support people with learning disabilities, in whatever setting they may work, is essential—hence, this new and updated edition of the Oxford Handbook is timely. Whereas there are a number of textbooks available, this new edition continues to adopt its unique approach. As with the 1st edition, it brings together key information in a readily accessible manner, addressing many practice-based queries and concerns. It also provides a starting point for further development through recommendations for additional reading. In a field of practice that continues to grow, develop, and expand, this book provides an essential point of reference for practitioners that will support them to provide the right care for people with learning/intellectual disabilities at the right time and in the right place.

Ruth Northway
Professor of Learning Disability Nursing
University of South Wales

References

Cullen C (1991). *Caring for People Community Care in the Next Decade and Beyond*. Department of Health, Mental Handicap Nursing: London.

Heslop P, Blair P, Fleming P, Hoghton M, Marriott A, Russ L (2013). *Confidential Inquiry into Premature Deaths of People with Learning Disabilities (CIPOLD)*. Norah Fry Research Centre: Bristol.

Scottish Government (2012). *Strengthening the Commitment. The Report of the UK Modernising Learning Disabilities Nursing Review*. Scottish Government: Edinburgh.

Dedication

In loving memory of Adam
Owen Barr

Acknowledgements

Owen Barr would like to thank his parents, as well as Marie, Shannágh, Shane, and Adam for all their support in his work, writing and reminding him of the important things in life. He would also like to acknowledge the insights gained from many people with intellectual disabilities and their families who continue to teach him many times about the importance of focusing on the individual person.

Bob Gates would like to thank Briege, Nicky, and Lucy, David, and Emily, Sean and Caiomhe, as well as all of their wonderful grandchildren for making the world a better place.

Our thanks also go to all the contributors, colleagues, and reviewers who have offered help and advice throughout the completion of this book. Finally, we thank the team at Oxford University Press for their continued help and hard work in bringing this 2nd edition to publication.

January 2018

Contents

Contributors

Owen Barr
Professor of Nursing and Intellectual Disabilities, Ulster University, Londonderry, UK
- 1: The nature of intellectual disability nursing
  - Principles and values of social policy and their effects on intellectual disability
- 2: Working with families
  - Defining families
  - People with intellectual disabilities as parents
  - Explaining intellectual disabilities to family members
  - The process of family adaptation
  - Resilience in families
  - Families at risk
  - Carer's assessment
  - Working with older carers
- 6: Physical health and well-being
  - Medicines management
- 8: Planning with people and their families
  - Undertaking a nursing assessment
  - Writing nursing care plans
  - Making best interests decisions
  - Direct care payments
  - Effective teamworking
  - Interagency working
  - Commissioning services
- 10: Accessing general health services
  - General hospital services
  - Radiology departments
  - Children's health services
  - Dental services
  - Maternity services
  - Planning for contact with general health services
- 14: Research and intellectual disability nursing
  - Involving people with intellectual disabilities in the research process
  - Mixed methods
- 16: Independent regulators of care quality
  - Regulation and Quality Improvement Authority: Northern Ireland

Jonathan Beebee
Chief Enablement Officer, PBS4, Southampton, UK
- 9: Therapeutic interventions
  - Positive behaviour support

Tina Bell
Managing Director, Artspace, Londonderry, UK
- 6: Physical health and well-being
  - People with profound and multiple learning disabilities
  - Hearing
  - Healthy skin
  - Personal and intimate care
  - Continence

- 9: Therapeutic interventions
  - Multisensory environments
  - Sensory integration
  - Complementary, integrated, and alternative therapies
  - Art, drama, and music
- 10: Accessing general health services
  - Continence advisors

Phil Boulter

Consultant Nurse in Learning Disabilities, Surrey and Borders Partnership NHS Foundation Trust, Surrey, UK

- 4: Assessment
  - Risk assessment
  - Quality of life
  - Life experiences
- 12: Lifestyles and intellectual disability nursing
  - Risk management

Aoife Bradley

Lead Genetic Nurse and Counsellor, Northern Ireland Regional Genetics Centre, Belfast, UK

- 1: The nature of intellectual disability nursing
  - Causes and manifestations of intellectual disability
  - Common conditions among people with intellectual disability
- 5: Changes across the lifespan
  - Antenatal screening and diagnosis

Rhona Brennan

Ward Sister, Erne, Muckamore Abbey Hospital, Antrim, UK

- 11: People with intellectual disabilities and forensic nursing
  - Forensic risk assessment and management
  - People who have offended in law
  - People in prison
  - Rights of victims
  - Rights of person offending
  - Rights to a solicitor
  - People with intellectual disabilities as witnesses
  - Admission for assessment
  - Admission for treatment
  - Emergency holding powers
  - Nurse's holding power
  - Mental Health Review Tribunal
  - Mental Health Act Commission
  - Use of restraint
  - Keeping yourself safe
  - Management in the community
  - Working with criminal justice agencies
- 18: Emergencies
  - Missing person
  - Risk of suicide

Jo Bromley

Consultant Clinical Psychologist, Manchester University NHS Foundation Trust, Manchester, UK

- 10: Accessing general health services
  - Child and adolescent services

Michael Brown
Professor, School of Nursing and Midwifery, Queen's University Belfast, Belfast, UK
- 6: Physical health and well-being
  - Cardiorespiratory disorders
  - Obesity
  - Nutrition
  - Mobility
  - Exercise
  - Diabetes
  - Thyroid
  - Cancer
  - Stopping smoking
  - Accidents
  - Sexual health and personal relationships
  - Gastrointestinal disorders
  - Constipation
  - Integration of sensory experiences
- 16: Independent regulators of care quality
  - Care regulation in Scotland

Julie Calveley
Associate of the Intensive Interaction Institute, UK
- 6: Physical health and well-being
  - Continence
  - Healthy Skin
  - Personal and intimate care

Steve Cartwright
Community Palliative Care Clinical Nurse Specialist, Walsall Palliative Care Centre, West Midlands, UK
- 5: Changes across the lifespan
  - End-of-life care, preferred place of care
- 6: Physical health and well-being
  - End-of-life care, preferred place of care
- 10: Accessing general health services
  - End of life
  - Palliative care

Eddie Chaplin
Professor of Mental Health in Neurodevelopmental Disorders, London South Bank University, London, UK
- 7: Mental health and emotional well-being
  - Introduction
  - Promoting assertiveness
  - Supporting people with intellectual disabilities in general mental health services
  - Primary care
  - Secondary care
  - Tertiary care
  - Self-harm
- 10: Accessing general health services
  - Mental health services

Rebecca Chester
Consultant Nurse for People with Learning Disabilities, Berkshire Health Care NHS Foundation Trust, Berkshire, UK
- 6: Physical health and well-being
  - Independent nurse prescribers in intellectual disability

Sue Colegrave
Consultant Clinical Psychologist, Manchester University NHS Foundation Trust, Manchester, UK
- 9: Therapeutic interventions
  - Family therapy

Maria Cozens
Lecturer in Learning Disability Nursing, University of West London, London, UK
- 1: The nature of intellectual disability nursing
  - Incidence and prevalence of intellectual disability
- 12: Lifestyles and intellectual disability nursing
  - Residential alternatives

Debbie Crickmore
Lecturer in Learning Disability, University of Hull, Hull, UK
- 5: Changes across the lifespan
  - Supporting people during transition
  - School-aged children
  - Adulthood
  - Preschool children

Caroline Dalton O'Connor
Lecturer, University College Cork, Cork, Ireland
- 6: Physical health and well-being
  - Dysphagia
  - Nasogastric feeding
  - PEG and PEJ feeding
  - Oral health

Jill Davies
Research Programme Manager, Foundation for People with Learning Disabilities, London, UK
- 17: Practice resources
  - Healthcare resources
  - National and international networks

Mary Dearing
Lecturer in Learning Disability, University of Hull, Hull, UK
- 5: Changes across the lifespan
  - Adolescence
  - Women and menopause
  - Puberty

Maurice Devine
Assistant Head, HSC Clinical Education Centre, Fern House, Antrim, UK
- 8: Planning with people and their families
  - Consent to examination, treatment, and care

Matt Dodwell
Head of Service, Kent Community Health NHS Foundation Trust, Gravesend, UK
- 4: Assessment
  - Risk assessment
  - Life experiences
  - Quality of life
- 12: Lifestyles and intellectual disability nursing
  - Risk management

Renée Francis

Senior Lecturer in Learning Disability Nursing, London South Bank University, London, UK

- 7: Mental health and emotional well-being
  - Introduction
  - Promoting assertiveness
  - Supporting people with intellectual disabilities in general mental health services
  - Primary care
  - Secondary care
  - Tertiary care
  - Self-harm
- 10: Accessing general health services
  - Mental health services

Bob Gates

Professor of Learning Disabilities, University of West London, Visiting Professor of Learning Disabilities, Institute of Education, University of Derby, Emeritus Professor, the Centre for Learning Disability Studies, University of Hertfordshire, and Editor in Chief, *British Journal of Learning Disabilities*.

- 1: The nature of intellectual disability nursing
  - Introduction
  - Diagnosing intellectual disability
  - The purist form of nursing
  - Holism and working across the lifespan
- 4: Assessment
  - Assessment of independence and social functioning
- 6: Physical health and well-being
  - Introduction
- 8: Planning with people and their families
  - Patient advice and liaison service
- 9: Therapeutic interventions
  - Advocacy
- 12: Lifestyles and intellectual disability nursing
  - Village communities
- 14: Research and intellectual disability nursing
  - Involving people with intellectual disabilities in the research process
- 16: Independent regulators of care quality
  - Care Quality Commission: England

Peter Griffin

Formerly Professional Lead in Learning Disability Nursing, Queen's University Belfast, Belfast, UK

- 8: Planning with people and their families
  - Client-held records
- 17: Practice resources
  - Children
  - Adults and older people

Lisa Hanna-Trainor

Formerly Research Associate, Ulster University, Londonderry, Northern Ireland

- 8: Planning with people and their families
  - Life planning
- 12: Lifestyles and intellectual disability nursing
  - Retirement
  - Retirement options

Kirsty Henry

Lecturer in Nursing Sciences (Learning Disabilities), University of East Anglia, Norwich, UK

- 8: Planning with people and their families
  - Independent Mental Capacity Advocates
- 18: Emergencies
  - Allergies
  - Adverse reactions to medications
  - Medication errors
  - Needlestick/sharps injuries

Neil James

Senior Lecturer in Nursing Sciences (Learning Disabilities), University of East Anglia, Norwich, UK

- 8: Planning with people and their families
  - Independent Mental Capacity Advocates
- 18: Emergencies
  - Allergies
  - Adverse reactions to medications
  - Medication errors
  - Needlestick/sharps injuries

Robert Jenkins

Former Principal Lecturer, Unit for the Development in Intellectual Disabilities, University of South Wales, UK

- 18: Emergencies
  - Self-harm
  - Self-injury
  - Unsafe standards of care
  - Recording and reporting
  - Complaints

Victoria Jones

Visiting Fellow, University of the West of England, Bristol, UK

- 8: Planning with people and their families
  - Advocacy
  - Circles of support
  - Child protection
  - Adult safeguarding
- 16: Independent regulators of care quality
  - Care and Social Services Inspectorate: Wales

Paul Michael Keenan

Assistant Professor of Intellectual Disability Nursing, Trinity College, Dublin, Ireland

- 15: National occupational standards and professional requirements
  - Nursing and Midwifery Council
  - Nursing and Midwifery Board of Ireland
  - Obtaining initial professional registration
  - Maintaining ongoing professional registration
- 16: Independent regulators of care quality
  - Health Information and Quality Improvement: Republic of Ireland

Chiedza Kudita

Public Involvement Coordinator and Lecturer, University of West London, London, UK

- 12: Lifestyles and intellectual disability nursing
  - Citizenship

Dorothy Kupara

Lecturer in Learning Disability Nursing, University of West London, London, UK
- 1: The nature of intellectual disability nursing
  - Defining intellectual disability nursing
- 12: Lifestyles and intellectual disability nursing
  - Supported living and home ownership

Elaine Kwiatek

Formerly Education Project Manager, NHS Education for Scotland, Edinburgh, UK
- 3: Communication
  - Developing accessible information
  - Communication passports
  - Objects of reference
  - Compiling life stories
- 8: Planning with people and their families
  - Care pathways
  - Care Programme Approach

Helen Laverty

Professional Lead Learning Disability Nursing, University of Nottingham, Nottingham, UK
- 2: Working with families
  - Principles of working collaboratively with families
  - Supporting siblings of people with intellectual disabilities
  - People with intellectual disabilities as parents
  - Family quality of life
  - Respite care
- 8: Planning with people and their families
  - Care management, case management, and continuing care

Kay Mafuba

Professor of Nursing, University of West London, London, UK
- 14: Research and intellectual disability
  - Qualitative approaches
  - Quantitative approaches
  - Ethical issues in research

Paul Maloret

Principal Lecturer, The Centre for Learning Disability Studies, University of Hertfordshire, Hatfield, UK
- 13: The law
  - Autism Act 2009

Lynne Marsh

Senior Lecturer, Queen's University Belfast, Belfast, UK
- 5: Changes across the lifespan
  - Personal relationships
  - Marriage and family life
  - Parents with intellectual disability
- 10: Accessing general health services
  - Parenting groups

Zuzana Matousova-Done

Manager of Residential Care, Glendale Home for the Intellectually Disabled, Cape Town, South Africa [this is Zuzana's affiliation]

- 9: Therapeutic interventions
  - Hydrotherapy
  - Conductive education
  - TEACCH (Treatment and Education of Autistic and related Communication-handicapped Children)

Damian McAleer

Nurse Education Consultant, HSC Clinical Education Centre, Fern House, Antrim, UK

- 8: Planning with people and their families
  - Vulnerability

Philip McCallion

Director of the School of Social Work, Temple University, Philadelphia, USA

- 5: Changes across the lifespan
  - Older people with intellectual disabilities
  - Older people with Down syndrome
- 7: Mental health and emotional well-being
  - Dementia (in people with intellectual disabilities)
- 10: Accessing general health services
  - Dementia nurse

Tanya McCance

Research Director, Nursing and Health Sciences, Ulster University, Newtownabbey, UK

- 8: Planning with people and their families
  - Person-centred planning

Mary McCarron

Dean of the Faculty of Health Sciences, Trinity College Dublin, Dublin, Ireland

- 5: Changes across the lifespan
  - Older people with intellectual disabilities
  - Older people with Down syndrome
- 7: Mental health and emotional well-being
  - Dementia (in people with intellectual disabilities)
- 10: Accessing general health services
  - Dementia nurse

Roy McConkey

Emeritus Professor, Ulster University, Newtownabbey, UK

- 12: Lifestyles and intellectual disability nursing
  - Productive work
  - Supported employment
  - Networks of support and friends
  - Encouraging friendships

Brendan McCormack

Head of the Division of Nursing, Queen Margaret University, Edinburgh, UK

- 8: Planning with people and their families
  - Person-centred planning

Garvin McKnight

Nurse Behaviour Therapist, Muckamore Abbey Hospital, Antrim, UK

- 11: People with intellectual disabilities and forensic nursing
  - Forensic risk assessment and management
  - People who have offended in law
  - People in prison
  - Rights of victims
  - Rights of person offending
  - Rights to a solicitor
  - People with intellectual disabilities as witnesses
  - Admission for assessment
  - Admission for treatment
  - Emergency holding powers
  - Nurse's holding power
  - Mental Health Review Tribunal
  - Mental Health Act Commission
  - Use of restraint
  - Keeping yourself safe
  - Management in the community
  - Working with criminal justice agencies
- 18: Emergencies
  - Missing person
  - Risk of suicide

Martina Meenan

Nurse Education Consultant, HSC Clinical Education Centre, CEC Altnagelvin, UK

- 8: Planning with people and their families
  - Vulnerability

Duncan Mitchell

Professor of Health and Disability, Manchester Metropolitan University, Manchester, UK

- 14: Research and intellectual disability nursing
  - Introduction
  - Defining areas for research
  - Undertaking a literature review
  - Audit
  - Evidence-based care

Ann Norman

Professional Lead for Learning Disability Nursing and Justice/Forensic Nursing, Royal College of Nursing, London, UK

- 11: People with intellectual disabilities and forensic nursing
  - Forensic risk assessment and management
  - People who have offended in law
  - People in prison
  - Rights of victims
  - Rights of person offending
  - Rights to a solicitor
  - People with intellectual disabilities as witnesses
  - Admission for assessment
  - Admission for treatment
  - Emergency holding powers
  - Nurse's holding power
  - Mental Health Review Tribunal
  - Mental Health Act Commission
  - Use of restraint
  - Keeping yourself safe
  - Management in the community
  - Working with criminal justice agencies

- 18: Emergencies
  - Missing person
  - Risk of suicide

Peter Oakes

Professor of Clinical Psychology, Staffordshire University,
Stoke-on-Trent, UK
- 1: The nature of intellectual disability nursing
  - Identifying intellectual disability
  - Degree of intellectual disability
  - Definition of intellectual disability

Edna O'Neill

Epilepsy Nurse Specialist, Thompson House Hospital, Lisburn, UK
- 6: Physical health and well-being
  - Epilepsy
  - Supporting people with epilepsy
- 10: Accessing general health services
  - Epilepsy nurse
- 18: Emergencies
  - Emergency management of person in a seizure

Sue Read

Professor of Learning Disability Nursing, Keele University, Newcastle, UK
- 5: Changes across the lifespan
  - End-of-life care, preferred place of care
- 6: Physical health and well-being
  - End-of-life care, preferred place of care
- 7: Mental health and emotional well-being
  - Responding to bereavement
- 9: Therapeutic interventions
  - Support associated with loss and bereavement
- 10: Accessing general health services
  - Tertiary care
  - Palliative care

Lesley Russ

Senior Lecturer in Learning Disabilities, Autism and Public Health,
University of the West of England, Bristol, UK
- 6: Physical health and well-being
  - Health inequalities
  - Principles of health promotion
  - Promoting public health
  - Promoting physical well-being of individuals
  - Physical health assessment of people with intellectual disability
  - Blood pressure, temperature, and pulse
  - Respiration and oxygen saturation levels
- 10: Accessing general health services
  - Primary care
  - General practitioners
  - Health visitors
  - District nurses
  - Community children's nurses
  - School nurses
  - Midwives
  - Dentists
  - Podiatrists
  - Audiologists
  - Dieticians
  - Physiotherapists
  - Occupational therapists
  - Optical care
  - Community nurses mental health

Jillian Scott

Health Facilitator, Learning Disability Team, Rathlea House, Coleraine, UK
- 10: Accessing general health services
  - Practice nurses

Margaret Sowney

Lecturer in Nursing/Subject Partnership Manager, Ulster University, Newtownabbey, UK
- 4: Assessment
  - Assessing pain
  - Assessing distress
  - Diagnostic overshadowing
- 10: Accessing general health services
  - Secondary care
  - Outpatient clinics
  - Emergency departments
  - Discharge planning

Mohammad Surfraz

Senior Lecturer/Continued Professional Development Lead, University of Hertfordshire, Hatfield, UK
- 4: Assessment
  - Purpose and principles of assessment
  - Framework of nursing assessment
- 9: Therapeutic interventions
  - Behavioural interventions
- 17: Practice resources
  - Behavioural management resources

John Swinton

Chair in Divinity and Religious Studies, University of Aberdeen, Aberdeen, UK
- 2: Working with families
  - Cultural, religious, and spiritual impact
- 6: Mental health and emotional well-being
  - Spirituality

Laurence Taggart

Reader, School of Nursing, Ulster University, Newtownabbey, UK
- 4: Assessment
  - Adaptive behaviour rating scales
  - Screening of mental problems
  - Measurement of IQ
- 7: Mental health and emotional well-being
  - Promoting emotional well-being
  - Prevalence rates
  - Factors contributing to mental health problems
  - Anxiety disorders
  - Psychotic disorders
  - Organic disorders
  - Substance misuse
- 9: Therapeutic interventions
  - Appropriate use of medication

Cath Valentine

Speech & Language Therapist for Adults with Learning Disabilities, Torbay & South Devon NHS Foundation Trust, Torquay, UK

- 3: Communication
  - Promoting effective communication
  - Verbal communication
  - Non-verbal communication
  - Providing information
  - Active listening
  - Principles in using augmentative and alternative communication (AAC)
- 9: Therapeutic interventions
  - Inclusive communication

Gaynor Ward

Nurse Consultant in Learning Disabilities & Mental Health, Derbyshire Healthcare NHS Foundation Trust, Derby, UK

- 7: Mental health and emotional well-being
  - Psychopathology
  - Autistic spectrum conditions

Michael Wolverson

Lecturer in Learning Disabilities, University of York, York, UK

- 9: Therapeutic interventions
  - Anger management
  - Cognitive behaviour therapies
- 13: The law
  - Mental Health Act 1983
  - Compulsory admission to hospital for assessment and treatment
  - Emergency holding powers
  - Mental Health (First Tier) Review Tribunals
  - The Equality Act 2010
  - Sexual Offences Act 2003
  - The Care Act 2014
  - Human Rights Act
  - European Convention of Human Rights
  - Dealing with abuse
  - Diversion from custody schemes
  - Appropriate adult
  - The Representation of the People Act (RPA) 2000
  - Consent to examination, treatment, and care
  - Mental Capacity Act 2005
  - Mental Capacity Act: Deprivation of Liberty Safeguards
  - Common law and duty of care
  - Safeguarding adults
  - Nurse prescribers
  - Physical assault
  - De-escalation
  - Use of restraint

Symbols and abbreviations

♂	male
♀	female
~	approximately
>	greater than
<	less than
≤	equal to or greater than
➔	cross reference
ℬ	website
°C	degree celsius
€	euro
®	registered trademark
™	trademark
©	copyright
AAC	augmentative and alternative communication
ABA	applied behavioural analysis
ABC	appropriate behaviour contract
ABG	arterial blood gases
ABMUHB	Abertawe Bro Morgannwg University Health Board
ABS	adaptive behaviour scales
AC	approved clinician
ACP	advance care planning
ADHD	attention-deficit/hyperactive disorder
ADR	adverse drug reaction
AED	antiepileptic drug
AET	Autism Education Trust
ANOVA	analysis of variance
ANP	advanced nurse practitioner
AOT	assertive outreach team
ARC	Association for Real Change
ASBO	antisocial behaviour order
ASC	autistic spectrum condition
AUDIT	Alcohol Use Disorder Identification Test
BILD	British Institute of Learning Disabilities
BMI	body mass index
BNF	British National Formulary

BSID	Bayley Scales of Infant Development
CAMHS	child and adolescent mental health services
CBF	Challenging Behaviour Foundation
CBT	cognitive behavioural therapy
CCG	clinical commissioning group
CCN	community children's nurse
CE	conductive education
ChA-PAS	Child and Adolescent Psychiatric Assessment Schedule
CIW	Care Inspectorate Wales
CLDT	community learning disability team
CMHT	community mental health team
CNMH	community nurse mental health
CNS	central nervous system
COAD	chronic obstructive airways disease
CPA	Care Programme Approach
CPD	continuing professional development
CPN	community psychiatric nurse
CPNP	community practitioner nurse prescriber
CQC	Care Quality Commission
CT	computerized tomography
CTR	care and treatment review
CVS	chorionic villus sampling
DC-LD	diagnostic criteria for psychiatric disorders for use with adults with learning disabilities/mental retardation
DDNA	Developmental Disabilities Nurses Association
DES	Directly Enhanced Service
DisDAT	Disability Distress Assessment Tool
DNA	deoxyribonucleic acid
DPII	Developmental Profile II
DRA	differential reinforcement of alternate responses
DRL	differential reinforcement of low-rates behaviour
DRO	differential reinforcement of other behaviour9
DSM-5	Diagnostic and Statistical Manual of Mental Disorders, 5th edition
DTP	deep touch pressure
ECG	electrocardiogram
ECHR	European Convention of Human Rights
ECI	Early Coping Inventory
ECT	electroconvulsive therapy
EDS	Equality Delivery System

EEG	electroencephalogram
EHC	Education Health and Care
EHCP	education healthcare plan
ELP	essential lifestyle planning
EMP	epilepsy management plan
EPIC	Equality, Participation, Influence, and Change
ESN	epilepsy specialist nurse
FAAR	family adjustment and adaptation response
FACE	Functional Analysis in the Care Environment
FFPWLD	Foundation for People with Learning Disabilities
FGM	female genital mutilation
FOC	fundamental of communication
FSA	Food Standards Agency
FSH	follicle-stimulating hormone
GAIN	Guidelines and Audit Implementation Network
GMC	General Medical Council
GORD	gastro-oesophageal reflux disorder
GP	general practitioner
h	hour
HaLD	Hearing and Learning Disabilities
HaLD SIG	Hearing and Learning Disabilities Special Interest Group
HAP	health action plan
HASI	Hayes Ability Screening Index
HCPC	Health and Care Professions Council
HEF	Health Equality Framework
HEI	Healthcare Environment Inspectorate
HF	health facilitator
HIQA	Health Information and Quality Authority
HIV	human immunodeficiency virus
HIW	Healthcare Inspectorate Wales
HOLD	home ownership for people with long-term disabilities
HPT	heat–pain threshold
HRA	Health Research Authority
HRT	hormone replacement therapy
HV	health visitor
HWB	Health and Wellbeing Board
IASSIDD	International Association for the Scientific Study of Intellectual and Developmental Disabilities
ICD-10	International Classification of Diseases, 10th revision
ICD-11	International Classification of Diseases, 11th revision

IDD	intellectual and developmental disabilities
IgE	immunoglobulin E
IhaL	Improving Health and Lives Learning Disabilities Public Health Observatory
IMCA	Independent Mental Capacity Advocate
IMHA	Independent Mental Health Advocate
IQ	intelligence quotient
IV	intravenous
JCHR	Joint Committee on Human Rights
JSNA	joint strategic needs assessment
kg	kilogram
L	litre
LARA	leave/absconding risk assessment
LD QOF	Learning Disability Quality of Outcomes Framework
LTP	light touch pressure
LUNSERS	Liverpool University Neuroleptic Side Effect Rating Scale
m	metre
MAPPA	Multi-Agency Public Protection Arrangements
MAPS	Making Action Plans
MAPS	McGill Action Planning System
MCA	Mental Capacity Act
MCADOLS	Mental Capacity Act Deprivation of Liberty Safeguards
MELAS	mitochondrial encephalopathy, lactic acidosis, and stroke-like episodes
MERRF	myoclonic epilepsy with ragged red fibres
MHA	Mental Health Act
MHRA	Medicines and Healthcare Products Regulatory Agency
MHRT	Mental Health Review Tribunal
mmHg	millimetre of mercury
MRI	magnetic resonance imaging
MSE	multisensory environment
NCAPC	Non-Communicating Adults Pain Checklist
NHS	National Health Service
NICE	National Institute for Health and Care Excellence
NIPT	non-invasive prenatal testing
NMBI	Nursing and Midwifery Board of Ireland
NMC	Nursing and Midwifery Council
NMP	Non-medical prescribing/prescriber
NOMS	National Offender Management Services
NPHS	National Public Health Service

NSF	National Service Framework
NVQ	National Vocational Qualification
OCD	obsessive–compulsive disorder
OT	occupational therapist
PACE	Police and Criminal Evidence Act 1984
PADS	Pain and Discomfort Scale
PALS	patient advice and liaison service
PAS-ADD	Psychiatric Assessment Schedules for Adults with Developmental Disabilities
PATH	Planning Alternative Tomorrows With Hope
PBS	positive behaviour support
PCP	person-centred profile
PEG	percutaneous endoscopic gastrostomy
PEJ	percutaneous endoscopic jejunostomy
PET	positron emission tomography
PFP	personal futures planning
PHCT	primary healthcare team
PHOF	Public Health Outcomes framework
PPI	public patient involvement
PRISMA	Preferred Reporting Items for Systematic Reviews and Meta-Analyses
PRN	*pro re nata* (as necessary)
QOF	quality outcomes framework
RCGP	Royal College of General Practitioners
RCSLT	Royal College of Speech and Language Therapists
RCT	randomized controlled trial
REC	research ethic committee
RNID	Registered Nurse in Intellectual Disability
RNLD	Registered Nurse in Learning Disability
RPA	Representation of the People Act
RQIA	Regulation and Quality Improvement Authority
s	second(s)
SCPHN	specialist community public health nurse
SD	standard deviation
SEN	special educational needs
SHC	Scottish Health Council
SHTG	Scottish Health Technologies Group
SI	sensory integration
SIB-R	Scales of Independent Behaviour: Revised
SIGN	Scottish Intercollegiate Guidelines Network
SIS-A	Supports Intensity Scale–Adult version

SLDO	Scottish Learning Disabilities Observatory
SLT	speech and language therapist
SMC	Scottish Medicines Consortium
SOAD	second-opinion appointed doctor
SOFI	Short Observational Framework for Inspection
SOPO	sex offender prevention order
SPOC	single point of contact
SPSP	Scottish Patient Safety Programme
STI	sexually transmitted infection
SUDEP	sudden unexpected death in epilepsy
T3	triiodothyronine
T4	thyroxine
TAC	team around the child
TAF	team around the family
TEACCH	Treatment and Education of Autistic and Related Communication-handicapped Children
TILII	*Tell It Like It Is*
TSH	thyroid-stimulating hormone
TTR	transition-to-retirement (programme)
UK	United Kingdom
USA	United States
UTI	urinary tract infection
VABS	Vineland Adaptive Behaviour Scale
VOCA	voice output communication aid
WHO	World Health Organization
yr(s)	year(s)

The nature of intellectual disability nursing

Introduction

In this chapter, the term intellectual disability is defined. It will be shown that intellectual disability is identified by the presence of *'a significantly reduced ability to understand new or complex information (impaired intelligence) along with a reduced ability to cope independently (impaired social functioning), and which occurred before 18yrs of age'.*[1]

The chapter outlines that there is general agreement that 3–4/1000 of the general population will have a severe intellectual disability, and that 25–30/1000 of the general population will have a mild intellectual disability.[2]

Also outlined are the various ways in which a diagnosis, or an assessment, of intellectual disability is made. A range of known causes and manifestations of intellectual disability will be provided.

Above all else, it will be emphasized that people with intellectual disability, regardless of the impact of their disabilities, share a common humanity with that of their fellow citizens in their communities and in the wider society in which they live. Most people desire love and a sense of connection with others; they wish to be safe, to learn, to lead a meaningful life, to be free from ridicule and harm, to be healthy, and to be free from poverty, and in this respect, people with intellectual disability are no different to any of us.

All health and social care workers, especially nurses in services for people with intellectual disabilities, have a professional responsibility to bring about their inclusion into their communities, by adhering at all times to a value base that respects them as fellow citizens.

This value base leads this chapter to conclude by articulating the nature of intellectual disability nursing and how this group of professionals works to support the whole person throughout their lives whenever they are in need of such support.

References

1 Gates B, Mafuba K (2016). Use of the term 'learning disabilities' in the United Kingdom: issues for international researchers and practitioners. *Learning Disabilities: A Contemporary Journal.* **14**: 9–23.
2 Hatton C, Glover G, Emerson E, Brown I (2016). *Learning Disabilities Observatory. People with Learning Disabilities in England 2015: Main Report.* Public Health England: London. ↗ healthwatchgateshead. co.uk/wp-content/uploads/2016/08/PWLDIE-2015-final.pdf (accessed 30 October 2017).

Identifying intellectual disability

It is essential to stress at the outset of this section that each person with an intellectual disability is a unique human being. Like everyone else, each person has their own personality, along with a profile of abilities and disabilities, that can only be understood in the context of their culture, history, and relationships. Intellectual disability manifests in a number of different ways for each individual.

Intellectual profile

Intelligence is understood as a general ability to make sense of the world. For a person with intellectual disability, the following intellectual abilities may be impaired but are still present to some degree.

Verbal abilities

- Learning quickly and learning from experience;
- Comprehension—understanding situations, knowing socially accepted norms, and being able to weigh up possible options;
- Language—vocabulary may be limited and some people may not understand words at all. Others may recognize words but struggle to understand more subtle meanings;
- Abstract thinking—people may find it hard to separate themselves from the thing they are thinking about. Hypothetical situations are particularly difficult;
- Reasoning, planning, and solving problems.

Non-verbal abilities

- Speed of processing—an individual may take a long time to work out what is going on in a situation;
- Reasoning—shapes, patterns, and numbers may be confusing and people can find it hard to put things in order;
- Coordination—there may be difficulty in coordinating movement or using fine motor skills.

Coping with everyday life

These difficulties in intellectual function can impact on a person's ability to cope with everyday life. This means that a person with intellectual disability may have a range of difficulties that require support in three main areas:

- Conceptual—language, reading and writing, number, including understanding money and time;
- Practical—including everything from getting up, washing, dressing, and cooking through to going to bed. This also includes staying safe, getting out and about, looking after health, and keeping some kind of routine;
- Social—getting on with people and managing social situations. It includes knowing how to avoid being victimized and having a sense of self-worth.

Aetiology and phenotypes

There are a number of people with specific syndromes, and these syndromes may be associated with a particular profile of strengths, limitations, and health needs. For example, people who are on the autistic spectrum are characterized by specific difficulties with social communication and information processing. Information about specific syndromes and the cause of intellectual disability (where known) therefore can be important in understanding and predicting possible manifestations of intellectual disability.

Additional needs

People with intellectual disability are more likely to have a range of additional needs. Of particular note are:

- Sensory impairments;
- Epilepsy.

Context

As mentioned previously on ➔ pp. 4–5, each person presents with a unique history, background, and set of important relationships. It is essential to understand these, alongside the immediate disabilities. People with intellectual disability are likely to be receiving support from their family, or from other carers, and these people will have a key role to play in any assessment or intervention.

Further reading

American Association on Intellectual and Developmental Disabilities (2010). *Intellectual Disability: Definition, Classification and Systems of Supports,* 11th edn. American Association on Intellectual and Developmental Disabilities: Washington DC.

World Health Organization (updated 2017). *The International Classification of Functioning, Disability and Health (ICF).* ⌘ www.who.int/classifications/icf/en/ (accessed 24 October 2017).

Degree of intellectual disability

As will be seen in ➲ Definition of intellectual disability, pp. 8–9, intellectual disability is defined by the presence of three criteria:

- The person has an intellectual ability that is significantly below average. This is generally measured by a standardized test of intelligence that gives a score (intelligence quotient, IQ) according to how far an individual is from the average of the population. An individual who consistently scores >2 standard deviations (SDs) below the mean on an IQ test, i.e. a measured IQ of <70, is said to meet the first criteria;
- There are also difficulties in social functioning. In other words, the person struggles to cope with everyday life;
- The difficulties began before the age of 18.

Intellectual disability has been divided or classified into a number of categories to reflect its nature and extent. These range from 'borderline' through 'mild', 'moderate' and 'severe', to 'profound'. It is essential that any classification is approached with caution and must be in the interests of the person with intellectual disability. Examples might include eligibility for services or support.

It is now considered more appropriate to see intellectual disability as an interaction between a person, the support they receive, and the environment in which they are.

For example:

> Andrew has very significant intellectual disabilities. He uses a wheelchair, he makes his needs known through sounds and facial expressions, and he is understood by people who know him well, but he cannot speak or understand words and he is not able to look after even his most basic needs. He needs a great deal of support to meet his basic care and understand what he is trying to communicate. He also needs an environment with special equipment, and opportunities to get out and meet new people—something he loves to do.

> Elizabeth has Down syndrome and can communicate very well with words. She looks after herself and can cope well in the community. She has to do things one at a time but can sometimes get overwhelmed if she feels there is too much to do. Elizabeth needs someone to visit her once a day to make sure she has remembered everything, including her epilepsy medication, and to make sure she is not getting overwhelmed. She needs an environment where she has just one task at a time to get through the day and the opportunity to meet her family at least once a week.

These examples show that each individual has a unique profile of intellectual disability that impacts on everyday life in different ways. Assessment of the degree of intellectual disability will identify the abilities and needs of the person as an individual, as well as the level of support they may need and the kind of environment and opportunities that will enable the person to make the most of their potential and achieve their personal goals.[3] There are a number of measures available to help people understand how much support a person needs in different areas of their life. These areas might include self-care, going out in the community, or engaging in work/leisure activities. The assessment will cover exactly what kind of support is needed, i.e. whether verbal prompts are sufficient or whether the person needs full physical support. It will also include how often the person needs support and perhaps how much time this will take.

To this is added an assessment of the kind of environment a person needs, and the opportunities that are important for them to be healthy, enjoy life, and achieve their personal goals. It is always important to remember that quality of life and relationships are very important to everyone, whatever the degree of intellectual disability.

References

3 American Association on Intellectual and Developmental Disabilities (2010). *Intellectual Disability: Definition, Classification and Systems of Supports*, 11th edn. American Association on Intellectual and Developmental Disabilities: Washington DC.

Definition of intellectual disability

Historically, intellectual disability has been understood from a number of different theoretical perspectives. Three key perspectives have led to modern definitions of intellectual disability:

- **Sociological**—people who fall outside accepted norms and expectations in society. From this perspective, intellectual disability can be seen as deviance where the task of services is to enable people to be included in community life. The alternative is to see intellectual disability as a subculture that is distinct and different from other groups in society. Here services are intended to empower and support the group;
- **Medical**—this focuses on the possibility that there is an underlying disease or pathology that might at some point be identified, understood, and treated as a medical condition. There is also a controversial notion that prevention of intellectual disability might be an important and valid aim;
- **Statistical**—here it is assumed that any aspect of human behaviour can be measured and will have a mean and SD. In the case of intellectual disability, there are two aspects of measurement—intelligence as measured by intelligence tests to arrive at an IQ, and adaptive behaviour (the ability to cope with the challenges of everyday life). People with intellectual disability are defined as those who fall below the mean on these measures.

These different perspectives have produced a common understanding that intellectual disability is defined as an interaction between the person and their environment.[4] A person may have significant deficits but cope well in the right environment and with the right support. Minor difficulties can be massively handicapping in a world where the person is isolated and unsupported.

These ideas have led to an accepted definition of intellectual disability. There are three main components:

- A significant lifelong difficulty in learning and understanding;
- A significant difficulty in learning and practising the skills needed to cope with everyday life;
- That there is evidence that these difficulties started before adulthood.[5-7]

These definitions have been worded very carefully from a political perspective, but they are not sufficiently precise for professional practice. It is important therefore to add the internationally accepted definition of intellectual disability, which is:

> 'Intellectual disability is characterized by significant limitations both in intellectual functioning and in adaptive behaviour as expressed in conceptual, social and practical adaptive skills. This disability originates before age 18.'[7]

Crucially, this definition is underpinned by five assumptions, each of which must be considered when using the definition. These assumptions include the importance of understanding people with intellectual disabilities in terms of what an ordinary life in the community might look like for a person of similar age and background. They stress the importance of linguistic and cultural diversity when making assessments, and the need to remember the strengths and gifts of the person, in addition to any limitations. One of the main reasons to assess intellectual disability is to identify the support a person needs, rather than to assign a category. Assessment is only to be carried out if it is of benefit to the person, and always remembering that, with good support, an individual's quality of life will generally get better.

References

4 Hatton C, Glover G, Emerson E, Brown I (2016). *Learning Disabilities Observatory. People With Learning Disabilities in England 2015: Main Report*. Public Health England: London. ℳ healthwatchgateshead. co.uk/wp-content/uploads/2016/08/PWLDIE-2015-final.pdf (accessed 30 October 2017).

5 Department of Health (2001). *Valuing People: A New Strategy for Learning Disability in the 21st Century*. Cm 5086. HMSO: London.

6 Scottish Executive (2000). *The Same as You: A Review of Services for People With Learning Disabilities*. Scottish Executive: Edinburgh.

7 American Association on Intellectual and Developmental Disabilities (2010). *Intellectual Disability: Definition, Classification and Systems of Supports*, 11th edn. American Association on Intellectual and Developmental Disabilities: Washington DC.

Incidence and prevalence of intellectual disability

Calculating the incidence of people with intellectual disability is difficult because there is no way of detecting the vast majority of those infants who have intellectual disability at birth. Therefore, to arrive at any estimate, one has to use cumulative incidence, and this has been calculated at 8yrs of age as 4.9/1000 for severe intellectual disability and 4.3/1000 for mild intellectual disability.[8]

It is only obvious manifestations of intellectual disability that can be detected at birth, e.g. Down syndrome (see ➜ Common conditions, pp. 16–17), and for these conditions, it is possible to calculate the incidence.

Therefore, it is more usual to refer to prevalence of intellectual disability, and where there is no obvious physical manifestation at birth, diagnosis must be delayed in order to await significant developmental delay, along with other manifestations, in order to diagnose intellectual disability, and this why it is more common to talk about prevalence.

Prevalence is concerned with an estimation of the number of people with a condition, disorder, or disease as a proportion of the general population.

If the IQ were used as an indicator of intellectual disability, then it could be calculated that some 2–3% of the population might have an IQ of <70. Given that a large proportion of people with such an IQ never come into contact with caring agencies, it is more common to refer to 'administrative prevalence', which actually refers to the number of people provided with some form of service from caring agencies.

Historically, there has been a general consensus that the overall prevalence of severe learning disabilities is ~3–4/1000 of the general population.[9]

The Department of Health has suggested that mild learning disability is quite common; prevalence has been estimated to be in the region of 20/1000 of the general population. In the United Kingdom (UK), it has been further calculated that, of the 3–4/1000 population with an intellectual disability, ~30% will present with severe or profound learning disabilities. Within this group, it is not uncommon to find multiple disabilities, including physical, and/or sensory, impairments or disability, as well as behavioural difficulties.

Emerson et al., drawing on extensive epidemiological data, have confirmed the estimation of prevalence for severe learning disabilities.[8] They state it to be somewhere in the region of 3–4/1000 of the general population. The prevalence rate Emerson et al. give for the intellectually disabled population referred to as having mild intellectual disability is much more imprecise. It is estimated that it might be 25–30 people/ 1000 of the general population. Estimates are constantly being revised. More current calculations suggest that there are 106 800 people with an intellectual disability in England. This includes 224 930 children and 900 900 adults, of whom 177 389 (20%) were eligible for an annual health check, 206 132 (23%) were known to general practitioners (GPs) as having an intellectual disability, and 429 530 (48%) were recorded by the Department of Work and Pensions as being entitled to received Disability Living Allowance or Attendance Allowance.[10]

It has been reported that there is a slight imbalance in the ratio of males to females in people with both mild and severe learning disabilities, with males having slightly higher prevalence rates. There is some evidence of slightly higher prevalence rates among some ethnic groups, and this includes black groups in the United States (USA) and South Asian groups in the UK.[8]

Finally, it is worth noting that there is no '*absolute*' number of people with intellectual disabilities, and this is the case internationally. This is because of different diagnostic systems, differences in terminology, and changing conceptualization of what intellectual disabilities actually means.

Further reading

BILD. *Need to Know Facts or Figures About Learning Disabilities?* ℘ www.bild.org.uk/resources/figures (accessed 30 October 2017).

Maulik PK, Mascarenhas MN, Mathers, CD, Dua T, Saxena S (2011). Prevalence of intellectual disability: a meta-analysis of population-based studies. *Research in Developmental Disabilities*. 32: 419–36.

Maulik PK, Mascarenhas MN, Mathers, CD, Dua T, Saxena S (2013). Corregendum to Prevalence of intellectual disability: a meta-analysis of population-based studies. *Research in Developmental Disabilities*. 34: 729.

Northern Ireland Assembly (2014). *Statistics on People with Learning Disabilities in Northern Ireland.* ℘ www.niassembly.gov.uk/globalassets/documents/raise/publications/2014/employment_learning/5014.pdf (accessed 30 October 2017).

Scottish Consortium for Learning Disability (2015). *Learning Disability Statistics Scotland, 2014.* ℘ www.scld.org.uk/wp-content/uploads/2015/08/Learning-Disability-Statistics-Scotland-2014-report.pdf (accessed 30 October 2017).

Welsh Government (2017). *Register of Persons with Learning Difficulties at 31 March.* ℘ statswales.gov.wales/Catalogue/Health-and-Social-Care/Social-Services/Disability-Registers/personswithlearningdisabilities-by-localauthority-service-agerange (accessed 30 October 2017).

References

8 Emerson E, Hatton C, Felce D, Murphy G (2001). *Learning Disabilities: The Fundamental Facts*. The Foundation for People with Learning Disabilities: London.

9 Department of Health (2001). Valuing People: A New Strategy for Learning Disability in the 21st Century. Cm 5086. HMSO: London.

10 Hatton C, Glover G, Emerson E, Brown I (2016). *Learning Disabilities Observatory. People with Learning Disabilities in England 2015: Main Report*. Public Health England: London. ℘ healthwatchgateshead.co.uk/wp-content/uploads/2016/08/PWLDIE-2015-final.pdf (accessed 30 October 2017).

Diagnosing intellectual disability

That this section concerns the diagnosis of intellectual disability would seem to imply that people with intellectual disability are the preserve of the medical model—this is not so. In the context of this section, it will be shown that identifying an intellectual disability is arrived at in a number of ways, and by different professionals; this may or may not include a medical diagnosis.

Diagnosing or identifying intellectual disabilities

The vast majority of parents will have no evidence that their child will have an intellectual disability before birth. Only a minority of parents have advance warning, possibly from screening investigations such as blood tests and ultrasound scans, or diagnostic investigations such as amniocentesis, chorionic villous sampling, or other tests undertaken because the parents are perceived as being at high risk.[11,12]

Unless a definite physical abnormality or characteristic signs (as in children with Down syndrome) are present at birth, or a traumatic delivery has taken place, intellectual disability is seldom suspected or diagnosed at birth. A diagnosis can vary from confirmation of the presence of a specific condition (e.g. Down syndrome) to a much broader diagnosis of developmental delay with no specific condition identified.

Intellectual disability is usually identified during childhood or sometimes later during adolescence, but in order to meet most international criteria for being classified as intellectually disabled, this should be before 18yrs of age, or if identified later in life, there should be sufficient evidence available that this commenced before 18yrs. Those children with severe or profound intellectual disability are likely to be noticed earlier as having an intellectual disability at a younger age than those with mild to moderate intellectual disability. Therefore, intellectual disability is most often diagnosed in early childhood when a child fails to reach 'normal' developmental milestones.

During this period, parents may have expressed concerns over the nature of their child's progress and suspect that a problem exists. It is unprofessional and potentially dangerous if those in contact with the parents at this time (e.g. GP, health visitor, paediatrician, or other nurses) dismiss parental concern and label them as 'over-anxious' or 'overprotective'. Such judgements are prejudicial and negate parents' concerns subsequently; they have no place in family-centred services. Rather a regular check should be kept on the child's progress, more frequently than the usual screening checks, and records kept. It is a relief to both parents and professionals, after a period of observation, to be able to show that their child is reaching normal milestones. The prospects of active family involvement will be damaged in the short term, and possibly for several years, when a diagnosis of intellectual disability is confirmed despite repeated concerns having been previously raised, only to be dismissed or largely ignored.

Finally, it is important to identify the nature and extent of intellectual disability and either exclude or include other more specific developmental disorders that are sometimes present, e.g. autistic spectrum condition (ASC), attention-deficit/hyperactivity disorder (ADHD), or dyspraxia (developmental coordination disorder).

Conclusion

Identification of the cause of intellectual disability and provision of an early diagnosis are crucial to:

- Identify the range of therapeutic approaches that may be used to ameliorate the effects of the condition, including mobilization of specific resources;
- Reduce the possibility of inadequate adaptation by the parents to their child and thereby hopefully avoid rejection;
- Limit the feelings of self-blame that may be experienced by some parents of children with intellectual disability;
- Understand the possible manifestation of the identified condition over a defined period of time;
- Establish, in some cases, the degree of risk to other family members of the condition reoccurring in their siblings and offspring.

Further reading

Harper P (2018). *Practical Genetic Counselling*, 8th edn. CRC Press: London.

References

11 Firth HV, Hurst JA (2017). *Oxford Desk Reference: Clinical Genetics*, 2nd edn. Oxford University Press: Oxford.
12 Nuffield Council on Bioethics (2017). *Non-Invasive Prenatal Testing: Ethical Issues*. ℗ nuffieldbioethics. org/wp-content/uploads/NIPT-ethical-issues-full-report.pdf (accessed 21 February 2018).

Causes and manifestations of intellectual disability

Intellectual disability is thought to affect an estimated 150 000 infants/year, either born with, or later diagnosed as having, an intellectual disability.[13] The reported frequency of intellectual disability varies across studies, but overall rates of 1–3% of the general population have been found, with a male:female ratio of 1.3:1, mainly attributed to X-linked intellectual disability.[14]

In 40–80% of individuals with intellectual disability, the cause cannot be determined.[13] Establishing the cause of intellectual disability can enable accurate information about any diagnosis reached to be imparted to patients and families, as well as assisting precise, rather than empiric, recurrence risks.[14] Recent progress in genetic testing, such as next-generation sequencing, has facilitated genetic diagnosis in unexplained cases of intellectual disability, developmental delay, and multiple congenital abnormalities with or without intellectual disability/developmental disabilities.[15] Discovering and diagnosing the molecular basis of rare genetic disorders and of intellectual disability, developmental delay, and multiple congenital abnormalities has provided valuable new insights into the mechanisms and treatment or management of disorders.[16] It has also provided information for affected families about disease prognosis, clarification of recurrence risks, access to disease-specific support groups, and new insights into the impact on parental quality of life of a diagnosis being made in previously undiagnosed conditions.[17]

Multiple congenital abnormalities can result from experiences in the prenatal environment that interfere with brain and central nervous system (CNS) development and functioning. Intellectual disability is a feature of numerous congenital conditions, but 5–15% are thought to result from genetic disorders. Abnormalities associated with chromosomes and/or genes can often disrupt physical and/or intellectual development.

Intellectual disability can result from a singular cause or insult during pregnancy or can arise from a combination of factors, as described next.

Genetic abnormalities

Genetic abnormalities may be subdivided into chromosomal, single-gene, multifactorial, mitochondrial, and/or somatic cell disorders. Recognized Mendelian patterns of inherited disorders include autosomal dominant, autosomal recessive, and X-linked (see ➔ Common conditions among people with intellectual disability, p. 17).

Exposure to environmental agents/teratogens

Environmental agents that cause disruption in normal prenatal development are known as teratogens. Fetal development can be disrupted by teratogenic exposure to chemicals, drugs, or diseases.

- *Chemicals*: examples of chemicals with known teratogenic effects include excessive radiation, smoking, and alcohol;

- *Drugs*: examples of drugs include so-called 'recreational' illegal substances and also prescribed drugs, which may have teratogenic effects (e.g. benzodiazepine, cocaine, or phenytoin);
- *Diseases*: examples of diseases with known teratogenic effects include toxoplasmosis, cytomegalovirus, or rubella.

It is now recognized that an embryo may be susceptible to virtually any substance if exposure to the substance is sufficiently concentrated. A number of broad generalizations have emerged from research on teratogens, e.g. some individual embryos and pregnancies are more *susceptible* to exposure, and/or there may be developmental periods which are *critical or sensitive* with regard to specific teratogen exposure.

Intrauterine or birth trauma

Where there is a clear biological cause of intellectual disability, e.g. oxygen deprivation at birth or placental insufficiency.

Prematurity

Intellectual disability caused by premature birth due to interruption of the normal course and duration of maturation in the uterine environment or due to trauma(s) experienced in the perinatal period following premature birth.

Postnatal developmental period

Intellectual disability may be caused in the immediate postnatal period, if there is interruption, disruption, or damage of a sufficient, significant level to the normal course of development. Examples would include infections such as meningitis, or trauma such as severe or intractable epilepsy or head injury.

Further reading

Harper P (2018). *Practical Genetic Counselling*, 8th edn. CRC Press: London.

References

13 Wynbrandt J, Ludman MD (2008). *The Encyclopedia of Genetic Disorders and Birth Defects*, 3rd edn. Facts on File Inc: New York.
14 Firth HV, Hurst JA (2017). *Oxford Desk Reference: Clinical Genetics*, 2nd edn. Oxford University Press: Oxford.
15 Vissers LE, de Ligt J, Gilissen C, et al. (2010). A de novo paradigm for mental retardation. *Nature Genetics*. 42: 1109–12.
16 Boycott KM, Vanstone MR, Bulman DE, MacKenzie AE (2013). Rare-disease genetics in the era of next-generation sequencing: discovery to translation. *Nature Review Genetics*. 14: 681–91.
17 Lingen M, Albers L, Borchers M, et al. (2016). Obtaining a genetic diagnosis in a child with disability: impact on parental quality of life. *Clinical Genetics*. 89: 258–66.

Common conditions among people with intellectual disability

Genetic diseases and disorders with associated intellectual disability may be subdivided into chromosomal, single-gene, multifactorial, and mitochondrial disorders. Recognized Mendelian patterns of inherited single-gene disorders include autosomal dominant, autosomal recessive, and X-linked inheritance.

Chromosomal disorders

The normal chromosome complement for humans is 46 chromosomes and these occur in pairs. Pairs 1 to 22 are called autosomes and are common to both genders. The 23rd pair are the sex chromosomes because they relate to gender. Thus, the normal male chromosome complement is 46 XY (see Fig. 1.1 for examples of normal karyotypes), whereas the female chromosome complement is 46 XX. An abnormal chromosome complement can be the result of loss, duplication, or rearrangement of genetic material.

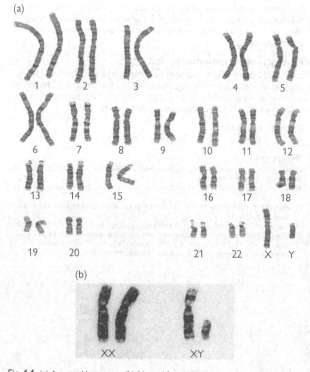

Fig. 1.1 (a) A normal karyotype. (b) Normal female XX and normal male XY.

Reprinted from Gardner, Sutherland, and Shaffer *Chromosome Abnormalities and Genetic Counselling* 4th ed. (2011) with permission from Oxford University Press.

Aneuploidy is a condition in which the chromosome number in the cells of an individual is not an exact number of the typical chromosome complement of 46 XX or 46 XY. There may be a full extra chromosome, called trisomy, or there may be a complete loss or absence of a chromosome called monosomy.[18] Examples of trisomy include trisomy 21 (Down syndrome), trisomy 18 (Edwards syndrome), or trisomy 13 (Patau syndrome). An example of monosomy that may be, but is not always, associated with intellectual disability is monosomy X (Turner syndrome).

Single-gene disorders

Genes located on the X chromosome are referred to as X-linked genes, and those on the autosomes as autosomal genes. Of each of the pairs in a chromosome set, one is derived from each parent, so each pair of chromosomes will have a comparable gene located at the same position on each chromosome pair, which may be referred to as alleles. Therefore, with the exception of the X and Y chromosomes in males, each gene is present in two copies, one from each parent. A gene mutation indicates a changed or altered gene.[19] These principles of dominant, recessive, and X-linked inheritance patterns reflect Mendelian laws of inheritance.[19]

- *Autosomal dominant*—a gene mutation in one of a pair of genes which produces an abnormal characteristic, despite the presence of the other normal or unaltered copy, is referred to as dominant. Examples of autosomal dominant disorders often associated with differing degrees of intellectual disability include Apert syndrome, myotonic dystrophy (early-onset and congenital cases frequently associated with intellectual disability, though adult-onset infrequently associated with intellectual disability), and tuberous sclerosis.
- *Autosomal recessive*—a gene mutation that causes an abnormal characteristic only when present in both copies of a gene is referred to as recessive. Examples of autosomal recessive disorders causing, or often associated with, differing degrees of intellectual disability include galactosaemia, Sanfilippo syndrome, Tay–Sachs disease, and phenylketonuria;
- *X-linked*—the sex chromosomes consist of two X chromosomes in a normal female, and one X and one Y chromosome in a male. Therefore, females have two copies of each X chromosome gene, one from each parent, but males have only one copy of each gene on the X chromosome. Mutations on the X chromosome may be described as dominant or recessive. X-linked dominant mutations may manifest obvious clinical effects in both males and females, whereas X-linked recessive mutations usually manifest in males but have minimal, or no, effect on (carrier) females. Examples of X-linked disorders causing, or often associated with, differing degrees of intellectual disability include fragile X syndrome, Coffin–Lowry syndrome, and adrenoleukodystrophy.

Multifactorial/polygenic disorders

In multifactorial/polygenic disorders, both genetic and environmental factors combine to influence the manifestation of the disorder. Such disorders, although frequently exhibiting familial clustering and raised recurrence risks in relatives, do not conform to Mendelian laws of gene transmission. Examples of multifactorial disorders include neural tube defects, orofacial clefting, and pyloric stenosis.

Mitochondrial disorders

Mitochondria of cells contain deoxyribonucleic acid (DNA), which has unique features that distinguish it from nuclear DNA. Mitochondrial DNA is exclusively maternally inherited, with few, very rare, exceptions. Paternal mitochondria enter the egg on fertilization only in miniscule proportions and are usually rapidly eliminated early in embryogenesis.[20] Examples of mitochondrial inherited disorders include myoclonic epilepsy with ragged red fibres (MERRF) and mitochondrial encephalopathy, lactic acidosis, and stroke-like episodes (MELAS).

Further reading

Harper P (2018). *Practical Genetic Counselling*, 8th edn. CRC Press: London.

References

18 Field RC, Stansfield WD (2013). *A Dictionary of Genetics*, 8th edn. Oxford University Press: Oxford.

19 Jones KL (2013). *Smith's Recognizable Patterns of Human Malformation*, 7th edn. Elsevier Saunders: Philadelphia, PA.

20 Firth HV, Hurst JA (2017). *Oxford Desk Reference: Clinical Genetics*, 2nd edn. Oxford University Press: Oxford.

Defining intellectual disability nursing

Nursing for people with intellectual disabilities is associated with supporting or caring for people with intellectual disability who have a broad range of health and social care needs and simultaneously supporting their families and carers. Registered Nurses Learning Disability or Intellectual Disability support people with intellectual disability, their families, and carers within a diverse range of settings, providing both generalist and focused nursing care.[21]

What do nurses for people with intellectual disabilities do?

The modern-day practice environment for nursing for people with intellectual disabilities is located in a landscape of complex service provision that includes residential care homes, independent living homes, supported living, and people with intellectual disability living in family homes. Some intellectual disability nurses work in specialist health and/or social care services such as assessment and treatment services and challenging behaviour services.[21]

Registered nurses for people with intellectual disabilities have an in-depth knowledge of the population they care for and a wide variety of skills, used to make a real and significant contribution to meeting the health needs of people with intellectual disability. They bridge a gap between primary, secondary, and tertiary care services.

The population of children, adults, and older people with intellectual disability is increasing and changing[22] due to improved preterm neonatal survival rates, and a growing number of adults with intellectual disability are living into older age.[23]

Also to be found are larger service configurations and/or very specialist settings such as treatment and assessment services or outreach community challenging behaviour services. They may also be found working in other specialist health or social care settings such as hospices or homes for older people, as well as acute hospitals in liaison roles.

Registered nurses for people with intellectual disabilities

Registered nurses specially educated to support people with intellectual disabilities currently work in various organizational settings that include: the National Health Service (NHS), local authorities, and private, statutory, and third sectors. Typically, they are likely to work in inter-professional teams and for multiple agencies. Recent changes are beginning to dictate a spectrum of new roles that are undertaken, e.g. nurses working in healthcare teams such as acute hospitals, mental health services, and primary care. In the UK and Ireland, the nurses' role include:

- Health facilitators, acute liaison nursing role,[23,24] annual health checks for people with intellectual disability;
- Assessing and responding to the diverse complex health needs experienced by people with intellectual disability[24] through assessing and treatment in inpatient, secure, and forensic services;
- Specialist roles in community teams for people with intellectual disability, criminal justice system, research, and advising on intellectual disability issues;

- Advising and providing a consultant nurse role;
- Academic/clinical career in higher education;
- Leadership—strategic roles in commissioning of services for people with intellectual disability.

Further reading

Department of Health (2014). *Strengthening the Commitment: One Year On: Progress Report on the UK Modernising Learning Disabilities Nursing Review.* Department of Health: London.

References

21 UK Chief Nursing Officers (2012). *Strengthening the Commitment: The Report of the UK Modernising Learning Disabilities Nursing Review.* Scottish Government: Edinburgh.

22 Hatton C, Glover G, Emerson E, Brown I (2016). *Learning Disabilities Observatory. People with learning disabilities in England 2015: Main Report.* Public Health England: London. ℘ healthwatchgateshead.co.uk/wp-content/uploads/2016/08/PWLDIE-2015-final.pdf (accessed 30 October 2017).

23 Royal College of Nursing (2014). *Learning from the Past—Setting Out the Future: Developing Learning Disability Nursing in the United Kingdom. An RCN Position Statement on the Role of the Learning Disability Nurse.* Royal College of Nursing: London.

24 Michael J (2008). *Healthcare for All: Report of the Independent Inquiry into Access to Healthcare for People with Learning Disabilities.* Department of Health: London.

The purist form of nursing

The context of nursing people with intellectual disabilities

The practice setting is located in complex landscapes of service provision. This includes, for example, residential care homes, independent living, supported living arrangements, as well as people with intellectual disability living in their own homes and family homes. There are also larger service configurations and very specialist settings such as assessment and treatment services, less commonly challenging behaviour units, as well as specialist health or social care settings such as hospices for children with life-limiting conditions, or homes for older people. Registered nurses for people with intellectual disabilities work with people from birth through to death, some of whom require a range of supports throughout their lives, ranging from minimal support through to intensive holistic nursing aimed at meeting their multidimensional needs. It is argued that this field of nursing practice is the 'purist' form of nursing; unlike our colleagues in other fields of nursing practice, they do not concentrate on specific manifestations of physical ill health or trauma, nor do they focus on mental health and well-being, or children or childbirth for that matter; rather they offer support to people with intellectual disability and their families that is all embracing, and quite literally from birth through to death.

The purist approach

In order to offer comprehensive nursing interventions that meet the multidimensional needs of people with intellectual disability, it is necessary to adopt a structured approach. A comprehensive needs assessment (physical, psychological, social, spiritual, and emotional) has to be completed. If a nurse is required to work with someone with intellectual disability and their families, it is necessary that their needs are assessed and incorporated into an individual care plan, taking their desires, wishes, and aspirations into account. The nurse must work closely with the client's family, care providers, and other professionals, as this broad approach may bring very important and essential information to light for assessment, as well as care plan development, its approach, delivery, and management. This is followed by construction of a written care plan that is then implemented and followed, with ongoing review and evaluation. It is this very structured approach, with partnership working, that ensures consideration of the multidimensionality of people. This, coupled with person-centred, co-produced planning, allows these nurses to claim, and validate, that what they do is the purist form of nursing.

A modelled approach

In response to social and political influences, the area of intellectual disability care models and that of care planning have changed considerably, so therefore has the practice of registered nurses for people with intellectual disabilities.[25] For example, during the last century, intellectual disability services were dominated by a medical model of care that emphasized the biological needs of people and the need to 'cure' physical problems in order to allow a person to function in society. Most people with intellectual disability have now moved out of long-stay hospitals, but there remains concern that the powerful effects of the medical model continue to influence care provided in smaller community-based residences. Klotz, for example, has argued that use of the medical model has pathologized and objectified people with intellectual disability, leading to them being seen as 'less human'.[26] Therefore, it is important that intellectual disability nurses use a nursing model to guide their care and support in practice, to ensure that what they offer is holistic. It must be remembered therefore that the use of such a model must hold the person with intellectual disability as central to the care-planning process and that the nurse must be mindful they use such a model to promote what is best for that person. There are numerous nursing models that can be adapted and used in a variety of health and social care settings. Some nursing models, such as Orem's self-care,[27] Roper's (2002) activities of daily living,[28] and Aldridge[29] are all well known and seemingly most used in intellectual disability nursing. It should be remembered that they may not be seen as relevant or ideal for all people with intellectual disability, but they can generally be adapted relatively easily, and then become ideal frameworks for the assessment of health, as well as more general needs.

References

25 Gates B (2015). The nature of learning disabilities and its relationship to learning disability nursing. In: B Gates, K Mafuba, eds. *Learning Disability Nursing: Modern Day Practice*. Taylor and Francis: London; pp. 1–26.

26 Klotz J (2004). Sociocultural study of intellectual disability: moving beyond labelling and social constructionist perspectives. *British Journal of Learning Disabilities*. **32**: 93–4.

27 Orem DE (1991). *Nursing: Concepts of Practice*. Mosby: St Louis, MO.

28 Roper N, Logan W, Tierney A (2002). *The Elements of Nursing*, 4th edn. Churchill Livingstone: Edinburgh.

29 Aldridge J (2004). Intellectual disability nursing: a model for practice. In: J Turnbull, ed. *Learning Disability Nursing*. Blackwell Publishing: Oxford; pp. 169–87.

Principles and values of social policy and their effects on intellectual disability

Across the UK and the Republic of Ireland, current policies underpinning services for people with intellectual disability have been in place since the early 2000s. Since 2000, each of the countries of the UK have published substantial reviews of their policy guiding the development and delivery of services.[30-34] These consistently highlight the importance of supporting people as individuals and giving due regard to their human, civil, and legal rights.

The key principles within these documents (outlined in the list below) are largely consistent, although at times slightly different language may be used to express similar ideas.

- **People should be valued**, and this should be reflected in them having the same legal and civil rights as all citizens of the country, and discrimination on all grounds, including disability, should be challenged.
- **People should be helped and supported to do everything they are able to.** The starting presumption should be one of maximizing independence, rather than dependence. Independence in this context does not mean doing everything unaided.
- **People should be actively included in a valued way in all aspects of society.** Often referred broadly under the principle of 'inclusion'. This is demonstrated by enabling people to do ordinary things, make use of all community, social, and health services, and be included fully in the local community.
- **People should be directly and actively involved in making decisions that affect them.** They should be asked about the services they need and wish to use, and be involved in making choices. This includes people with severe and profound disabilities who, with the right help and support, can make important choices and express preferences about their day-to-day lives. People should access independent advocacy services.
- **People should have services that take account of their individual age, abilities, and other needs.** General services are required to make 'reasonable adjustments' to maximize the accessibility and positive outcomes for people using these services. When necessary, people should have access to high-quality specialist social, health, and educational services.
- **People with intellectual disabilities should have full access to services that demonstrably improve their physical and mental health.** It is recognized that many people with intellectual disabilities continue to have poorer health than other members of the general population and less access to health promotion. In addition, it has been found that, despite some improvements to general health services and services for people with intellectual disabilities, many people with intellectual disabilities continue to have less accessibility and poorer quality of services.[35] There is emphasis for all general health services, including primary care, general hospital, mental health services, and palliative care, to ensure the services they provide are fully accessible to people with intellectual disabilities.

Alongside this, there is a need for intellectual disabilities services to recognize their limitations and to effectively collaborate with general health services, including the need to become more skilled at looking after physical and mental health promotion and care of people with intellectual disabilities.

Room for improvement

Despite the national policy documents and a wide range of supporting more specific documents, progress to implementing the principles underpinning these policies has been patchy and limited in many places.

Repeated investigations into services for people with intellectual disabilities (look at website of care regulators in your respective jurisdistion) have concluded people with intellectual disabilities continue to be marginalized, have limited access to general services in their local communities, and continue to be at risk for abuse within services and local communities.

These limitations have often been linked to a lack of proactive steps to promote the rights of people with intellectual disabilities as citizens of the country. This is further compounded by poor governance and safeguarding within the leadership and management of services.

Nurses should seriously consider the need to implement these principles and use them as important guidelines in all aspects of decision-making and their actions in working with people with intellectual disabilities. In considering your professional practice, professional and care regulators will expect you to explain how you took these into account.

References

30 Scottish Executive (2000). *The Same as You? A Review of the Services for People with Learning Disabilities*. Scottish Executive: Edinburgh.
31 Department of Health (2001). *Valuing People. A New Strategy for Learning Disability for 21st Century*. Department of Health: London.
32 Welsh Office (2001). *Fulfilling the Promises*. Welsh Assembly: Cardiff.
33 Department of Health, Social Services, and Public Safety (2005). *Equal Lives*. Department of Health, Social Services, and Public Safety: Belfast.
34 Inclusion Ireland (2012). *Information Pack: A Guide to Disability Law and Policy in Ireland*. ℭ www.inclusionireland.ie/sites/default/files/documents/information_pack-final.pdf (accessed 30 October 2017).
35 Heslop P, Blair P, Fleming M, Hoghton M Marriott A, Russ L (2013). *Confidential Inquiry into Premature Deaths of People with Learning Disabilities (CIPOLD)*. Norah Fry Research Centre: Bristol. ℭ www.bris.ac.uk/cipold/ (accessed 30 October 2017).

Holism and working across the lifespan

Holistic nursing for health

Holistic approaches to nursing seek to promote nursing interventions that adopt a whole-person approach or what is now increasingly referred to as a person-centred approach. This means providing nursing that responds to the various dimensions of being, and these typically include attention to the physical, emotional, social, economic, and spiritual needs of people ($\rightarrow$ see Person-centred approach, pp. 26–7).

Working holistically across the lifespan

Being healthy is a positive state of being that we all seek. We are constantly exposed to factors throughout our lives that have the potential to compromise our health. The health of people with intellectual disability is likely to be compromised by inequity and inequality, and thus they are susceptible to health loss. To seek health gain and health maintenance for people with intellectual disabilites will sometimes require the support of a registered nurse specifically educated in this field of nursing practice. This can occur throughout the lifespan from childhood to old age, and in end-of-life care. Nurses must remember that holistic co-produced care plans and delivery form an essential part of their everyday practice. They can enable people with intellectual disability to obtain good-quality care. In order to do this, they must reflect on their practice and use the best possible evidence to meet their multidimensional needs—thus providing person-centred holistic care. They have many dimensions and responsibilities to their role; however, supporting people with intellectual disability to reach their goals by living their lives as fully and independently as possible is by far the most vital. As registered nurses, they have a duty of care and they have to act within the best interests of their clients at all times. This necessarily includes planning and delivery of care that attends to the holistic nature of the people they are supporting.

Further reading

Journal of Holistic Nursing. journals.sagepub.com/home/jhn (accessed 21 February 2018).

McCormack B, McCance T, eds. (2016). *Person-Centred Practice in Nursing and Healthcare*. Wiley Blackwell: Oxford.

Working with families

Defining families

Families of people with intellectual disabilities can be major influences in their lives, and in many situations, they provide most of the care and support to family members. The need for nurses to work collaboratively with family members is integral to current government policy within services, and a key professional requirement by the Nursing and Midwifery Council (NMC) and the National Nursing and Midwifery Board of Ireland (NMBI).

In using the word 'family', there is often a perceived common understanding of what we mean by the term. There is common language used when talking about family members and relatives within the wider family. The nature of these relationships, however, and the importance attached to them can differ considerably between different individuals within the same family, and people across different families. Although considerable variation may occur between family structures, overall the family unit is still recognized as a core unit within society that has a major influence on the development and overall functioning of its individual members, as well as on local communities.[1]

The meaning of what a family is has altered considerably since the 1970s. Although most children, including those with intellectual disabilities, grow up within a family environment, the stereotypical definition of a family of two married parents and two children growing up together no longer reflects the range of possible family structures within the current society in the UK or the Republic of Ireland.

As a consequence, defining the nature of families is not as straightforward as it may first appear. There are a growing number of possible differences to be considered, for instance: number of parents present, marital or legal relationships between parents, biological and legal relationships between children and adults within the family, gender of parents, number of children, and number of generations present within the one family unit as defined by family members, and cultural backgrounds. Given the considerable evolution of the nature of families, it is reasonable to expect that there will be further developments in the structure and function of families over the years to come.

However, despite variations in family structures and the roles of members, it is generally accepted that a family involves the following key components:
- A defined membership;
- Agreed group values;
- Relationships between members;
- Roles;
- Structure;
- Functions;
- Stability over time.

Nurses need to learn the legal definitions of families and family relationships, such as next of kin, partners, parental responsibility, civil partnerships, and marriage used within the jurisdiction in which they are working, and consider the practical implications of these and how they should be applied within their role. Such definitions can be found in mental health legislation, children-based legislation such as the relevant Children's Act or Order, as well as in guidance on consent, safeguarding, and child protection. Nurses should make time to review and remain up-to-date with these definitions, because often when you need to make decisions, for instance about the role of parents or other family members in relation to consent or admission to care or safeguarding issues, there may be limited opportunity to consult legal documents or seek a legal opinion at that time.

Nurses working with people with intellectual disabilities need to be aware of the changing nature of the demography of people with intellectual disabilities, and the structure and membership of families. There is growing diversity of family arrangements, spanning from small nuclear family groups to more extended networks, and the social, cultural, and religious factors that may influence these arrangements. It is also important to be alert to the potential differing rules and roles within families, yet treat all families with respect and not to discriminate against families or the members within them due to their differing family structures and functioning.

References

1 Haralambos M, Holburn M (2013). *Sociology. Themes and Perspectives*, 8th edn. Collins Educational: London.

Family members of people with intellectual disabilities

Family membership—a lifetime bond?

All people with intellectual disabilities are born into families of some description. It is accepted that the composition and structure of the families may vary considerably, depending on the number of parents living together, other siblings, and extended family networks, together with other social and cultural influences. However, most people recognize themselves as family members, with the roles and responsibilities that brings during their life. It is important to acknowledge that a person with intellectual disabilities may also be a brother, sister, cousin, grandchild, aunt, uncle, and increasingly parents. In situations when a person with intellectual disabilities is adopted or fostered, they will usually still see themselves as 'belonging' to a family.

Furthermore, just like most people who do not have intellectual disabilities, individuals with intellectual disabilities will normally view themselves as family members, even after they have left home and possibility moved some miles away. Likewise, other family members will continue to see the person with intellectual disabilities as a family member and will often wish to continue to maintain contact and may wish to be involved in providing some ongoing support.

Nurses need to recognize that family members will provide most of the support for people with intellectual disabilities during their lifetime, and that successful collaborative working arrangements with family members is key to being able to provide effective professional support. Furthermore, while it is accepted that working with family members can at times be difficult, the need to seek ways to work effectively with families is a professional requirement for all nurses and is never an optional extra.[2,3]

Impact of having family member(s) with intellectual disabilities

Much has been written about the impact of having a family member with intellectual disabilities, and the picture that emerges from the research is very mixed. Depending on the literature you are reading and the focus of the research undertaken, nurses could, at times, almost be forgiven for believing that the impact on other family members is almost universally negative.

However, this is not an accurate picture and is, in many ways, more reflective of the research focus taken and the pathological view of families held by some professionals. This is not to deny that, at times, families may have difficulties, but consider how many families of people with intellectual disabilities manage very well most of the time, and with limited need for ongoing professional support.

For many families, the impact is mixed, a combination of positive and negative experiences. At times, extra challenges may arise as a consequence of having a person with intellectual disabilities in the family, for instance, additional physical care needs, concerns over further education and development, and reduced opportunities for flexibility in family activities. In contrast, parents have reported positive impacts, including increased knowledge and skills, increased confidence, and stronger family cohesion.[4]

The impact on the family is evolving and will change as the abilities and needs of other family members and the person with intellectual disabilities change. For example, as parents get older, they may require more support; on some occasions, the person with intellectual disabilities may play an important role in supporting other family members. In seeking to develop effective collaboration with family members, nurses need to take time to understand the strengths and challenges for each family and avoid making stereotypical judgements about the support that all families may need. While nurses cannot always 'make things better' for families, and most family members understand that, we should always seek not to make things worse by our actions or omissions.

Acknowledging family membership

In acknowledging the person with intellectual disabilities as a family member, nurses should seek to support the person with intellectual disabilities to maintain contact with other family members. Practical examples may include knowing the birthdays of other family members and supporting the person to send a card if they wish, supporting them to be included in important family events such as birthday parties, wedding ceremonies, and other family celebrations of a religious or cultural significance.

It is also important to recognize the other roles people with intellectual disabilities may have in the family such as aunt, uncle, or cousin. Many people may wish to have the opportunity to 'maintain contact' with dead family members, and for this reason, it is also important they have the opportunity if they wish to remember anniversaries and visit burial sites, as is culturally appropriate.

References

2 Nursing and Midwifery Council (2015). *The Code: Standards of Conduct, Performance and Ethics for Nurses and Midwives*. Nursing and Midwifery Council: London.

3 Nursing and Midwifery Board of Ireland (2014). *Code of Professional Conduct and Ethics for Registered Nurses and Registered Midwives*. Nursing and Midwifery Board of Ireland: Dublin.

4 Families Special Interest Research Group of IASSIDD (2014). Families supporting a child with intellectual or developmental disabilities: the current state of knowledge. *Journal of Applied Research in Intellectual Disabilities*. **27**: 401–92.

Explaining intellectual disabilities to family members

Changing understandings and terminology

To some degree, the changing names used to describe people with intellectual disabilities reflect a developing understanding of the nature of intellectual disabilities, as it becomes more understood as a condition that could be ameliorated by education, support, and effective healthcare, in contrast to a previous view that a child or an adult would learn little and have little chance of becoming independent, with many people going to live in large hospitals or other congregated living settings. Indeed, in planning this book, much discussion took place on the title and terminology to be used, as noted in ➡ Preface, p. vi. However, for people not familiar with the history of these debates and discussions of the fine differences between terms, their understanding of intellectual disabilities may be quite varied, with a mixture of previous understandings and terms being used. It is likely that new terms will become used in the years to come as further debates and discussions occur, such as 'intellectual and developmental disabilities'. Some conditions that have previously been linked to intellectual disabilities may be viewed as separate with separate legislation, for instance, autism, Asperger's syndrome, and cerebral palsy, as intellectual disabilities is not always a key feature of these conditions, although developmental disabilities may be.

Need for a common understanding

Given the potential for debate about the meaning of terms, a useful starting point in explaining the nature of intellectual disabilities is the definitions largely used within current policy documents.[5] Within the UK, the Republic of Ireland, and internationally, the term 'intellectual disabilities' has three key components:

- A significantly reduced ability to understand new or complex information (impairment of intelligence);
- A reduced ability to cope independently (impaired social functioning);
- Started before adulthood, with a lasting effect on development.

The need for an explanation

Despite having a largely agreed policy-based definition, this will not be familiar to many parents or other family members of children with intellectual disabilities. In fact, even the term intellectual or learning disability may have limited agreed understanding across family networks, even after a diagnosis has been provided. It is important therefore to provide opportunities for further discussion about what such terminology means, so that parents, siblings, other family members, and professionals are all using the term to mean the same thing. It is necessary to tailor any explanation to the audience, be that mothers, fathers, parents together, siblings, or members of the extended family. Although nurses will largely be involved in discussions with members of the immediate family, the words and explanations that parents and siblings may use with other people can be a useful investment of time. Although parents may be aware of the terminology and have received a diagnosis, how effectively a diagnosis and an explanation are provided can have lasting effects on the future relationships parents and other family members may have with professionals.

Key points to remember

- Family members' concerns should be fully discussed and investigated—they know their child best. Their concerns must not be dismissed as being 'over-anxious' or fobbed off as 'each child developing at different rates', or 'sometimes people with intellectual disabilities do things like that'.
- Not being told should not be mistaken for not knowing; just because a confirmed diagnosis has never been provided does not mean parents are not aware that some difficulties may exist, even if they have never mentioned them.
- At times, more detailed explanations of complex conditions are necessary in relationship to origins and care needs, and nurses should work collaboratively with other professionals, such as geneticists, if required. An assessment of family members' understanding and possible training needs should be undertaken in relation to caring for the person with intellectual disabilities, and this is used as a basis for further information provision and skills teaching. Be aware that mothers, fathers, and siblings may have quite different understanding and different informational needs.
- The potential of any individual to learn is largely influenced by the opportunities they have to learn; therefore, any explanation should include hope that individuals will continue to learn and avoid categorical statements about final outcomes such as 'he/she will never … '
- Siblings need explanations in a language they can understand; it is often helpful to explain this as people learning slower and may be having different abilities from each other. Balance against confidentiality of personal information.
- Adult siblings may need further explanations as the care of the person may change, and parents may have provided limited detailed explanation of their sibling's condition or future care needs as an adult.
- Provide opportunities for grandparents to ask questions; they may not have had a reason or an opportunity to update their previous views towards intellectual disabilities and understanding of interventions.
- Never lose sight of the fact that the person with intellectual disabilities is still first and foremost a family member—a son, daughter, brother, sister, or grandchild—build on strengths.

Further reading

Down's Syndrome Association. ℘ www.downs-syndrome.org.uk (accessed 23 February 2018).
Foundation for People with Learning Disabilities. ℘ www.learningdisabilities.org.uk (accessed 23 February 2018).
Mencap. ℘ www.mencap.org.uk (accessed 23 February 2018).

References

5 Department of Health, Social Services and Public Safety (2005). *Equal Lives*. Department of Health, Social Services and Public Safety: Belfast.

The process of family adaptation

Parents and other family members (on the news of a pregnancy within the family) often start planning the birth of a child well in advance of the day it is born. Even with the developments in antenatal screening, very few families expect the birth of a child with, or the subsequent diagnosis of, intellectual disabilities.

The diagnosis of a condition linked to intellectual disabilities can be made within a few weeks of birth only in a small number of conditions with clearly recognized syndromes and diagnostic tests available. For most parents, the presence of intellectual disabilities becomes visible over a period of months, often years, before a diagnosis is confirmed.

Bereavement reaction—a note of caution

Previously, a comparison has been made between the bereavement process and the birth of a child with intellectual disabilities, the rationale being that parents and other family members 'grieve' the loss of the expected child without intellectual disabilities. Although parents have reported shock and a sense of loss at the diagnosis of a child with intellectual disabilities, caution is needed when using a bereavement model to explain the process of family adaptation.

A fundamental difference exists in that when a child with intellectual disabilities is born, no child actually dies and the parents and other family members have the task of caring for, and supporting, the child who was born. Following on from this, parents do not reach an end-stage of 'acceptance', as outlined in earlier bereavement models, rather they continue to work through a process of adaptation as the abilities and needs of the child and other family members change. Therefore, nurses and other professionals need to be very careful about what they mean if they choose to use the word 'acceptance' of the birth or diagnosis of intellectual disabilities in a child.

Adaptation as a process

The diagnosis of intellectual disabilities does come as a shock to parents and other family members, whether this information was suspected during pregnancy, confirmed during pregnancy, or when the child was a few weeks, months, or years old. Over the past 30 years, several models have been presented to explain the stages parents may go through in seeking to adapt. While some differences exist in the terminology used and the number of stages within individual frameworks, the overall process outlined is largely similar.

One four-stage model, developed by Miller and mothers of children with a range of disabilities, although written several years ago, still provides important understandings and is supported more by recent research findings.[6,7]

- The first stage is that of 'surviving' and is characterized by mixed emotions of shock, fatigue, feelings of weakness, fragility, vulnerability, grief, helplessness, confusion, self-doubt, shame and embarrassment, resentment, and feelings of betrayal. Parents may find themselves preoccupied with their child, worrying about the uncertainty of the future, asking questions that appear to have no answers.

- The second stage has been called 'searching' and often involves a focused search of a more confirmed diagnosis and a 'label' for the condition beyond intellectual disabilities, while at the same time parents are gaining increased knowledge and skills in caring for their child. Parents may also find that they reconsider their priorities in life and start to ask more realistic questions about their child's abilities, without giving up hope.
- With the realization that there are no quick answers or cures, parents enter a stage of 'settling in', during which they recognize the progress their child has made and you become aware of regular progress and realize that some questions they have been asking do not have answers. Parents may also make further adjustments to their own life goals, continue to develop knowledge, skills, and flexibility, and start to know what works for them in supporting and caring for their child.
- Finally, as parents move to the next stage, they start to give over some control to the child and others, admitting that they cannot make the disability go away, and yet take pride in seeing their child achieve goals. This stage is called 'separating'.

One important limitation of this model is it focuses on mothers; therefore, it is important to consider the role of fathers, particularly as it appears many fathers have differing journeys from mothers.[7] It is also important to be aware of changes within the functioning of the wider family systems.[8]

Supporting the process of adaptation
In seeking to support the effective adaptation process for families, nurses need to remember:
- No two families will follow exactly the same journey; factors inside and outside each family will influence it;
- The model presented is a broad framework, and not a rigid structure; parents do not experience all emotions;
- Progression through the stages is not linear—it may be two steps forward and one back at times;
- Both parents and each family member is an individual, and they will often go through the process at different speeds;
- There is a need to recognize where each parent is in the process and provide relevant tailored support; there is no point in assuming 'settling in', if parents are clearly still 'surviving'.

References
6 Miller NB, Burmester S, Callahan DG, Dieterle J, Niedermeyer S (1994). *Nobody's Perfect*. Paul H Brookes: Baltimore, MD.
7 Davys D, Mitchell D, Martin R (2016). Fathers of people with intellectual disability. A review of the literature. *Journal of Intellectual Disabilities*. 21: 175–96.
8 Seligman M, Darling R (2009). *Ordinary Families, Special Children*. Guildford Press: New York, NY.

Resilience in families

Resilience

Resilience is the ability to adapt successfully to challenges in the face of ongoing adversity. Initially, the study of this area focused on the ability of individuals, but since the mid 1990s, there has been growing recognition of the ability of families to adapt successfully and an acknowledgement of the internal and external factors that may assist in that process.[9]

The changing view of families of people with intellectual disabilities

Until the 1990s, much of the literature about the families of people with intellectual disabilities portrayed the family and its members within a largely pathological frame of reference. Much of the research investigated the 'burden' on families and the negative emotional impact such as 'chronic grief', stress in families, and difficulties for siblings. While some of this type of research continues, it is now somewhat balanced by studies and personal accounts of relatives about the way they have successfully managed to adapt and cope with challenges.

Such a view is often evident, in my experience, when you ask professionals an open question: 'What do you think the impact of having a family member with intellectual disabilities is?' In my experience over the past 25 years, almost every time I ask this question to a group of professionals working in intellectual disabilities services, ten or more negative attributes are called out before any potentially positive aspects are noted. On the rare occasions that a positive aspect is noted within the first ten comments, a family member of a close relative with intellectual disabilities has been in the group. Nurses and other professionals need to be careful that they recognize the full range of abilities and needs of families of people with intellectual disabilities and do not become restricted to seeing families as always 'in need'. They need to recognize that although this may be reflective of the families with whom they, as professionals, may come in contact, many families with whom they do not have regular contact manage well within their family and social support networks.

A revised view of families now recognizes that many families of people with intellectual disabilities manage successfully most of the time and largely require support at times of particular difficulty, for instance in the early stages of adapting, during key transition points to and from school, and when the ability of the family to continue providing care is challenged due to changes within the family.[10,11] Effective service planning seeks to recognize the potential difficulties for families at these times and to work with them to plan ahead.

It is not the presence of a person with intellectual disabilities in the family that causes difficulties for families, but rather the reaction of family members, friends, and members of the local community that may present the biggest challenges. The stress of family members can be added to considerably by having contact with professionals, particularly if they feel they have to 'fight for services'.

Supporting families to develop and maintain resilience

Increasing the view of families is about their resilience and ability to adapt if given the opportunities and support. Patterson has developed a model known as the family adjustment and adaptation response (FAAR) model to explain how services can effectively support families.[12]

Within the first phase of this model, families work through the process of adjustment, during which time demands on the family outweigh their coping resource. The emphasis of intervention is to increase individual, family, and community resources in order to facilitate families to develop, establish, and maintain successful coping behaviours. The focus is on developing strength and resilience within families and their communities, rather than dealing only with crises that may arise for families.

As families increase their range of coping behaviours, the demands on the family are dealt with successfully, and equilibrium between demands and resources is achieved. Professionals and family members work together to achieve their 'increased ability to meet the needs and goals while maintaining autonomy and integrity'.[11] Through this partnership working, both family members and professionals can develop new understanding and skills.

The last words ...

The importance of supporting families developing and maintaining their abilities to respond successfully is captured in the words of a mother who, on reflecting on her experience of what helped in a real way, noted that: '*the journey has been made easier for us by friends and professionals who took time to listen to what I was saying, knowing I only wanted the best for Peter, and attempting to find it for me. By friends who allowed me to cry when I needed, and to rejoice when he achieved some particular goal no matter how small. By the school and its teachers who have kept on working with Peter over the years and watch with satisfaction his achievements ... '*[13]*

References

9　McCubbin H, Thompson E, Thompson A, Futrell J, eds (1999). *The Dynamics of Resilient Families.* Sage: Thousand Oaks, CA.

10　Families Special Interest Research Group of IASSIDD (2014). Families supporting a child with intellectual or developmental disabilities: the current state of knowledge. *Journal of Applied Research in Intellectual Disabilities.* 27: 401–92.

11　McConnell D, Savage A (2015). Stress and resilience among families caring for children with intellectual disability: expanding the research agenda. *Current Developmental Disorders Reports.* 2: 100–9.

12　Patterson J (1995). Promoting resilience in families experiencing stress. *Pediatric Clinics of North America.* 42: 47–63.

13　Maxwell V, Barr O (2003). With the benefit of hindsight: a mother's reflection on raising a child with Down's syndrome. *Journal of Learning Disabilities.* 7: 51–64.

* Maxwell V, Barr O (2003). With the benefit of hindsight: a mother's reflection on raising a child with Down's Syndrome. *Journal of Learning Disabilities.* 7(1) 51–64.

Families at risk

This term is increasingly applied to families with multiple disadvantages in the UK. Among these families are children and parents with intellectual disabilities who, like others placed in this group, are said to experience multiple disadvantages. Families at risk of social exclusions may experience five or more disadvantages; these include low income (below 60% of the median) and family cannot avoid to buy a number of items of food or clothing, at least one parents with long-standing limiting illnesses or disabilities, the mother with mental health problems, poor quality or overcrowded housing, and parental unemployment and limited qualification.[14] The children of such families are said to be at great risk of social exclusion and at risk of this being perpetuated into adulthood.

In 2008, the Social Exclusion Task Force published a policy entitled 'Think Family: Improving the Life Chances of Families at Risk'.[15] This highlighted the need to provide coordinated services that would improve the coordination of services for children, young people, and families with additional needs and provide specific services and approaches to tackle social exclusion among people facing multiple and complex issues. Though a minority of this group have intellectual disabilities, like others, they may place themselves at risk and, in some cases, heighten the risks to those around them. Service provision is expensive when people require support from several services and becomes most expensive and less effective if support is uncoordinated between services or they drop through safety nets, often not receiving the help they need until a crisis is reached.

What is often distinctive about 'families at risk' is that they often face multiple problems which cross several agencies and professional groups, with long-term issues such as homelessness, mental health problems, childhood abuse, and addictions, combined perhaps with relationship breakdowns or loss of social supports. Think family[15] *'means being alert to considering the impact of any event on other family members and alert to engaging with the person's circle of support. It involves coordinating services and support so that they work around the family. This means breaking down professional barriers and achieving changes in culture that mean practitioners work across organisations and service providers to achieve the best outcomes for the whole family.'* An increasing number of services now recognize the importance of a coordinated interdisciplinary and inter-agency service to support families, particularly when at risk of social exclusion. However, there is a need to develop more specific outcome measures in order to demonstrate the impact and increased resilience in families and more coordinated services.

Work has also been undertaken to support adults facing chronic exclusion, and an evaluation report of these projects found that projects were effective in supporting people.[16] In particular, it was noted these projects supported people to make more appropriate use of health and social care services and less use of emergency services, and people received support at key transition points, in particular in relation to changes in accommodation, which resulted in more integrated and cost-effective working across services.[17]

Nurses and other health and social care professionals working with families and individuals who are at risk of social inclusion should:

- 'Think family';
- Familiarize themselves with current policy relating to their country—often outside traditional health knowledge and practice zones.
- Contribute to the monitoring of targets to ensure that people with intellectual disabilities are included in society and are not excluded or neglected because they have a lower profile than many other excluded groups;
- Demonstrate a committed interagency approach to their work to improve processes of collaboration, but with a strong and well-developed sense that it is the outcome of this collaboration that is important, and not just the process;
- Be aware of the multiple meanings of risk.

References

14 Department of Health (2015). *The Care Act and Whole-Family Approaches*. HM Government: London.
15 Social Exclusion Task Force (2008). *Think Family: Improving the Life Chances of Families at Risk*. Social Exclusion Task Force: London.
16 Cattell J, Mackie A, Gibson K, et al. (2011). *Simple but Effective: Local Solutions for Adults Facing Multiple Deprivation*. Department for Communities and Local Government: London.
17 Day L, Bryson C, White C, et al. (2016). *National Evaluation of the Troubled Families Programme. Final Synthesis Report*. Department for Communities and Local Government: London.

Carers' assessment

Introduction

Carers are crucial to the support of people who have acute or longer-term health needs; this includes people caring for family members, relatives, and friends. The importance of their role is formally recognized in their right to a carer's assessment. This right was established in legislation across the four countries of the UK[18–20] and has been updated and reinforced since it first appeared in the mid 1990s. Carers, including young carers who provide 'regular and substantial care' (although this is not clearly defined), are entitled to an assessment of their needs on their request, and health and social care authorities have a duty to inform carers of their right to an assessment of their needs. This assessment should be separate from the needs of the person they are caring for, and local health and social care providers should develop a plan of care that arises from their carers' assessment for carers and have to provide support for carers.

What does a carer's assessment involve?

A carer's assessment should cover the carer's perceptions of the situation, the carer's relationship with the person they support, the caring tasks, the carer's willingness and ability to continue to provide care, their other commitments, and their coping strategies. If appropriate, this will lead to a care plan that is monitored and reviewed, with agreed and identified outcomes. Local authorities can delegate their powers of carers' assessments to health service staff (in Northern Ireland, these may be undertaken by health service staff, as joint health and social services structures exist). Despite carers' assessments being a right for over 20 years, in some parts of the UK, there are still challenges in translating the assessment outcomes into action to support carers, the willingness and ability of professionals 'to have the courage to tease out difficult issues with carers',[21] and improving communication before, during, and after assessments.[22] Nurses working with carers throughout the UK should ensure:

- They provide information leaflets about carers' assessment and are familiar with the process and are confident in explaining the purpose of carers' assessments;
- They are encouraging of carers' rights to an assessment (even if the person they are supporting refuses to be assessed) and they understand local definitions of regular and substantial, and can challenge misinformation;
- They are sensitive to the needs and wishes of a carer to being assessed separately and in private, away from the person they are supporting;
- They are able to discuss with carers their desired outcomes from such assessments;
- They record the existence of a carer's assessment in their documentation and use it to influence their work;
- They are sensitive to the possible anxieties surrounding the term 'assessment' as making judgements upon someone and carers' possible worries about involvement with social services (adults' or children's departments or social work services) for fear of stigma;

- They encourage carers to make sure that they receive written copies of their assessments and care plans;
- They offer assistance with, or explanation of, if required, elements of the assessment that involve self-completion by the carer;
- They are aware of the circumstances in which carers may be at risk of additional stress, e.g. at times of illness, when the person for whom they care is first diagnosed, if his or her condition deteriorates suddenly, if a person is being discharged from hospital, or if he or she becomes terminally ill. They recommend carers ask for a review if needs change or circumstances alter;
- They are aware of the nature and extent of the support systems that the carer has and their care plans reflect these.

At system level, processes for starting a carer's assessment should be incorporated into strategic documents such as local Carers' Strategies. Joint information may be a useful product of collaboration between agencies. Joint (interagency and interdisciplinary) training around carers' assessment may foster closer collaboration. Carers with experience of assessment may be important contributors to training, information provision, and auditing. Nurses therefore have a key role in working with carers to promote their rights in acknowledging their expertise and in using aggregated information to inform local commissioning of services.

Further reading

Care Information Scotland (2017). *Carer's Assessment.* ℘ www.careinfoscotland.scot/topics/how-to-get-care-services/carers-assessment/ (accessed 26 February 2018).

Carers NI (2014). *Assessments. Your Guide to Getting Help. Factsheet.* ℘ www.carersuk.org/images/Factsheets/Factsheet_NI1020_Assessments_-_guide_to_getting_help.pdf (accessed 26 February 2018).

NHS Choices (2015). *Carer's Assessments.* ℘ www.nhs.uk/Conditions/social-care-and-support-guide/Pages/carers-assessment.aspx (accessed 26 February 2018).

References

18 Northern Ireland. *Carers and Direct Payments Act (2002).* ℘ www.legislation.gov.uk/nia/2002/6/contents (accessed 23 February 2018).

19 Scottish Government. *Carers (Scotland) Act (2016).* ℘ www.gov.scot/Topics/Health/Support-Social-Care/Unpaid-Carers/Implementation/Carers-scotland-act-2016 (accessed 2 March 2018).

20 England and Wales. *The Care Act (2014).* ℘ www.legislation.gov.uk/ukpga/2014/23/contents/enacted (accessed 23 February 2018).

21 Skills for Care (2013). *Carers Assessments: Workforce Development Opportunities Based on Carers Experiences.* Skills for Care: London.

22 Gamiz R, Tsegai A (2013). *Carer's Assessment and Outcomes Focused Approaches to Working with Carers.* Centre for Research on Families and Relationships/Institute for Research and Innovation in Social Services: Edinburgh.

Principles of working collaboratively with families

Introduction

'The family is the natural and fundamental group unit of society and is entitled to protection by society and the State' (United Nations, 1948). Since this statement was written, the nature of family structures has evolved considerably, from the more traditional view of a family of a mother, father, and children to including families headed by single parents, same-sex couples, blended families from previous relationships, married couples, cohabiting couples, and wider kinship networks.[22,23] Unfortunately, at times, policy documents still have a restricted view of what a family structure should be.

The family is a basic unit of society that represents racial, ethnic, cultural, and socio-economic diversity. It is also important to reinforce that people grow both individually and as part of a family. Therefore, families will use a whole raft of coping strategies and expect (or not) partnership/collaboration at different levels.

It is also important to acknowledge that, within a digital age, the way families choose to interact and stay in contact is very different from the picture even 20 years ago.

Working in partnership

Nurses and other health and social care professionals are expected to work collaboratively with family members, and this expectation is also reflected in policy documents.[24,25]

While some developments, such as Partnership Boards, have brought about some real empowerment in the lives of individuals who have intellectual disabilities, the principles of working collaboratively with families need further exploration. Such partnerships need to recognize that parents and other family members can often be important informal and formal educators of professionals in their training and in practice. Professionals need to learn to listen to the views of parents and learn from their experience, avoiding the belief that they have all the answers as professionals. This can be particularly critical when people with intellectual disabilities are accessing healthcare services.[26]

The essential principles of collaborative working have their roots and origins firmly linked to the principles of beneficence and non-maleficence (i.e. the duty to produce good and avoid harm). The essence of these principles is integrated into the following discussion on the principles of working collaboratively with families.

Relationship building—a positive goal or outcome will only be achieved if the professional establishes a firm base for the relationship. This could involve setting a time frame; being clear about what it is possible to achieve, by not making unrealistic promises; being willing and proactive to try non-traditional ways of working; listening, accepting, and responding to the other party's points of view; and valuing the other members of the partnership as equals, who have worth and a valid opinion.

Needs-based services/approaches—demonstration of a willingness to listen to the needs of the individual and their family, responding appropriately to expressed abilities and needs by family carers, while making accessible the focus of the professional's intervention.

Care decisions have to be based in the 'families' world, not just in services. Families need to be clear about the role a professional will take in the seamless web of care provided to a relative. Individuals need a benchmark by which they can assess the success of the partnership.

Independence—the ultimate aim of any professional intervention should be to promote an individual level of independence with the person in receipt of care. To do this collaboratively, families and people with intellectual disabilities should be given the opportunity to develop their own sustainable solutions through appropriate packages of education.

Further reading

Blacher J, Knight E, Kramer BR, Feinfield KA (2016). Supporting families who have children with intellectual disability. In: A Carr, G O'Reilly, P Noonan Walsh, J McEvoy, eds. *The Handbook of Intellectual Disability and Clinical Psychology Practice*. Routledge: London; pp. 283–310.

Chadwick DD, Mannan H, Garcia Iriarte E, et al. (2013). Family voices: life for family carers of people with intellectual disabilities in Ireland. *Journal of Applied Research in Intellectual Disabilities*. 26: 119–32.

References

22 Pillitteri A (2013). *Maternal and Child Health Nursing Care of the Childbearing and Childrearing Family*, 7th edn. Lippincott Williams & Wilkins: Philadelphia, PA.

23 Department of Health (2001). *Valuing People: A New Strategy for Learning Disability in the 21st Century*. Cmnd 5086. HMSO: London.

24 Nursing and Midwifery Council (2015). *The Code: Standards of Conduct, Performance and Ethics for Nurses and Midwives*. Nursing and Midwifery Council: London.

25 Nursing and Midwifery Board of Ireland (2014). *Code of Professional Conduct and Ethics for Registered Nurses and Registered Midwives*. Nursing and Midwifery Board of Ireland: Dublin.

26 Heslop P, Blair P, Fleming P, Hoghton M, Marriott A, Russ L (2013). *Confidential Inquiry into Premature Deaths of People with Learning Disabilities (CIPOLD) Final Report*. Norah Fry Research Centre: Bristol. ♒ www.bris.ac.uk/cipold/ (accessed 30 October 2017).

Supporting siblings of people with intellectual disabilities

Is there a need for specialist sib groups?

Over the past 10yrs, there has been a growing awareness that there is a need to effectively support the siblings of individuals who have intellectual disabilities. The growing interest in the stories of people who have a 'looked-after' life has heightened recognition of the needs of these brothers and sisters. This is becoming increasingly important to understand, as siblings often become the carers for adults with intellectual disabilities.[27,28]

The experience of being a sibling of a person with intellectual disabilities can be mixed, and no two siblings should be viewed as the same. While the experience of siblings can be difficult at times, depending on how the wider family reacts to, and manages, the presence of a person with intellectual disabilities, there can be positive impacts also. Professionals should remember this when seeking to provide holistic support to siblings. Siblings may have a range of feelings.

Mia Goleniowska,[29] with the help of her mother, guides a new sibling through an introduction to Down syndrome which details a loving story, but professionals must acknowledge that this is not always the case. Another perspective is given in the comment that: 'I can feel like a stranger to my brother. He can feel almost unreachable, devoid of emotion or a capacity to regard me as a sister who he might love ... but ultimately, despite the strain, nothing could replace it.'[30]

Such stories offer insights into family life, but those that detail the resentment very rarely get an airing.

- *Isolation*—there is often a belief that the brother or sister is the only one in this situation; no one else has ever had a sibling who has such an impact on the way a family lives their lives.
- *Fear*—will the other kids at school think it's catching? What if they want to come to my house? If they come what'll I do if my sibling acts out? A 'major concern from the teen's perspective is to be accepted by peers; above all, they don't want to be 'different.'
- *Burden*—anecdotal evidence from a professional's experience demonstrates that there is often an unspoken belief that the non-disabled sibling will assume some responsibility for the sibling with intellectual disabilities, whether that is in providing a home, financial responsibility, or emotional/social responsibility. Parents often reinforce to the non-disabled sibling their 'duty' to always care for the brother or sister.
- *Guilt*—the concept of 'why wasn't it me?' needs considering in the psychological welfare of the sibling, in particular of the sibling whose brother or sister has acquired their intellectual disabilities after birth, coupled with the isolation experienced by parents and the guilt of leaving home and starting a life independent of the family of origin.
- *Loss of childhood*—the need to be always the sensible sibling, the one who 'minds' the less able member of the family group. The one who

misses out on family days out because one parent has to stay at home with the sibling who reacts badly in crowds or to loud noises.

- *Resentment*—why are they described as special and I am not? It is important to acknowledge that siblings who require support and consideration with the person-centred process are not always children.

However, it is equally important to recognize that the impact of having a sibling with intellectual disabilities can have a positive impact, such as:

- *Confidence*—some siblings develop a clear understanding of their brother's or sister's abilities and needs, and become confident in interacting with them and with professionals;
- *Caring skills*—over the years of growing up, siblings are often involved in providing day-to-day support, and at times physical and emotional care, to their younger siblings. This can increasingly become the situation for adult siblings;
- *Increased communication skills*—siblings can become very adept at understanding their brother's or sister's non-verbal communication. These skills are often transferable to working with other people, in particular the confidence and ability to communicate with someone who cannot communicate verbally;
- *Understanding of difference*—siblings have often witnessed the range of difficulties in acceptance that their brother or sister had, and how they were treated differently by others. These insights often encourage recognition of the impact of treating people differently due to a disability and encourage a greater acceptance of the diversity in people.

Remember, just because one sibling has intellectual disabilities does not mean that the other will like them any more than if they did not; by the same token, some siblings remain close and attached for all their lives. The key feature in offering support to siblings has to be that the support is what the individual says they need, not what we believe they want/need, and individuals grow both within, and independently of, their family of origin. Support should make the sibling feel valued and not reinforce negative feelings; it should be personalized and tailor-made. How this may be achieved? Can you suggest three or four key points?

Further reading

Blacher J, Knight E, Kramer BR, Feinfield KA (2016). Supporting families who have children with intellectual disability. In: A Carr, G O'Reilly, P Noonan Walsh, J McEvoy, eds. *The Handbook of Intellectual Disability and Clinical Psychology Practice*. Routledge: London; pp. 283–310.

References

27 Jacobs P, MacMahon K (2017). 'It's different, but it's the same': perspectives of young adults with siblings with intellectual disabilities in residential care. *British Journal of Learning Disabilities*. 45: 12–20.

28 Coyle CE, Kramer J, Mutchler JE (2014). Aging together: sibling carers of adults with intellectual and developmental disabilities. *Journal of Policy and Practice in Intellectual Disabilities*. 11: 302–12.

29 Goleniowska H, Goleniowska M (2014). *I Love You Natty: A Sibling's Introduction to Down's Syndrome*. Downs Side Up UK.

30 Jones A (2014). Sister to Autism. ℘ www.huffingtonpost.co.uk/alice-jones/autism-and-siblings_b_5524267.html (accessed 30 October 2017).

People with intellectual disabilities as parents

The ethical dilemma

The idea of adults with intellectual disabilities becoming parents often causes us moral and professional difficulties—particularly in our thought process.

- Firstly, the historical notion of the individual who has intellectual disabilities is seen to have a looked-after life, e.g. the Wolfensberger[31] concept of deviancy reinforces the eternal child notion, and therefore the need for that individual to be 'looked after'; in today's climate, most modern social policy reinforces the 'label' of vulnerable adult, into which most people who have intellectual disabilities fall and therefore have some level of service intervention in the day-to-day running of their lives.
- Secondly, we are not always comfortable with the idea of people with intellectual disabilities having a sexual identity, let alone engaging in consensual sexual activity.
- Thirdly, the concept of pregnancy does not feature prominently in health action plans or healthy living programmes; much of the limited literature concentrates on safe sex and therefore avoiding pregnancy.
- Fourthly, who is going to be left holding the baby? Not many adults who have intellectual disabilities get the opportunity to demonstrate that they are poor parents, let alone the opportunity to learn and demonstrate good parenting skills. For most parents with intellectual disabilities, the high risk of having their children taken away from them is almost constant.

It is important that nurses seek to understand the perspectives, abilities, and challenges of parents with intellectual disabilities and make their decisions about future services to parents and their children from an informed basis.[32,33] Therefore, if little is known about the long-term outcomes of these children, surely the starting point should be how to support adults with intellectual disabilities to become 'good enough' parents. After all, there is no model of good parents that is inherent in all theories on family life; this is often the unspoken benchmark of professionals, rather than a reality based on actual of 'good enough parenting' for each given situation.

So how is this supported by practice-based evidence? Some parents with intellectual disabilities may feel that their opportunity for family life is constantly under threat, yet adequate support services geared to their needs are almost non-existent; the number of parents with intellectual disabilities who have their parental rights taken away far exceeds the number of those parents who do not have intellectual disabilities. While it is accepted that risks may exist, it is also clear that some parents with intellectual disabilities can be successful parents with varying degrees of support.[32,34]

Some examples of positive support[34,35] for parents have been documented and highlight the need for:

- Good, clear, and accessible information for the professionals offering the support—a geographical audit on local support services; holistic assessment of the coping strategies on the individuals; networking across non-traditional boundaries; and a willingness to find sustainable solutions grounded in the real world, not just in services;

- A commitment from services to discuss abilities, conflict, and difficulties openly and proactively. Remember that meetings are de-signed to discuss the way forward, not the difficulties a service is having at a macro-operational level;
- Being proactive and avoiding crisis-driven services/responses;
- Trust—especially between parents and the interdisciplinary team members, and between different agency professional staff;
- A recognition of the right to family life that acknowledges parents, children, and grandparents;
- Holistic family health being incorporated into healthy living programmes, to include relationship building and preconception care;
- Remembering that there is choice involved in becoming a parent, and that choice belongs to that adult, not the 'system'.

References

31 Wolfensberger W (1991). *A Brief Introduction to Social Role Valorization as a High-order Concept for Structuring Human Services.* Syracuse University Training Institute: Syracuse, NY.

32 Chinn D (2012). *Enabling Parenting with Support: Effective Working with Parents with Learning Disabilities.* Pavilion Publishing: Brighton.

33 Emerson E, Llewellyn G, Hatton C, et al. (2015). The health of parents with and without intellectual impairment in the UK. *Journal of Intellectual Disability Research.* 59: 1142–54.

34 Tarleton B (2015). A few steps along the road? Promoting support for parents with learning difficulties. *British Journal of Learning Disabilities.* 43: 114–20.

35 Noray Fry Research Centre (2009). *Supporting Parents with Learning Disabilities and Learning Difficulties. Stories of Positive Practice.* Noray Fry Research Centre: Bristol.

Family quality of life

It has long been accepted that families experience a higher quality of life, both individually and collectively, when their needs are met.[36] Recognition of those collective and individual needs being met could include families that enjoy spending time together, alongside being supported to be independent and do things that are important to them. Factors that influence family quality of life are community participation, friendships, family interaction, parenting, emotional well-being, alongside access to support mechanisms that promote health, and opportunities for financial well-being. This is no different for the family who has a member with intellectual disabilities. With this in mind, while it is recognised that many families of people with intellectual disabilities encounter additional challenges, it should not be assumed that their life is always a burden.

Pillitteri described the key factors of family-centred practice:[37]
- 'The family is the basic unit of society;
- Families represent racial, ethnic, cultural, and socioeconomic diversity;
- Children grow both individually and as part of a family.'

So how can family quality of life be measured?

'Quality of life has received much attention in recent years as a method of determining general well-being. Consequently, a wide range of tools now exist measuring quality of life in a variety of ways. However, family quality of life has received not nearly the same level of attention despite its crucial role in shaping our young lives. For this reason, the Family Quality of Life Scale (FQOL) was developed by Hu et al., 2011.'*[38,39]

Parenthood is a major transition, and therefore, the way a family forms and views itself relates to that transition. It is important to acknowledge that transitions occur both on and off time, and in relation to the family who has a member with a diagnosed extra-special need, this is no different (see ➔ The process of family adaptation, pp. 34–5). It is very easy for families and professionals to latch on to a notion that everything that happens in a family is related to the intellectual disabilities with which one member lives. However, it is important to acknowledge that systems and services often create 'disabled families', rather than acknowledging that one member of the family has a disability.

It is widely acknowledged (particularly in illness-related literature) that the measurement of family quality of life cannot relate solely to the perceived 'burden' of a disability or illness, and that issues of independence, resilience (see ➔ Resilience in families, pp. 36–7), and hope have to be taken into consideration. There is no one definitive checklist that the professional can take into an assessment and measure the quality of life a family is experiencing; what is intolerable for one family is an everyday occurrence for another, and when exploring family quality of life, the key factor to remember is that families and the individuals who live in them are not part of a homogenous group.

* Reprinted from Hu X. et al (2011) The quantitative measurement of family quality of life: A review of available instruments. Journal of Intellectual Disability Research. 55, 1098–1114 with permission from John Wiley.

Family quality of life has the same key domains as individual quality of life. These are:

- 'Physical well-being;
- Emotional well-being;
- Interpersonal relationships;
- Social inclusion;
- Personal development;
- Material well-being;
- Self-determination;
- Human and legal rights'.[36]

In seeking to gain an understanding of a family's quality of life, it is necessary to consider the degree to which the domains listed above result in families being able to have meaningful life experiences that they value, and the degree to which life domains contribute to a full and interconnected life.

It is important for professionals to recognize and acknowledge that the way an individual with intellectual disabilities lives their life within a family is ordinary for them, and our response is not to be judgemental and subjective; we are often the ones that describe that way of living as out of the ordinary, even when families consider they are coping well.

Further reading

Caples M, Sweeney J (2011). Quality of life: a survey of parents of children/adults with an intellectual disability who are availing of respite care. *British Journal of Learning Disabilities*. 39: 64–72.

Schalock RL, Keith KD, Verdugo MA, Gomez LE (2010). Quality of life model development and use in the field of intellectual disability. In: R Kober, ed. *Quality of Life: Theory and Implementation*. Sage: New York, NY; pp. 17–32.

References

36 Schalock RL (2000). *Outcome-Based Evaluation*, 2nd edn. Kluwer Academic: New York, NY.

37 Pillitteri A (2013). *Maternal and Child Health Nursing Care of the Childbearing and Childrearing Family*, 7th edn. Lippincott Williams & Wilkins: Philadelphia, PA.

38 Hu X, Summers JA, Turnbull A, Zuna N (2011). The quantitative measurement of family quality of life: a review of available instruments. *Journal of Intellectual Disability Research*. 55: 1098–114.

39 Measurement Instrument Database for the Social Sciences. *The Family Quality of Life Scale (FQOL)*. www.midss.org/content/family-quality-life-scale-fqol (accessed 31 October 2017).

Respite care

This discussion works on the premise that respite is a 'gift of time'; it should be planned and have purpose for both the individual in receipt of care and the people left at home, which, in turn, supports the philosophy that planned care is a right for those who live a looked-after life. For modern twenty-first century services to people who have intellectual disabilities, the more traditional idea of what respite is can be considered largely out-of-date.

Adults and children who have intellectual disabilities today receive a far more creative and proactive gift of time—respite in the community for a set period of hours to undertake a specific activity usually related to leisure, or respite in the home of another person who is an approved carer and registered under a scheme such as 'adults supporting adults'.

However, the recognition of respite provided by family carers such as grandparents has been acknowledged through the use of individual direct care payments and should no longer remain hidden.

Since the development of the Care Act (2014), changes to funding and arrangements have made life both easier and more complex to 'plot' the way through a myriad of policy to access respite services and funding:

> 'In April 2015, The Care Act 2014 replaced most recent law regarding carers and people being cared for. It outlines the way in which local authorities should carry out both needs assessments and Carer's assessments; how local authorities should decide who is eligible for support; how local authorities should charge for both residential and community care; and places new responsibilities on local authorities.
>
> The Care Act is primarily for adults in need of care and support, and their adult carers. There are limited provisions for the transition of children in need of care and support, parent carers of children in need of care and support, and young carers. However, the main provisions for these groups before the transition period are covered by the Children and Families Act 2014.'*

There is often a misconception that all care away from the home of origin for a fixed period of time has to be considered as respite, and with this in mind, practitioners need to remain cognisant that assessment and treatment services are not respite facilities and the advent of care and treatment reviews (CTRs) has highlighted many of these anomalies for adults.[40]

So why is respite offered as, and often considered, the panacea of all 'ills'? It may be useful for the reader to consider respite services that they have knowledge of under the following points:

- What is the purpose of the respite?
- Is the service offered the most appropriate?
- What could be an alternative?
- What has influenced your thoughts?
- Does anyone benefit from this service?
- What is the way forward?

It is also necessary to consider some key differences between the services offered to children and adults. Often respite for children, unless they have complex health needs or behaviour that challenges and/or a life-limiting diagnosis, is delivered within generic 'share the care' schemes (National Children's Home). Children and families become used to relating to one type of service/provider, and then the reality of the caring experience at the point of transition to adult-orientated services is often very different; perhaps in the advent of such advances in medical technology, one of the questions that should have prominence in service planners' and commissioners' minds is 'how and where to provide care for children who live into adulthood and for longer than initially anticipated'.[41]

There is presently limited robust research and literature that shows respite care is more than a rest period for parents and siblings, or from the perspective of the person with intellectual disabilities receiving it. Respite care provided is often for the benefit of the primary carers, rather than the individual who is in receipt of the care. Although a break in caring for parents or other family carers is, for many carers, a major help, further research is required to demonstrate how to maximize the benefit of respite care for the person with intellectual disabilities and their families. Respite needs to be proactive and planned and have purpose if it truly is to be a 'gift of time'.

Further reading

Blacher J, Knight E, Kramer BR, Feinfield KA (2016). Supporting families who have children with intellectual disability. In: A Carr, G O'Reilly, P Noonan Walsh, J McEvoy, eds. *The Handbook of Intellectual Disability and Clinical Psychology Practice*. Routledge: London; pp. 283–310.

Carers UK. *What is the Care Act?* www.carersuk.org/help-and-advice/practical-support/getting-care-and-support/care-act-faq#q1 (accessed 30 October 2017).

NHS Choices (2018). *Carers' Break and Respite Care*. www.nhs.uk/conditions/social-care-and-support-guide/pages/breaks-for-carers-respite-care.aspx (accessed 30 October 2017).

Wayman S (2016). *Home Sharing: Valued Respite for People with Intellectual Disability*. www.irishtimes.com/life-and-style/health-family/home-sharing-valued-respite-for-people-with-intellectual-disability-1.2879619 (accessed 30 October 2017).

Wilkie B, Barr O (2008). The experiences of parents of children with an intellectual disability who use respite services. *Learning Disability Practice*. 11: 30–6.

References

40 NHS England. *Care and Treatment Reviews*. www.england.nhs.uk/learning-disabilities/care/ctr/ (accessed 23 March 2018).

41 Together for Short Lives. *Help for Professionals*. www.togetherforshortlives.org.uk/professionals/care_and_best_practice (accessed 23 March 2018).

Working with older carers

The number of older carers of people with intellectual disabilities is growing, as life expectancy of people with intellectual disabilities increases. The number of older carers of people with intellectual disabilities poses new challenges for health and social care services who seek to support them, alongside their sons and daughters with intellectual disabilities.[42] It has been argued that there is a new generation of older people with intellectual disabilities and ageing carers, as the number of people with intellectual disabilities living with their ageing parents continues to grow.[43,44] This changing demography among people with intellectual disabilities and their ageing carers presents major challenges for individual practitioners, services, and overall policy development.

Older carers of people with intellectual disabilities

Older carers have a very important role in the lives of their son or daughter with intellectual disabilities, and integral to their personal identity is often their role as a carer. Many of older carers are lone carers, often mothers, and have considerable concerns for the future care provision for their son or daughter with intellectual disabilities.

In addition, many have poor physical and mental health. At times, this results in a mutually dependent caring relationship between the person with intellectual disabilities and their parent, which can add to the complexity of the care situation.[43,44] This interdependence may restrict willingness and opportunities to plan for the future, both because their carer needs their support and/or the son or daughter with intellectual disabilities does not wish to leave their parent as they know the support they provide is required. Even when planning for the future is desired by ageing carers, it may be discouraged by professionals if the caring relationship appears to be stable due to the complexities involved and the perceived lack of resources for alternative arrangements. All too often, these positive developments of an increased life expectancy for people with intellectual disabilities and normal ageing of their parents continue with no future planning by the older carer or professionals, until a crisis arises and emergency actions are required when the health of an older carer changes.[45]

It is important for professionals to recognize that older carers may have had difficult experiences with service provision over their lifetime. They may have well-placed fears from their perspective of professionals, as many will have been provided with limited support when their son or daughter was younger and they may have had limited ongoing contact with professionals over many years. Older carers have often lost trust in professionals being helpful and providing high-quality services. Recent inquiries into the quality of services in the UK and the Republic of Ireland may reinforce their concerns through highlighting the major failings of care provision. This can reinforce the need for ageing parents to continue to look after their son or daughter, because they believe professional services are not willing to do it, will not do it well, or cannot do as well as them. This can result in older carers living from day to day and not seeking to actively plan for the future. This challenging situation has been described as older carers' 'tolerating uncertainty'[45]—they know that future plans need to be addressed but are often reluctant how to do this.

Supporting future planning

When working with ageing carers, it is important to listen to, and recognize, their concerns, which, no matter how unrealistic you feel they may be, can be very real for the ageing carer. Staff should engage in open, transparent, and realistic discussions about future planning, being honest about opportunities and challenges that may be present.

It is important to provide ageing carers with the opportunity to learn about and, if possible, visit high-quality local services that their son or daughter may use in the future. Sharing information about future planning with ageing carers and people with intellectual disabilities that will help them consider possible opportunities can help people to start to plan for the future.[46]

Staff should work with ageing carers to support them to move forward together, mindful of their concerns as well as the wishes and needs of their son or daughter with intellectual disabilities, also ensuring ageing carers receive information about how their future care needs can be met and providing the opportunity for a separate assessment of their needs (see ➔ Carers' assessment, pp. 40–1).

Further reading

Care Alliance Ireland. ℘ www.carealliance.ie/index (accessed 26 February 2018).
Carers UK. ℘ www.carersuk.org (accessed 26 February 2018).

References

42 Ryan A, Taggart T, Truesdale-Kennedy M, Slevin E (2013). Issues in caregiving for older people with intellectual disabilities and their aging carers: a review and commentary. *International Journal of Older People Nursing*. **9**: 217–26.

43 Walker C, Ward C (2013). Growing older together: ageing, people with learning disabilities and their family carers. *Tizard Learning Disability Review*. **18**: 112–19.

44 Taggart L, Truesdale-Kennedy M, Ryan A, McConkey R (2012). Examining the support needs of aging family carers in developing future plans for a relative with an intellectual disability. *Journal of Intellectual Disabilities*. **16**: 217–34.

45 Pryce L, Tweed A, Hilton A, Priest HM (2017). Tolerating uncertainty: perceptions of the future for ageing parent carers and their adult children with intellectual disabilities. *Journal of Applied Research in Intellectual Disabilities*. **30**: 84–96.

46 Towers C (2015). *Thinking Ahead. A Planning Guide for Families*. Foundation for People with Learning Disabilities: London. ℘ www.mentalhealth.org.uk/sites/default/files/thinking-ahead-planning-guide-23042013-D2143.pdf (accessed 30 October 2017).

Cultural, religious, and spiritual impact

Increasingly, healthcare professionals need to be responsive and sensitive to the cultural needs of people with intellectual disabilities who come from minority ethnic backgrounds. The preferred approach to cultural care is ethnicity, cultural diversity, and nursing practice. This may include spiritual care according to the needs of clients. Spiritual care is distinct from religious care, but religious care may be part of cultural and spiritual needs. It is important to make no assumptions about people's ethnicity, culture, spirituality, and religion. It is always best to be guided by clients, their next of kin, or their representatives about their individual preferences with regard to the above dimensions of care. In the absence of personal preferences, for reasons of incapacity to express wishes, cultural and religious fact files are consulted, but these should be used thoughtfully as cultural and religious preferences may or may not be fixed or permanent.

Ethnicity

Ethnicity is the preferred term to explain race and culture. It is a fluid term that is used by individuals to assert aspects of their identity at particular points in life. The use of the term 'ethnicity' in nursing and healthcare encourages individuals to exercise people's choice to locate themselves in whatever categories with which they wish to be identified. Such an approach treats clients as individuals and invites them to determine their cultural and spiritual preferences. It avoids the essentialist assumption that the cultural identities of individuals are fixed and frozen in time. It is important to appreciate and acknowledge that individuals negotiate and move between ethnic, cultural, and spiritual identities and affiliations as part of their life course transitions. Various trajectories in life affect an individual's experience of identity, ethnicity, culture, and spirituality.

Cultural diversity

The literature acknowledges that the UK is regarded as one of the most ethnically diverse countries in Europe. Globalization, communication and Internet revolutions, transnational corporations, global migration, asylum seeking, diasporas, international studentships, sports, and European Union ascension and integration have all contributed to the diversity in the UK. It is within this ethnically diverse society that healthcare providers must deliver a service that is culturally sensitive and appropriate to meet specific needs.

Spirituality

Spirituality contains a multiplicity of meanings to an extent that the ambiguity of the concept can allow for deep misunderstandings as well as misuse. Spirituality refers to those aspects of our life that provide us with a sense of meaning, purpose, hope, value, and love. For some, but not for all, spirituality relates to a person's ongoing relationship with God. Our spirituality gives us a sense of personhood and individuality. It provides us with a sense of wholeness, stability, wellness, security, hope, and peace. Spirituality often comes into focus at critical junctures in our lives when we face emotional stress, physical illness, or death.[47]

Religion

Religions usually have to do with people's relationship with God or some kind of divine force. It comprises a system of beliefs, a comprehensive code of ethics or philosophy, and a prescribed set of rituals and practices. Religions are often associated with institutional and symbolic things such as places of worship, religious artefacts, prayer, and so on. Many people use religion as a medium to express their spirituality, although spirituality is a broader concept.

Cultural care framework for practice

The **ACCESS** model, derived from Narayanasamy,[48] could be used as a framework for delivering culturally sensitive care:

- *Assessment*—focuses on cultural aspects of clients' lifestyle, health beliefs, and health practices to create a life story file;
- *Communication*—focuses on cultural variations with respect to verbal and non-verbal aspects of clients' communication;
- *Cultural negotiation and compromise*—pays special attention to other people's culture;
- *Establishing respect and rapport*—a therapeutic relation that portrays genuine respect for clients' cultural beliefs and values is required;
- *Sensitivity*—delivers diverse, culturally sensitive care to culturally diverse groups;
- *Safety*—enables clients to derive a sense of cultural safety. Its strategy is to avert actions that diminish, demean, or disempower the cultural identity and well-being of an individual.

Further reading

Watts G (2011). Intellectual disability and spiritual development. *Journal of Intellectual Development Disability.* **36**: 234–41.

References

47 Harshaw J (2016). Finding accommodation: spirituality and people with profound intellectual disabilities. *Journal of Disability and Religion.* **20**: 140–53.
48 Narayanasamy A (2006). *Spiritual Care and Transcultural Care Research.* Quay: London.

Chapter 3

Communication

Promoting effective communication

Overview

Human communication can be extremely complex; it is an essential part of our experience of forming and building relationships, making choices, and expressing thoughts, opinions, and emotions (including discomfort or pain). This consequently affects the control we have over our own life and impacts on our mental health. Communication is dynamic; we adapt what we are saying by negotiation, and also how we say things in response to what and how another person communicates with us. Negotiation goes on throughout the interaction and, when successful, can lead to multifaceted meaning that is understood by both parties. The history of communications between people (what each one knows about the other and about communicating with the other), as well as what is currently happening around us, how we are feeling at that moment, and our reasons for communicating will all impact on the effectiveness of our communication.

Communication disabilities

Up to 80% of people with intellectual disabilities have communication difficulties, with half having significant difficulties, and many people with profound and multiple intellectual disabilities having extremely limited communication skills which may be restricted to eye gaze and changes in facial expression.[1] It should be remembered that all humans communicate, whether or not it is intentional. Common areas of difficulty are as follows:[2]

- Understanding spoken and written words, as well as symbols, and interpreting environmental sounds;
- Having a sufficient vocabulary to express a range of needs, wants, thoughts, or emotions;
- Being able to construct meaningful sentences;
- Maintaining focus and concentration in order to communicate;
- Dysfluency, e.g. stammering;
- Being able to articulate clearly (this may be due to related physical factors);
- Social skills (which may impede positive interactions with others).

People with intellectual disabilities are at risk of not being asked their opinions due to their communication difficulties. There are many day-to-day tasks and events from which people are excluded, as well as a risk of not being properly represented. This is because consultation with people with intellectual disabilities is difficult to achieve effectively.

Recognizing people's communication strengths and needs

Most of us think of speech as fundamental to human communication, but many people with intellectual disabilities can learn to communicate well without necessarily relying on speech. They may use actions, objects, photos, pictures, symbols, and signing, as well as or instead of speech. However, they often rely on others to pick up and interpret these signals. They may also need help with using these methods, not least in having reasons and opportunities to communicate, provided by others. Their communication partners will also need to amend their way of talking and use augmentative methods in order to promote understanding.

Interaction styles used by communication partners

Those paid to support people with intellectual disabilities do not always communicate effectively. For instance, we may:

- Overestimate the ability of people to understand what we are saying to them (i.e. our language is too complicated);
- Fail to adjust to the comprehension of the person's level, even where this is known;
- Not recognize the person's non-verbal signals;
- Underestimate the amount and complexity of our own speech;
- Overly rely on using speech, even when communicating with predominantly non-verbal individuals;
- Underestimate the level of hearing impairment (40%).

Staff in residential services do not always adopt optimal strategies when communicating with people with intellectual disabilities.[3] Furthermore, hospital staff not recognizing or supporting patients' communication has been highlighted as a major factor failure in service provision for people with intellectual disabilities by the NHS.[4]

Person-centred service provision

The Royal College of Speech and Language Therapists has published *Five Good Communication Standards*,[2] which are reasonable adjustments to communication that individuals with intellectual disabilities and/or autism should expect:

- **Standard 1**: there is a detailed description of how best to communicate with individuals;
- **Standard 2**: services demonstrate how they support individuals with communication needs to be involved with decisions about their care and their services;
- **Standard 3**: staff value and use competently the best approaches to communication with each individual they support;
- **Standard 4**: services create opportunities, relationships, and environments that make individuals want to communicate;
- **Standard 5**: individuals are supported to understand and express their needs in relation to their health and well-being.

References

1 Kelly A (2000). *Working with Adults with a Learning Disability*. Winslow Press: Bicester.
2 Royal College of Speech and Language Therapists (2013). *Five Good Communication Standards*. ℔ www.rcslt.org/news/docs/good_comm_standards (accessed 30 October 2017).
3 Healy D, Walsh PN (2007). Communication among nurses and adults with severe and profound intellectual disabilities. *Journal of Intellectual Disabilities*. 11: 127–41.
4 Heslop P, Blair P, Fleming M, Hoghton M Marriott A, Russ L (2013). *Confidential Inquiry into Premature Deaths of People with Learning Disabilities (CIPOLD)*. Norah Fry Research Centre: Bristol. ℔ www.bris.ac.uk/cipold/ (accessed 30 October 2017).

Verbal communication

The term 'verbal communication' is used here to mean the use of language to send and receive messages. This can involve written or spoken words. Speech, language, and communication are essentially interlinked yet can occur in isolation, so that it is possible to have:

• Language without speech (e.g. sign language or written words);
• Speech without language (when words are used without meaning, e.g. some people with intellectual disabilities and autism may apply rote-learnt or echoed words in certain situations, without necessarily understanding what those individual words mean);
• Communication without speech or language (i.e. non-verbal communication; see ➲ Adaptive behaviour rating scales, pp. 84–5).

What is language?

There are over 3000 languages and major dialects currently spoken around the world. Humans typically start life with an inherent ability to learn any language, and the one(s) they acquire will depend on the culture into which they are born. Language consists of socially shared rules that specify:

• The meaning of established words;
• How to create new words;
• How to string words together to form an inestimable variety of sentences and paragraphs.

Most of us are capable of creating language to express anything and everything we may wish to say in any situation. Within the language of a person's culture, difficulty in understanding others (receptive language) or in sharing needs, wants, ideas, and emotions (expressive language) is known as a language disorder. This may be caused developmentally or acquired through brain injury.

What is speech?

Speech is the means by which most of us use language to communicate on a daily basis. It consists primarily of:

• *Articulation*—how different speech sounds are made through a coordination of rapid movements of the articulators (primarily the tongue, jaw, soft palate, teeth, and lips). There are a variety of mouth shapes and placements of the articulators, as well as different ways of producing sounds within the human vocal tract. This is done in combination with *voice* and a sustained release of air from the lungs. There are 44 speech sounds in the English language, which are typically acquired in a developmental order;
• *Voice*—use of the vocal folds to produce vibrations in the outgoing airstream, which then reverberate in the oral and nasal (possibly also pharyngeal and thoracic) cavities. The 'voice' (vibrations) can be switched on or off, so that sounds are either voiced or voiceless.

Other aspects of speech do not convey language (i.e. what we are saying), rather they add meaning to the words and express notions such as sarcasm, innuendo, humour, and emotions (i.e. how we are saying something).

- *Fluency*—the rhythm of speech (hesitations, blocking, repetitions, stuttering. or stammering);
- *Pitch*—how high or low our voice is (women are usually higher-pitched than men, and pitch tends to go up when we are anxious);
- *Intonation*—how the pitch of speech is altered across a sentence to emphasize certain words or indicate some aspect of meaning (e.g. going up at the end to indicate a question);
- *Rate*—the speed with which speech is delivered (e.g. fast often means anxious or excited);
- *Volume*—how loud or quiet we are (e.g. loud often means angry).

Likely problems in verbal communication for people with intellectual disabilities

For many people with intellectual disabilities, difficulties in understanding and producing language can form part of their global developmental disabilities and some people will never develop language. Others might use a few single words and/or short phrases in combination with non-verbal signals. Some may talk in fluent sentences yet still have difficulty understanding and using language for complex concepts such as emotions, time, and money. Only 5–10% of people with intellectual disabilities have recognized literacy skills, and most are not able to access standard written information.[5] They might also need more time to process what someone else is saying and then to formulate a response. This needs to be considered, particularly for decision- and choice-making where capacity to consent (or to refuse consent) is likely to be misinterpreted unless communication, especially understanding of information, has been maximized for the person using inclusive communication strategies.

Many people (particularly those with autism) may have difficulty with the rules of how to apply language to interaction with others (pragmatic difficulties).

Difficulties with language production may be compounded by hearing impairment or by problems in combining speech sounds to form words due to poor motor sequencing (dyspraxia). Also, as acquisition of the phonological (sounds) system is aligned with cognitive development, some people with intellectual disabilities may not achieve a full range of speech sounds. This may affect the intelligibility of their speech, particularly to people who do not know them well. They may use signs (e.g. Makaton) to back up their speech and/or other augmentative means. People with muscle coordination problems (e.g. cerebral palsy) often have dysarthria, which leads to difficulties in clearly articulating sounds for speech. They may use alternative or augmentative systems of communication.

Further reading

Royal College of Speech and Language Therapists (2013). *Five Good Communication Standards.* ℘ www.rcslt.org/news/docs/good_comm_standards (accessed 30 October 2017).

References

5 All-Party Parliamentary Group for Education (2011). *Report of the Inquiry into Overcoming the Barriers to Literacy.* (As cited in Royal College of Speech and Language Therapists (2013). *Five Good Communication Standards.*)

Non-verbal communication

The term 'non-verbal communication' is used here to mean the use of any signals that do not contain language to send and receive messages. This is often referred to as 'body language' but also includes aspects of our speech (how we speak, rather than what we say) and other sounds we produce that carry meaning (e.g. laughing, crying, screaming, etc.).

Pre-intentional (or unconscious) communication

Initially, babies are not aware that they can influence other human beings through what they do—they do not understand *cause and effect* and they have yet to learn to send messages that intentionally signal meaning to another person. A baby will cry in a particular way and the parent may interpret this as meaning she is hungry and feed her. Long before the development of speech, she will learn to cry like this on purpose to indicate hunger, and also to signal in different ways intentionally to indicate other needs. Some adults with intellectual disabilities may still be at the pre-intentional stage of communication development. They rely on us to interpret their signals and to support them to develop intentional communication, if at all possible.

Development of human communication

As Fig. 3.1 shows, we develop recognition of objects before we can recognize photographs. Only then can we develop the skill of recognizing pictures, and finally symbols (or icons) that represent a word or an idea. Similarly, we develop situational understanding (taking meaning from what is going on around us) and functional understanding (e.g. that a cup is for drinking from) before we go on to understand what words mean. Unless we understand what words mean, we cannot use words to express ourselves. Some people with intellectual disabilities may totally rely on situational understanding (including others' non-verbal signals) to know what is happening, and these people are likely to express themselves wholly or primarily through non-verbal means.

Even where people are verbal, non-verbal communication plays a significant role in carrying meaning—after all, we all tend to believe how people tell us things, rather than what they are saying, should the messages be in any way conflicting.

So what are non-verbal communication signals?

Head signals Eye contact can be essential in effective communication; frequent eye contact can put people at ease, show interest, and help maintain the interaction, but staring can be seen as rude or threatening. Facial expressions (e.g. smiling, frowning, and grimacing) are very effective in relaying our emotions. Head nods (positive or negative) are an integral way of expressing 'yes' and 'no' and also play a role in maintaining interaction (we move our heads almost constantly during conversation).

Hand signals Gestures are used to describe, emphasize, demonstrate, and give directions or instructions. Most of us would be lost without the use of our hands while talking. Signs (e.g. Makaton) can be used instead of speech or to augment speech. Touch is another important aspect to human communication and can be positive or negative.

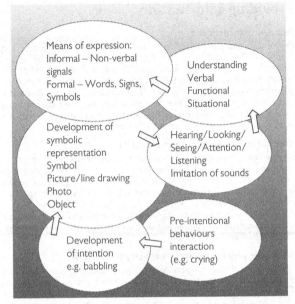

Fig. 3.1 Typical communication development involves progress through developmental stages to learn increasingly more complex means of communication.

Whole body signals
- Posture, e.g. slumped and arms folded (bored);
- Orientation, e.g. facing each other (interest) or turning away;
- Distance—how near or far you are from another;
- Appearance—clothing (e.g. uniform), personal grooming.

Vocal signals. Intonation, rate, volume, and fluency of speech (see ➔ Framework of nursing assessment, pp. 82–3) add meaning to what we say. Remember, it is not what you say, it is the way that you say it.

Further reading

Chan ZC (2013). A qualitative study on non-verbal sensitivity in nursing students. *Journal of Clinical Nursing*. 22: 1941–50.

Griffiths C, Smith M (2016). Attuning: a communication process between people with severe and profound intellectual disability and their interaction partners, *Journal of Applied Research in Intellectual Disabilities*. 29: 124–38.

Providing information

Accessing healthcare

People with intellectual disabilities can have significant difficulties accessing healthcare. This can be, in part, due to problems with reading written health promotion materials or invitations for health screening (and consequently missing appointments). Furthermore, people with communication difficulties may not be able to effectively tell a medical professional what the problem is nor be able to understand the advice/treatment options being offered. A hospital passport detailing particular communication needs can assist staff to know how best to pitch their communication.[1]

The nurse's role and communication

Services for people with intellectual disabilities generally promote access to generic healthcare services wherever possible. In addition, some nurses are employed within commissioning teams as care managers who assess for, and devise, service plans—this involves supporting people to make important decisions about what happens in their life. Both roles require nurses to consider how to provide information effectively in a format that will facilitate them to have the best chance of participating in the decisions which affect them.

Assessing and maximizing capacity to consent

Understanding the information that has been provided forms a major part of a person's capacity to consent to assessment and intervention (see ➋ Mental capacity and decision making, pp. 102–3). It is our legal responsibility to ensure that a person's capacity is maximized by providing pertinent information in whatever means appropriate to each individual. Where a best interests pathway is followed, the person must be informed as far as possible regarding what is to happen to them. As decisions need to be made regularly about the capacity to consent when working with people with intellectual disabilities, care should be taken when note-writing to include not just what was said to the person, but also *how* it was communicated (e.g. that certain gestures, signs, or symbols/pictures/photos were used, including a description and/or copy of any easier-read materials).

Pitching language to match the level of understanding

It can be difficult to know how far to simplify information to help someone with intellectual disabilities to understand, as a person's level of understanding is not always apparent. People with intellectual disabilities have often learnt through experience to appear to understand when, in fact, they are not sure what you mean. Think of yourself in a foreign language situation where you are catching key words and nodding and smiling, and hoping that you will get the meaning soon or at least the person will appear satisfied with your minimal response and go away. For many people with intellectual disabilities, it may well be a similar experience when you are talking to them, especially if you are using medical jargon and/or if they are anxious or in pain. Also remember that visual or hearing impairment may not be obvious.

Whereas no one wants to appear patronizing by unnecessarily over-simplifying, there is a real danger in making assumptions about how much language a person can understand. You cannot be effective if you cannot communicate with the person—it is your responsibility to get your message across as far as possible. If you are unsure, assessment of a person's level of understanding and advice for that individual can be requested from speech and language therapy.

General guidelines

In reality, we make judgements about others' communication all the time—we say something, wait for a response, and then adjust what we say next. Some general guidelines are:

- Wherever possible, plan how you are going to communicate in advance. Consider which visual resources you might need—pictures, photos, signs, written information, videos (see ➜ Principles in using augmentative and alternative communication (AAC), pp. 68–9);
- Consider the person's attention span—maybe short bursts of information are better (repeat visits?);
- Make reasonable adjustments to allow for any problems with hearing or vision;
- Reduce background noise and other distractions (e.g. switch off the TV);
- Allow processing time—do not talk too quickly;
- Use short, straightforward sentences (one or two ideas at a time);
- Use easy words (reduce jargon/long words/abstract ideas);
- Watch the person—be prepared to repeat/rephrase;
- Check they have understood—ask them to confirm what you said.

Autism and communication

People with autism often have a literal understanding of language (see ➜ Autistic spectrum conditions, pp. 254–5), with difficulties understanding figurative language and also reading others' non-verbal signals. It is important for you to say what you mean and to describe things precisely. Providing visual information (pictures, photos, written words as appropriate), along with your spoken words, may be essential (see ➜ TEACCH (Treatment and Education of Autistic and related Communication-handicapped Children), pp. 334–5). Also, because new social situations (or perhaps the ones for which there are existing negative connotations such as visiting the dentist, having injections, having a haircut, or meeting new people) can induce anxiety, it is important to explain exactly what is to happen and why. Social Stories™ can be very effective in supporting the person to predict and prepare for what is to happen and are easy to write with a little guidance. Please see the website ℛ carolgraysocialstories.com/social-stories/and/or request help from your local speech and language therapist (SLT).

References

6 Bell R (2012). Does he have sugar in his tea? Communication between people with learning disabilities, their carers and hospital staff. *Tizard Learning Disability Review*. 17: 57–63.

Active listening

Active listening is taking into account the tone of voice, body language, and other non-verbal signs, and not only listening to the words someone uses, in order to gain a fuller understanding of what they are actually communicating.[7] The application of active listening principles to people with intellectual disabilities means giving the person space for personal expression by observing whatever communication signals the person is sending. It is about genuinely hearing the message the person is telling us, rather than merely part of this message, or some version of it that better suits our own needs, and then verifying the message with the person (letting them know they have been heard).

Active listening can be tiring as it takes effort, especially when the person has communication difficulties. For nurses, it involves taking the time to develop a rapport with the person before engaging in assessment or intervention. You must 'tune into' the person and be sensitive to their communication needs if you are to understand their point of view and to prevent communication breakdowns. This will enable you to know how much to do at any one time—when to start, when to take a break, when to encourage someone into doing a little bit more, and when to stop. It is about finding the right balance between listening, hearing, allowing time, and responding.

An important part of promoting expressive communication (so that you can actively listen to them) is to ensure that you maximize their understanding of what is being communicated to them (see ➡ Providing information, pp. 64–5). To effectively listen to others, you must first recognize and own the communication signals you are sending out to others, making adjustments as necessary.

Strategies to hear what the person is telling you

- Remaining calm and showing patience—putting the person at ease.
- Allowing processing time for the person to think about what to communicate to you and also to get that message across.
- Encouraging the person to say it another way if they get stuck ('Show me?'; see ➡ Principles in using augmentative and alternative communication (AAC), pp. 68–9).
- Commenting (providing statements, rather than questions) or asking open questions (e.g. 'How are you feeling?'), rather than closed ones ('Do you feel sad?'), to draw out the person's own opinions.
- Focusing questions down ('Is it x or y?') if the person is struggling with comments or open questions.
- Encouraging elaboration by keeping quiet and indicating that we are listening (head to one side, leaning forward, eye contact, nodding, smiling, 'uh-huh' type of vocalizations, words of encouragement, etc.).
- Rephrasing what we have understood—checking this with the person.

Barriers to communication

Sometimes what we say or do (however inadvertently) can have a negative effect on the person's expressive communication capabilities. At times, especially when we are busy and already focusing on what we need to do next, we may all be guilty of:

- Not actually listening (very off-putting);
- Rushing the person;
- Providing reassuring clichés or stereotyped comments;
- Giving advice (we do not always know what is best);
- Expressing approval/disapproval (making value judgements);
- Requesting an explanation (asking why? Just accept what they say);
- Defending ('I'm sure he didn't mean that');
- Belittling feelings ('Now, now, don't cry! It's not that bad');
- Changing the subject (perhaps when the topic is difficult).

Cultural differences

Having English as a second language may exacerbate communication difficulties. In addition, cultural differences in the use of both verbal and non-verbal communication will need to be taken into account if the person comes from a different ethnic background to yourself (you may need to seek advice on this—do not make assumptions). Active listening occurs when you treat people as they would want to be treated, not as you yourself would necessarily want to be treated.

Supporting choices and decision-making

It is your responsibility to ensure a person's capacity to communicate is maximized by supporting each individual to communicate in whatever means is appropriate to them and to actively listen to their response. This will often need to involve use of inclusive communication strategies, e.g. facilitating the person to use signing or photos, as well as any speech (see ➲ Inclusive communication, pp. 308–9). Talking Mats[8] can also be a powerful tool, providing a safe concrete arena to share thoughts and ideas using pictures, symbols, and/or written words.

Sharing information about communication with others

When writing reports or clinical notes, we should include *how* the person communicates, not just what we heard the person communicate. Written records should provide documentation of the person's status and intervention in order to ensure continuity of care, as well as serving as legal documentation. If a person has communication difficulties, it is important to share known strategies for listening to, and supporting, communication for that person with any other potential communication partners. This can be done simply through the use of a communication profile and/or a communication passport (see ➲ pp. 72–3) for each person.

References

7 Ivanovic A, Collin P (2006). Active listening. In: A Ivanovic, P Collin, eds. *Dictionary of Human Resources and Personnel Management*. A&C Black: London.

8 Talking MATS. ⌕ www.talkingmats.com/ (accessed 30 October 2017).

Principles in using augmentative and alternative communication (AAC)

What is AAC?

This refers to ways of communicating, in addition to speech (augmentative) or instead of speech (alternative), bearing in mind that speech could be in sentences, phrases, single words, or parts of words. A broad classification of AAC systems would be as *aided* [e.g. voice output communication aid (VOCA), which produces speech when the person activates it, and low-tech devices such as symbols boards used to point to] and *unaided* (e.g. manual sign systems).

The person's level of communication development (outlined in ➔ Non-verbal communication, pp. 62–3) must be considered, and this may need formal assessment by an SLT. However, applying basic principles described in this section should promote communication on a day-to-day basis. Used in conjunction with appropriate modifications to the way we provide information (see ➔ Providing information, pp. 64–5) and active listening (see ➔ Active listening, pp. 66–7), AAC should result in inclusive communication and promote effective participation.

Objects

Objects of reference are used where people are just beginning to understand symbolic representation (see ➔ Objects of reference, pp. 74–5). However, we all take meaning from objects quite readily because they are concrete, so we understand these before we hear words. The other advantage is that we can show people the action associated with the object. Showing someone a cup and miming taking a drink is likely to be more effective than merely using the word 'drink'.

Pictures and drawings

Most of us think we are pretty useless at drawing, but with a little effort, we can all manage simple line drawings (try 'stick people' and ideas from any symbols you have seen). Having a pad of paper and a pen handy may be all that is needed to overcome communication breakdown at times and, if you use it to show what you mean, maybe the other person will join in and use drawings too. Thinking about how to draw what you are explaining will really help you to stick to easier words.

Photographs and video

So long as the person is able to take meaning from photos, you can use photos of their possessions, of friends and family, or of the person doing an activity, or to show favourite places. This can make for a truly effective and person-centred communication tool; you can inform the person of coming events, explain everyday/service/intervention options, and support decision-making. The person can use photos to express opinions and choices, make jokes, tell stories, and pass on information. If the person owns a smartphone or tablet, then that can be used to take photos and videos and then to show to other people—either directly or within a visual story using a photo story App (e.g. *Book Creator*).

Symbols

A potential problem with photos is that they may contain extraneous detail which could distract from the message. Symbols may be preferred, as they tend to be iconic representations of general concepts, rather than of specific people, actions, or objects. This may be particularly important for people with autism. There are a number of symbol sets used around the globe (with or without written words); some examples are Picture Communication Symbols,[9] Widgit,[10] and Makaton.[11] Symbols can be used at an individual or environmental level, e.g. on signage for buildings, for easier-read versions of health information leaflets, for personalized communication books, or for visual timetables. PhotoSymbols[12] are a crossover between symbols and photos.

Natural gestures and signing

Many people with intellectual disabilities will find it easier to understand what you are saying if you augment your speech with gestures and/or sign key words. This is not the same as using sign languages, which are totally different to spoken languages and based in a different linguistic culture. However, some people may have partly learnt a sign language such as British Sign Language. Makaton[11] is a developmental language programme integrating speech, manual signs, and symbols. Many people sign key words along with speech. If you sign key words, it will help you to slow your speech down a little and to think carefully about which words you are using.

Voice output communication aids (VOCAs)

There is a huge range of VOCAs whereby pictures, symbols, or typed words may be used to generate speech, which may be digitized or recorded:

- Single-message output devices (you record and re-record one message at a time and press to play it);
- Devices with a defined number of messages (4, 9, 12, 32, 64, etc.) where there is a message for each keypad and you may be able to switch between overlays to get a separate set of messages;
- Hi-tech devices that are multilayered and can be used to produce highly complex language. These VOCAs can be accessed directly (by pressing the keypad) or via head pointing, tracking, or eye gaze.

In addition to bespoke VOCA devices, there are communication Applications (Apps) for smartphones and tablets (e.g. iPad), although because these have been designed for people who do not have any difficulty in using their hands, they may presently have limited use for people who need alternative access due to physical disabilities.[13]

References

9 Mayer-Johnson. ♫ www.mayer-johnson.com/ (accessed 30 October 2017).
10 Widgit. ♫ www.widgit.com/ (accessed 30 October 2017).
11 The Makaton Charity. ♫ www.makaton.org (accessed 30 October 2017).
12 Photosymbols. ♫ www.photosymbols.com/ (accessed 30 October 2017).
13 Bradshaw J (2013). The use of augmentative and alternative communication apps for the iPad, iPod and iPhone: an overview of recent developments. *Tizard Learning Disability Review*. **18**: 31–7.

Developing accessible information

Why do we need accessible information?

People with, and particularly those with severe, intellectual disabilities often do not acquire effective speech. They may also have difficulty in processing written or visual information.

These communication difficulties mean that people with intellectual disabilities may find the experience of accessing healthcare frightening and confusing.[14] It is suggested that providing information in an accessible format will make healthcare journeys for people with intellectual disabilities easier to manage and less frightening.

What is available?

Books Beyond Words

Whether supporting somebody with an intellectual disability or communication difficulty, their products and services empower through the use of pictures (see 🖰 www.booksbeyondwords.co.uk).

The titles include the *Health Care Mini Set*:

- *Going to the Doctor*;
- *Going into Hospital*;
- *Going to Out-Patients*.

They have also recently developed a BW Story App. This is a fast and straightforward way to access pictures that will help enable people to explore and understand the world.

Royal National Institute of Blind People

The Royal National Institute of Blind People produces both booklets and tapes and gives advice on a range of eye conditions which could be modified for people with intellectual disabilities (see 🖰 www.rnib.org.uk).

Talking Mats

Talking Mats 'improve the lives of people with communication difficulties by increasing their capacity to communicate effectively about things that matter to them'. They have now developed a New Talking Mats digital which can be used on any tablet or computer (see 🖰 www.talkingmats.com).

Pain assessment tools

The Disability Distress Assessment Tool (DisDAT) is designed to capture the ways in which someone with intellectual disabilities presents when feeling content and when distressed. Subtle changes in a person's presentation can be objectively recorded on the tool. The DisDAT tool can be accessed at 🖰 prc.coh.org/PainNOA/Dis%20DAT_Tool.pdf (see ➔ Assessing pain, pp. 90–2).

Creating accessible information

The patterns of mortality and morbidity of people with intellectual disabilities vary from the general population.[15] Also as the communication ability of people with intellectual disabilities varies, it means that often the information required for an individual's personal healthcare journey needs to be created on an individual basis.

Considerations when developing accessible information

It has been suggested that creating individualized information packages is not without its pitfalls. The person who requires the information should be assessed carefully to identify if they would benefit most from plain English, symbols, pictorial images, or photosymbols. It would be good at this point to liaise and take advice from the SLT.

Creating your own accessible information

There are now many symbol systems that either substitute for speech or provide help for those with linguistic issues. The common symbol systems that can be accessed and used to create individualized accessible information are:

- Rebus Communication System;
- Picture Exchange Communication System;
- Boardmaker;
- Blissymbolics;
- Bonnington Symbol System.

Many websites offer free downloads of symbols or photographs, and these could be used to develop individual accessible information.

Benefits of accessible information

The development and use of accessible information might lead to:

- Seamless approach to care;
- Better understanding of information;
- Reduced anxiety and distress;
- Increased ability to consent;
- Reduction in risks;
- Increased choice;
- Increased participation of people in their own care.

Further reading

Horn JH, Moss D (2015). A search for meaning: telling your life with learning disabilities. *British Journal of Learning Disabilities.* **43**: 178–85.

References

14 NHS Education for Scotland (2016). *Equal Health*. NHS Education for Scotland: Edinburgh.
15 Scottish Government (2013). *The Keys to Life*. Scottish Government: Edinburgh.

Communication passports

Communication passports can provide an efficient way of sorting and presenting accessible information about an individual. The information contained within the passport can enable healthcare professionals to communicate with the person with intellectual disabilities, and also to ensure that the person's individual needs, likes, and dislikes are taken into account. They gather important and complex information about the person and make this accessible to others.

Types of communication passports

Type 1—personal communication passports
This type of passport contains information about all aspects of the person's life and is used as a tool in enabling the person to have a say and to make choices.

Type 2—personal communication passports
This type of passport is usually 4–5 pages used to facilitate and support access between different services to try and ensure the necessary reasonable adjustments are made. It is a snapshot of the person's life and individual needs at the time of access. This type of passport tends to concentrate on the health needs or health profile of the person at a particular point in time, and therefore they will require review and updating at each point of access.

Type 3—combination of types 1 and 2
This type of passport is a combination of types 1 and 2. This type then includes all the personal information of the type 1 passport plus the health profile information of the type 2 passport.

Features of passports

All types of passports present highly personal information, in an empowering and positive manner. They usually contain information on:
• Personal contact details;
• Professional contact details (e.g. social worker, community nurse);
• Medical history;
• Communication details;
• Language;
• Spirituality;
• Likes and dislikes;
• Current medication;
• Allergies;
• How to support a person to maximize their capacity and consent.

Depending on an individual's level of communication, the passports may use plain English, symbols, or photographs. They should be bright, attractive, and easy to use.

Benefits of passports

Passports are a positive way of supporting, enabling, and empowering people with intellectual disabilities who have communication problems. The benefits can include:

- Ensuring continuity of care;
- Supporting the person to be actively involved in decisions about their care;
- Orientating new staff about possible reasonable adjustments that may be required;
- Empowering the person;
- Enabling more competent observation;
- Enhancing relationships between the person and health staff;
- Providing a focus for discussion about health issues;
- Enabling quicker access to suitable care;
- Responding to the person's individual need;
- Improving treatment and care.

Constraints of passports

Passports do not have any legal status, although their use is recommended. This could pose some ethical problems for healthcare professionals. They contain highly personalized information about the person and their health needs. It is suggested that healthcare professionals use the passports to make decisions about future treatment and care; however, this can be problematic if the information in the passport is flawed or out-of-date. It is important therefore that healthcare professionals check out the information contained within the passports with the individual and relevant others. All passports should be reviewed regularly, and updated information within these should also be dated and signed.

Further reading

FIND. *The Benefits of Communication Passports.* ℘ www.findresources.co.uk/communication-passports (accessed 30 October 2017).

Scope (2014). *Communication Passport Template: A Scope Guide to Making Communication Passports.* ℘www.scope.org.uk/Scope/media/Images/Support/Scope-communication-passport.docx (accessed 30 October 2017).

University of Edinburgh. *Personal Communication Passports.* ℘ www.communicationpassports.org.uk/Home/ (accessed 30 October 2017).

Objects of reference

People with intellectual disability have a wide range of communication abilities and needs. Some will be able to communicate verbally, while others may learn how to use symbols or photos. Others will not be able to grasp that a symbol means something. In these cases, objects of reference may be useful.

Definition

The term 'objects of reference' refers to the use of tangible objects as a method of communication.[16]

Using objects of reference

Objects of reference are tangible items that are used in a systematic way with people with intellectual disabilities and additional communication difficulties. The objects are items that have meaning for the individual and they help with identifying what is going to happen next or in making choices between two different activities. The objects are real items that are used every day by the person. So a toothbrush may be used to signify teeth cleaning, or a spoon to indicate eating.[16]

Much of the literature identifies that each individual should have their own unique objects of reference. This can be time-consuming for professionals, however, and may also be confusing. Studies where the same objects of reference are used in a group, rather than an individual, basis suggest that using objects in this way is beneficial both for people with intellectual disabilities, who mostly progressed in the use of objects as a means of communication, as well as care staff, in that they could use the same objects for a number of people.

Constraints of using objects of reference

It should be noted that the objects themselves are representations of activities and they tend to be chosen by the healthcare professional or the educationalist. Goldhart et al.[17] suggest that this may be problematic, because the object chosen may be a commonsense choice to the professional but may be meaningless to the person with intellectual disabilities.

It is also identified that objects of reference are only used to order or represent utilitarian activities of daily routine like eating or having a bath, and are not used for ordinary social communication. Thus, Park argues that objects of reference are rarely used for activities such as play.[18]

How is success achieved?

It is argued by Goldhart et al.[17] that, in order to be successful, referencing is dependent on the collaboration between the speaker and the listener. They identified that analysis of the discourse of interaction shows that both verbal and non-verbal communication is actively negotiated across the referencing task. These findings have implications for professionals, in that they are suggesting that successful use of objects of reference is best achieved through close relationships.

Interactive storytelling

Park[18,19] has explored the success and use of objects of reference in more detail. He suggests that the use of interactive storytelling enables people with intellectual disabilities to share experiences in which they choose or negotiate the object of reference. He believes that this empowers the individual at the same time as enhancing their early communication skills.

Further reading

Blair J (2011). Care adjustments for people with learning disabilities in hospitals. *Nursing Management.* 18: 21–4.

References

16 Harding C, Lindsay G, O'Brien A, Dippe L, Wright J (2011). Implementing AAC with children with profound and multiple disabilities: a study in rational underpinning intervention. *Journal of Research in Special Educational Needs.* 11: 120–9.

17 Goldhart J, Cadwick D, Buell S (2014). Speech and language therapists' approaches to communication intervention with children and adults with profound and multiple learning disability. *International Journal of Language and Communication Disorders.* 49: 687–701.

18 Park K (2001). Oliver Twist: An exploration of interactive storytelling and object use in communication. *British Journal of Special Education.* 28: 18–23.

19 Park K (2002). Macbeth: a poetry workshop on stage at Shakespeare's Globe Theatre. *British Journal of Special Education.* 29: 14–19.

Compiling life stories

People with intellectual disabilities are not a homogenous group. Even people with a similar diagnosis, e.g. Down syndrome, have different abilities and needs. Enabling individual people to compile their individual life story can be empowering for the individual, but it also gives the healthcare, social care, or educational professional opportunities to glimpse the cultural and social aspects of the lived experience of the person.

Life stories provide sensitive individual accounts of the person with a disability and are contextualized by the environment within which the person lives, the community of which the person is part, and the wider society.

Recording personal histories

Facilitating people with intellectual disabilities to record their life stories can be challenging. Guidance on creating life stories is provided by Anchor. This guidance is mainly related to people with dementia, but the concepts could also be used for people with intellectual disabilities.[20]

Some people have the ability to recall and record their own narrative, whereas others will need communication aids, which will make this process more accessible for them. It is suggested that Talking Mats could be a useful tool. This is an interactive resource that concentrates on 13 life-planning topics (see ➔ Developing accessible information, pp. 70–1). Other life-planning tools may also be of use in this process (see ➔ Person-centred planning, pp. 26–7). These would include all of the following:

- Person-centred planning;
- Personal future planning;
- Essential lifestyle planning;
- Planning Alternative Tomorrows with Hope (PATH);
- Making Action Plans (MAPS).

Many people with intellectual disabilities have been empowered to develop their life stories by becoming involved in an advocacy group or by having an individual advocate. It is suggested by NHS Education for Scotland[21] that all people with intellectual disabilities in Scotland should be given the opportunity to develop their own life story.

Possible benefits of compiling life stories alongside the person with intellectual disability

- Empowerment;
- Emancipation;
- Coming to terms with the past;
- Understanding the present;
- Looking to the future;
- Increasing self-identity;
- Increasing the capacity to consent.

Benefits of compiling life stories for healthcare professionals

- Better understanding of patterns of behavioural distress;
- Better understanding of the effects of service redesign;
- Limiting possibilities of past mistakes being replicated;
- Increasing empathy;
- Creating a basis for communication;
- Creating a basis for future person-centred planning.

Further reading

Boodle A, Ellem K, Chenoweth L (2014). Anna's story of life in prison. *British Journal of Learning Disabilities*. **42**: 117–24.

Horn JH, Moss D (2015). A search for meaning: telling your life with learning disabilities. *British Journal of Learning Disabilities*. **43**: 178–85.

Wilson H, Bialk P, Freeze TB, Freeze R, Lutfiyya ZM (2012). Heidi's and Philip's stories: transitions to post-secondary education. *British Journal of Learning Disabilities*. **40**: 87–93.

References

20 Anchor. *Creating a Life Story*. ℘ www.anchor.org.uk/sites/default/files/media_centre_sub_section/pdfs/creating-a-Life-Story.pdf (accessed 31 October 2017).

21 NHS Education for Scotland (2016). *Equal Health*. NHS Education for Scotland: Edinburgh.

Chapter 4

79

Assessment

Purpose and principles of assessment

Purpose of assessment

In the context of intellectual disabilities, nursing assessment refers to a process where the abilities and needs of a person are identified in a structured process. This is generally followed by planning for support, implementing an agreed intervention plan, and evaluating the outcomes by comparing changes to the baseline assessment. Assessment is based on learning through shared action, reflection, and refining, and should be seen as a team effort that involves people with intellectual disabilities and significant others. Assessment is an ongoing process, rather than a one-off event. It should be part of an overall support cycle that leads to planning of interventions, if needed, implementation of an individualized support plan, and evaluation of intended goals/outcomes. The overall purpose of assessment of a person with intellectual disabilities is essentially to:

- Investigate the current 'bio-psycho-social' status of the person;
- Determine the level of abilities and needs at that time (and also looking into the future);
- Establish priorities for the development of a support plan and intervention.

The rationale for assessment of a person should address the following questions:

- What is the reason for undertaking such an assessment?
- Who will act and benefit from the information provided by the assessment?
- What issues and questions one is trying to address through the assessment process?

Areas of assessment

Assessment of a person with intellectual disabilities should be holistic and follow a structured approach such as a model of nursing or other agreed format. The initial assessment should include an initial assessment of their physical, emotional, and social health. Following this, it may be helpful to undertake additional secondary and more detailed assessments in areas that have been highlighted in the initial assessment. Such areas may include aspects such as specific physical health conditions, mental/psychological/ emotional health, challenging behaviour, offending behaviour, risk to the person and others, engagement in activity/training programmes, mobility, finance, housing, employment, respite, social engagements, spiritual needs, level of support required, and overall quality of life.

Principles of assessment

The nature of assessment

- Objective[1]—such as measurement of factual data such as blood pressure and weight;
- Subjective—such as considering how a person feels and thinks about their current situation;
- Reliable—if repeated, would similar results be found?

- Efficient—will it lead to positive outcomes?
- Valid—offers an accurate indication of issues at stake;
- Useful—fulfils a worthwhile purpose for the person.

Person-centred approach

One of the key principles of assessment of a person with intellectual disabilities is it must be undertaken using person-centred values (see ➲ Undertaking a nursing assesssment, pp. 264–5). A person-centred assessment will:

- Emphasize the abilities and needs expressed by the person or advocate, rather than those imposed by carers, professionals, and services;
- Link with a range of informal support networks available to the person, as well as the formal support available from services;
- Establish current strengths and needs as a baseline to evaluate the progress of intervention and support;
- Identify areas for support/development/intervention, and strengths and possible contribution/participation of the person;
- Focus on support necessary to achieve identified goals;
- Identify potential difficulties of intervention/support, and agree how best to manage them;
- Facilitate building a good rapport with the person/significant others;
- Ensure information gathering addresses the person as a whole, and not just concentrate on problem areas.

Sources of information

Information can be gathered from a range of people and sources. This will include the individual and their families/relatives, observation, and discussion with the person, families, carers, professionals, and agencies, as well as examining existing written records. Assessment by a professional (e.g. nurse) usually forms part of a wider interdisciplinary assessment; this makes it important that all assessment data are analysed and coordinated effectively through regular liaison and communication forums. Professional assessments should be an integral part of an overall life plan agreed with the person.

Reasonable adjustments

The assessment of people with intellectual disabilities may need to be adapted or adjusted to meet their needs and abilities. Some people with intellectual disabilities may have communication difficulties, and the use of creative strategies, such as picture cards, sign language, video, or other forms of symbolic communication, will assist in assessment.

Further reading

Potter PA, Perry AG, Stocker P, Hall A (2012). *Fundamentals of Nursing*, 8th edn. Elsevier: London.
Wilson SF, Giddens JF (2016). *Health Assessment for Nursing Practice*. Elsevier: London.

References

1 Barrett D, Wilson B, Woollards A (2009). *Care Planning: A Guide for Nurses*. Pearson Education Limited: Harlow.

Framework of nursing assessment

Nursing process and nursing models

The nursing process is a problem-solving approach to nursing care, providing a systematic way of investigating care and support needs in order to plan interventions for resolving issues identified in the assessment. Whereas the nursing process is critical to care delivery, it is only a cyclical process with four stages of how to deliver individualized care. It is not a conceptual framework/model offering practitioners with underpinning values and dimensions on which to base their nursing assessments and care delivery.[2]

Conceptual models of nursing

A conceptual nursing model can guide nurses when they are engaged with the nursing process, and the use of a model is viewed as a practical way of putting the nursing process into action. There are numerous nursing models[3] (e.g. Peplau, 1952; Roy, 1976; Roper, Logan, and Tierney, 1980; Orem, 1991) that have been developed over the years to enhance nursing practice. Nursing models are used to guide nursing practice and enhance standards of nursing care by providing a framework for nursing interventions through the use of specific approaches to assessing, planning, implementing, and evaluating nursing care.

Each model makes clear statements about the nature of people, health, the environment, and nursing.[3] To understand the potential utility of a nursing model, it is important that practitioners are aware of these core areas. Conceptual frameworks vary from those that have a more physical health-orientated emphasis and focus on care provision, through to those that are more focused on developing independence and self-care. A key decision for the nurses is to match the selection of a nursing model with their understanding of the likely abilities and needs of the person with intellectual disabilities they are supporting. Nurses should have a wide working knowledge of nursing models; they should resist the idea that one nursing model alone is suitable for all people with intellectual disabilities. Nursing models are not ideal for all people with intellectual disabilities.

A model for intellectual disability nursing

Aldridge (2004) developed the *Ecology of Health Model*,[4] designed specifically for intellectual disability nursing practice. The framework uses the concept of the person's health and independence as an ecological system. The latter explores all aspects of the individual's health, and the person with intellectual disabilities is seen as having physical and psychological dimensions existing within a social environment. The model guides nurse practitioners to investigate causative, as well as stabilizing, factors affecting an individual's health.[4] This model provides a structured framework for intellectual disability nursing and has a clear synergy with the values underpinning services for people with intellectual disabilities.

Using nursing models across all stages of the nursing process

The majority of nurses for people with intellectual disability work within a wider interdisciplinary group of staff, some within structured teams, and the role of the nurse needs to be integrated with the work of other team members, and vice versa. Therefore, it is important for nurses to be aware of how the proposed nursing model for their assessment, planning, implementation, and evaluation relates to any wider interdisciplinary assessments and care planning being undertaken. The relationship between the nursing model and the wider planning process is normally complementary, with the nurse using a model of nursing to undertake their nursing assessment and then feed this information into care planning discussions.

Once the input of the nursing team member has been identified, the nurse will then be able to use the structure of the nursing model to plan, implement, and evaluate their interventions. This is an important point, as too often nursing models are used for assessment only and can be limited to a checklist, without following this through to planning, implementing, and evaluating nursing care. This may result in the care plan bearing little attention to the model of nursing, and hence the focus of nursing interventions within that model. Regardless of the model used, it is critical to consult with the person with learning disability about who will be present.

Opportunities and cautions in developing new nursing models

As already noted, nursing models are 'conceptual frameworks' which have specific views about four key areas (people, health, environment, and nursing). There is a wide variety of nursing models already in existence, and more can be developed if people wished to do so. It is important when developing new 'models' that clear statements are made on at least the four key areas outlined in this section. Simply adding additional items to the list of areas for assessment does not make it a 'new' nursing model. Indeed, doing so may compromise the integrity of the existing nursing models as originally developed and risks people focusing on the assessment as a checklist only.

Further reading

Fawcett J, DeSanto-Madeya S (2013). *Contemporary Nursing Knowledge: Analysis and Evaluation of Nursing Models and Theories*, 3rd edn. FA Davis Company: Philadelphia, PA.

References

2 Brooker C, Waugh A (2013). *Nursing Practice: Fundamentals of Holistic Care*. Mosby Elsevier: London.

3 McKenna H, Pajnkihar M, Murphy F (2014). *Fundamentals of Nursing Models, Theories and Practice*, 2nd edn. Wiley-Blackwell: London.

4 Aldridge J (2004). Learning disability nursing: a model for practice. In: J Turnbull, ed. *Learning Disability Nursing*. Blackwell Publishing: Oxford; pp. 169–87.

Adaptive behaviour rating scales

The diagnosis of intellectual disabilities must include significant deficits in adaptive functioning and cannot be made on an IQ score alone. Adaptive functioning relates to the skills required for a person to cope successfully with the daily tasks involved in living from day to day, linked to a person's chronological age. These adaptive functioning skills include: communication, self-care, home living, social, community use, self-direction, health and safety, leisure, and work.

Purpose of adaptive behaviour rating scales

Adaptive behaviour rating scales will help nurses and professionals to:
• Obtain a prompt and accurate picture of the level of ability in people with intellectual disabilities and who also have autism, communication deficits, and other developmental delay (i.e. functional skills impairment);
• Aid in determining the person's eligibility for the appropriate supports;
• Plan a socially valid and effective intervention package of care;
• Evaluate intervention outcomes and demonstrate if the person has returned to their optimal level of functioning as they were before they became ill.

Measurement of adaptive functioning

Adaptive behaviour rating scales are standardized tests based upon measurement from large samples of populations. There are a number of adaptive behaviour rating scales commercially available for nurses and other professionals to use to measure a person's adaptive functioning. Some of these include:
• Developmental Profile II (DPII);
• Early Coping Inventory (ECI);
• Bayley Scales of Infant Development (BSID);
• Scales of Independent Behaviour: Revised (SIB-R);
• Adaptive behaviour scales (ABS);
• Vineland Adaptive Behaviour Scale (VABS).

Vineland Adaptive Behaviour Scale

The most widely used tool within the field of intellectual disabilities is the VABS.[5] This scale measures the personal and social skills of a person from birth to adulthood. It can be used in clinical settings, for education, and in home settings. It uses a questionnaire format and has 213 questions/items. A teacher, parent, or nurse who knows the person well indicates whether the individual has mastered the skill in question.

The VABS assesses a wide range of adaptive behaviours:
• *Communication*—receptive, expression, written, and the ability to listen;
• *Daily living skills*—personal, domestic, and community;
• *Socialization*—interpersonal relationships, play and leisure time, and coping skills;
• *Motor skills*—gross and fine motor skills.

With the VABS, there are standardized and normative scores where the person's scores can be compared, based upon age and gender. This scale has very strong internal consistency, test–retest reliability, and inter-rater reliabilities.

Vineland Adaptive Behaviour Scale-III

More recently, the VABS has been redeveloped and is now called VABS-III[6] (see ➲ Assessment of independence and social functioning, pp. 98–9). Along with the earlier benefits of the VABS, it has been updated with new norms, expanded age ranges, and improved items. In addition to assessing the four areas listed under ➲ Vineland Adaptive Behaviour Scale-III, pp. 98–9 within the original VABS, the latest edition has a fifth category of assessment: Maladaptive Behaviour Index—internalizing, externalizing, and other. The VABS-III can now measure adaptive behaviour of people with:

- Intellectual disabilities.
- Autistic spectrum;
- ADHD;
- Post-traumatic brain injury;
- Hearing impairment;
- Dementia/Alzheimer's disease.

Using the adaptive behaviour rating scales

Learning more about the person's adaptive behaviours will help nurses to gain a broader picture of the individual, of what they can and cannot do. When completing an assessment with an individual, you should identify an informant who knows the person well (i.e. parent or teacher). If there is no sufficient information to score the form, return again and continue with the assessment and/or seek information from other members of the interdisciplinary team. Also ensure the person is offered a range of opportunities to demonstrate the skills that are required to achieve a score on the form.

Ensure the person is physically and emotionally well and performing at their best. If the person is unwell, it may be better to return another day to complete the assessment. Be confident and competent in scoring and interpreting the behaviour rating scale, as these scores will be compared with people of similar age and gender, which will then be used to develop an appropriate care plan for this person.

References

5 Sparrow SS, Cicchetti DV, Saulnier CA (2016). *Vineland Adaptive Behavior Scales, 3rd edn (Vineland-3)*. Pearson Assessments: Livonia, MN. ℒ www.pearsonclinical.co.uk/Psychology/ChildMentalHealth/ChildAdaptiveBehaviour/vineland-3/vineland-adaptive-behavior-scales-third-edition-vineland-3.aspx (accessed 2 March 2018).
6 Sparrow S, Cicchetti D, Saulnier C (2016). *Vineland Adaptive Behavior Scales (Vineland-III)*, 3rd edn. Pearson Education: San Antonio, TX.

Health checks

The term 'health checks' refers to an important service that people with intellectual disabilities are eligible to access, which is provided by their own GP. It is the information that comes from health checks that forms the basis of the individual's health action plan (see ⊋ Health action plans and health facilitation, p. 155). The development of health checks is in response to the considerable research-based evidence identifying that, relative to the general population, people with intellectual disabilities have higher rates of unmet health needs, yet access health services less often.[7] Research has shown that such checks do result in previously unrecognized health needs being identified.

Various frameworks for annual health checks exist[7] and there can be variation in local services. It is likely that an annual health check will include certain core areas as a matter of routine such as:

• History of illness in the individual's family and associated health risks;
• Review of current medication;
• Immunization history and current status;
• Height, weight, and blood pressure;
• Assessing levels of fitness and advice about exercise;
• Take up of health screening services available to members of the general public;
• Access to health promotion messages such as those concerning healthy eating.

Where necessary, the following health checks may also be undertaken:
• Eye test (optometry);
• Hearing test (audiometry);
• Monitoring long-term conditions such as epilepsy, asthma, and coronary heart disease;
• Sexual health;
• Guidance, where necessary, regarding drugs and alcohol;
• Elimination and continence;
• Investigating any reports of behaviour that other people find of concern;
• Assessing mental health and emotional needs;
• Assessing mobility and posture;
• Oral and dental health.

A GP or senior nurse (such as a practice nurse) should take responsibility for implementing the programme of health checking, ensuring that accurate records are kept and any health action plans completed. Depending on the need of the individual concerned, other professionals or carers will be required to assist with aspects of the process. For example, community nurses in intellectual disability services may assist the practice to identify which of their patients are priorities for health checking, e.g. as follows:
• Individuals with severe or profound impairments;
• Individuals in transition from young person to adult services;
• Individuals who have complex health needs;
• Individuals at risk of developing health needs (e.g. those missing important health promotion or health education messages);
• Individuals named on the local authority register.

It is now considered good practice to name a registered nurse from the local community intellectual disability team to link with the practice to support the health check process. Nurses are well placed to alert healthcare professionals to the particular needs of people with intellectual disabilities (e.g. with regard to communication) and to support individuals to understand their right to a health check. They can also have a role in encouraging and advising people who may be reluctant to attend. Nurses should also be involved in health facilitation (see ➔ Health action plans and health facilitation, p. 154), as this is fundamental to ensuring that the health action plan is implemented.

It is important to remember that service providers share a responsibility for the health and well-being of people in their care. If health checking is not happening automatically as it should (i.e. that people are being invited annually), it may sometimes be necessary to prompt a local GP to provide the health check as required. This advocacy can be fundamental in ensuring that health needs are met. Sometimes advocacy will also be needed to ensure an individual gains access to the healthcare intervention identified as required, especially when resources are limited (e.g. dialysis). Service providers who see people on a day-to-day basis must be vigilant in their observation of those with whom they have contact. The early reporting of any signs or symptoms of ill health or change in health status of people can result in earlier health interventions, and as a result an improved prognosis.

Further reading

Emerson E, Turner S (2011). *Health Checks for People with Learning Disabilities: An Audit Tool*. Improving health and lives: The Learning Disabilities Public Health Observatory. Department of Health: London.

Royal College of General Practitioners (2010). *A Step by Step Guide for GP Practices: Annual Health Checks for People with a Learning Disability*. Royal College of General Practitioners: London.

Royal College of Psychiatrists (2015). *Outcomes Framework for Improving the Quality of Services for People with Intellectual Disability*. Royal College of Psychiatrists: London. ℞ www.rcpsych.ac.uk/pdf/FRID07.pdf (accessed 30 October 2017).

References

7 Royal College of General Practitioners. *Learning Disabilities*. ℞ www.rcgp.org.uk/learningdisabilities (accessed 30 October 2017).

Screening of physical health

Physical health screening is a proactive intervention, which seeks to detect any possible sign of ill health before it has fully developed. Health screening is a central tenet of health promotion activity, as its aim is that ill health is prevented. It is important that people with intellectual disabilities have access to all national health screening programmes that are available to other citizens of the same age and gender, e.g. cervical screening, breast screening, bowel screening, diabetic retinopathy screening, and abdominal aortic aneurysm screening.[8]

All people with intellectual disabilities should be offered health screening in the same way as other citizens, e.g. routine invitations to women 50yrs and over to have breast screening (mammography); however, in practice, this has not always happened.

In recent years, there has been a growing concern about the unmet health needs of people with intellectual disabilities. Screening (and health checking; see **>** Health checks, p. 155) can help to identify otherwise undetected conditions, which may have remained hidden for various reasons, e.g.:

- The signs and symptoms of ill health may be masked by the presence of intellectual disabilities. This is sometimes referred to as diagnostic overshadowing (see **>** Diagnostic overshadowing, pp. 110–11).
- Low rates of self-reporting health problems by people with intellectual disabilities.
- Polypharmacy can mask signs and symptoms of ill health.
- Additional obstacles to people with intellectual disabilities accessing physical health screening have included (see **>** Physical health and well being, p. 154):
  - Ineffective means of communicating health screening information to this client group;
  - The knowledge and attitude of staff who support people with intellectual disabilities;
  - Lack of time and specialist equipment;
  - Concerns about a person's ability to consent to treatment;
  - Lack of confidence and experience of medical professionals to work with people with intellectual disabilities;
  - Anxiety and fear of individuals, based on previous negative experiences of the NHS.

Equality legislation means that people with intellectual disabilities should have equal access to health services, and this includes the right to have physical health screening. For example, the care standards outlined in national standards such as the National Service Frameworks (NSFs) in England, or the equivalent in other countries within the UK and the Republic of Ireland, for cancer, coronary heart disease, older people, renal disease, and diabetes apply equally to people with intellectual disabilities as they do to the rest of the population.

Where service users themselves are unable to do so, staff working with people with intellectual disabilities will need to ensure appointments for health screening are made when necessary. A requirement for these may be prompted via the routine annual health check conducted by the person's GP, practice nurse, or health facilitator (see **>** Health action plans and health facilitation, pp. 86–7). People may access current national screening programmes (as referred to earlier in this section). Others may be referred for non-routine screening, as their health needs determine.

This may include:

• Faecal occult blood (for colorectal health);
• Bone density scan;
• Urinalysis;
• Electrocardiogram (ECG);
• Blood tests for thyroid function, cholesterol levels, diabetes, etc.;
• Eye and hearing tests.

It may be necessary to advocate on behalf of people you support to ensure that they receive the screening to which they are entitled. Once the appointment has been made, it is advisable also to plan ahead and allow enough time to ensure the person understands the process and is able to give informed consent. Double-time appointments may be necessary, and good liaison beforehand with the service providers should ensure that the experience for the person is more positive.

There is also now a wide range of accessible teaching and advice materials which have been developed to help prepare people with intellectual disabilities understand the benefit to them of health screening. These also help explain the process that the person will need to go through and can be used effectively to prepare people for screening well in advance of the appointment.

Further reading

Cancer Research UK. *Cervical Screening for Women with Learning Disabilities*. ℘ www.cancerresearchuk.org/about-cancer/type/cervical-cancer/about/cervical-screening-for-people-with-learning-disability#more (accessed 27 February 2018).

Easyhealth (examples of accessible information about a range of health screening). ℘ www.easyhealth.org.uk (accessed 27 February 2018).

Marriott A, Turner S, Ashby S, Rees D (2015). Cancer screening for people with learning disabilities and the role of the screening liaison nurse. *Tizard Learning Disability Review*. **20**: 239–46.

References

8 Turner S, Giraud-Saunders A, Marriott A (2013). *Improving the Uptake of Screening Services by People with Learning Disabilities Across the South West Peninsula. A Strategy and Toolkit*. National Development Team for Inclusion: Bath. ℘ www.ndti.org.uk/uploads/files/Screening_Services_Strategy_Toolkit_final.pdf (accessed 27 February 2018).

Assessing pain

Pain is considered to be a subjective experience, which is multidimensional, presenting itself in many ways. The pain experience and the individual's reaction to it are influenced by their developmental stage, cognitive ability, and cultural factors. Describing felt pain is difficult and is particularly challenging for a young child or for an individual who has cognitive impairment or communication difficulties.

Pain is experienced more often in people with intellectual disabilities than those without, particularly in individuals with profound multiple disabilities, as their increased health care needs are often accompanied with pain.[9] Yet pain is often undetected, and therefore untreated, and it has been suggested that this group of people are prescribed less analgesia than those with no cognitive impairment.[10] The under-recognition of pain increases their risk of harm, diagnostic overshadowing, and potential delays in the diagnosis of serious medical conditions, which can have devastating consequences.[11]

Challenges in assessing pain

Cook et al. (1999)[12] identify the following four factors in poor pain assessment, shown in Fig. 4.1.

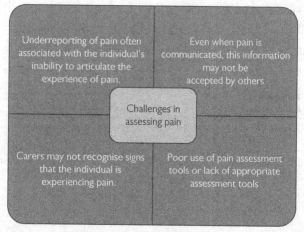

Fig. 4.1 Challenges in assessing pain.

Adapted from Cook AKR, Nevin CA, Downs MG (1999) Assessing pain of people with cognitive impairment. *International Journal of Geriatric Psychiatry.* **14**, 421–425 with permission from Wiley.

Expressions of pain

Pain is expressed in various ways in people with intellectual disabilities. In addition to the physiological signs of pain, it may also be demonstrated through unusual or changed behaviours, as outlined in Box 4.1.

Box 4.1 Unusual or changed behaviours

- Vocalizations;
- Grimacing;
- Reduced limb mobility;
- Change in behaviour;
- Withdrawal;
- Self-injurious behaviour;
- Sweating;
- Inappropriate laughing;
- Holding of a body part.

Assessing pain

The assessment is informed by perceptive observation and interpretation of the individual's communicative behaviour and evidence from carers, followed by sound clinical judgements.[13] Vital to the assessment is the nurse's recognition that challenging behaviour does have a communicative function and nurses must assess if the presenting behaviour is a person's way of communicating 'I am in pain'. Nurses need to participate in frequent pain assessment for people with communication difficulties and by using a comprehensive holistic approach in that pain can be detected and treated appropriately in people with intellectual disabilities. This holistic approach should be informed by the nurse's understanding:

- That pain is often under-recognized and therefore undertreated in this population;
- That factors such as the environment, situations, and emotions can influence both perception and response to pain;
- Of the risks and causes of pain and the potential consequences of under-diagnosis and treatment;
- Of the various pain assessment tools available and their use, in order to be able to select the tool that will be most useful in the care of the person;
- An awareness of how the experience of pain may be verbalized and demonstrated in people with intellectual disabilities;
- That the nurse's attitude to pain can influence appropriate assessment and subsequent management of an individual's pain;
- And respect the role of the families and carers in the assessment process.

Some pain/distress assessment tools

- Pain and Discomfort Scale (PADS);
- Heat–Pain Threshold (HPT);
- Non-Communicating Children's Pain Checklist-Revised;
- DisDAT;
- Non-Communicating Adults Pain Checklist (NCAPC);
- Visual Analog Scale and Faces Pain Scale-Revised.

References

9 Findlay L, Williams AC de C, Scior K (2014). Exploring experiences and understandings of pain in adults with intellectual disabilities. *Journal of Intellectual Disability Research.* **58**: 358–67.

10 Boerlage AA, Valkenburg AJ, Scherder EJ, et al. (2013). Prevalence of pain in institutionalized adults with intellectual disabilities: a cross-sectional approach. *Research in Developmental Disabilities.* **34**: 2399–406.

11 Mencap (2012). *Death by Indifference: 74 Deaths and Counting. A Progress Report 5 Years On.* Mencap: London.

12 Cook AKR, Nevin CA, Downs MG (1999). Assessing pain of people with cognitive impairment. *International Journal of Geriatric Psychiatry.* **14**: 421–5.

13 Zaballa M (2016). Pain assessment: a relevant concern to increase quality of life in people with intellectual disabilities. *Journal of General Practice.* **4**: 231.

Assessing distress

Distress, pain, and suffering are descriptions of unpleasant experiences that individuals perceive and experience. Like pain and suffering, distress is perceived and experienced differently in individuals and may be felt as emotional, psychological, or physical in nature, and just like pain and suffering, its impact on the individual needs to be recognized and validated.

Defining distress is not easy, yet it is a term used frequently within nursing and is associated with discomfort which can be physical, emotional, or psychological in nature. Ridner (2004) describes distress as 'a non-specific, biological or emotional response to a demand or stressor that is harmful to the individual'.[14] It is essential that nurses identify the signs of distress, validate its existence, identify possible causes, and deal appropriately with it. Early recognition of distress can help alleviate some of the unpleasant feelings associated with it, avoiding a potential crisis. But stress is difficult to assess in people with intellectual disabilities, and particularly so in those with profound and multiple disabilities.

Increased experience of distress

People with intellectual disabilities are likely to experience more distress than others for a number of reasons, including:

- A lack of response to their rights to inclusion, choice, friends, and freedom;
- An increased risk of their needs not being recognized or validated, thus left untreated;
- A greater incidence of both acute and chronic illness, thus more episodes of pain;
- Greater risk of both accidental and non-accidental injury.

Expressing distress

Early recognition of distress can help alleviate some of the unpleasant feelings associated with it. To avoid a potential crisis, it is important that health professionals know the difference between pain and distress. However, distress is difficult to assess in people with intellectual disabilities, and particularly so in those with profound and multiple disabilities. Approximately 40–50% of people with intellectual disabilities have communication difficulties; the degree of difficulty increases with the severity of the intellectual disability. Consequently, communicating perceptions or experiences of distress are often expressed through behavioural cues, posture, expressions, or vocalizations and often are similar to those used to identify pain. While signs of distress are often recognized by families, communicating this information to others is challenging. Distress recognition is likely to be an implicit, rather than explicit, act; however, pattern recognition (connected pieces of information) used to identify stress in palliative care is now adapted in people with intellectual disabilities.[15]

Assessing distress

Although distress and pain are often used synonymously, they are not the same. Distress often accompanies pain; however, it is important to note that distress is not always caused by pain. While there are a number of pain assessment tools that may be used with people with intellectual disabilities, there are, however, few tools to assess distress, which can be caused by various factors, equally as disturbing as pain.

DisDAT, a comprehensive distress assessment tool (not a scoring tool), seeks to present an accurate representation of an individual's language that 'denotes distress'. Regnard et al. (2007) note that signs of distress are specific to individuals, and not specific to its cause.[15] Furthermore, they stress that teams using this tool are more likely to pick up distress signals than an individual using it and it is easy for carers to use.

This assessment tool helps to:
- Identify distress in people with cognitive impairment and communication difficulties;
- Record changes in behaviour and other signs that are demonstrated by the person when they were seen to be content, so that changes in behaviour indicating distress would be more easily recognized;
- Provide a checklist of the possible causes for the distress, while taking account of the context in which the behaviour was demonstrated;
- Provide an accurate outline of the signs and behaviours of the individual, so that other carers, within different environments, have a clear understanding of the meaning of these, which can help guide their plan of individualized care).[15]

Further reading

McKenzie K, Smith M, Purcell A-M (2013). The reported expression of pain and distress by people with an intellectual disability. Journal of Clinical Nursing. 22: 1833–42.

Taylor I, Conway V, Knight A (2014). Measuring and addressing pain in people with limited communication skills: The "I hurt help me" pain management project. Journal of Pain Management. 9: 129–36.

References

14 Rinder SH (2004). Psychological distress concept analysis. Journal of Advanced Nursing. 45: 536–45.

15 Regnard C, Reynolds J, Watson B, Matthews D, Gibson L, Clarke C (2007). Understanding distress in people with severe communication difficulties: developing and assessing the Disability Distress Assessment Tool (Dis DAT). Journal of Intellectual Disability Research. 51: 277–92.

Screening of mental health problems

Aims of assessment

Assessment is a core role of the nurse and has a number of important functions:

- To identify the underlying reason(s) for the person's behaviours;
- To identify patterns of normative behaviours and the changes in these behaviours (baseline distortion);
- To clearly describe the person's explicit behaviours in terms of quality of life, life events, gender, and social mores;
- To diminish any other explanations for the presenting behaviours, thereby formulating a 'working hypothesis' or suspected reasons for the behaviour(s);
- To develop a socially valid and effective intervention programme;
- To determine whether the person is eligible for particular supports and who will provide these supports;
- To provide a basis, so the implemented care can be evaluated/reassessed.

Structured frameworks

In undertaking a comprehensive assessment, based upon a bio-psycho-social model, as proposed by the International Association for the Scientific Study of Intellectual and Developmental Disabilities (IASSIDD),[16] it is important that a structured approach to assessment is used. Some of the key areas to assess are:

- Interview with carers to seek information on the person's baseline behaviours, developmental history, social history (i.e. employment/education status, friends/relationships, routines, likes/dislikes, quality of life), forensic history, family functioning, and how they manage the person's behaviours, and also presenting behaviours;
- Interviews with other professionals within the person's life;
- Direct observation of the person, and also a functional behavioural analysis of his/her behaviours;
- Via the GP or medical officer to obtain a medical history, physical examination, and list of medications and side effects. Also, if needed, laboratory tests such as blood levels of medication and toxicology levels;
- Unstructured psychiatric interview aided by standardized mental health screening scales [i.e. Psychiatric Assessment Schedules for Adults with Developmental Disabilities (PAS-ADD), Glasgow Depression Scale].

Use of screening tools

Within general psychiatry and psychology, a number of screening tools have been developed to help nurses to recognize mental health signs and symptoms, thereby aiding in the assessment process. Some of these screening tools include Beck's Depression Inventory and Hamilton Anxiety Inventory. People with borderline to mild intellectual disabilities, with good comprehension, may be able to complete these tools with assistance; however, many more people with intellectual disabilities will be unable to score in these and subsequently rely upon third-party informants or their carers to inform professionals about the person's behaviours. Recent developments have seen the introduction of the PAS-ADD schedules.

- *The PAS-ADD Checklist*[17] is a 27-item screening instrument examining affective/neurotic disorders, organic conditions and psychotic disorders. No formal training is required to use this tool, although knowledge and awareness of mental health in people with intellectual disabilities is an important benefit.
- *The Mini PAS-ADD Interview*[17] is a 66-item screening instrument that probes a wider range of mental health symptoms [depression, anxiety and phobias, hypomania, obsessive–compulsive disorder (OCD), psychosis, and unspecified] using a glossary. Specific training of half a day is required for the practitioner to effectively use this tool.
- *The PAS-ADD 10 Interview*[17] is a more detailed semi-structured clinical interview designed for the person with intellectual disabilities and/or informants. Specific training of 1 day is required to use this tool.
- *The ChA-PAS (Child and Adolescent Psychiatric Assessment Schedule Interview)* is a 97-item screening instrument that assesses mental health problems in children and adolescents with intellectual disabilities. This tool examines depression, anxiety, ADHD, compulsions, conduct issues, psychotic disorders, and ASC. Specific training of 1 day is required to use this tool.

For information on screening in relation to dementia among people with intellectual disabilities, see ➡ Dementia (in people with intellectual disabilities), pp. 138–9.

As medical officers and psychiatrists draw significantly on reports from nurses in making a diagnosis, it is important that nurses are skilled in identifying and reporting the typical and atypical signs and symptoms displayed by this population, as well as the shift from the person's usual pattern of behaviour (baseline).

Further reading

Cooper SA, McLean G, Guthrie B, et al. (2015). Multiple physical and mental health comorbidity in adults with intellectual disabilities: population-based cross-sectional analysis. *BMC Family Practice*. 6: 110.

Dykens EM, Shah B, Davis B, Courtney B, Fife T, Fitzpatrick J (2015). Psychiatric disorders in adolescents and young adults with Down syndrome and other intellectual disabilities. *Journal of Neurodevelopmental Disorders*. 7: 9.

Luckasson R, Schalock RL (2015). Standards to guide the use of clinical judgment in the field of intellectual disability. *Intellectual and Developmental Disabilities*. 53: 240–51.

References

16 International Association for the Scientific Study of Intellectual and Developmental Disabilities (2001). *Addressing the Mental Health Needs of People with Intellectual Disabilities*. ⌖ www.iassid. org/ (accessed 27 February 2018).

17 Moss S (2002). *PAS-ADD Schedules*. Pavilion Press: Brighton.

Assessment of independence and social functioning

The need to assess independence and social functioning

Social competence and social functioning have long been used as a functional means of contributing to a decision as to whether a person has intellectual disabilities. This is because these concepts relate to an individual's ability to develop skills of independence, as well as living as independently as possible as a member of society. However, it should be remembered that impairment/s in social competence are not exclusively shown by people with intellectual disabilities and may be due as much to lack of opportunity as to intellectual functioning.[18] More recently, health and social policy in the UK and Ireland has reinforced the need for people to develop independence as an entitlement (see ➲ Principles and values of social policy, pp. 24–5). Adaptive behaviour might be considered as a collection of conceptual, social, and practical skills that are learnt and performed by people in their everyday lives.[19] These include, e.g.:

- 'Conceptual skills—language and literacy; money, time, and number concepts; as well as self-direction;
- Social skills—interpersonal skills, social responsibility, self-esteem, gullibility, level of naivety, social problem-solving, and an ability to follow rules/obey laws and to avoid being subject to mate/hate crime;
- Practical skills—activities of daily living, occupational skills, healthcare, travel/transportation, schedules/routines, safety, use of money, use of the telephone.'[19]

Standardized tests can be used to determine limitations in adaptive behaviour. Two examples of those currently available are briefly outlined below.

Vineland Adaptive Behaviour Scale-III

VABS-III[20] is a comprehensive assessment scale of US origin and covers personal and social skills from birth to adulthood. These are broken down into the following domains and subdomains:

- Communication—receptive, expressive, and written;
- Daily living skills—personal, domestic, and community;
- Socialization—interpersonal relationships, play and leisure time, coping skills;
- Motor skills—fine motor, gross motor;
- Maladaptive behaviour index (optional)—internalizing, externalizing, other.

A range of assessment forms are available:

- Survey Interview Form and Expanded Interview Form—assessment using a semi-structured interview format;
- Parent/Caregiver Rating Form—assessment using a rating scale format;
- Teacher Rating Form—assessment in school or day-care setting using a questionnaire format.

VABS-III Survey Forms ASSIST is a computer software program designed to calculate scores and print report forms. To order or for more information on VABS-III, see ✎ www.pearsonclinical.com/psychology/products/100001622/vineland-adaptive-behavior-scales-third-edition--vineland-3.html.

The Supports Intensity Scale–Adult version (SIS-A)

The SIS-A is available in both English and French and is widely used in North America as well as internationally.[21] This assessment scale has been designed for use with people with intellectual and/or developmental disabilities who are aged 16 or over. The scale identifies and measures the supports needed by individuals to participate in various activities. The scale is conducted through an interview process every 3 years. The SIS includes three sections, each of which measures a particular area of support need. Section 1 comprises 49 life activities that are grouped into six domains that includes:

• Home living;
• Employment;
• Lifelong learning;
• Community living;
• Health and safety;
• Social activities.

Sections 2 and 3 include protection and advocacy issues, as well as health and behaviour needs assessment. As such, the scale enables measurement across time of these support needs, recognizing that the needs of some people with intellectual disabilities require an increase in support over time. There is also a similar scale available for children.

References

18 Gates B (2015). The nature of learning disabilities and their relationship to learning disability nursing. In: B Gates, K Mafuba. *Learning Disability Nursing: Modern Day Practice*. Taylor and Francis: London; pp 6–8.

19 American Association on Intellectual and Developmental Disabilities (2010). *Intellectual Disability: Definition, Classification, and Systems of Supports*, 11th edn. American Association on Intellectual and Developmental Disabilities: Washington, DC.

20 Sparrow S, Cicchetti D, Saulnier C (2016). *Vineland Adaptive Behavior Scales (Vineland-III)*, 3rd edn. Pearson Education: San Antonio, TX.

21 Thompson JR, Bryant BR, Schalock RL, et al. (2015). *Supports Intensity Scale—Adult Version (SIS-A) User's Manual*. American Association on Intellectual and Developmental Disabilities: Washington, DC.

Measurement of IQ

The IQ test is the main method used today for measuring a person's intelligence or mental ability. It measures a variety of different types of ability such as:
• Verbal;
• Mathematical;
• Spatial;
• Memory;
• Reasoning.

In 1905, a French psychologist by the name of Alfred Binet, working with a physician associate Theodore Simon, developed the Binet Simon Test designed to measure intelligence. Debate surrounds the validity of the IQ test, as well as the cultural and linguistic problems in developing and completing such a test.

Many see IQ tests as an assessment of a person's problem-solving ability, rather than general intelligence. However, IQ tests are not even a comprehensive test of someone's mental ability. Although they may assess analytical and verbal aptitude well, they are not an accurate test of creativity, practical knowledge, and other skills involved in mental ability. Despite this, IQ tests today are still widely used to assess people's intelligence.

Obtaining IQ scores

The IQ test has been conducted on a large sample that is representative of the wider population. The average or mean score of the population has been found to be approximately 100. This indicates that about half of the population's IQ scores fall below the mean, and likewise half of the population's IQ scores fall above the mean. When the IQ scores of a representative population are pictorially drawn, this graph takes on a 'bell shape' appearance—known as the 'bell shape curve'. The majority of people are distributed around the mean, indicating average intelligence, and few people are at the extreme ends of the curve. This is also known as the 'normal distribution curve'.

As previously identified, the mean IQ score is 100, and variations from the mean are measured in standard deviations (SDs). There are 3 SDs below the mean and 3 SDs above the mean; 1 SD equals 15 points.

Classification of intellectual disability

In addition to IQ, intellectual disability must also be assessed by significant deficits in adaptive functioning. The concept of these adaptive/social functioning competencies relates to everyday life and how the person copes with the demands of his/her own environment (see → Adaptive behaviour rating scales, pp. 98–9). This assessment identifies the degree of assistance required by the person in providing the appropriate care and support to live in his/her own social environment. Consequently, classification systems universally agree that three core criteria should be used in making a diagnosis of intellectual disabilities.[22,23]

These are:
• Significant impairment of intellectual functioning;
• Significant impairment of adaptive/social functioning (of at least two or more adaptive skills, i.e. communication, self-care, home living, social skills, community use, health and safety, leisure, and work);
• Age of onset before 18yrs.

Levels of intellectual disability

According to International Classification of Diseases, 11th revision (ICD-11) and Diagnostic and Statistical Manual of Mental Disorders, 5th edition (DSM-5), there are four levels of intellectual disabilities; these are based on standardized IQ scores (i.e. at least 2 SDs below the mean).[22,23] Adaptive behaviour should also be included in making the classification.

- Mild intellectual disabilities—IQ 50–70;
- Moderate intellectual disabilities—IQ 35–49;
- Severe intellectual disabilities—IQ 20–34;
- Profound intellectual disabilities—IQ <20.

It is important to remember, however, that the level of one's intelligence does not decide what a person can learn but may give an indication of how fast they may learn it. It is largely the opportunities for learning presented to people that determine what they will learn.[24]

References

22 World Health Organization (2015). *ICD-11 Classification of Mental and Behavioural Disorders: Clinical Descriptions and Diagnostic Guidelines.* World Health Organization: Geneva.

23 American Psychiatric Association (2015). *Diagnostic and Statistical Manual of Mental Disorders,* 5th edn. American Psychiatric Association: Arlington, VA.

24 Emerson E, Einfeld SL (2013). *Challenging Behaviour.* Cambridge University Press: London.

Mental capacity and decision-making

When making decisions related to the receipt of health and social care, the right of the service user to choose is supported and protected in a number of ways. It is protected and nursing practice guided by specific capacity legislation in England, Wales, and Scotland.[25,26] Within Northern Ireland and the Republic of Ireland, the right to choose and make decisions is protected via common law and by healthcare policy.[27,28] It is important to note that although specific capacity legislation is not yet formally in place, in Northern Ireland or the Republic of Ireland, new capacity-based legislation is going through a process of implementation. Professional standards also direct that nurses must practice within the parameters of the legislation and/or guidance within one's specific jurisdiction.[29,30]

Consequently, the most fundamental legal principle that is expected across all of UK and Republic of Ireland jurisdictions is that all adults (over 16/18yrs) should be presumed to have capacity to make their own health and social care decisions and choices, unless it can be proven that they do not have capacity and there is need for capacity to be considered in relation to each decision. Mental illness, acquired brain injury, intellectual disability, and other disorders that affect the functioning of the mind and/or brain should never, in themselves, override the presumption that the individual has the capacity to make decisions.

What is mental capacity?

In the delivery of health and social care, having the mental capacity to make decisions is most often considered within the context of giving consent. Consent may be required for examination, treatment, and care, and range from day-to-day interventions such as what to wear or what to eat, to specific hands-on activity, such as taking a blood pressure or providing support with personal care, or to more intrusive care such as surgery under general anaesthesia. In ALL of these circumstances, for consent to be legal and valid, it is necessary that the person has 'sufficient' mental capacity to accept or refuse the care or intervention that is being offered to them. As there is a presumption of capacity, and capacity is required to be decision-specific, this means that no person with intellectual disabilities can be presumed to not have capacity. Therefore, it is essential that nurses attempt to obtain consent, making reasonable adjustments within the process, and only if it is established during this process that the person is experiencing difficulties, should their capacity be questioned. For consent to be valid, health or social care professional must have a reasonable belief that the person is able to:
• Comprehend and retain the information provided to him/her;
• Weigh it in the balance and arrive at a choice;
• Communicate his/her choice.

The determination of capacity

The assessment and determination of capacity is everyone's business. While there will be circumstances where very specialist and expert assessments of capacity are required, in the day-to-day delivery of health and social care, every nurse will be required to make judgements related to the capacity of the service users with whom they are working. As outlined earlier, it is important to always presume capacity and seek consent. If, when doing so, it is suspected that the capacity of the service user is compromised at that time, it is first of all important to be able to provide sufficient evidence that demonstrates a reasonable belief that the person does not have the capacity to make the decision in question. This evidence will be provided via an assessment of capacity. Such assessments may be very informal (e.g. the person demonstrates a clear rationale for a one-off refusal to accept a blood pressure check) or a more formal assessment of capacity that would be necessary if someone refused lifesaving cardiac surgery. All assessments of capacity should be documented. Capacity can be temporarily affected for a number of reasons, and if this be the case, then it may be prudent to wait until the person regains capacity, if possible.

The capacity to make decisions must always be decision-specific. Therefore, if a person is assessed as lacking capacity to make one decision, that does not mean that this assessment can apply to another decision. Professionals are expected to take reasonable steps to maximize a person's capacity and their opportunity for involvement in decision-making, e.g. providing information in an easy-read format, smaller chunks of information, or more time for decision-making.

How to proceed if the person lacks capacity?

Specific capacity legislation and common law provide a legal safeguard to provide care and/or intervention to someone who lacks capacity, as long as it can be demonstrated that the care/intervention provided is in their best interests. Best interests decisions should take a range of factors into account and should never be solely considered on the basis of 'what will benefit the service user medically'. Decisions should be made which are identifiable in the best interests of the person with intellectual disabilities. Members of the health/social care team should be involved in this decision-making and be able to show it is in the person's best interests. When it is not possible to reach an agreement, consideration should be given to the involvement of the appropriate legal professionals/courts who can be asked to determine what is in the person's best interests.

References

25 *Mental Capacity Act* (2005). HMSO: London.
26 Scottish Executive (2000). *Adults with Incapacity (Scottish) Act*. HMSO: Edinburgh.
27 Ireland Department of Health, Social Services and Public Safety (2003). *Good Practice in Consent: Consent for Examination, Treatment or Care. A Handbook for the HPSS*. HMSO: Belfast.
28 Health Service Executive (2014). *National Consent Policy*. Department of Health: Dublin.
29 Nursing and Midwifery Council (2015). *The Code: Standards of Conduct, Performance and Ethics for Nurses and Midwives*. Nursing and Midwifery Council: London.
30 Nursing and Midwifery Board of Ireland (2014). *Code of Professional Conduct and Ethics for Registered Nurses and Registered Midwives*. Nursing and Midwifery Board of Ireland: Dublin.

Risk assessment

Context

Within risk assessment, risk is widely recognized as having two key components, firstly that the likelihood that an event may occur and secondly that if the event does occur, it may have negative consequences. However, it is also important to recognize that much or our learning experiences have involved risk-taking, albeit carefully managed risk-taking. Therefore, taking risks may provide an opportunity for learning.[31] However, exposure to risk will only benefit people where there is a systematic approach to identifying through assessment and managing any potentially harmful outcomes within a person-centred way. This will not occur if people with intellectual disabilities are exposed to unacceptable risks, risks of discrimination, risk of poor health access and care, risk of premature death, and risk of abuse. The recent publication NICE/Winterbourne Concordat *'Positive and Safe'* addressed concerns around the way people were supported such as the use of locked doors, use of antipsychotic medication, and restrictive practice.

'Transforming Care'[32] has changed the focus of care for some people with intellectual disabilities, and more people are being supported within local communities, rather than large congregated settings, although it is not without the risks associated with everyday living.

Nurses needs to be confident in challenging practices where they pose a risk to a person with intellectual disabilities, e.g. reporting unsafe and abusive practices, challenging inequality, and promoting understanding of safeguarding practices in order to protect people's rights.

Key perspectives in risk assessment

Systemic approaches to personalized risk assessment must be done in collaborative partnership and demonstrate positive links to an individual's Positive Behaviour Support Plan. It should include balancing the risk of everyday living using the least restrictive approaches to ensure good quality of life outcomes for people. All staff have a duty of care to ensure risks are communicated with all stakeholders and appropriate training is provided.

Key principles of risk assessment

- Organizations should have clear procedures for assessing and managing risk within a person-centred planning process.
- Training should be provided to enable those supporting people to be competent and practise safely when assessing risk.
- Staff supporting people need to be able to identify possible risks.
- People are entitled to make decisions that staff may not agree with or make ourselves; the role of nurses is to ensure the individual has the information in an accessible format and the capacity to understand the consequences of their actions and the impact on others.
- People need to be supported in making decisions about the risks in their lives, involving family, carers, and partners when necessary.
- Staff should always assume that the person has capacity until demonstrated otherwise.

- Regular planned evaluation and updating of the risk plans in accordance with how best they work for the person. These need to reflect changes in the person's mental or physical health.
- Clearly document all discussions and decisions.

Risk assessment

When undertaking a risk assessment, individual organizations may have their own assessment criteria/assessment tool to support the risk assessment process. There are a number of recognized assessment tools being used, e.g. HCR20[33] (Historical, Clinical, Risk management), Functional Analysis in the Care Environment (FACE)[34] tool associated with Care Programme Approach (CPA), and the Modified Sainsbury Tool.[35]

The key principle must be that this is conducted in a person-centred way. People involved in working with people with intellectual disabilities may encounter varying degrees of risks for the people whom they support. This may include risks of everyday living (road safety, access to kitchens/bathrooms, lifestyles), and risk of poor health conditions (including long-term conditions—epilepsy, dysphagia), compounded by inequalities in accessing general healthcare services. Other risks may arise from personal relationships (and lack of), poor mental health, or offending behaviours or exploitation due to vulnerability.

Good risk assessment is underpinned by involvement of both the person and their families and/or significant others. The nurse needs to be mindful in ensuring the practice of risk assessment reflects the mental capacity of individuals and, where the person lacks capacity, that best interests decision-making processes are followed. Therefore, the consequences will also vary in degree, according to the identified risk. They should never start from the point that the identified activity poses too many risks and therefore will not be considered. People's lives should not necessarily be restricted, as we all take risks as part of everyday living; a life without risk may be impoverished and may prevent a person from living a fulfilling life. However, when supporting someone, we cannot ignore the identified risks that may cause harm to the individual or others but need to support them in determining the associated risks, in order to explore new opportunities.

References

31 Robertson JP, Collinson C (2011). Positive risk taking: whose risk is it? An exploration in community outreach teams in adult mental health and learning disability services. *Health, Risk and Society*. **13**: 147–64.
32 Local Government Association (2015). *Transforming Care, Building the Right Support*. NHS England: London.
33 imosphere (2006). *Functional Analysis in the Care Environment (FACE)*. ℘ www.imosphere.co.uk (accessed 30 October 2017).
34 Douglas KS, Hart SD, Webster CD, Belfrage H (2013). *HCR-20V3: Assessing Risk of Violence – User Guide*. Mental Health, Law, and Policy Institute, Simon Fraser University: Burnaby. ℘ hcr-20.com (accessed 2 March 2018).
35 Stein W (2005). Modified Sainsbury tool: an initial risk assessment tool for primary care mental health and learning disability services. *Journal of Psychiatric and Mental Health Nursing*. **12**: 620–33.

Quality of life

Context

Over the past 5 years, there has been an increased focus on service delivery and outcomes. The publications post-Winterbourne View—*Transforming Care, Building the Right Support, Driving Up Quality, Health Equality Framework*—are all very much focused on embedding service change and improving the quality of life for people with intellectual disabilities. These publications are in keeping with the principles of government policies for services with people with intellectual disabilities. The recurring principles within these policy documents[36-39] across the UK and Ireland highlight the need to promote a high quality of life for people with intellectual disabilities, with an emphasis on inclusion in decision-making and full participation in society. There is recognition that services sometimes have failed people in relation to their physical and mental healthcare and social care needs. The focus is rightly on moving people out of hospital provision into skilled community-based provision and ensuring reasonable adjustments are made so people can access general services. Nurses need to ensure that the quality of all services meet the requirements of the healthcare regulator in the country. Abuses and lack of care have occurred over the past 30 years, ranging from Sutton and Merton to Cornwall right through to Winterbourne View, and most recently, the Mazars report[39] scrutinized the role of the nurse and quality of life issues. This can be in all settings, so we need to ensure that the support needs are tailored to meet the individual needs of the person through the process of robust assessment and effective care planning, including risk management, regular reviews, and evaluation involving the individual and their family.

There is now also an increased focus on improving the physical health of people with intellectual disabilities. The Health Equality Framework (HEF), and now the HEF+, was developed on the basis of a series of systematic reviews of health inequalities experienced by people with intellectual disabilities, which identified and described the five key determinants of health inequalities in this population:

- Social;
- Genetic and biological;
- Communication difficulties and reduced health literacy;
- Personal health behaviour and lifestyle risks;
- Deficiencies in access to, and quality of, health provision.

It is clear, from the evidence, the greater exposure to these determinants, the greater the likelihood of experiencing otherwise avoidable negative health outcomes, which would lead to an impoverished quality of life.

Transforming Care[38] found failings in quality around how we care for people with intellectual disabilities and/or autism with complex needs. The report identified important quality of life outcomes for individuals as:

- 'Being safe;
- Being treated with compassion, dignity, and respect;
- Being involved in decisions about care;
- Knowing those around them and looking after them are well supported;
- Making choices in their daily life;
- Receiving good-quality general healthcare'.

Evidence-based approach

When considering tools to assess a person's quality of life, it is critically important that the nurse adopts an evidence-based approach and also involves families, friends, other professionals, and agencies. When adopting a person-centred approach, the nurse should be aware of all the evidence available that supports this (see Fig. 4.2).

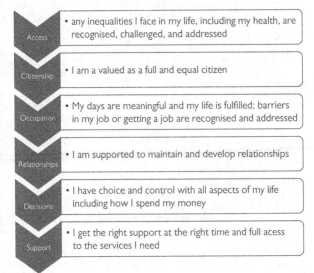

Access
• any inequalities I face in my life, including my health, are recognised, challenged, and addressed

Citizenship
• I am a valued as a full and equal citizen

Occupation
• My days are meaningful and my life is fulfilled; barriers in my job or getting a job are recognised and addressed

Relationships
• I am supported to maintain and develop relationships

Decisions
• I have choice and control with all aspects of my life including how I spend my money

Support
• I get the right support at the right time and full acess to the services I need

Fig. 4.2 ACHORD—the authors' approach to assessing the quality of life for people with intellectual disabilities (see also Local Government Association (2015). *Transforming Care, Building the Right Support.* NHS England: London.)

Further reading

Brown I, Hatton C, Emerson E (2013). Quality of life indicators for individuals with intellectual disabilities: extending current practice. *Intellectual and Developmental Disabilities.* 51: 316–32.

Townsend-White C, Pham AN, Vassos MV (2012). A systematic review of quality of life measures for people with intellectual disabilities and challenging behaviours. *Journal of Intellectual Disability Research.* 56: 270–84.

References

36 Department of Health (2012). *Winterbourne View Hospital: Department of Health Review and Response.* Department of Health: London.

37 Department of Health (2007). *Valuing People Now. From Progress to Transformation.* Department of Health: London.

38 Local Government Association (2015). *Transforming Care, Building the Right Support.* NHS England: London.

39 Green B, Bruce MA, Finn P, et al. (2015). *Mazers Report: Independent Review of Deaths of People with a Learning Disability or Mental Health Problem in Contact with Southern Health NHS Foundation Trust April 2011 to March 2015.* NHS England: London. ✆ www.england.nhs.uk/south/wp-content/uploads/sites/6/2015/12/mazars-rep.pdf (accessed 30 October 2017).

Life experiences

Following the exposure of the recent abuses[40,41] in care, it is clear there is still a lot of work to do to ensure that these individuals with intellectual disabilities have the same rights to an ordinary life and to being treated as equal citizens. It is essential that the focus must be linked to opportunities for a greater range of life experiences, including positive health, social activities, and meaningful activities. Good physical and mental health is a key outcome to ensuring that people with intellectual disabilities can enjoy a full range of life experiences.

There is a clear focus in services on personalization, recognizing that each person is unique, with different hopes and aspirations for a fulfilling life, and that they have the right to shape and control this with support from others as they choose. The seven key elements of personalized support, as identified in the section on quality of life (⮕ Quality of life, pp. 106–7), will be instrumental in supporting individuals in leading a fulfilling life. An obstacle to enhancing the life experiences of people with intellectual disabilities can be the perceived risks associated with ordinary living and the opportunity to experience new things. Facilitation to support individuals with a focus on positive risk-taking is essential. It is important to ensure that personalization facilitates and promotes enhancing life experiences and reducing any restrictions.

Putting people in control

One of the main complaints of people who receive services was that they have little, if any, control over what services they are to receive and how these services are to be delivered, with a prevailing attitude that the professional or public servant knows best.[42]

The guiding principle for nurses supporting individuals is to approach their care with the central aim of ensuring that the individual is in control of all that happens for them and to them. A key model to facilitate this should be the use of person-centred approaches. When assessing a person's abilities and needs, the nurse should ensure that all aspects of the individual's life are included. For example, there have been a number of publications which have identified that people with intellectual disabilities have poor life experiences in relation to the health and care they receive.[43] Also, people encounter hate crime and difficulties with getting a job, with shocking reports in 2016 of 88% of people with intellectual disabilities experiencing hate crime.[44]

There are a number of models and guiding principles in supporting nurses to ensure that they take a person-centred approach to assessing people's life experiences (see Box 4.2).

Box 4.2 Guiding principles to supporting people in their life experiences

- Be full and equal citizens.
- People should be supported to have a good and meaningful everyday life.
- People have choice and control.
- People should have a choice of where and with whom they live.
- People should get good support from all services when they need them, including the NHS, social care, criminal justice system (where needed), etc.
- Reasonable adjustments are put in place to reduce inequality.

Data sourced from *Transforming Care Building the Right Support* (2015) and including Human Rights Act (1998) and Equality Act (2010) Personalised Support (2010).S

Further reading

Equality and Human Rights Commission (2010, updated 2016). *Equality Act Guidance.* ℘ www.equalityhumanrights.com/en/advice-and-guidance/equality-act-guidance (accessed 30 October 2017).

Human Rights Act (1998). ℘ www.legislation.gov.uk/ukpga/1998/42/contents (accessed 30 October 2017).

References

40 Department of Health (2012). *Winterbourne View Hospital: Department of Health Review and Response.* Department of Health: London.
41 Inclusion Ireland (2016). *Aras Attracta?* ℘ www.inclusionireland.ie/aras-attracta (accessed 23 March 2018).
42 Poll C, Duffy S, Hatton C, Sanderson H, Routledge M (2006). *A Report on In Control's First Phase.* In Control Publications: London.
43 Heslop P, Blair P, Fleming M, Hoghton M Marriott A, Russ L (2013). *Confidential Inquiry into Premature Deaths of People with Learning Disabilities (CIPOLD).* Norah Fry Research Centre: Bristol. ℘ www.bris.ac.uk/cipold/ (accessed 30 October 2017).
44 Learning Disability Today (2016). *Government Hate Crime Action Plan Does not Go Far Enough to Protect People with Learning Disabilities.* Pavilion Publishing and Media Ltd: Brighton.

Diagnostic overshadowing

The term 'diagnostic overshadowing' is used to describe instances when a healthcare professional makes an association of presenting signs with a previously diagnosed major condition. Consequently, there is the potential for failure to recognize and treat another new condition and, as such, this increases the risk of harm to patients.[45–48] For a person with intellectual disabilities, diagnostic overshadowing is seen to occur when healthcare professionals make an assumption that the presenting signs and symptoms and/or behaviour is related only to the presence of intellectual disabilities and fails to consider other more likely physical, mental, or social causes.[45]

Factors influencing diagnostic overshadowing

People with intellectual disabilities experience greater ill health with regard to both acute and chronic illness, and their attendance at general hospitals is greater than that of the general population, although they are often discharged earlier than the general population. Although they are high users of general health services, evidence shows that healthcare professionals within general hospitals have little understanding of the nature of intellectual disability nor do they have experience working with people with intellectual disabilities.[45]

The risk of diagnostic overshadowing increases where there is a lack of knowledge and understanding of the nature of intellectual disabilities, the healthcare needs of this population, and a poor recognition that the presentation of illness may be different in this group of people. Indeed, a diagnosis of intellectual disability in itself can inadvertently lead staff to fail to notice some fundamental explanations of the new presenting signs and symptoms.

Up to 50% of people with intellectual disabilities experience problems communicating, which increases their difficulties expressing their health needs, and in addition healthcare professionals experience challenges communicating with those people effectively.[46] For people with severe or profound intellectual disabilities, their main means of communicating may be through vocalizations, facial expressions, postural movements, or other behaviours. While families and close carers often recognize intuitively signs of distress, they may experience problems explaining their intuition to health professionals and therefore have difficulty advocating for the individual.

Consequences of diagnostic overshadowing

If signs of distress or physiological signs and symptoms are unrecognized, or not validated, being attributed to the fact that the person has intellectual disabilities, then the risk of harm to the patient increases significantly. When diagnostic overshadowing occurs, unrecognized health problems remain untreated and the subsequent consequences can be very serious, even fatal.[45,46,49]

The term 'differential diagnosis' is the term used to describe the range of possible clinical diagnoses that may result from the patient's history; so if a full history is not sought and the full range of potential causes of illness is not investigated, there is a risk of wrong diagnosis, which may also have serious consequences for the individual.

Reducing the risk of diagnostic overshadowing

Patient safety in healthcare is a priority, and healthcare professionals must ensure that an individual's right to remain safe while receiving care is respected. If a person is presenting with a new behaviour, or an existing behaviour has intensified:

• See the individual first, before the intellectual disability. Ask yourself, 'What would I think caused this if the person did not have intellectual disabilities?'
• Know that all behaviour is communicative and is telling us something;
• Appreciate that the presentation of illness may be different in a person with intellectual disability;
• Seek the most effective way to 'hear' from, and to communicate with, the individual;
• Recognize the role of the family and carers, and listen to their information regarding the history of the individual.

Assess for:

• Physical problems—pain or discomfort. People with intellectual disabilities experience the same range of health problems as the general population, from toothache to oesophagitis;
• Possible psychological distress and mental health problems;
• Social causes such as a change in carers, bereavement, or abuse;
• Utilize the appropriate assessment tools in their assessment such as pain and distress assessment tools;
• Seek consent to examination, treatment, and care, using appropriate guidelines to aid decision-making;
• Recognize also that people with intellectual disabilities are at risk of over-investigation due to poor communication, which can impact on their safety. Be clear about the need for all investigations, and explain this to the person with intellectual disabilities in order to maximize their cooperation.

References

45 Michael J (2008). *Healthcare for All: Report of the Independent Inquiry into Access to Healthcare for People with Learning Disabilities*. Department of Health: London.
46 Mencap (2012). *Death by Indifference: 74 Deaths and Counting. A Progress Report 5 Years on*. Mencap: London.
47 Department of Health (2012). *Department of Health Review: Winterbourne View Hospital. Interim Report*. Department of Health: London.
48 The Westminster Commission on Autism (2016). *A Spectrum of Obstacles: An Inquiry into Access to Healthcare for Autistic People*. Westminster Commission on Autism: Huddersfield.
49 Heslop P, Blair P, Fleming M, Hoghton M, Marriott A, Russ L (2013). *Confidential Inquiry into Premature Deaths of People with Learning Disabilities (CIPOLD)*. Norah Fry Research Centre: Bristol. ℜ www.bris.ac.uk/cipold/ (accessed 30 October 2017).

Changes across the lifespan

Antenatal screening and diagnosis

Prenatal programmes aimed at the general population use ultrasound scanning and biochemical analysis as screening tools to identify pregnancies at high risk of chromosomal disorders or polygenic disorders such as neural tube defects. There have been many developments in screening for genetic disorders in pregnancy. Whether such screening programmes are deemed successful or not depends on consideration of the appropriate aims and outcomes of these programmes. If the primary aim is to reduce the birth frequency of a serious medical disorder, then some can be considered to have been a 'success', but if the aim is to provide maximum choice, information, and support to women, couples, and/or their families, then outcomes are perhaps more questionable.[1]

In any form of intellectual disabilities associated with a genetic condition or disorder, unless a specific diagnosis has been made for the cause of intellectual disabilities, no specific prenatal diagnostic testing for the condition will be available. If laboratory based genetic diagnosis in the presenting affected family member or a known carrier of the disorder has identified the causative gene change or alteration (gene mutation) for the condition, specific prenatal diagnostic tests are likely to be available to the family. If the causative gene mutation in the family has been found and identified, prenatal diagnosis by chorionic villus sampling (CVS) or amniocentesis is possible. However, both CVS and amniocentesis are invasive procedures, with an associated risk of miscarriage of 1–2%, regardless of whether the pregnancy is affected or unaffected.

In the case of X-linked intellectual disabilities where no mutation has been identified, if precise prenatal testing is not available, it may be possible to offer sex selection, by CVS or amniocentesis, and termination of ♂ offspring. However, the fact that such testing cannot distinguish between affected and unaffected ♂, and the possible risks of an affected ♀ child, should be explained carefully to individuals seeking testing for sex selection.[2] Parents should also have the opportunity, through effective genetic counselling, to explore ethical aspects that may be relevant to them in relation to sex selection and other decisions, including the continuation of pregnancy.

Further reading

Antenatal Results and Choices (ARC). ℘ www.arc-uk.org (accessed 30 October 2017).
Gen-Equip Project. ℘ www.primarycaregenetics.org/?page_id=109&lang=en (accessed 30 October 2017).
Newlife the Charity for Disabled Children (formerly Birth Defects Foundation). ℘ www.bdfnewlife.co.uk (accessed 30 October 2017).
Nuffield Council on Bioethics (2017). *Non-invasive Prenatal Testing: Ethical Issues*. ℘ nuffieldbioethics.org/wp-content/uploads/NIPT-ethical-issues-full-report.pdf (accessed 30 October 2017).

References

1 Clarke A (2018). *Harper's Practical Genetic Counselling*, 8th edn. CRC Press: London.
2 Firth HV, Hurst JA (2017). *Oxford Desk Reference: Clinical Genetics*, 2nd edn. Oxford University Press: Oxford.

Supporting people during transition

Being part of someone's circle of support as they experience transition should be viewed as a privilege. Although a dictionary definition of transition—a passage or change from one state or set of circumstances to another—could be seen as neutral, associations between transition, the imposition of change, and loss may contribute to negative perceptions of what is essentially a universal human process. Recognizing that both the passage of time and change are inevitable could reframe transition as an opportunity to be embraced. Positive synonyms to support this suggested shift include transformation, metamorphosis, adaptation, and adjustment.

Many of the rites of passage experienced in contemporary Western cultures remain atypical for people with intellectual disabilities, e.g. entering into a relationship (civil ceremony, marriage), having children, securing paid work, or living to an age, either to retire or comparable to peers without intellectual disabilities. Conversely, they also face transitions on a daily basis which may give them concern, e.g. the passage from day to night, moving on from a familiar activity, or leaving home for school. Such micro-transitions may impact disproportionately, with significant effects, and should be considered within the range and multiplicity of the spectrum of transition which is uniquely experienced.

Spectrum of transition with examples

Transitions may involve one or more of the following (descriptions are not mutually exclusive):

- Experiences universally recognized or personal to the individual:
  - Leaving school or moving from natural to harsh fluorescent light.
- Imposition, inevitability, or choice:
  - Moving home due to parental bereavement or choosing to attend residential college post-16.
- Loss or gain:
  - Successive, cumulative, or multiple loss; identity, possessions, relationships, or weight lost by someone previously identified as obese, leading to gain in energy or self-esteem.
- Change that is distressing in the short or longer term or transformational:
  - Historical decommissioning of long-stay hospitals; contemporary policy on reducing inpatient beds.[3]
- Factors internal or external to the individual, impacting directly or indirectly:
  - General healthcare or psychiatric hospital admission; changes in household composition.
- Physical, psychological, social, environmental, age, and gender issues:
  - Puberty, mental ill health, changes in support, residential campus to community, menopause in women.

Transition in relation to people with intellectual disabilities tends to focus on the journey between childhood and adulthood (see ➲ School-aged children, pp. 120–1). Imposed, rather than being a choice, this is largely steered by administrative and legislative structures of age and organization of services, rather than centring on the individual and their readiness for change. It is perhaps therefore unsurprising that this transition is often cited negatively by parents and professionals—an ordeal to be faced, rather than an achievement to be celebrated. The introduction of the prom (formal dance) by some special schools may offer some balance to those experiencing it first-hand.

Whereas the advent of mental capacity legislation in the UK and Ireland has provided important protection for those judged unable to make their own decisions, in relation to individual transitions, it has also proved difficult for some parents who now find themselves not the only ones to be consulted regarding what may be in the best interests of their adult child. Information and support should therefore be extended at transition to all involved parties, including where there are differences of opinion or safeguarding concerns.

Components of a 'transition toolkit'
- Support to understand, seek, or accept change;
- Provision of accessible information;
- Help to express views and feelings;
- Involvement in planning change;
- Personalizing services, use of person-centred resources, e.g.:
  - One-page profiles; individual responses to change, how best to help;
- Use of transitionary objects, e.g. photograph on key fob;
- Multimedia life story work;
- Encouraging advocacy, responding to and influencing policy, e.g.:
  - Easy News;
  - Parliament's Adults with Learning Disabilities (ALD) Programme.

All people, including those perceived as, and considering themselves to be, independent, exist within a milieu in which family, friends, communities, and, where required, professional supports can share in teaching and learning, skills development, and positive risk-taking at times of transition.

Further reading
Easy News. ℘ www.unitedresponse.org.uk/easy-news (accessed 30 October 2017).
One-page Profiles. ℘ onepageprofiles.wordpress.com/ (accessed 30 October 2017).
Parliament UK. *Adults with Learning Disabilities (ALD) Programme: EMPOWER.* ℘ www.parliament.uk/get-involved/education-programmes/learning-disabilities-programme/ (accessed 30 October 2017).

References
3 Brittain K (2016). *Time for Change: The Challenge Ahead.* Association of Chief Executives of Voluntary Organizations: London.

Preschool children

While focusing on the period between birth and entering full-time education typically identified in the UK as 0–5 years, it must be recognized that children in contemporary society often access regulated environments during this time, e.g. local government, private or voluntary nursery provision, and childminders. This not only means that responsibility for supporting children whose intellectual disabilities has been established is shared between family and others, but also that recognizing delays in a child's development—or illnesses and accidents that have potential to influence future development—is not confined to home. Early years, foundation phase, or stage frameworks (see Welsh Government, 2015[4] for examples and links to other searchable government websites) support the progress review of children in receipt of such services with shared action planning, should preschool developmental issues emerge. In addition, routine surveillance and response to specific parental concerns by primary health services, e.g. health visitors (see ⟳ Health visitors, pp. 366–7) and GPs should be recorded in the Personal Child Record Health.

Influencing factors with reference to intellectual disabilities

Even where intellectual disability is a feature of a condition that can be recognized at or around birth, such as Down syndrome, the future ability of an individual child cannot be known. Powerful parent-led responses to the diagnosis of Down syndrome are gaining prominence, fuelled by use of social media, e.g. the Cornwall Down's Syndrome Support Group gift *Looking Up*, a beautiful book of photographs to new parents to help them see beyond the wealth of factual information they are often given to focus on real children in the context of their families.

Hayley Goleniowska,[5] founder of Down's Side Up, advocates from her personal experience that midwives adopt particular approaches.

The Down's Syndrome Association is also providing *Tell It Right, Start It Right* training, accredited by the Royal College of Midwives. Such initiatives need to reach all families and professionals likely to benefit.

In explaining prenatal screening tests and results, a small, but significant, shift in the use of language to 'chance', rather than 'risk', has been welcomed and may be considered particularly relevant following the recently announced recommendation to phase in non-invasive prenatal testing (NIPT) in England.

Latest UK guidance on alcohol consumption in pregnancy (no level of alcohol being considered safe in relation to alcohol-related birth defects) and publication of the *Valproate Patient Guide*[6] provide a reminder of the potential for the child of any woman known to have consumed alcohol or have epilepsy or mental ill health—both conditions more likely in women with intellectual disabilities—treated with the drug valproate during pregnancy to have intellectual disabilities.

Prematurity and/or difficulties during birth may also indicate a need for a watching brief.

In many cases, however, continuing delay in a child's overall (global) or area-specific development may be a trigger for referral for more formal assessment, rather than previous history. It may also be indicated where a child's development has been straightforward then either arrests or falls back. This may follow from an accident or illness or may represent emergence of a genetic regressive or progressive condition such as Rett syndrome or Sanfilippo disease, respectively.

Examples of intellectual disabilities seen in a preschool child

These may be as a result of (not an exhaustive list):
- A genetic condition, investigated prenatally and/or recognized at/or around birth;
- Maternal consumption during pregnancy;
- Prematurity or difficult birth;
- Accident or illness, a regressive or progressive genetic condition in a child previously developing typically.

It is possible some may not be established until school age or that a physical, sensory, or more generic diagnosis may be offered, e.g. autistic spectrum (see ➲ Autistic spectrum conditions, pp. 254–5) or cerebral palsy, where intellectual disabilities may or may not be a feature.

However, regardless of the cause, a comprehensive assessment of the child's abilities and needs is key to providing individualized support to promote future development and avoid emergence of secondary issues, both for them and their family. The involvement of a range of professions and agencies may be best coordinated by a lead professional, supported by a team around the child and/or family, which may be referred to as a TAC or TAF, respectively; other acronyms for this role include SPOC (single point of contact).

It is also important to include the circle of support that currently surrounds the child, parents, and siblings—grandparents, aunts, uncles, cousins, friends, and community networks—as a basis for the future and to focus, wherever possible, on regular early childhood needs (e.g. consistency, affection, security, play, healthy sleep patterns, regular mealtimes, toilet routines), rather than the diagnosis.

Further reading

Cornwall Down's Syndrome Support Group (CDSSG). ℘ www.cdssg.org.uk/ (accessed 30 October 2017).
Government of Ireland. ℘ www.gov.ie/ (accessed 28 February 2018).
Northern Ireland Executive. ℘ www.northernireland.gov.uk/ (accessed 28 February 2018).
UK Government. ℘ www.gov.uk/ (accessed 28 February 2018).

References

4 Welsh Government (2015). *Foundation Phase Framework*. Welsh Government: Cardiff; Scottish Government (2009). *Early Years Framework*. Scottish Government: Edinburgh.
5 Goleniowska H (2012). *What to Say When a Baby is Born with Down's Syndrome*. ℘ www.downssideup.com/2012/01/what-to-say-when-baby-is-born-with.html (accessed 30 October 2017).
6 Medicines and Healthcare products Regulatory Agency (MHRA) (2016). *Valproate Patient Guide*. MHRA: London. ℘ www.medicines.org.uk/emc/RMM.421.pdf (accessed 30 October 2017).

School-aged children

Full-time education is required from the age of 5, with school-leaving in the UK and Ireland focused at around age 16, though the detail is determined by country.[7] Whereas life for any child within this age range is multifaceted, it is likely to be dominated by education, not least where intellectual disabilities is present.

Context of education for children with intellectual disabilities

Baroness Mary Warnock is widely credited with revolutionizing education for children with intellectual disability (among other groups) when she chaired the *Committee of Inquiry into the Education of Handicapped Children and Young People*, reporting eponymously in 1978. It introduced the term special educational needs (SEN), recommending a five-stage assessment process culminating in the issuing of Statements (of SEN) to identify the educational needs of individual children with more severe disabilities and ensure they received appropriate resources to make progress. It also recognized that the many children with less severe disabilities already receiving their education in mainstream settings should be identified and their SEN provided for by expanding advisory and support services.

Over time, this has been variously interpreted and, as Warnock herself observed in 2010,[8] inaccurately reported as, 'all children should be taught under the same roof or ... special schools should be abolished'. While the original intent was for only a small number of children to need special schools, Warnock later felt the system of funding additional help to children in mainstream schools came to be abused, leading some to mistakenly suggest she was reneging on ideals of integration.

Inclusion remains an aim of contemporary education for children with intellectual disabilities in England, Ireland, and the devolved administrations of the Northern Ireland Executive, Scottish Government, and Welsh Assembly. Although the detail of processes involved may vary, involvement of the child and family and the route to securing additional support can be illustrated with reference to the most recent changes in England.

The Children and Families Act 2014

Currently steering a transition to embed a new SEN assessment process, this could be seen in England as an imposition for which elements of a transition toolkit may be useful (see ➔ Supporting people during transition, pp. 116–7). From September 2014, Education Health and Care (EHC) assessments and plans are available for children and young people aged up to 25 who need more help than SEN support. As is clear from the title, EHC plans identify not only educational, but also health and care, needs and set out the additional support to meet them, recognizing the whole person, rather than a single aspect.

Children who previously received support through School Action or School Action Plus will move to SEN support. One-page Profiles have been suggested as a vehicle for supporting this. Children with existing Statements will move to an EHC plan by April 2018, normally at a planned review or when moving school.

The Local Offer

Another aspect of the reforms which every local authority must make widely available. It contains information about services, including education, health, leisure, transport, financial assistance, and help towards independence. Feedback on the Local Offer from children and their families is essential; EPIC (Equality, Participation, Influence, and Change), the Department for Education's young people's advisory group, provides an opportunity to more strategically influence the reform agenda.

EHC assessment and plans

- Parents, young persons aged 16–25, and anyone else who thinks an assessment may be necessary (including doctors, teachers, family friends) approach the local authority.
- Relevant information should accompany the request, e.g. reports from the school, doctor's assessment, parent's letter.
- The local authority confirms within 16 weeks whether an EHC plan will be made.
- If so, the local authority creates a draft EHC plan, supplies it to the child and family who have 15 days to comment, including asking for a special school; the local authority has 20 weeks from the date of assessment to issue the final EHC plan.
- The local authority can be challenged about a decision to not carry out an assessment or not create an EHC plan/the special educational support or school named in the EHC plan.
- If no resolution, you have redress to the tribunal.
- Personal budgets may be available if the child has an EHC plan.
- Independent support is available to help through the process.

Edward Timpson, then Children and Families Minister in the Conservative and Liberal Democrat Coalition government, said of the Children and Families Act 2014, *'Our reforms to special educational needs will see a system introduced which is designed around the needs of children and will support them up to the age of 25.'*

The passage of time will bear witness to its impact.

References

7 Gov.uk (2015). *School Leaving Age.* ℳ www.gov.uk/know-when-you-can-leave-school (accessed 30 October 2017).
8 Warnock M Baroness (2010). *The Cynical Betrayal of my Special Needs Children.* ℳ www.tele-graph.co.uk/education/educationnews/8009504/Baroness-Mary-Warnock-The-cynical-betrayal-of-my-special-needs-children.html (accessed 30 October 2017).

Adolescence

The transition from childhood to adulthood is the stage of life defined as adolescence. This period of development is a complex interaction which comprises biological change (see ➔ Puberty, p. 124) and psychological transition shaped by a social context.[9] For people with intellectual disabilities this transition may include developing their individuality, their independence, and forming new attachments with friends or sexual partners, as they journey towards adulthood. However, this transition is often marked with family conflict, as teenagers develop greater emotional autonomy.[10] For other teenagers with intellectual disabilities who are dependent on family and carers, this transition becomes more complex, as autonomy and sexual and occupational identity become more difficult goals to achieve.

During adolescence, the limbic system, which is responsible for emotion and the exploration of new behaviour, develops rapidly; however, the frontal lobe, which is responsible for self-regulation, does not develop as quickly. Therefore, research suggests this is why adolescents take more risks and seek greater rewards.[11] Additionally, adolescents may have unusual sleep patterns related to circadian temperature regulation and melatonin rhythms which contribute to the onset of sleep.[12] In parallel, adolescents are more likely to engage with technology, e.g. social media and mobile phones, which may influence bedtime routines. Therefore, rebelliousness and mood swings are common causes of conflict with others, as adolescents come to terms with their personal identity.

The challenges of adolescence

Identity

Throughout adolescence, young people continue to tussle with identity. The opportunity to make decisions about sexuality and relationships has been grasped by some people with intellectual disabilities, as they strive to gain control of their lives. Often the challenge faced is that their primary diagnosis dominates their sexual identity, as their carers and society inhibit sexual exploration in order to manage risk.[13] This is further compounded by going through puberty, changing school, and the possibility of losing long-established peer relationships.

The role of the Registered Nurse in Intellectual Disability (RNID) is to encourage opportunities to explore fears and anxieties with the individual, while simultaneously supporting families to comprehend and contextualize changes.

Maintaining health

During adolescence, nutritional intake is important, as a balanced diet promotes optimal health, growth, and cognitive development.[14] Research suggests that this transitional period is often associated with unhealthy dietary changes. Energy needs may vary, according to gender, age, and puberty (see ➔ Puberty, p. 124). Additionally, medication and opportunity for physical activity will also influence weight management.[15] Physical health, e.g. mobility, may be compromised due to accelerated growth spurts which are related to growth hormone released during sleep.

The RNID should encourage a healthy lifestyle by promoting exercise and a balanced diet. Additionally, the RNID should provide a holistic assessment on the impact medication (antiepileptic and antipsychotic) may have on appetite and to assess for the impact body image has on self-esteem.

Behaviour

Risk-taking is often regarded as a normal stage of adolescence, and recent research indicates that young people with intellectual disabilities actually engage more regularly in some high-risk activities such as drug use, delinquency, and acts of aggression, as adolescents become more aware of their differences.[16]

For those individuals with severe intellectual disabilities, promoting positive mental health and resilience is also important to improve the quality of their future lives.

The RNID's involvement can become complex, as they balance the continuum between empowerment and protection. Therefore, assessment of risk and promotion of positive risk-taking become important, e.g. encouraging independent travel. Additionally, the nurse may be required to support and help families to develop strategies, as the adolescent continues to dispute boundaries and family rules.

References

9 Beckett C, Taylor H (2016). *Human Growth and Development*, 3rd edn. SAGE Publications Ltd: London.

10 Story M, Stang J (2005). Nutrition needs of adolescents. In: J Stang, M Story, eds. *Guidelines for Adolescents Nutritional Services*. Centre for Leadership, Education and Training in Maternal and Child Nutrition: Minneapolis, MN; pp. 21–34.

11 Music G (2011). *Nurturing Natures: Attachment and Children's Emotional, Sociocultural and Brain Development*. Psychology Press: Hove.

12 Wiggins SA, Freeman JL (2014). Understanding sleep during adolescence. *Pediatric Nursing*. 40: 91–8.

13 Wilkinson VJ, Theodore K, Raczka R (2015). As normal as possible: sexual identity development in people with intellectual disabilities. *Sexuality and Disability*. 33: 93–105.

14 World Health Organization (2003). *Diet, Nutrition and the Prevention of Chronic Disease: Report of a Joint WHO/FAO Expert Consultation*. WHO Technical Report 916. World Health Organization: Geneva.

15 Lobstein T, Baur L, Uauy R (2004). Obesity in children and young people: a crisis in public health. *Obesity Reviews*. 5: 4–85.

16 McNamara JK, Willoughby T (2010). A longitudinal study of risk-taking behavior in adolescents with learning disabilities. *Learning Disabilities Research and Practice*. 25: 11–24.

Puberty

Definitions

Puberty is an intricate process which includes changes in the physical, psychological, and emotional health of young people as a result of alterations in hormonal activity. The word puberty was originally derived from the Latin *pubertas*, which means the age of man, and is therefore associated with sexual maturation. However, simultaneous to these rapid changes, other changes are occurring to the heart and the cardiovascular, respiratory, and muscular systems, which all impact on the well-being of the young.[17] It is therefore important for all young people with intellectual disabilities to be prepared for these changes, so they know what to expect and hence reduce anxiety.

Onset

Puberty commences when the hypothalamus begins to release gonadotropin-releasing hormone. This hormone then triggers the pituitary gland to release luteinizing hormone and follicle-stimulating hormone (FSH).[18] This process can occur in ♂ as early as 9yrs or as late as 15yrs, and in ♀ from 7yrs to 14yrs. It is commonly characterized by the onset of menstruation in ♀ and testicular enlargement in ♂. For most young people with intellectual disabilities, these changes will occur at similar ages to their peers, but for others, these changes may occur earlier (precocious puberty) or later (delayed puberty). However, the emotional changes may be delayed by several years. Precocious puberty is more prevalent in ♀, and delayed puberty is more prevalent in ♂. These may be seen in specific genetic conditions such as Turner, Klinefelter, and Noonan syndromes.[19]

Biological

During puberty, numerous physical changes occur in both ♂ and ♀.

Male

- Testicles and scrotum become enlarged.
- Pubic hair develops.
- Penis increases in length and circumference.
- Growth and weight spurt occurs.
- Spermarche occurs (first ejaculation).
- Body and facial hair develops.
- Shoulders become wider and muscles develop.
- Body odour and acne can become noticeable.
- Larynx becomes bigger and voice becomes deeper.

Female

- Breast buds develop under one or both nipples.
- Growth and weight spurt occurs.
- Body hair develops.
- Two years after breast development commences, menarche (first menstruation) is experienced.
- Body shape alters and the waist appears smaller, as body fat becomes stored on the hips, buttocks, and legs.
- Body odour and acne can become noticeable.
- Menstruation becomes regular, as ovaries mature and production of eggs regulates.

Psychological

Both ♂ and ♀ may have difficulties adapting to physical and emotional changes resulting in:
- Increased reports of aggressive behaviour and mood swings due to hormonal changes, as some adolescents begin to test boundaries,[20] while others feel unsure of how to deal with the emotional changes that are occurring.
- Self-esteem may be affected by changes to physical appearance, e.g. acne and changes to body weight.[21]

Social

Physical changes often occur at a similar chronological age. However, difficulties with social interaction may occur, as individuals with intellectual disabilities may lack the accompanying maturity and hence may feel different to their peers.[22]
- Changes to family dynamics occur, as some adolescents may strive towards independence.
- Mood regulation as a result of hormone changes may impact on the quality of the parent–child relationship.[23]
- Hormonal changes stimulate the need to seek out personal relationships.

Considerations for the RNID
- Provide advice on hygiene as skin changes occur.
- Encourage individuals to maintain a healthy body mass index (BMI), the statistical measure of the weight of a person according to height.
- Provide appropriate material and support parents in educating their children on body changes and sexual development.

References

17 Coleman J (2014). *The Nature of Adolescence*, 4th edn. Psychology Press: New York, NY.
18 Perry M (2012). Development of puberty in adolescent boys and girls. *British Journal of School Nursing*. 6: 275–7.
19 Gwee A, Rimer R, Marks M (2015). *Paediatric Handbook*, 9th edn. Wiley Blackwell: Chichester.
20 Manoharan B (2008). Adolescence and associated behavioural problems. *InnovAiT*. 1: 743–9.
21 Story M, Stang J (2005). Nutrition needs of adolescents. In: J Stang, M Story, eds. *Guidelines for Adolescents Nutritional Services*. Centre for Leadership, Education and Training in Maternal and Child Nutrition: Minneapolis, MN; pp. 21–34.
22 Rosen D (2004). Physiology growth and development during adolescence. *Paediatrics in Review*. 25: 194–20.
23 Marceau K, Dorn LD, Susman EJ (2012). Stress and puberty-related hormone reactivity, negative emotionality. *Psychoneuroendocrinology*. 37: 1286–98.

Adulthood

Society often associates adulthood with the adoption of responsibilities, commitments, and autonomy.[24] This may mean a change of circumstances, with some people adopting new responsibilities, living independently, or moving from their family home, making autonomous decisions which will influence their lives. For other people with intellectual disabilities, these aspirations may remain a challenge.

'Nothing about us without us'

This historical mantra was adopted in 2001 by the Service Users Advisory Group in its report to the English government as part of the *Valuing People* strategy for people with intellectual disabilities; People First Scotland reprised it to celebrate their 25th anniversary in 2014.[25] Learning Disability Wales 'actively supports the slogan';[26] its influence can also be seen in the '*Telling It Like It Is*' (TILII) project of the Association for Real Change (ARC) in Northern Ireland[27] and in the active involvement of a panel of people with intellectual disabilities as advisors to Senator Zappone's Private Member's Bill to reform criminal law on sexual offences in Ireland.[28] It represents the necessity to include, involve, and engage people who use services in their development, running, and evaluation, and promote control over their lives.

Examples of this in relation to adults with intellectual disabilities can be seen at several levels from the individual to the more strategic:

• Parents involved in the development and dissemination of a care planning application (App) to better support their adult son with profound and multiple disabilities, and services co-delivering his complex care;
• Primary health well-being service where Graham and Colleen volunteer to develop easy-read material and co-facilitate GP training to improve provision of annual health checks;
• Individuals who recently attended a student nursing conference for the UK and Ireland—*Positive Choices*—to promote their work with NHS England as expert advisors by experience in CTRs;[29]
• Organizations like Yorkshire-based Purple Patch Arts which recently produced a short animation *Present in My Past*, illustrating a social history of intellectual disabilities, part-narrated by Emily and Rachel who had been supported to research and better understand their heritage;
• Regulators of services, e.g. Health Inspectorate Wales, engaging volunteer lay reviewers with disabilities as part of inspection and review teams.

Potential physical health gain to individuals and carers could be seen in the App development, from better recognition of—and therefore the ability to treat—epilepsy through to lower risk of injury associated with moving and handling. Psychological and emotional health may be positively impacted by feedback from primary health staff or knowing others may be helped by your actions.

Promoting health

Evidence suggests there are issues for adults with intellectual disabilities accessing public health initiatives[27] (see ➲ Promoting public health, pp. 150–1); they often experience health inequalities associated with poorer living conditions, rather than their level of cognitive ability.[28] The RNID needs to be proactive and responsive to the public health needs of people with intellectual disabilities.

The public health agenda has made substantial gains in population health and longevity over the past century, and nurses have been advised that every interaction with an individual is seen as an opportunity to promote health and prevent illness.[30]

This has been emphasized across the UK, e.g. with prevention in England's *Five Year Forward View* and Scotland's *2020 Vision*. The focus of these strategies is to prevent, promote, and protect health by encouraging individuals to:

• Stop smoking;
• Eat healthily;
• Maintain a healthy weight;
• Drink alcohol within recommended daily limits;
• Undertake the recommended amount of physical activity;
• Improve their health and well-being.

In order for people with intellectual disabilities to achieve optimum health, it is essential that wider determinants, e.g. housing and financial support, are also considered. The World Health Organization (WHO)[31] supports an inclusive approach but notes disability-specific services will also be required. Therefore, it is the role of the RNID to support individuals to access general health services and specific services where appropriate.

References

24 Blatterer H (2007). Adulthood: the contemporary redefinition of a social category. *Sociological Research Online.* 12: 3.

25 People First Scotland (2015). *Nothing About Us Without Us.* ⅏ peoplefirstscotland.org/files/2012/10/PF-25th-anniversary-May-15.pdf (accessed 30 October 2018).

26 Learning Disability Wales (2013). *What We Do.* ⅏ www.ldw.org.uk/who-we-are/what-we-do.aspx#.Vyt-Nk32bq4 (accessed 30 October 2017).

27 ARC Northern Ireland (nd). *TILII.* ⅏ arcuk.org.uk/northernireland/influence-voice/telling-it-like-it-is/ (accessed 30 October 2017).

28 Zappone Senator K (2014). *Bill to Change Sexual Offenses in the Criminal Law: Summary in Every Day Language.* ⅏ www.inclusionireland.ie/sites/default/files/attach/basic-page/1218/summaryineverydaylanguagesexoffencesbill2014.pdf (accessed 7 March 2018).

29 NHS England. *Care and Treatment Reviews.* ⅏ www.england.nhs.uk/learningdisabilities/ctr/ (accessed 30 October 2017).

30 Wood R, Douglas M (2007). Cervical screening for women with learning disability: current practice and attitudes within primary care in Edinburgh. *British Journal of Learning Disabilities.* 35: 84–92.

31 World Health Organization (2011). *World Report on Disability.* World Health Organization: Geneva.

Personal relationships

Many people with intellectual disabilities aspire to have friends, and this is achieved largely through the development of personal relationships, which is no different to every person within society. Personal relationships are essential in improving quality of life, as it gives a sense of purpose and meaning and add a richness to one's life, irrespective of intellectual disabilities. While there has been an increased awareness that personal relationships are essential for growth and development, there is still an apprehension within society that some people with intellectual disabilities are not capable of developing a personal relationship outside of their immediate families. As a consequence, many people have fewer opportunities to socialize and/or develop personal relationships that would encourage the formation of such relationships. Certainly, the majority of people with intellectual disabilities have limited opportunities for socializing with friends outside of services, so personal relationships would be a rarity, rather than a normality.[32] However, with the development of person-centred planning, people's needs are better understood and respected more and there has been a move to provide the opportunity for people to make choices, develop personal relationships, and be involved within their local community, which, for many people, had never occurred before, because services sought to protect people from the harshness of life.

Time spent with friends and family, laughing, enjoying local amenities, and being involved within the community are the very things which make life rich for us all. A life without personal relationships can be very limiting, and these aspects of a person's life with intellectual disabilities may at times not be fully understood, or ignored. A recent study by Lafferty et al. (2013) in Northern Ireland with eight couples with intellectual disabilities found that relationships were very important in their lives but support by staff and family was required to facilitate opportunities.[33] Within the same study, the benefits of forming close personal relationships included comradeship, a sense of contentment, availability of mutual support, coping with the ups and downs of relationships, and a continuing commitment.[33]

What are the barriers to developing or maintaining relationships?

- Lack of support by families and staff to facilitate opportunities—a person may need to be brought to meet their friend, as they may not be able to travel independently;
- No opportunities outside of services to meet peers;
- Over-reliance on immediate family and extended family as friends;
- Lack of money—the costs of travelling and social functions can be prohibitive;
- Parents and/or staff—fear of being taken advantage of and/or abused (physically/emotionally/sexually/financially);
- A person's family may have problems with travelling or live too far away. This should always be taken into consideration when people move away from home or move into residential/assessment or treatment services;
- Not enough time—people working and/or have other family commitments;

- Not enough support—a person with high support needs may need extra support to be able to go out, as they need help with toileting or need more than one person to support them;
- People cannot get out or are too ill to be able to leave the home;
- People are afraid to get out or leave the home;
- Loss of older carers' independence due to ill health/frailty.

What could you do differently?

- Always seek to support and maintain friendships and relationships with family members; ensure that this is part of the person-centred plan.
- Always think about what would be in the person's best interests when a care home move is being considered.
- Support the person to maintain contact with family and friends; this might be by supporting writing letters or sending photographs, video clips, text messages, or emails.
- Recognize that every individual, irrespective of intellectual disabilities, aspires to belong, and forming personal relationships is essential to an improved quality of life.
- Listen to, and hear, the person when/if they express the need to form personal relationships.

References

32 Weafer J (2010). *Independent and Community Living: Focus Group Consultation Report.* National Disability Authority: Dublin. ℜ nda.ie/Publications/Social-Community/Independent-and-Community-Living-Focus-Group-Consultation-Report/ (accessed 30 October 2017).
33 Lafferty A, McConkey R, Taggart L (2013). Beyond friendship: the nature and meaning of close personal relationships as perceived by people with learning disabilities. *Disability and Society.* 28: 1074–88.

Marriage and family life

According to the United Nations Convention on the Rights of Persons with Disabilities (2006),[34] people with intellectual disabilities of marriageable age have the right in law to marry and decide freely and responsibly if they wish to have a family or not. A person who is at least 18yrs can legally marry without parental consent, providing the registrar or minister is satisfied that they understand what marriage means (the capacity to consent). If a person is 16–17yrs, permission needs to be sought from the person's parents/legal guardian. However, there is a clear acknowledgement that fewer people with intellectual disabilities marry and/or have families, compared to the general population.

Can anyone refuse to marry a person with an intellectual disability?

The registrar or clergy can refuse to marry someone, but only if they believe that either of the intending spouses does not have the capacity to understand the consequences of their actions.

What could the intellectual disability nurse do?

- Offer support and guidance to the person(s) regarding choices, rights, and their legal standing specific to marriage and family.
- Discuss the implications and consequences with the person(s) concerned.
- Assess the help and support the person(s) may need, including marriage counsellors and parenting groups.
- Only involve the parents with the person's consent (parents' support in any marriage is helpful; starting married life without this support would be difficult for many).
- Educate the wider community regarding the negative myths and stereotypical assumptions that people with intellectual disabilities are not capable of entering into marriage and should/could not be good parents.

Remember

- Having an intellectual disability does not mean that the person is unable to have a happy or successful marriage.
- Nor does it mean that a couple with intellectual disabilities cannot plan a family.
- Just because one or both parents have an intellectual disability, a child will not automatically be separated from his/her parents against their wishes.
- While every person believes that their marriage will last forever, there are no guarantees, and this is the same for people with intellectual disabilities.
- Marriage should be entered into only with the free and full consent of the intending spouses.[35]

There are occasions, however, when people with intellectual disabilities have been forced into marriage by harassment, trickery, assault, kidnapping, and blackmail. On occasion, family members have been the perpetrators of forced marriages, and the person with intellectual disabilities may have no one to whom to turn for support outside of the family.[36] Having an intellectual disability can cause difficulties for the person, as they may be fearful of reporting abuse and may inevitably remain in the marriage. If the marriage is abusive, they may be subjected to repeated abuse and/or even rape, inevitably affecting their mental, physical, and emotional health. As a result, they may find it difficult to remove themselves from a difficult or abusive relationship, because they may be dependent on others for the care they need. In addition, a person may be subject to unwanted sexual acts and become pregnant as part of an abusive relationship.[37]

What are the warning signs?

- The person is accompanied to appointments by people who restrict their opportunities to talk freely and in confidence to a health professional;
- Withdrawal of the person from social networks;
- Unreasonable financial control;
- Inability to attend outside activities;
- Changes in behaviour (e.g. anxiety, self-harm, mental illness, eating disorders, suicide attempts).

What to do?

Take any concerns raised seriously, and speak to your supervisor/manager as soon as is practicable; contact the child or adult protection services (depending on the age of the person).

Further reading

Beber E, Biswas A (2009). Marriage and family life in people with developmental disability. *International Journal of Culture and Mental Health.* 2: 102–8.

ℜ www.complexneeds.org.uk/ChooseModule.aspx (accessed 7 March 2018) (see Module 4.2 on safeguarding).

References

34 United Nations (2006). *United Nations Convention on the Right of Persons with Disabilities.* ℜ www. un.org/disabilities/documents/convention/convoptprot-e.pdf (accessed 30 October 2017).

35 United Nations (1948). *The Universal Declaration of Human Rights.* General Assembly. Article 16 (2).

36 Foreign and Commonwealth Office (2007). *Dealing with Cases of Forced Marriage: Practice Guidelines for Health Professionals.* Foreign and Commonwealth Office: London.

37 Rauf B, Saleem N, Clawson R, Sanghera M, Marston G (2013). Forced marriage: implications for mental health and intellectual disability services. *Advances in Psychiatric Treatment.* 19: 135–43.

Parents with intellectual disability

Contrary to what some people might think, people with intellectual disabilities can become parents and can be very good parents, given the right support. Becoming a parent is a significant life-changing event for any individual, but if a person has intellectual disabilities, there are generally negative assumptions within our society about their capacity to parent. As a consequence, it is more likely that their child will be placed on an '*at-risk register*' or taken '*into care*', and it is more likely that they will have to prove their ability to parent before they can keep their child. Therefore, there needs to be an acknowledgement that people with intellectual disabilities have the right to be parents and when they have children, they may need extra support to ensure that they can remain together as a family. Regrettably, recent studies have highlighted that between 40% and 50% of parents with intellectual disabilities do not have their children living with them, and possible reasons include low levels of literacy, difficulties with communication, poverty, poor mental health, lack of supports (both formal and informal), and social isolation. Additionally, many people are not asking for help for fear their parenting will be scrutinized. Therefore, professionals and services need to communicate better in terms of offering advice, support, and education to keep the family intact in as far as possible.

Possible barriers to successful parenting for people with intellectual disability

- Poor societal attitudes (primarily negative assumptions that people with intellectual disabilities cannot parent);
- A real lack of understanding of how to work with people with intellectual disabilities who become parents;
- Being watched at all times by different people and agencies;
- Too many people being involved;
- Conflicting advice/poor liaison between professionals and agencies;
- Inadequate/poor housing;
- May have smaller support networks;
- Poor money management skills;
- Lack of knowledge of entitlements (children's allowance, GP/medical cards);
- Less likely to have good wage-paying jobs;
- Lack of knowledge, skills, or capacity;
- Lack of opportunities to develop new knowledge and skills required;
- Having to be the perfect parent at all times;
- Lack of confidence in own parenting skills.

What can help?

- Early identification of pregnancy;
- Support during the pregnancy (e.g. attendance at antenatal classes, education around body changes during pregnancy);
- Early identification of the person's needs (e.g. wish to breastfeed, use of pain relief during labour);

- Respectful communication with the parent with intellectual disabilities and building trusting relationships with the person, their partner, and family members;
- Positive attitudes (not making assumptions about their ability to parent);
- Skills training (e.g. preparation of feeds, changing diapers, bathing, bed/sleep routines);
- Help in the home/parenting groups;
- Education on child development (i.e. what a parent should expect in terms of milestones; health surveillance);
- Agencies and staff working together;
- Involving family members in support;
- Keeping the information clear and straightforward; providing easy-to-read and accessible information to the person on all aspects of parenting. This is especially important at child protection proceedings or involvement with the courts;
- Education for staff (e.g. how to communicate effectively with people with intellectual disabilities);
- Education (reviewing attitudes and values of staff members about the rights of a person with an intellectual disability to be a parent).

Who can help?

There are a number of people from a variety of agencies that can help a person to parent (see ➲ Principles of working collaboratively with families, pp. 42–3). This includes midwives, health visitors, community nurses, psychologists, SLTs, occupational therapists, social workers and care officers, and advocacy and voluntary services. These services range from assessing a person's ability to parent to providing day-to-day hands-on support. There are also a number of very useful publications[38,39] available as well for healthcare professionals that provide guidance in terms of support.

It needs to be recognized that these services may be needed long term, supporting the mother (parents) through the pregnancy, in the early days/months, and thereafter as the child grows, and particularly during the normal childhood difficulties, i.e. 'terrible 2s', going to school, at puberty, etc.

Further reading

CHANGE. *You and Your Baby 0-1*. CD-ROM. Available from: ℵ www.changepeople.co.uk (accessed 1 March 2018).

Llewellyn G, Hindmarsh G (2015). Parents with intellectual disability in a population context. *Current Developmental Disorders Report*. 2: 119–26.

Morris J, Wates M (2006). *Supporting Disabled Parents and Parents with Additional Support Needs*. Social Care Institute for Excellence: Bristol.

Tarleton B (2015). A few steps along the road? Promoting support for parents with learning difficulties. *British Journal of Learning Disabilities*. 43: 114–20.

References

38 Spencer M (2016). Parenting with intellectual disability. What does it take to make it work? *Frontline*, 10 October 2016. ℵ frontline-ireland.com/parenting-intellectual-disability-take-make-work/ (accessed 7 March 2018).

39 Scottish Consortium for Learning Disability (2015). *Scottish Good Practice Guidelines for Supporting Parents with Learning Disabilities*. ℵ www.scld.org.uk/publications/scottish-good-practice-guidelines-for-supporting-parents-with-learning-disabilities/ (accessed 30 October 2017).

Women and menopause

Definition

Menopause can be defined as the spontaneous cessation of menstrual periods due to the permanent ending of ovarian function, usually diagnosed retrospectively after 12 months of amenorrhoea (an absence of menstruation).[40]

Perimenopause is the period immediately before the menopause. Endocrinological, biological, and clinical features of approaching menopause become evident and continue for at least the first year after menopause.

Onset

Menopause onset usually occurs when women are aged late 40s to early 50s. Research suggests that menopause occurs earlier in women with intellectual disabilities than in the general population, and up to 2yrs earlier in women with epilepsy and earlier still in women with Down syndrome.[41] Diagnosis is usually made by a GP on presentation of symptoms. A blood test to measure FSH levels can be undertaken, but as hormone levels fluctuate daily, this is not a reliable indicator. However, good practice suggests that screening for type 2 diabetes, depression, and thyroid disorders are essential to preclude a differential diagnosis.

Symptoms

Women with intellectual disabilities may not understand the concept of menopause.[42] Therefore, education to empower women to recognize symptoms is vital. Symptoms are generally associated with the decline in oestrogen levels and can include the following.

Biological

- Vasomotor symptoms (hot flushes and night sweats);
- Urogenital symptoms (vaginal dryness);
- Dry skin;
- Stress incontinence;
- Osteoporosis, particularly in women who have low bone mineral density related to age, use of antiepileptics, immobility, and diagnosis of Down syndrome.

Psychological

- Weight gain, increase of facial hair, and thinning of hair can impact on women's self-esteem;
- Depression;
- Irritability;
- Poor memory.

Social

- Lethargy and sleep disturbance can impact on social life and decision-making processes.

Treatments

Hormone replacement therapy (HRT) can offer symptom relief and improved quality of life for perimenopausal women.[43] HRT usually comprises two hormones: oestrogen and progestogen. Women who have had a hysterectomy can safely take oestrogen on its own. However, oral HRT cannot be recommended for women with epilepsy, as studies have shown that HRT reduces the effects of antiepileptic medication, particularly lamotrigine.[44]

Additional considerations

- Women who experience premature menopause have a significantly increased risk of cardiovascular disease.
- Women prescribed antipsychotics may need medication adjusting, as changes occur in the absorption and metabolism of drugs at menopause. Medications such as clozapine induce excessive sweating and therefore may exacerbate symptoms.[45]

The role of the registered nurse for people with intellectual disabilities

- Enable women to live healthily; promote and encourage annual health checks.
- Prepare women for potential menopausal changes, using images and other visual aids.
- Encourage women to live active and meaningful lives to promote their self-esteem.
- Act as a resource to other health professionals to ensure symptoms of menopause are not misrepresented or misdiagnosed in women with intellectual disabilities.

References

40 Melville C (2015). *Sexual and Reproductive Health at a Glance*. Wiley Blackwell: Chichester.
41 Schupf N (2003). Onset of dementia is associated with age at menopause in women with Down's syndrome. *Annals of Neurology*. 54: 433–8.
42 Willis D, Wishart JG, Muir WJ (2011). Menopausal experience of women with intellectual disability. *Journal of Applied Research in Intellectual Disabilities*. 24: 74–85.
43 Bostock-Cox B (2015). Focus on women's health: the menopause. *Practice Nurse*. 45: 10–14.
44 Sveinsson O, Tomson T (2014). Epilepsy and menopause: potential implications for pharmacotherapy drugs. *Aging*. 21: 671–5.
45 Seeman MV (2012). Treating schizophrenia at the time of menopause. *Maturitas*. 72: 117–20.

Older people with intellectual disabilities

There have been marked changes in the life expectancy of people with intellectual disabilities, but their life expectancy still remains less than that of the general population. Data from the Republic of Ireland show a steady increase in the number of people with intellectual disabilities >35yrs.[46] In 1974, 28.5% of registered persons were >35yrs, and in 1996 38%, with a projected increase by 2014 of 48.7% (41.2% actual prevalence). However, there are questions as to whether this is about more people living to a more advanced age, rather than the length of lives continuing to increase.[47]

Health status of older people with intellectual disabilities

Individuals with intellectual disabilities are reported to have 2.5 times the health problems of other persons.[48] Common concerns include: hypertension, obesity, respiratory disease, cancer, gastrointestinal disorders, diabetes, chronic urinary tract infections (UTIs), oral diseases, musculoskeletal conditions, osteoporosis, thyroid disease, hypothermia, pneumonia, vision impairment, and hearing impairment. Poor nutrition and polypharmacy, social disadvantage, syndrome-specific disorders, and improved survival rates for those with profound and severe disabilities increase such risks.[49]

Psychological health

In a review of available studies, Parry reported that depending on the instruments and definitions of old age used, 20–40% of older persons with intellectual disabilities have a mental health problem.[50] Social, cultural, environmental, and developmental factors, gender issues, and polypharmacy are all of concern and, in old age, may contribute to sedation, increased confusion, constipation, postural instability, falls, incontinence, weight gain, endocrinological or metabolic effects, impairments of epilepsy management, and movement disorders.[51]

The health service needs of older people with intellectual disabilities

People with intellectual disabilities are more likely to lead unhealthy lifestyles; their health problems are often not recognized and they have less access to health promotion and health screening services, compared to non-disabled peers. There are additional access barriers because many people with intellectual disabilities are reliant on health management by proxy. People often experience discrimination, inequality, and barriers (e.g. attitudinal and physical) when using healthcare. For people with intellectual disabilities who are terminally ill, concerns have been raised about a lack of specialist knowledge and training among frontline nurses, as well as a lack of experience among specialist palliative care staff who work with this population (see End of life, pp. 218–9).[52]

Living situations

Better health has been reported for those in community settings, compared to those living in nursing homes, and quality of life increases when people move from homes with institutional features to community settings. Living with the family may also have the benefit of a community-based lifestyle, natural social networks, continuity, and consistency in care, familiarity of environment, greater acceptance by family members, and greater respect for the needs of the older person and the contribution of the person with intellectual disabilities to activities of daily living.[53–56] More work is needed to better understand if these findings hold true for all.

References

46 Kelly C (2015). *Annual Report of the National Intellectual Disability Database Committee 2014*. Health Research Board: Dublin.

47 McCarron M, Carroll R, Kelly C, McCallion P (2015). Mortality rates in the General Irish population compared to those with an intellectual disability from 2003–2012. *Journal of Applied Research in Intellectual Disabilities*. **28**: 406–13.

48 van Schrojenstein Lantman-De Valk HM, Metsemakers JF, Haveman MJ, Crebolder HF. Health problems in people with intellectual disability in general practice: a comparative study. *Family Practice*. **17**: 405–7.

49 Burke E, McCarron M, McCallion P, eds. (2014). *Advancing Years, Different Challenges: Wave 2 IDS-TILDA. Findings on the Ageing of People with an Intellectual Disability*. School of Nursing and Midwifery, University of Dublin: Dublin.

50 Parry JR, ed. (2002). *Overview of Mental Health Problems in Elderly Persons with Developmental Disabilities*. NADD Press: Kingston, NY.

51 McCarron M, Swinburne J, Burke E, McGlinchey E, Carroll R, McCallion P (2013). Patterns of multimorbidity in an older population of persons with an intellectual disability: results from the Intellectual Disability Supplement to the Irish Longitudinal Study on Ageing (IDS-TILDA). *Research in Developmental Disabilities*. **34**: 521–7.

52 McCarron M, McCallion P, Fahey-McCarthy E, Connaire K (2010). The role and timing of palliative care in supporting persons with intellectual disability and advanced dementia. *Journal of Applied Research in Intellectual Disabilities*. **24**: 189–98.

53 Hamelin JP, Frijters J, Griffiths D, Condillac R, Owen F (2011). Meta-analysis of deinstitutionalisation adaptive behaviour outcomes: research and clinical implications. *Journal of Intellectual and Developmental Disability*. **36**: 61–72.

54 Chowdhury M, Benson BA (2011). Deinstitutionalization and quality of life of individuals with intellectual disability: a review of the international literature. *Journal of Policy and Practice in Intellectual Disabilities*. **8**: 256–65.

55 Amado AN, Stancliffe RJ, McCarron M, McCallion P (2013). Social inclusion and community participation of individuals with intellectual/developmental disabilities. *Intellectual and Developmental Disabilities*. **51**: 360–75.

56 McCausland D, McCallion P, Cleary E, McCarron M (2016). Social connections for older people with intellectual disabilities in Ireland. Results from Wave One of IDS-TILDA. *Journal of Applied Research in Intellectual Disabilities*. **29**: 71–82.

Older people with Down syndrome

Life expectancy for people with Down syndrome has improved dramatically from reports of death at 9yrs and 12yrs through the 1940s, to 30yrs by the early 1970s, to late 50s by the 1990s, and anecdotal reports today of some people living to their 9th decade.[57]

Longevity appears influenced by the active treatment of two issues in people with Down syndrome: upper respiratory tract infection and heart anomalies.[57] There is some suggestion that perimenopausal women with Down syndrome are particularly prone to heart problems, given pre-existing heart anomalies. Nurses must be observant for the complications associated with these heart and respiratory conditions and make prompt referrals to appropriate primary or secondary healthcare services.

It is also likely that living in the community, greater quality of life, and opportunities for self-determination have made important contributions to longevity. People with Down syndrome will therefore be more likely to maintain good health and quality of life if nurses work to support both continued living in the community and the opportunity for such lives for those currently in more restrictive settings.

A popular myth that adults with Down syndrome will not exercise is not true. Systematic programmes offering exercise and health education improve attitudes to exercise and offer better exercise outcomes, improved life satisfaction, and lower depression. Attention to exercise by nurses therefore offers an opportunity for people with Down syndrome to be active partners in the pursuit of their own good health.

Old age will not always be without health complications. Comorbid health conditions are of particular concern in older adults with Down syndrome. Many of these health issues, even those associated with ageing in the general population, appear to begin in earlier years. There are also high levels of obesity, low levels of exercise, and poor nutritional intake.[58] By 50yrs:

• 40% of people with Down syndrome have developed a thyroid disorder;
• There are sensory losses in 40–80%;
• 28% have hip disease;
• 50% have adult-onset epilepsy;
• Diabetes, osteoporosis, and depression are more prevalent;
• Dementia occurs at higher rates than in the general population.[58]

Dementia is reported to be present in 15–45% of people with Down syndrome over 40yrs old,[59] increasing with age, and there is also evidence that people with Down syndrome experience an early and more abrupt decline in memory, behaviour, and day-to-day functioning and work skills. There is also a danger that all health concerns and symptoms in people with Down syndrome will be misattributed to dementia. This can prevent people with Down syndrome from having these symptoms being appropriately treated when they have not been appropriately attributed to other treatable conditions. This approach also fails to recognize that people with Down syndrome and dementia are also prone to other conditions. Among people with Down syndrome and dementia, epilepsy is reported to be as high as 80%, and compared with those without dementia, there are:

• Higher levels of depression;
• Higher levels of arthritis, gastric problems, and immobility;
• Higher levels of balance problems, falls, gastrointestinal disorders, night-time incontinence, diarrhoea, malnutrition, and musculoskeletal disorders.[60]

Failure to recognize that other conditions are present means that those conditions will be not be treated effectively, decreasing the quality of life for older people with Down syndrome and increasing the likelihood of premature death. Therefore, screening for dementia among people with Down syndrome and other people with intellectual disabilities is important and more likely to be accurate when using assessments specifically designed for use with these populations, rather than generic screening tools.[61]

Important roles for nurses in intellectual disability services are:

• Monitoring for likely health concerns;
• Screening for dementia symptoms;
• Advocating for community maintenance and self-determination;
• Ensuring appropriate treatment of health concerns;
• Supporting care if dementia is present and progresses.

Above all, the risk that health concerns and dementia may lead to long-term residential care must be recognized, and nurses must work with interdisciplinary team members to address treatable health concerns and to modify expectations programmes and living situations to ensure successful ageing in their community residence for as long as possible.

References

57 Bittles AH, Glasson EJ (2004). Clinical, social and ethical implications of changing life expectancy in Down syndrome. *Developmental Medicine and Childhood Neurology*. **46**: 282–6.
58 Burke E, McCarron M, McCallion P, eds. (2014). *Advancing Years, Different Challenges: Wave 2 IDS-TILDA. Findings on the Ageing of People with an Intellectual Disability*. School of Nursing & Midwifery, University of Dublin: Dublin.
59 Prasher VP, Krishnan VHR (1993). Age of onset and duration of dementia in people with Down's syndrome. *International Journal of Geriatric Psychiatry*. **8**: 923–7.
60 McCarron M, McCallion P, Reilly E, Mulryan N (2014). A prospective 14-year longitudinal follow-up of dementia in persons with Down syndrome. *Journal of Intellectual Disability Research*. **58**: 61–70.
61 Jokinen N, Janicki MP, Keller S, McCallion P, Force LT (2013). Guidelines for structuring community care and supports for people with intellectual disabilities affected by dementia. *Journal of Policy and Practice in Intellectual Disabilities*. **10**: 1–24.

End-of-life care, preferred place of care

Planning for the future

On approaching the end of life, it is important to consider preferences regarding where people wish to be cared for. Most people would prefer to die at home, but many do not and are admitted to hospital in the last few days or hours of life.[62] Reasons for this in the general population are complex but are compounded in marginalized groups (such as people with intellectual disability) who may lack the ability to fully understand, make informed personal choices, or articulate their own needs and wants at this difficult time.

End of Life Care Programme

Patients who are dying should have access to palliative care and opportunities for a good death in the place of their choosing. The Department of Health *End of Life Care Programme* recognizes the importance of patient involvement in aiming to reduce the number of unnecessary admissions to hospital. It supports nationally recognized tools for end-of-life care, including the five key priorities of care,[63] which remain important if death is likely to be imminent. The five key priorities include:

- A recognition and communication that death is imminent, with decisions made in accordance with the person's needs and wishes;
- The use of sensitive communication to the patient and family;
- Active involvement of the patient and those important to them in any decision-making process, as directed by the patient themselves;
- The needs of families and others important to the patient are explored, respected, and met wherever possible;
- An individual care plan is agreed, coordinated, and delivered, including the support of eating, drinking, symptom assessment, and management, psychological, social, and spiritual support.

Such key priorities should be '*relevant and accessible to everyone*' and are supported by the National Institute for Health and Care Excellence (NICE) (2015) guidance.[64]

Advance care planning (ACP)

The ACP is a tool to record patient preferences and priorities in relation to care and place of death. Belonging to the patient, the ACP recognizes that views are likely to change. The ACP is a generic tool and does not easily translate across to those who may have communication impairments such as people with intellectual disabilities. The ability of care staff involved to facilitate the ACP process and the person's ability to communicate clearly need to be assessed. Patients should be supported to make informed (often difficult) choices about sensitive issues. Communication at this level should be facilitated in the most appropriate manner suitable for each person and their circumstances. Those closest to the person can be supported by palliative care professionals to sensitively record the needs of the individual at this time in the ACP or other appropriate document.

Issues for people with intellectual disabilities

Marginalized groups, such as people with intellectual disabilities, have an increased risk of disenfranchised death, resulting from a lack of autonomy and choice and social exclusion, particularly at the end of life.[65] Challenges to reciprocal communication, processing complex information, and limited writing skills can make end-of-life choices around patient preferences difficult both for the staff and the patient. A multidisciplinary team using a person-centred approach[66] and supporting the carers will facilitate the expression of options for that individual. In domiciliary settings, the team usually consists of community nurses, specialist nurses, matrons, and the patient's GP. People with intellectual disabilities may have already expressed their options to those closest to them or have been engaged in processes where they have reflected on their own losses and formed an opinion about their future care.

Person-centred approaches

Discussions with people with intellectual disabilities should not be left until death is imminent, but held as early as possible following a diagnosis or prognosis. Person-centred approaches to care planning promote inclusion, civil rights, and independence for people with intellectual disabilities (see Fig 5.1). Person-centred planning and palliative care share similar philosophies: adopting a holistic approach, placing the person at the centre of the palliative care process, and incorporating active listening throughout. Health action plans and essential lifestyle plans are well suited to providing holistic palliative or end-of-life care.[67]

Compassionately supporting people with intellectual disabilities to make choices at the end of life may not be easy. Shared values across different professional groups will promote collaborative working to support and help individuals to die in places of their own choosing. Further research around this topic should inform a sound evidence base for future development and support.

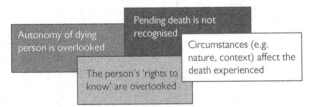

Pending death is not recognised

Autonomy of dying person is overlooked

Circumstances (e.g. nature, context) affect the death experienced

The person's 'rights to know' are overlooked

Fig. 5.1 Features of disenfranchised death.

Further reading

European Association for Palliative Care (EAPC) Taskforce on People with Intellectual Disabilities. *Consensus Norms for Palliative Care of People with Intellectual Disabilities in Europe.* ℰ www.eapcnet. eu/LinkClick.aspx?fileticket=lym7SMB78cw%3D (accessed 7 March 2018).

picTTalk. Communication tool to support and facilitate conversations about ill health, loss, and bereavement. Free to download from: ℰ itunes.apple.com/gb/app/picttalk-communicating-people/id951053318?mt=8 (accessed 30 October 2017).

References

62 Higginson IJ (2003). *Priorities and Preferences for End of Life Care in England, Wales and Scotland.* National Council for Palliative Care: London.

63 Leadership Alliance for the Care of Dying People (2014). *One Chance to Get it Right.*

64 National Institute for Health and Care Excellence (2015). *Care of Dying Adults in the Last Days of Life.* ℰ www.nice.org.uk/guidance/ng31 (accessed 30 October 2017).

65 Read S (2006). Communication in the dying process. In: S Read, ed. *Palliative Care for People with Learning Disabilities.* Quay Books: London; pp. 93–106.

66 Department of Health (2001). *Valuing People: A New Strategy for Learning Disability for the 21st Century.* Department of Health: London.

67 Read S, Elliott D (2006). Care planning in palliative care for people with intellectual disabilities. In: B Gates, ed. *Care Planning and Delivery in Intellectual Disability.* Blackwell Publishing: Oxford

Physical health and well-being

Introduction

Physical ill health and challenges to well-being are common in people with intellectual disabilities. Consequently, it is important that they have early access to assessment, treatment, and interventions, thereby maintaining physical health and well-being, reducing complications, and leading to an improved quality of life.

As a population, children, adults, and older people with severe intellectual disabilities all have higher health needs, compared with those of the general population. They also have a different pattern of physical health needs and high comorbidity, and many of their health needs go unrecognized and remain untreated. However, in the absence of a specific syndrome, the health profile of people with mild intellectual disabilities is likely similar to that of the general population once socio-economic factors are taken into account, although they may experience more difficulty in accessing health promotion and primary and secondary care services. Such difficulties may contribute to increased health problems for some individuals.

As a result of a range of factors, which include unmet health needs, many die unnecessarily at a premature age. This chapter provides comprehensive coverage of the very many factors that can compromise the health and well-being of people with intellectual disabilities, along with a range of strategies that registered nurse for people with intellectual disabilities can adopt to provide effective support.

Further reading

Heslop P, Blair P, Fleming M, Hoghton M, Marriott A, Russ L (2013). *Confidential Inquiry into Premature Deaths of People with Learning Disabilities (CIPOLD)*. Norah Fry Research Centre: Bristol. ℐ www.bris.ac.uk/cipold/ (accessed 30 October 2017).

Norah Fry Research Centre (2018). The Learning Disabilities Mortality Review (LeDeR) Programme Annual report December 2017. NHS England/University of Bristol. ℐ www.hqip.org.uk/resource/the-learning-disabilities-mortality-review-annual-report-2017/#.WvMuni-ZNE6 (accessed 9 May 2018).

Health inequalities

Definition

Health inequalities may be described as the gap in access to care, or in the health status, between individuals and discrete populations. These populations may include people from different ethnic communities and social groups, as well as people with intellectual disabilities or people living in defined geographical localities. Many people with intellectual disabilities are known to experience persistent and multiple factors that can result in health inequalities and social exclusion.

The Improving Health and Lives Learning Disabilities Public Health Observatory (IHaL) identified four broad determinants of health inequalities for people with intellectual disabilities:[1]

- 'Social determinants of poorer health such as poverty, poor housing, unemployment, and social disconnectedness;
- Physical and mental health problems associated with specific genetic and biological conditions;
- Communication difficulties and reduced health literacy;
- Personal health behaviour and lifestyle risks such as diet, sexual health, and exercise.'[1]

Tackling health inequalities

Reducing health inequalities for people with intellectual disabilities is considered a priority for all countries within the UK. Following the four UK learning disability policies, more recent documents have focused on the evidence base describing the inequalities faced[2,3] and recommendations for action.[4] The Learning Disability[5] Mortality Review (LeDeR) Annual Report 2017 reported that men died 22.8 years earlier and women died 29.3 years earlier compared to the general population. Forty-two per cent of deaths were assessed as being premature, many early deaths linked to inequalities of access to high-quality healthcare. While national public health agencies collate evidence and produce strategic guidance on tackling health inequalities, the focus of delivery is often directed at a local level. Within England, Health and Wellbeing Boards have a key role in tackling health inequalities.

What are Health and Wellbeing Boards (HWBs)?

HWBs were established under the Health and Social Care Act 2012 to act as a forum for leaders from local health and social care agencies to work together to address health inequalities and to improve the health and well-being of their local population. They are a formal committee of local authorities and charged with promoting greater integration and partnership working between the NHS, public health, local government, and voluntary groups. They have a statutory duty, with clinical commissioning groups (CCGs), to produce and publish joint strategic needs assessments (JSNAs), outlining evidence of needs of the local population, and a joint health and well-being strategy.

Tackling health inequalities in people with intellectual disabilities

Everyone working with people with intellectual disabilities, whether in general or specialist health, social care, leisure, or housing, has a role to play in reducing health inequalities in this population. The HEF[6] presents an outcomes framework, based on the determinants of health inequalities, which enables any service to measure the effectiveness of their role in addressing health inequalities.

The following three principles underpin how health inequalities may be tackled in practice.

Inclusive and accessible national policies and local services

Intellectual disabilities flagging within cancer screening and general health programmes. Making accessible information available on all chronic health conditions, health treatment, housing tenancies, and employment contracts. Confronting staff attitudes by using people with intellectual disabilities to train staff. Making reasonable adjustments to accommodate wider service delivery and job recruitment processes.

Preventing inequalities by addressing underlying causes of ill health

Supporting the introduction and delivery of high-quality annual health checks and health action plans to all people with intellectual disabilities. Providing individual/group education on health conditions to improve personal knowledge, locus of control, and health ownership. Building evidence on national and local health needs assessment and best practice outcomes.

Finding new ways of meeting needs, particularly in areas that are resistant to change, and targeting interventions at these

Working with commissioners to develop acute liaison or prison nurse posts. Collecting and publishing evidence on the health needs and numbers and causes of death of people at a local level. Working with the police in training them to understand the needs of people with intellectual disabilities, in relation to bullying and the management of local hate crime.

References

1 Emerson E, Baines S, Allerton L, Welch V (2011). *Health Inequalities and People with Learning Disabilities in the UK*. Public Health England: London.
2 Black LA (2013). *Health Inequalities of People with a Learning Disability*. Northern Ireland Assembly: Belfast.
3 Emerson E (2015). *The Determinants of Health Inequities Experienced by Children with Learning Disabilities*. Public Health England: London.
4 The Scottish Government (2013). *The Keys to Life*. ℡ www.gov.scot/resource/0042/00424389. pdf (accessed 30 October 2017).
5 Norah Fry Research Centre (2018). The Learning Disabilities Mortality Review (LeDeR) Programme Annual report December 2017. NHS England/University of Bristol. ℡ www.hqip. org.uk/resource/the-learning-disabilities-mortality-review-annual-report-2017/#.WvMuni-ZNE6 (accessed 9 May 2018).
6 Atkinson D, Boulter P, Hebron C, Moulster G (2013). *The Health Equalities Framework (HEF) UK Learning Disabilities Consultant Network*. ℡ www.ndti.org.uk/uploads/files/The_Health_Equality_Framework.pdf (accessed 30 October 2017).

Principles of health promotion

Health promotion comprises a broad span of activities that work towards achieving the positive health and well-being of individuals, groups, and communities. The focus of health promotion work includes health education, lifestyle, and preventative approaches, alongside environmental, legal, and fiscal measures.

Key health promotion principles for healthy settings

- Equity;
- Participation;
- Partnership;
- Empowerment;
- Sustainability.[7]

What health promotion barriers do people with intellectual disabilities experience?

- Lack of informed choices due to limited staff communication skills and poor use of resources to deliver accessible information;
- Inequality in access to high-quality health promotion;
- A limited range of published quality evidence on health needs;
- A lack of defined policy on health for the population;
- Reduced access to health screening and health education;
- Low priority given to the health of the population;
- Reduced health ownership and control, with less opportunity for decision-making and informed choice.

Everyone who works with people with intellectual disabilities has a role to play in tackling health inequalities through health promotion activities. Health promotion comprises complex and wide-ranging activities, which at times may require innovative thinking. It facilitates opportunities to focus on developing choice, promoting independence and rights, and enabling inclusion. Health promotion activities may take place with individuals or collectively within small or large groups. It may be necessary, in order to meet the needs of people with intellectual disabilities to the same level as those of the general population, to adopt different kinds of solutions. Reasonable adjustments may need to be made to ensure equality of access.

The following list identifies five key principles of health promotion that may be used in work relating to people with intellectual disabilities.

Equity

- Promote the need for, and supporting, GPs and their staff in developing and introducing good-quality annual health checks.
- Highlight and work with all sector employers in raising the need for job carving and developing an accessible application process to help people with intellectual disabilities to apply for, and get, jobs.
- Keep up-to-date with new developments at a local level. Work with staff in education, housing, health, and leisure services to help make all services accessible to people with intellectual disabilities.

- Ensure that people with intellectual disabilities have equal access to national health programmes, such as flu vaccines or cancer screening, with necessary reasonable adjustments.
- Ensure equal access to activities promoting positive physical and mental well-being, including healthy walking groups or use and supported application of tools such as the 5 Ways to Wellbeing.

Participation

- Inform and educate people with intellectual disabilities on the role of Health Watch and other local health advocacy groups.
- Support membership, attendance at meetings, and service quality checking.
- Employ people with intellectual disabilities as co-trainers in the delivery of training to health, local authority, and public health training programmes.
- Involve people with intellectual disabilities in recruitment.
- Ensure meetings and any minutes are accessible.

Partnership

- Work in partnership with councillors and members of neighbourhood partnerships, developing inclusive local services and policies.
- Work across service boundaries to ensure the needs of people with intellectual disabilities are incorporated into local services, e.g. older people's services, sexual health, drug, alcohol, mental health.
- Work with health visitors and midwives in the delivery of training to staff on the needs of parents with intellectual disabilities.

Empowerment

- Promote and use person-centred approaches to care.
- Organize and deliver health education-related activities, either individually or in groups.
- Consult with user-led groups, e.g. transgender or black and minority ethnic groups, on their needs in local service development.
- Involve people with intellectual disabilities in the service commissioning strategy.
- Work jointly in evidence gathering/co-chairing strategic groups.

Sustainability

- Develop and use accessible health education resources to help people understand and take greater control of their health.
- Undertake inclusive research activities (see ➜ Involving people with intellectual disabilities in the research process, pp. 538–9).
- Support self-advocacy groups run health-related activities.
- Be innovative in the collection of evidence to promote the need for new service developments.
- Ensure feedback from people with intellectual disabilities is included in any disability equality schemes or the Equality Delivery System (EDS).

References

7 World Health Organization. *Healthy Settings*. ℛ www.who.int/healthy_settings/en/ (accessed 31 October 2017).

Promoting public health

Definition

The Faculty of Public Health (℘ www.fph.org.uk) describes public health as, '*The science and art of preventing disease, prolonging life and promoting health through the organized efforts of society*'. Public health is about helping people to stay healthy and protecting them from threats to their health.

Overview

The role of public health is strongly driven towards reducing health inequalities. Public health may be considered from four different approaches. These are:

- A multidisciplinary profession, whose wide range of skills are focused on, predominantly, proactive work, directed towards improving the health of the population;
- A set of diverse skills, including specific skills in working with populations, as well as collecting, interpreting, and using evidence to direct and develop programmes of service delivery, to meet identified needs;
- A range of desired outcomes originating from both individuals and populations, relating to the aim of achieving lasting improvements across mainstream health service delivery;
- Factors that contribute to health and illness, focused on tackling the root causes of ill health. These include addressing personal lifestyle issues such as diet, exercise, and smoking, as well as wider determinants, which may include housing or the quality of healthcare.

Public health delivery

Within England, in April 2013, the responsibility for planning and delivery of public health at a local level moved from the NHS into local authorities. National guidance and oversight is provided by Public Health England. The public health team plays a key role in influencing local authority staff and other key partners in identifying key priorities for local action and supporting in practice initiatives that meet priority needs. Local evidence is collated and published in a JSNA. National priorities for action are identified and measured by a Public Health Outcomes framework (PHOF).

What is the Public Health Outcomes framework?

The PHOF is a data tool comprising of a number of key indicators that is developed and collated by Public Health England. It has a close relationship with both the NHS and social care outcomes frameworks. All are reviewed 3-yearly, the latest refresh being in May 2016.

The PHOF has two key outcomes that include increased life expectancy and reduced differences in life expectancy between communities. Each of these outcomes contains indicators collected within four domains, including:

- Improving the wider determinants of health, e.g. employment for adults with intellectual disabilities;
- Health improvement, e.g. excess weight in adults;
- Health protection, e.g. treatment completion for tuberculosis;
- Preventing premature mortality, e.g. suicide rates.

Public health in practice

People working in public health consider their role and application in three domains:
- Health protection and prevention;
- Improving health and social care;
- Health improvement.

Public health departments should not be considered the only agency responsible for health inequalities of people with intellectual disabilities. Making Every Contact Count is operated by local authorities and health services to promote the importance of recognizing everyone's role in promoting healthy lifestyles, to support behaviour change, and to contribute to reducing risk of chronic disease.

Health protection and prevention
- Facilitating accessible sex education to children and adults;
- Educating services and supporting people to access *Chlamydia* testing and breast, bowel, and cervical screening;
- Providing education on home/community safety;
- Promoting and supporting annual health checks;
- Working with the police in education on, and prevention of, bullying, harassment, and hate crime.

Improving health and social care
- Developing and auditing quality standards in primary/acute hospitals or in day/residential services;
- Conducting local needs assessments to inform JSNAs and local service delivery;
- Facilitating groups to enable people to understand local service provision and contribute to local consultation;
- Undertaking research, reporting, and publishing findings.

Health improvement
- Ensuring availability of accessible health resources;
- Developing accessible health, housing, employment projects;
- Influencing/working with public health specialists to ensure intellectual disabilities are included in local strategies.

Further reading

Walker C, Beck CR, Eccles R, Weston C (2016). Health inequalities and access to health care for adults with learning disabilities in Lincolnshire. *British Journal of Learning Disabilities*. **44**: 16–23.

Promoting physical well-being of individuals

Good health is the foundation on which a good quality of life can be built. Good physical well-being, that includes a sense of health ownership and a personal locus of control, is strongly linked with positive mental well-being. People with intellectual disabilities experience many barriers in the achievement of optimum physical health. Multiple sources of evidence from the UK, and wider, have found that people with intellectual disabilities die prematurely and experience worse physical health, due to many different factors. In addition, they receive inequitable treatment from health services, with both primary care and secondary hospital system failures. It is also widely acknowledged that insufficient staff training or service priority is given in addressing the specific health needs of this population.

What do we know about the health of people with intellectual disabilities?

- They have an increased risk of early death and have a different picture of health needs, compared to the general population.
- Some syndromes (e.g. Down syndrome, Prader–Willi syndrome) are accompanied by an increased range of specific health conditions.
- They have significant levels of unmet physical and mental health needs and higher rates of specific long-term health conditions, e.g. epilepsy.
- They have higher rates of vision and hearing impairments and are less likely to have received regular physical health, dental, vision, and hearing checks.
- Women with intellectual disabilities are much less likely to access breast, bowel, or cervical screening.
- They are more likely to experience mental ill health.
- They are less likely to have access to health education or to live healthy lives, and they have reduced ownership and control of their personal health needs.

People with intellectual disabilities need to access a health service designed around their individual assessed needs. They require equitable high-quality accessible care, delivered locally and with access to flexible support, as required.

Practical steps to consider when promoting physical well-being

Individual

- Make reasonable adjustments in the delivery of care. This may mean that to offer equal services, they may need to be different.
- Make every contact count. Be proactive in promoting healthy lifestyles in all working roles and care environments.

- Ensure information is delivered in an accessible format to facilitate each individual making informed decisions on health treatments, health screening, and lifestyle choices.
- Enable each individual to select someone they know and trust to be their health facilitator (HF), to support them in thinking about their health and building knowledge, health ownership, and responsibility.
- If not initiated by the local GP practice, the HF should support each individual to arrange and attend an annual health check. This should help each person to identify individual health needs and consider how these will impact on their wider lifestyle aspirations and future plans.
- Work with the individual; record the needs identified by the health check. Consider how these needs will be met, by whom, and in what timescale. Support the person to put these into a plan, where possible, in a style and format accessible to the individual. This may be known as a health action plan (HAP) that should link directly with a wider lifestyle or person-centred plan.
- Plan and prepare for any health or hospital visits, where possible, in advance. Write any special requirements down in a patient passport, to share and leave with medical staff.

Organizational
- Raise the health profile of people with intellectual disabilities across commissioning, health, social, and voluntary agencies at local levels. Offer support and initiate partnership working with local primary care teams, acute hospitals, and dental and other health agencies.
- Ensure any plans to develop a new local health strategy involves multi-agency input and includes an equality impact assessment.
- Employ people to deliver intellectual disabilities awareness training across the organization. Ensure resources are in place to train staff, and to implement and audit the use of the Mental Capacity Act (MCA).
- Develop a resource base that contains a wide range of accessible resources on physical health conditions, health screening, and medical procedures. Make these resources, or the links to them, easily available to all. Also build a local resource of examples of HAPs, to support training, and work in partnership with self-advocacy groups in building health knowledge in people with intellectual disabilities.
- Link with national networks to share and learn from best practice.
- Develop surveys, research, audit, or other approaches that record and publish evidence on local health needs.

Further reading

Norah Fry Research Centre (2018). The Learning Disabilities Mortality Review (LeDeR) Programme. Annual Report December 2017. NHS England/University of Bristol: London. www.hqip.org.uk/resource/the-learning-disabilities-mortality-review-annual-report-2017/#.WvMuni-ZNE6. (accessed 9 May 2018).

Heslop P, Blair P, Fleming M, Hoghton M., Marriott A, Russ L (2013). *Confidential Inquiry into Premature Deaths of People with Learning Disabilities (CIPOLD)*. Norah Fry Research Centre: Bristol. www.bris.ac.uk/cipold/ (accessed 30 October 2017).

Michael J (2008). *Healthcare for All: Report of the Independent Inquiry into Access to Healthcare for People with Learning Disabilities*. Department of Health: London.

Physical health assessment of people with intellectual disability

People with intellectual disabilities experience a wide range of inequalities in relation to their physical health. These include an increased prevalence of a number of specific health conditions that may, or may not, be associated with an identified syndrome and an increased number of conditions associated with lifestyle or reduced health education and choices, along with poor health outcomes. Other evidence suggests that they are less likely than the general population to self-identify health changes or deteriorating health or to proactively access regular health checks or health screening. These differences lead to higher rates of health conditions, late diagnosis of ill health, and poor health outcomes. Proactive annual health checks are one approach to addressing this issue. There is growing research evidence that when health checks are of good quality, they can detect previously unrecognized, and potentially treatable, health conditions and can lead to targeted actions to address these health needs. As it is not compulsory for GP practices to offer annual health checks, they may be considered to be a reasonable adjustment to general health services, an anticipatory duty introduced by the Equality Act 2010 to help overcome the disadvantage experienced due to having an intellectual disability.

> **What is physical health assessment?**
> Physical health assessment is the process of gaining a fuller understanding of the health needs of an individual, in order to detect, treat, and manage any health conditions.

Supporting people with intellectual disabilities in understanding, managing, and taking responsibility for their health should be the responsibility of all carers working with this population, not just health staff. National recommendations are that physical health assessment may be best managed in people with intellectual disabilities in the delivery of annual GP-led health checks. There is variation in the way health checks are offered and delivered across the UK, and there is no measure of their quality built into the check, so the quality is variable too. Within England, annual health checks are offered by GP practices to all adults on their Learning Disability Quality and Outcomes Framework (LD QOF) practice registers. Not all GP practices hold comprehensive GP registers; however, most are likely to be aware of adults with moderate to severe intellectual disabilities. Annual health checks are commissioned by NHS England in a contract called a Directly Enhanced Service (DES). These contracts are not compulsory; therefore, not all practices have signed up to deliver annual health checks. In 2014, Public Health England reported that, in the previous year, ~60% of adults known to GPs in England received an annual health check. In order to improve child/adult transition, from 2016, the DES annual health check contract was extended to include children aged 14 and older.

Preparing people with intellectual disabilities for a health check

People with intellectual disabilities may need support in preparing to have a health check, so that they can attend and give informed consent for it. This may require preparation by informing them when a letter of invite arrives, using accessible health information resources to build their awareness on procedures offered in the health check, and checking that the practice is aware and can deliver any reasonable adjustments required. Guidance from the Royal College of General Practitioners (RCGP) suggests that the health check may require two appointments, the first for blood tests and the second a week or so later to complete the comprehensive check. Most annual health checks are completed using a systematic approach following the Cardiff Health Check. A copy of this and the GP guidance can be found at ℘ www.rcgp.org.uk/learningdisabilities.

Any person attending an annual health check should be offered support to attend. This support might be offered by a HF. On completion, each person should have an increased awareness of their health status and have an accessible plan of actions to achieve optimum health, to add to any HAP.

What areas of physical health warrant assessment in a health check?

- Family history and risk factors;
- Immunization record;
- Weight, height (BMI), and dietary review;
- Lifestyle choices, including smoking, exercise, illegal drug, and alcohol use;
- Vision and hearing;
- Review of chronic illness, including epilepsy;
- Physical examination, including skin condition, mobility, and posture;
- Syndrome-specific check;
- Medication review;
- Oral health;
- Sexual health;
- Engagement with cancer screening programmes;
- Continence.

Further reading

McConkey R, Taggart L, Kane M (2015). Optimising the uptake of health checks for people with intellectual disabilities. *Journal of Intellectual Disabilities*. **19**: 205–14.

Robertson J, Roberts H, Emerson E (2010). *Health Checks for People with Learning Disabilities: A Systematic Review of Evidence*. Department of Health: London.

Blood pressure, temperature, and pulse

Blood pressure

Blood pressure is a measure of the levels of force exerted on the walls of blood vessels, due to the flow of blood from the heart. Blood pressure is dynamic and varies from minute to minute. It is measured by an instrument called a sphygmomanometer, a gauge that measures the pumping (systolic) and resting (diastolic) stages of the heart. Readings of blood pressure may be performed by trained health staff but increasingly may be self-measured by patients in GP waiting rooms, using portable machines or by self-purchased wrist/arm cuffs.

Blood pressure is influenced by a large number of factors. These include temperature, respiration, environmental noise, pain, fear, anxiety, exercise, smoking, excessive eating, and drinking. Body position can also affect blood pressure readings.

High blood pressure is known as hypertension, and low blood pressure is hypotension. Consistent readings of 140/90 mmHg and above are likely to be associated with hypertension. Hypertension is an increasing medical concern, being commonly associated with obesity, diabetes, and high levels of fat in blood. If left untreated, a combination of the above can lead to cardiovascular (heart) disease, stroke, kidney failure, dementia, and early death. Treatment is usually based on lifestyle changes and drug interventions.

People with intellectual disabilities are known to have higher rates of obesity than the general population and receive fewer health checks. In meeting the health needs of people with intellectual disabilities, carers have a key role in the prevention, detection, and management of hypertension. This can be difficult to detect without measuring blood pressure; therefore, blood pressure measurement is required in any regular health check. In preparing a person for the procedure, people need to be aware of the discomfort of a tightening cuff on the upper arm—distraction interventions may help. There are a number of less uncomfortable wrist readers, but these are less accurate.

Preventative lifestyle measures include healthy eating, eating a well-balanced, low-salt diet, maintaining a healthy weight, regular exercise, low alcohol intake, reduced caffeine intake, stopping smoking, stress reduction, and learning free relaxation techniques.

Temperature

Body temperature varies from person to person—the normal range is 36–37.5°C. It is always useful to have a record of each individual's normal temperature, as what may be a normal temperature for one person may be high or low for another. Normal body temperature is slightly lower in the morning than in the evenings.

A wide range of factors influence body temperature. These include age, exercise, circadian rhythms, hormonal actions, stress, and environmental factors. Hypothermia, or low body temperature, develops when the body temperature becomes too cold and when the usual body mechanism of heat production cannot maintain a thermal balance. This is most often seen in older people or people overly exposed to very low temperatures for a long time. A high temperature, known as pyrexia or hyperthermia, is symptomatic of infection, neurological injury, extreme drug reaction, or heat exhaustion.

Body temperature is recorded using a thermometer. There are different types of thermometer, including glass thermometers, tympanic (ear) battery-operated devices, fever brow (chemical disposable strips), and electronic readers. Hospitals now generally use tympanic ear thermometers; however, these can be less accurate in people who get ears blocked with ear wax.

The most commonly used thermometer, in the home, is the glass thermometer. Under the tongue, in the mouth, is the most commonly used site for recording temperature. The mouth, however, should never be used for infants, small children, people who have poorly controlled epilepsy, or people with intellectual disabilities who are confused or have poor cognitive understanding. In these situations, the thermometer should be placed, and held, in the axilla (armpit), or another type of thermometer should be used. On rare occasions, body temperature may be taken using a special rectal thermometer.

Pulse

The measurement of pulse rate is another aspect of a person's health assessment, closely associated with temperature, respiration, and blood pressure. Taking a pulse reading is one common technique used to assess how well the heart is working, and therefore to assess the general health of the patient. A pulse reading measures the force of blood pumped from the ventricle, in the left side of the heart, into the aorta, the main artery that then sends blood around the body. Pulse points are places in the body where an artery can easily be felt when pressed against a bone. There are ten common pulse points, the most common being the wrist (radial pulse), the neck (carotid pulse), and the inner arm of the elbow (brachial pulse). Placing a finger or a stethoscope over a pulse point is referred to as 'taking a pulse'. This gives information on the number of times the heart beats in a minute, the rhythm and regularity of the pulse, and its strength. If taken over several pulse points, it can also measure the consistency of blood flow throughout the body.

A normal adult pulse rate is 60–100 beats/min. Depending on the age, a child's pulse rate is significantly faster. Exercise, temperature, anxiety, pain, body posture, and drugs or medication can all influence the pulse rate.

Further reading

Dougherty L, Lister S (2015). *The Royal Marsden Hospital Manual Nursing Procedures*, 9th edn. Wiley-Blackwell Publishing: Oxford.

Respiration and oxygen saturation levels

Respiration

When a body is at rest, and the person is in good general health, respiration, or breathing, should be regular, require minimal effort, and be quiet. By discreetly observing a patient's respiration, much can be indicated relating to general health. The measurement of respiration involves counting the rate, depth, and pattern of chest wall movement. Breathing rates are extremely variable, being influenced by age, emotion, and pain. The normal adult respiratory rate is 12–18 breaths/min.

> **What is respiration?**
> Respiration is another word for breathing. It involves a process of gaseous exchange in the lungs. This involves air constantly moving in and out of the lungs, bringing oxygen into the body and removing carbon dioxide.

The observation of respiration is something that can be done by anyone working with people with intellectual disabilities and may be the first observation to identify physical ill health. Changes in respiration may include coughing, either dry or productive; that may be different at different times of the day or in different postural positions. This could indicate the presence of infection, asthma, or allergy. Coughing during eating or drinking may suggest that the person is aspirating (inhaling) food or liquid into their lungs and should be referred to the GP as a matter of urgency. In observing seizures in epilepsy, particular attention needs to be given to ensure that the airway to the lungs does not become blocked. Halitosis, bad smelling breath, may indicate poor oral hygiene, infection, or severe constipation. Sweet smelling breath may indicate diabetes.

Oxygen saturation levels

The body cannot function well without high levels of oxygen in the blood. Oxygen is carried in the haemoglobin of red blood cells, which take oxygen to all parts of the body. Levels of blood gases may be monitored using a non-invasive method of pulse oximetry, in which a probe is placed on the end of a finger, covering the fingernail. If more detailed information is required, a blood test known as arterial blood gases (ABG) is undertaken to measure oxygen, carbon dioxide, and acidity levels of blood. These levels relate to how well body organs, predominantly the lungs, are working.

An ABG test is carried out on blood taken from an artery. It is likely to be requested to:
- Check for breathing problems in lung disease such as asthma, cystic fibrosis, or chronic obstructive airways disease;
- Check how well lung treatments are working;
- Check whether more oxygen is needed if the person is on oxygen treatment;
- Measure the acid levels in the blood of people with heart failure, uncontrolled diabetes, severe infections, or drug overdoses.

Further reading

Dougherty L, Lister S (2015). *The Royal Marsden Hospital Manual Nursing Procedures*, 9th edn. Wiley-Blackwell Publishing: Oxford.

Epilepsy

Epilepsy is a neurological disease where there is a continuing tendency to have seizures resulting from a primary change to the electrical activity in the brain, caused by a disruption to the electrical and chemical balance of brain cells. The type of seizure experienced depends on the part of the brain in which the activity originates and how it spreads.

Diagnosis of epilepsy

Primarily a clinical diagnosis, it relies on a description of the episode from the individual, if possible, and/or an eyewitness. Detailed information is essential and should include: *before*—what the person was doing, the environment, the time of the day, how they felt/appeared, focal onset, any trigger; *during*—sudden onset, fall, movements, eyes open/closed, incontinence, gum/tongue bite, level of consciousness, behaviour, duration; and *after*—level of consciousness, tiredness, confusion, behaviour, recovery time, injury. Video recording can assist diagnosis. Investigations—ideally the following are needed: electroencephalogram (EEG), magnetic resonance imaging (MRI), ECG, and blood screening to rule out other causes and may support a diagnosis of epilepsy. Epilepsy syndrome: defined by seizure type, EEG findings, age of onset, family history, and response to treatment; allows for more targeted treatment and provides information on prognosis.

Main seizure types

Focal (partial) seizures

Arise within an area confined to one hemisphere of the brain, differing depending on the area affected. Normally last 1–3min but can be longer. Types are related to the level of consciousness:

Without impairment of consciousness/awareness: can recall event

- Localized motor signs, e.g. twitching of the mouth which may spread to other areas, head turning, lip smacking, rhythmic jerking of one part of body;
- Special sensory symptoms, e.g. taste, smell, tingling, light flashes, sound;
- Autonomic symptoms, e.g. epigastric sensation, pallor, sweating, flushing;
- Psychic symptoms, e.g. déjàvu, distortion of time, fear, anger, dreamy state.

With impairment of consciousness/awareness: no memory of event

- Repetitive movements—automatisms;
- Strange behaviours;
- Picking up objects for no reason or fiddling with clothing;
- Chewing or lip-smacking movements;
- Muttering or repeating words that do not make sense;
- Wandering around in a confused way;
- Making a loud cry or scream;
- Strange postures or movements such as cycling or kicking;
- A feeling of numbness or tingling;
- A sensation that an arm/leg feels bigger or smaller than it actually is;
- Visual disturbances, e.g. coloured or flashing lights;
- Hallucinations;
- Uncontrollable laughing.

Focal seizure activity can spread to all parts of the brain, evolving into a secondary generalized seizure.

Generalized seizures: originate within both hemispheres, rapidly spread across neuronal networks on both sides

- *Absence seizures*—brief loss of consciousness, will stop what they are doing and stare; may be some mild motor movements, e.g. eye blinks, mouth/finger movements. Last <10s, quick recovery;
- *Atypical absence*—similar to above but last longer and motor movements are more pronounced. Seen in particular epilepsy syndromes;
- *Myoclonic seizures*—very quick muscle jerks usually of arms, legs, or trunk, may be one-sided or both sides, frequently happens soon after waking;
- *Tonic seizures*—sudden stiffening of all body, will fall if standing, lasts seconds, can cause injury, fairly quick recovery;
- *Atonic seizures*—sudden loss of muscle tone, person drops to the floor, lasts a few seconds, can cause injury, quick recovery;
- *Tonic–clonic seizures*—may be preceded by focal seizure. May experience a 'prodrome', feeling unwell for some hours/days before (may be recognized as behaviour change). Tonic stage: sudden contraction of muscles, will fall if standing, may cry as air is expelled from lungs, may bite gum or side of tongue. Intermittent relaxation and contraction of muscles follows. Clonic stage: rhythmical jerking of body. Person may become blue around the lips, exaggerated by dilation of blood vessels in the face caused by pressure from contraction of the chest. There may be excess saliva; snorting noises may be heard, and the person may lose bladder and/or bowel control. Also periods of relaxation become more prolonged; eventually, contractions stop, usually within 1–2min. Full consciousness may not return for 10–60min; confusion and tiredness may persist for hours or days. Person may experience headache and/or muscle ache post-seizure.

Unclassified seizures

- Seizures may present which are unclassifiable.

Treatment of epilepsy

Antiepileptic drugs (AEDs) are the mainstay of treatment; the aim is to gain complete seizure control without drug-related side effects; 70% of newly diagnosed have a good outcome with AEDs. Choice of AED depends on seizure type and individual circumstances, including age, gender, and physical and mental comorbidities. Monotherapy is preferable, but >1 AED may be required. Published guidelines provide recommendations for AED treatment.[8] If AEDs fail to work, vagal nerve stimulation, ketogenic diet, and surgery may be considered. Non-pharmacological approaches to the management of epilepsy include psychological and alternative therapies and avoidance of obvious triggers for seizures. Generally, a healthy lifestyle approach is recommended to help seizure control; consideration should be given to diet, exercise, and compliance with medication, along with a regular sleep pattern and controlled alcohol intake.

Further reading

Dougherty L, Lister S (2015). *The Royal Marsden Hospital Manual Nursing Procedures*, 9th edn. Wiley-Blackwell Publishing: Oxford.

National Institute for Health and Care Excellence (2012). *Epilepsies: Diagnosis and Management.* ℛ www.nice.org.uk/guidance/cg137 (accessed 30 October 2017).

References

8 Royal College o1f General Practitioners (2012, updated 2016). *Clinical Guideline Epilepsies: Diagnosis and Management*. Royal College of General Practitioners: London.

Supporting people with epilepsy

Approximately 25% of people with intellectual disabilities have epilepsy, compared with about 1% of the general population; the more severe the person's intellectual disabilities, the higher the prevalence of epilepsy. The aim of treatment is to control seizures without drug-related side effects.

Epilepsy management plan (EMP)

Individual EMPs help carers support people in managing their epilepsy on a day-to-day basis. The EMP should include the following:

- Description of seizure/s—what happens before, during, and after the seizure (see ➋ Epilepsy, pp. 160–1). Name of specific seizure type should be avoided;
- Usual duration of seizure—care should be taken to detail the time of actual seizure activity and recovery period separately;
- Management of seizure—first aid required for particular seizure type and individual's unique presentation (see ➋ First aid for seizures, p. 162);
- Emergency management—generally advised to call emergency services if the person has a prolonged single seizure of >5min or recurrent seizures. Alternatively, if prescribed emergency medication, this should specify when it is to be administered—a separate EMP may be agreed (see ➋ Emergency management of a patient in a seizure, pp. 588–9). If seizures controlled for some years, then advised to call emergency services immediately as there may be underlying health problem;
- Other relevant information—frequency of seizures, time of day, any particular environment, any triggers, and how these can be avoided.

First aid for seizures

- Focal (partial) seizures—vary widely; note the time, stay with the person, speak calmly and reassuringly. It is important to recognize that touching the person may be misinterpreted as aggression, and they may respond aggressively; however, guide from danger if necessary. Keep others from interfering. Reassure when seizure stops—may recover quickly or may need to rest. If the seizure is unusually prolonged, seek medical advice.
- Absence seizures—if walking, may require guidance and reassurance.
- Myoclonic seizures—usually so short-lived that little can be done, reassure when over; may be unbalanced, help to steady them, check for injury.
- Tonic and atonic seizures—are brief, therefore little can be done during the seizure; adhere to manual handling guidance; check for injury which may need medical attention; stay with the person and reassure.
- Tonic–clonic seizures—note time, assess danger to self and client, only move if in danger; adhere to manual handling guidance. Protect from injury; move or cushion objects that may cause injury, loosen tight clothing, remove glasses. Let the seizure run its course. When seizure stops/jerking stops, if unconscious place in recovery position. Monitor breathing and skin colour post-seizure. Wipe away excess saliva; do all you can to minimize embarrassment, quietly reassure, keep others from gathering around if in public. Assess for injury. May be confused and agitated; do not restrict or restrain as they may hit out in confused state. Check for potential triggers; seek medical review if appropriate. Allow to rest if needed. Inform carer where appropriate.

Maximizing seizure control and quality of life

- Correct diagnosis—people with intellectual disabilities with suspected seizures should be seen by a specialist. Observe and secure a detailed description of seizures for correct diagnosis; involve the individual and family, and consider video recording. Challenging behaviour, repetitive stereotyped behaviour, and behaviour relating to mental health can make diagnosis difficult; monitor and record; behavioural analysis may be required. Communication difficulties and complex health needs may further complicate diagnosis and treatment.
- Review—review seizure records and the use of emergency medications, if prescribed; seek specialist review if changes or AED side effects observed.
- Medication—adherence: consider education and support appropriate for individual's cognition, use of alarms, mobile applications, pill dispensers; timing and slow-release preparations help adherence and independence. Also consider choice, capacity, and consent issues. Side effects: may be transient during titration, start low/go slow, may be changes in cognition/behaviour. Long-term effects: bone health, hyponatraemia. Blood checks and serum level monitoring for some AEDs appropriate.
- Identifying and managing triggers—detailed assessment; consider pain, pyrexia, constipation, lack of sleep, stress, missed medications, alcohol, drugs (prescribed and illegal), and hormonal impact in women.
- Comorbidity—complex physical/mental health effects on seizure control, including drug effects/interactions. Impact of seizures on health.
- Complementary therapies—may reduce stress as a trigger.
- Lifestyle choices—a healthy lifestyle approach helps seizure control, including diet, exercise, regular sleep pattern, structured routine, avoidance of drugs, and controlled alcohol intake.
- Education/training/support—individuals, family, and support staff. Voluntary organizations; helpline, groups, web-based support.
- Minimizing risk—all the above and having relevant EMPs in place will collectively reduce risk. Specific risk assessments may be required. A balanced approach is needed to minimize risk and maximize quality of life. There can be a tendency to overprotect; individual choice, capacity, and consent need to be considered. A multidisciplinary approach is recommended, with a regular review of risks and measures agreed to manage risks.

Status epilepticus—see ➲ Emergency management of a person in a seizure, pp. 588–9.

Sudden unexpected death in epilepsy (SUDEP)—this is when a person with epilepsy dies suddenly and unexpectedly and no obvious cause of death can be found at post-mortem.

Further reading

Heslop P, Blair P, Fleming M, Hoghton M, Marriott A, Russ L (2013). *Confidential Inquiry into Premature Deaths of People with Learning Disabilities (CIPOLD)*. Norah Fry Research Centre: Bristol. ℛ www.bris.ac.uk/cipold/ (accessed 30 October 2017).

Robertson J, Hatton C, Emerson E, Baines S (2015). Prevalence of epilepsy among people with intellectual disabilities: a systematic review. *Seizure*. 29: 46–62.

van Schrojenstein Lantman-de Valk HM, Walsh PN (2008). Managing health problems in people with intellectual disabilities. *BMJ*. 337: a2507.

Cardiorespiratory disorders

Some people with intellectual disabilities' experience may be a consequence of the underlying comorbid conditions related to their disability. People with Down syndrome, for example, can experience tetralogy of Fallot, ductus arteriosus, mitral valve disorder, and aortic insufficiency. Some may go on to experience pulmonary hypertension as a consequence of their cardiac disorder, with associated complications such as heart failure. It is important therefore that cardiorespiratory disorders are assessed effectively and managed across their lifespan; this is important as they are now living into older age.

Respiratory disease is the most common cause of death for people with moderate or severe intellectual disabilities.[9] This point is significant and is a major factor in the premature death of some people with intellectual disabilities. Nurses who practise in all care settings should recognize this and develop care plans to detect and minimize risks. For example, gastric aspiration is associated with swallowing, specific nutrition, and feeding problems—and this is experienced by some in this population. Gastro-oesophageal reflux disorder (GORD) is common and is experienced by some 70% of people with intellectual disabilities.[10,11] As can be seen in ➲ Gastrointestinal disorders, pp. 186–7, this may lead them to regurgitate the acidic gastric contents back up the oesophagus, and inhalation into the lungs may result in inflammation of the respiratory tract that, in turn, leads to infection and, if untreated, pneumonia. Another example is illustrated in a recent study that identified respiratory disorders as common reasons for hospital admission for people with Prader–Willi syndrome.[12]

Cardiovascular disease is another leading cause of death in people with moderate or severe intellectual disabilities.[13] Congenital heart diseases are common in people with intellectual disabilities, and as this population is now living longer, it is anticipated that more will experience complications of cardiovascular disease associated with the ageing process. As a consequence, some people with intellectual disabilities will experience conditions such as hypertension, vascular dementia, myocardial infarction, diabetes, dyslipidaemia, and cerebrovascular accident.[14] Therefore, it is important for nurses working in primary care, general hospitals, and specialist intellectual disabilities assessment and treatment services to be aware of an increased likelihood of these physical disorders being present.

As a consequence of these physical disorders, children, adults, and older people with intellectual disabilities will be regular users of primary care and general hospital services.[15] Nurses working in these care environments must familiarize themselves with the distinct needs of people with intellectual disabilities in their care to ensure that their needs are appropriately addressed.

Some people with intellectual disabilities who have cardiorespiratory disorders will also require assessment and treatment from specialist intellectual disabilities health services, because of the nature of their complex health needs. Nurses practising in such services need to be familiar with the physical health problems that can be experienced by people with intellectual disabilities in their care. They have an important contribution to make in supporting them during the assessment and treatment of their physical healthcare, and have a responsibility to liaise and communicate effectively with colleagues in primary and general hospital care settings to ensure that support needs related to communication, behaviours, mental illness, and ASC are reflected within care plans.

References

9 Tyrer F, McGrother C (2009). Cause-specific mortality and death certificate reporting in adults with moderate to profound intellectual disability. *Journal of Intellectual Disability Research*. 53: 898–904.

10 Galli-Carminati G, Chauvet I, Deriaz N (2006). Prevalence of gastrointestinal disorders in adult clients with pervasive developmental disorders. *Journal of Intellectual Disability Research*. 50: 711–18.

11 Glover G, Ayub M (2010). *How People with Learning Disabilities Die*. Improving Health and Lives: Learning Disabilities Public Health Observatory: London.

12 Thomson A, Glasson A, Bittles A (2006). A long-term population-based clinical and morbidity review of Prader–Willi syndrome in Western Australia. *Journal of Intellectual Disability Research*. 50: 69–78.

13 Emerson E, Hatton C, Baines S, Robertson J (2016). The physical health of British adults with intellectual disability: cross sectional study. *International Journal for Equity in Health*. 15: 11.

14 Wee LE, Koh GC-H, Auyong LS, et al. (2014). Screening for cardiovascular disease risk factors at baseline and post intervention among adults with intellectual disabilities in an urbanised Asian society. *Journal of Intellectual Disability Research*. 58: 255–68.

15 Melville C, Cooper SA, Morrison J, et al. (2006). The outcomes of an intervention study to reduce the barriers experienced by people with intellectual disability accessing primary healthcare services. *Journal of Intellectual Disability Research*. 50: 11–17.

Obesity

Obesity is a growing public health concern in developed countries. The level of obesity is higher in people with intellectual disabilities than in the general population.[16] There are a range of factors that contribute to this situation, which include limited physical activity, poor nutritional practices, lack of nutritional knowledge, and poor knowledge of families and carers of the contributing factors and preventative actions that collectively result in a population that is overweight.[17] Obesity is a contributory factor in people with intellectual disabilities for the development of coronary heart disease, cardiovascular disease, cerebrovascular accident, hypertension, and type 2 diabetes. Obesity results in a decrease in life expectancy and an increase in health needs.[18] Obesity is also linked to genetic conditions such as Prader–Willi syndrome and women with Down syndrome. Men with Down syndrome have been found to be obese, but less so than in people with intellectual disabilities without Down syndrome. In recognition of the increasing life expectancy of people with intellectual disabilities, obesity is a significant health issue that needs to be addressed.[19]

Inactivity and lack of regular physical activity play an important part in contributing to obesity in the intellectual disabilities population. People with intellectual disabilities lead more sedentary lifestyles, when compared with the general population, and have limited opportunities to participate in regular physical activity. Many people with intellectual disabilities are dependent on a family member or carer to provide everyday living support. Studies have found that people who receive care in care homes and from family carers are more likely to be overweight and have limited access to physical activity.[20] Evidence further suggests that increasing the amount of daily physical activity, reducing carbohydrate intake, and improving the daily diet by way of fruit and vegetables can bring about health benefits and reduce weight.[21]

Following assessment that includes identifying dietary habits and other risk factors, it is necessary to monitor and record weight regularly and to jointly agree weight parameters appropriate to the individual. Treatment needs to include a focus on providing education for carers and others involved in the care. There is opportunity to work collaboratively with people with intellectual disabilities and their carers to effect longer-term change.

Primary care has an important role in assessing diabetes, hypertension, and cardiovascular disease. Preventative strategies are important, and effectiveness is increased when delivered in partnership with staff in intellectual disabilities services such as nurses, physiotherapists, and dieticians. Nurses have an important role in working in partnership with dieticians to provide support, advice, and regular monitoring, thereby enabling reduction or maintenance of weight. Medications used to treat mental illness need to be reviewed, as they can contribute to obesity. Structured, accessible services and access approaches need to be in place, including the development of weight management services that can provide a focus for supporting weight maintenance and, where possible, weight reduction.[22]

References

16 Spanos D, Melville CA, Hankey CR (2013). Weight management interventions in adults with intellectual disabilities and obesity: a systematic review of the evidence. *Nutrition Journal*. **12**: 132.

17 McGuire BE, Daly P, Smyth F (2007). Lifestyle and health behaviours of adults with an intellectual disability. *Journal of Intellectual Disability Research*. **51**: 497–510.

18 Rimmer JH, Yamaki K, Davis Lowry M, Wang E, Vogel LC (2010). Obesity and obesity-related secondary conditions in adolescents with intellectual/developmental disabilities. *Journal of Intellectual Disability Research*. **54**: 787–94.

19 Melville CA, Boyle S, Miller S, et al. (2013). An open study of the effectiveness of a multi-component weight-loss intervention for adults with intellectual disabilities and obesity. *British Journal of Nutrition*. **105**: 1553–62.

20 Bartlo P, Klein PJ (2011). Physical activity benefits and needs in adults with intellectual disabilities: systematic review of the literature. *American Journal of Intellectual and Developmental Disabilities*. **116**: 220–32.

21 Sohler N, Lubetkin E, Levy J, Soghomonian C, Rimmerman A (2009). Factors associated with obesity and coronary heart disease in people with intellectual disabilities. *Social Work Health Care*. **48**: 76–89.

22 Heller T, McCubbin JA, Drum C, Peterson J (2011). Physical activity and nutrition health promotion interventions: What is working for people with intellectual disabilities? *Intellectual and Developmental Disabilities*. **49**: 26–36.

Nutrition

Food plays an important part in everyone's life. Food has a central role in relation to socialization and is generally an enjoyable experience. Nutrition plays an important part in the lives of people with intellectual disabilities, and there are growing concerns about the high rates of obesity, when compared with the general population.[23] Obesity contributes to a range of important risk factors such as the development of coronary heart disease, reduced mobility, hypertension, musculoskeletal problems, and diabetes.[24] This emphasizes the need to develop opportunities for people with intellectual disabilities to improve their diet, participate in community activities, and experience regular physical activity. Providing accessible information to help improve health and well-being is important when supporting people with intellectual disabilities and their carers to make informed choices. Early intervention and prevention that includes addressing nutrition issues that impact on the lives of people with intellectual disabilities are of importance, as the population ages and more live into old age.[25]

Whereas there is clear evidence of the prevalence of obesity within the intellectual disabilities population, for others, particularly those with profound disabilities and other impairments, there is a risk of being underweight or malnourished.[26] The prevalence of being underweight increases with the severity of intellectual disabilities and is common in conditions such as cerebral palsy. People with profound and multiple intellectual disabilities are at increased risk of swallowing and feeding problems such as choking, regurgitation, vomiting, and gastric aspiration.[27,28] As a consequence, a comprehensive assessment is required of the gastro-oesophageal tract and swallowing mechanism, and of nutritional needs to maintain weight and appropriate hydration.

Nurses have a role to play in providing additional support during hospitalization when investigations are necessary. The issue of consent to treatment is important, particularly in those with profound intellectual impairment and where capacity may be lacking. Effective individual nutrition plans are required to minimize the possibility of dehydration, gastric aspiration, and pneumonia. The prevention of aspiration pneumonia is important, as it is the highest cause of death in this population, and, with appropriate assessment and management, can be prevented. Nurses have an important role in working collaboratively with people with intellectual disabilities and their families and carers, to promote healthy lifestyles that include a focus on improving nutrition and physical activity wherever possible.

References

23 Jinks A, Cotton A, Rylance R (2011). Obesity interventions for people with a learning disability: an integrative literature review. *Journal of Advanced Nursing*. 67: 460–71.

24 Rimmer JH, Yamaki K, Davis Lowry M, Wang E, Vogel LC (2010). Obesity and obesity-related secondary conditions in adolescents with intellectual/developmental disabilities. *Journal of Intellectual Disability Research*. 54: 787–94.

25 Heller T, McCubbin JA, Drum C, Peterson J (2011). Physical activity and nutrition health promotion interventions: what is working for people with intellectual disabilities? *Intellectual and Developmental Disabilities*. 49: 26–36.

26 Bhaumik S, Watson J, Thorp C, Tyrer F, McGrother C (2008). Body mass index in adults with intellectual disability: distribution, associations and service implications: a population-based prevalence study. *Journal of Intellectual Research*. 52: 287–98.

27 Galli-Carminati G, Chauvet I, Deriaz N (2006). Prevalence of gastrointestinal disorders in adult clients with pervasive developmental disorders. *Journal of Intellectual Disability Research*. 50: 711–18.

28 Mansell J (2010). *Raising Our Sights: Services for Adults with Multiple and Profound Learning Disabilities*. Department of Health: London.

Mobility

There are high rates of mobility problems experienced by people with intellectual disabilities. Some mobility problems will be evident such as those experienced by people with cerebral palsy and more severe forms of intellectual disabilities. Mobility may be reduced as a consequence of falls and injuries that result in deformity and pain which impact on the ability and confidence to mobilize. Some antipsychotic and antiepileptic medication can impair mobility, thereby contributing to falls and injuries.[29,30] People with intellectual disabilities participate in lower levels of physical activity, well below those recommended to protect and improve health. As a result, there is an increased prevalence of obesity in people with intellectual disabilities. Physical activity, as part of a structured preventative approach, has the potential to increase life expectancy and improve health and well-being.[31]

In people with severe physical disabilities and those in older age, the role of postural management is relevant and plays an important role in minimizing and preventing deformities and breathing difficulties in order to maximize mobility potential.[32] Providing appropriate access to assessment and management by specialists such as intellectual disabilities nurses, physiotherapists, occupational therapists, and specialist services, contributes to promoting and maintaining mobility.[33] Ensuring regular attendance at podiatry services is important because of a higher prevalence of foot and toenail problems in this population. Access to, and use of, specialist footwear may also be required. Addressing these issues all help to reduce pain and falls and accidents, and offers people with intellectual disabilities increased mobility, which, in turn, creates the opportunity to participate in physical activity and community activities.[29,34]

Some people with intellectual disabilities experience visual and hearing disorders that can be treated easily, which helps to improve mobility and self-confidence.[35] Nurses have a role to play in facilitating access to audiology and ophthalmology services, orthotics, and wheelchair clinics, and acquiring the necessary aids to promote mobility. Regular review of medication used to treat mental ill health and epilepsy is important in this population to minimize possible side effects impacting on mobility.

Further reading

Courtenay K, Murray A (2015). Foot health and mobility in people with intellectual disabilities. *Journal of Policy and Practice in Intellectual Disabilities.* **12**: 42–6.

Kleiner AFR, Galli M, Albertini G, et al. (2015). Context-dependency of mobility in children and adolescents with cerebral palsy: optimal and natural environments. *Journal of Policy and Practice in Intellectual Disabilities.* **12**: 288–93.

References

29 Finlayson J, Morrison J, Jackson A, Mantry D, Cooper SA (2010). Injuries, falls and accidents among adults with intellectual disabilities. Prospective cohort study. *Journal of Intellectual Disability Research.* **54**: 966–80.

30 McGrowther C, Bhaumik S, Thorp C, Hauck A, Branford D, Watson J (2006). Epilepsy in adults with intellectual disability: prevalence, associations and service implications. *Seizure.* **15**: 376–86.

31 Hamilton S, Hankey C, Miller S, Boyle S, Melville C (2007). A review of weight loss interventions for adults with intellectual disability. *Obesity Reviews.* **8**: 339–45.

32 Mansell J (2010). *Raising Our Sights: Services for Adults with Multiple and Profound Learning Disabilities.* Department of Health: London.

33 Willgoss TG, Yohannes AM, Mitchell D (2010). Review of risk factors and preventative strategies for fall-related injuries in people with intellectual disabilities. *Journal of Clinical Nursing.* **19**: 2100–9.

34 Cox CR, Clemson L, Stancliffe RJ, Durvasula S, Sherrington C (2010). Incidence of and risk factors for falls among adults with an intellectual disability. *Journal of Intellectual Disability Research.* **54**: 1045–57.

35 Robertson J, Hatton C, Emerson E, Baines S (2014). The impact of health checks for people with intellectual disabilities: an updated systematic review of evidence. *Research in Developmental Disabilities.* **35**: 2450–60.

Exercise

Regular physical activity and exercise are important for everyone and bring about positive benefits to both physical and mental well-being. Undertaking regular exercise increases community visibility and presence and offers opportunities to establish and develop new relationships and friendships.

Ensuring that people with intellectual disabilities of all ages have access to, and participate, in regular physical activity has become an issue of increasing importance and concern.[36] As a population, people with intellectual disabilities are more likely to be unhealthy and overweight and to undertake limited exercise.[37] Increasing physical activity with people with intellectual disabilities offers an effective way to improve health and well-being. Inactivity is common within this population, and there is lack of light, moderate, and vigorous exercise.[38]

As a result of their health conditions and restrictions resulting from living environments, the opportunity for people with intellectual disabilities to undertake exercise regularly can be limited.[39] Many people with intellectual disabilities live in supported living or with families and may continue to attend congregated day activities where there may be limited opportunities for physical activity.[40] As the population ages and increases in number, there is an opportunity to develop and incorporate physical activity within the supports and services offered to older people with intellectual disabilities. This is important, because few people with intellectual disabilities achieve the recommended daily level of physical activity.[38-40]

Nurses and others working with people with intellectual disabilities have an important part to play in supporting the development of healthy lifestyle choices. It is important to ensure that regular physical activity appropriate to the individual is incorporated within their daily activities. Identifying opportunities to participate in local leisure and exercise activities offers the potential to bring about the benefits of regular exercise, which, in the longer term, impacts on physical and mental health and well-being. Developing collaborations with people with intellectual disabilities and their carers and co-producing opportunities whereby people with intellectual disabilities can be supported and enabled to undertake regular daily physical activity are vital in promoting and improving their overall health and well-being and minimizing health complications as a consequence of lack of exercise.[41]

References

36 Hinckson EA, Dickinson A, Water T, Sands M, Penman L (2013). Physical activity, dietary habits and overall health in overweight and obese children and youth with intellectual disability or autism. *Research in Developmental Disabilities*. 34: 1170–8.

37 Heller T, McCubbin JA, Drum C, Peterson J (2011). Physical activity and nutrition health promotion interventions: what is working for people with intellectual disabilities? *Intellectual and Developmental Disabilities*. 49: 26–36.

38 Bartlo P, Klein PJ (2011). Physical activity benefits and needs in adults with intellectual disabilities: systematic review of the literature. *American Journal of Intellectual and Developmental Disabilities*. 116: 220–32.

39 Hamilton S, Hankey C, Miller S, Boyle S, Melville C (2007). A review of weight loss interventions for adults with intellectual disability. *Obesity Reviews*. 8: 339–45.

40 Rimmer JH, Chen M-D, McCubbin JA, Drum C, Peterson J (2010). Exercise intervention research on persons with disabilities: what we know and where we need to go. *American Journal of Physical Medicine and Rehabilitation*. 89: 249–63.

41 Haveman M, Heller T, Lee L, Maaskant M, Shooshtari S, Strydom A (2010). Major health risks in aging persons with intellectual disabilities: an overview of recent studies. *Journal of Policy and Practice in Intellectual Disabilities*. 7: 59–69.

Diabetes

Diabetes is an endocrine disorder affecting glucose metabolism. In diabetes, the pancreas produces little or no insulin and, for reasons that are poorly understood, the body cannot effectively use the insulin that is produced. Insulin is a hormone produced by the islets of Langerhans in the pancreas and is necessary for the uptake of glucose by cells. Glucose is required for normal body functioning and circulates in blood where it is used by cells and muscles as energy. In diabetes, there is a build-up of glucose in the bloodstream, which is excreted by the body in the urine.

There are two main forms of diabetes: type 1 and type 2. People with type 1 diabetes have difficulty manufacturing insulin; it is more common at a younger age. In type 1 diabetes, insulin is required for treatment. In type 2 diabetes, there is an inadequate amount of insulin produced by the cells in the pancreas to enable glucose metabolism. This form of diabetes is more common in adults, particularly those who are overweight. The common clinical features of diabetes can include fatigue, an increase in micturition, glycosuria, and an increase in thirst and hunger.

There are a range of risk factors associated with the development of diabetes, including obesity, coronary heart disease, and poor diet.[42] The link with sedentary lifestyles, limited physical activity, and obesity and the development of type 2 diabetes is clear; these are significant issues for many people with intellectual disabilities. The intellectual disabilities population is increasing and ageing, and evidence further points to many of the population developing long-term health conditions, such as diabetes, which contribute to a reduction in their life expectancy and increases the risk of associated health complications. Diabetes is more common in the intellectually disabled population, with some 10% experiencing the condition.[42,43] It is important therefore to recognize the possibility of diabetes within the intellectual disabilities population and enable access to health screening, appropriate management, such as weight reduction and increased physical activity, and, if required, medication or insulin treatment.[44] Within the intellectual disabilities population, where diagnostic overshadowing is possible, the existence of diabetes may be overlooked, and therefore go untreated.

Effective prevention and management of diabetes are therefore an important issue for many people with intellectual disabilities and require coordinated support and interventions.[44] Interventions include the need to ensure that there are effective and systematic health screening programmes that identify the need for health prevention programmes such as weight reduction, access to physical activity, healthy eating, and behavioural interventions.[45] There is an important role for people with intellectual disabilities and their families and carers in the prevention and management of diabetes, and specific education and support need to be available for them.[46] Nurses also have an important role in supporting people with intellectual disabilities and their family and carers to enable weight reduction as a means to reduce possible consequences of diabetes, coronary vascular disease, and obesity. Where diabetes is diagnosed, it is necessary to ensure that the treatment regimens in place are adhered to, and this could include compliance with hypoglycaemic medication such as metformin and insulin. There is also a need to ensure effective monitoring and recording of weight, urinalysis, and blood results to ensure effective management.[44] Effective management of diabetes can therefore require a coordinated approach to care, and this must include the person with intellectual disabilities, their family and carers, primary care services, specialist diabetes services, and staff for intellectual disabilities health services.

Further reading

Diabetes UK. *Improving Care for People with Diabetes and a Learning Disability.* ℘ www.diabetes.org. uk/Professionals/Resources/Resources-to-improve-your-clinical-practice/For-patients-with-learning-disability/ (accessed 30 October 2017).

Scott J (2013). *Type 2 Diabetes. Pictorial Information about Type 2 Diabetes for People with a Learning Disability.* Northern Health and Social Care Trust: Coleraine. ℘ www.northerntrust.hscni.net/pdf/Diabetes_booklet_for_those_with_a_learning_difficulty.pdf (accessed 30 October 2017).

References

42 Taggart L, Brown M, Karatzias T (2014). Diabetes. In: L Taggart, W Cousins, eds. *Health Promotion for People with Intellectual and Developmental Disabilities.* Open University Press: London; pp. 69–76.

43 MacRae S, Brown M, Karatzias T, *et al.* (2015). Diabetes in people with intellectual disabilities: a systematic review of the literature. *Research in Developmental Disabilities.* **47**: 352–74.

44 Taggart L, Coates V, Truesdale-Kennedy M (2013). Management and quality indicators of diabetes mellitus in people with intellectual disabilities. *Journal of Intellectual Disability Research.* **57**: 1152–63.

45 Shireman T, Reichar A, Nazir N, Backes J, Pharm D, Griener A (2010). Quality of diabetes care for adults with developmental disabilities. *Disability and Health Journal.* **3**: 179–85.

46 Dysch C, Chung MC, Fox J (2012). How do people with intellectual disabilities and diabetes experience and perceive their illness? *Journal of Applied Research in Intellectual Disabilities.* **25**: 39–49.

Thyroid

The thyroid gland is an organ that forms part of the endocrine system and is responsible for producing thyroid hormones, which is responsible for regulating some of the physiological functions of the body. The gland is situated behind the thyroid cartilage below the larynx in the neck. It comprises a right and a left lobe, joined in the middle by an isthmus. The thyroid gland produces the hormones thyroxine (T4) and triiodothyronine (T3), which are responsible for the regulation of metabolism and growth. T3 and T4 hormones are regulated by thyroid-stimulating hormone (TSH), which is released by the pituitary gland in the brain.

Thyroid disorders commonly take the form of hypothyroidism (myxoedema) where there is underproduction of thyroid hormones, or hyperthyroidism (thyrotoxicosis) where there is overproduction of thyroid hormones. Hyperthyroid disease can result in conditions such as Graves' disease, characterized by goitre (a swelling in the neck), tachycardia, arrhythmias, exophthalmus, overactivity, sweating, and non-pitting oedema of the lower limbs.

The clinical features associated with an underactive thyroid gland include:
• Tiredness;
• Lethargy;
• Dry skin;
• Weight gain;
• Depression;
• Reduced concentration;
• Memory impairment;
• Constipation.

Diagnosis of thyroid disorders is made by measuring TSH, T3, and T4 levels in blood and, in some cases, by biopsy.

In people with intellectual disabilities, hypothyroidism may not be detected until the later stage of the disease, and screening and diagnosis are important to enable treatment to minimize the effects of the condition and prevent further complications.[47–49] Hypothyroidism is more common in people with Down syndrome, and the incidence of this condition increases with age.[47–50] Treatment is with levothyroxine tablets, and annual screening is recommended in people with Down syndrome.[51]

Nurses have an important role to play in the possible detection of hypothyroidism. A detailed history obtained from families and carers familiar with the person with intellectual disabilities can provide useful insight and background information regarding their usual behaviours and presentation, and changes that have occurred over a period of time. Regular recording of weight can indicate an increase, which, when coupled with other symptoms, may indicate the need for screening by primary care services. Health screening should include blood tests to check thyroid functioning, and ongoing monitoring and review are required for those with active hypothyroidism and for older people with Down syndrome in whom the condition is more common.[48,49,51]

References

47 van Schrojenstein Lantman-de Valk HM (2005). Health in people with intellectual disability: current knowledge and gaps in knowledge. *Journal of Applied Research in Intellectual Disability*. **18**: 325–33.

48 Määttä T, Määttä J, Tervo-Määttä T, Taanila A, Kaski M, Iivanainen M (2011). Healthcare and guidelines: a population-based survey of recorded medical problems and health surveillance for people with Down syndrome. *Journal of Intellectual and Developmental Disability*. **36**: 118–26.

49 McCarron M, Gill M, McCallion P, Begley C (2005). Health co-morbidities in ageing persons with Down syndrome and Alzheimer's dementia. *Journal of Intellectual Disability Research*. **49**: 560–6.

50 McCarron M, Swinburne J, Burke E, McGlinchey E, Carroll R, McCallion P (2013). Patterns of multimorbidity in an older population of persons with an intellectual disability: results from the intellectual disability supplement to the Irish longitudinal study on aging (IDS-TILDA). *Research in Developmental Disabilities*. **34**: 521–7.

51 Prasher V, Gomez G (2007). Natural history of thyroid function in adults with Down syndrome: 10-year follow-up study. *Journal of Intellectual Disability Research*. **51**: 312–17.

Cancer

Cancer comprises a large number of diseases where abnormal cells divide uncontrollably and infiltrate normal body tissue. Cancer can spread throughout the body from the primary source and is a disease that is found across all age groups and both genders. It is recognized that there are risk factors associated with the development of cancers such as smoking, harmful chemicals such as asbestos, family history, and conditions such as ulcerative colitis. Tumours may be benign or malignant. Malignant tumours can involve the invasion of tissues throughout the body, resulting in metastastic spread. Leukaemia is a cancer that involves blood, the bone marrow, the lymphatic system, and the spleen and does not form into a tumour.

People with moderate or severe intellectual disabilities experience a different cancer pattern, compared with the general population, that contributes to their mortality.[52–54] In the general population, respiratory cancer is the leading cancer for men and women, with breast cancer being prevalent in women and prostate cancer in men. People with intellectual disabilities experience lower levels of prostate, respiratory, and urinary tract cancers, with evidence suggesting an increased risk of stomach, oesophageal, and gall bladder cancers.[54–56] Cancers of the stomach and oesophagus may be related to the high prevalence of gastrointestinal disorders, and in particular GORD and *Helicobacter pylori*.[55,56]

White blood cells have an important role to play in protecting the body from infection. Leukaemia is a cancer of white blood cells, and there are two main types: lymphocytic leukaemia and myeloid leukaemia. Lymphocytic leukaemia affects the lymphocytes, and myeloid leukaemia arises from immaturity of the myeloid stem cell. People with Down syndrome are at risk of leukaemia, with rates being significantly higher than in the general population.[55] People with Prader–Willi syndrome are at increased risk of myeloid leukaemia.[57]

Cancers are diagnosed by examining the biopsy of a tumour, blood analysis, computerized tomography (CT) scan, or mammography. A range and combination of treatments may be used, including surgery, bone marrow transplants, chemotherapy, and radiotherapy.

Cancer detection and prevention is important. Ensuring that all people with intellectual disabilities have support to access national cancer screening programmes, such as for bowel screening, is important, and women with intellectual disabilities may need support to access national cervical and breast screening services, as uptake is poor. Nurses have an important role in ensuring adjustments to care are made to help obtain consent and to ensure cooperation. Men with intellectual disabilities may need support and advice to assist with testicular self-examination. Screening for *H. pylori* should be undertaken, and treatment initiated. Some patients may require admission to hospital for further investigations such as endoscopy. GORD should be treated with proton pump inhibitors.

For those diagnosed with a cancer, additional support and information are required during investigations, diagnosis, and treatment.[58] The issue of capacity to consent to treatment needs to be considered, and communication needs identified and addressed. With the population of people with intellectual disabilities, there is a need to consider and identify their information and support needs, as some will require end-of-life care as a consequence of their cancer or other life-limiting conditions.

References

52 Hollins S, Attard MT, von Fraunhofer N, McGuigan S, Sedgwick P (1998). Mortality in people with learning disability: risks, causes, and death certification findings in London. *Developmental Medicine and Child Neurology*. **40**: 50–6.

53 Patja K, Molsa P, Livanainen M (2001). Cause-specific mortality of people with intellectual disability in a population-based, 35-year follow-up study. *Journal of Intellectual Disability Research*. **45**: 30–40.

54 Heslop P, Blair PS, Fleming P, Hoghton M, Marriott A, Russ L (2014). The Confidential Inquiry into premature deaths of people with intellectual disabilities in the UK: a population-based study. *The Lancet*. **383**: 889–95.

55 Emerson E, Baines S (2011). Health inequalities and people with learning disabilities in the UK. *Tizard Learning Disability Review*. **16**: 42–8.

56 Haveman M, Heller T, Lee L, Maaskant M, Shooshtari S, Strydom A (2010). Major health risks in aging persons with intellectual disabilities: an overview of recent studies. *Journal of Policy and Practice in Intellectual Disabilities*. **7**: 59–69.

57 Davies H, Leusink G, McConnell A, et al. (2003). Myeloid leukemia in Prader–Willi syndrome. *Journal of Pediatrics*. **142**: 174–8.

58 Tuffrey-Wijne I, Bernal J, Hollins S (2010). Disclosure and understanding of cancer diagnosis and prognosis for people with intellectual disabilities: findings from an ethnographic study. *European Journal of Oncology Nursing*. **14**: 224–30.

Stopping smoking

People with intellectual disabilities smoke less than the general population, and the incidence is even lower in people with moderate or severe intellectual disabilities.[59,60] This may, in part, be attributed to social and occupational factors, which could account for the lower rates. Of those that do smoke, it is more common in older people with intellectual disabilities and is also linked to asthma and increased BMI. Even though the overall level of cigarette smoking appears lower, some people with intellectual disabilities are cigarette smokers, and they require access to information, education, interventions, and support to assist them to stop.[61,62]

Information available for the general population about the risks of cigarette smoking may be inaccessible to people with intellectual disabilities who may have difficulty reading. Therefore, developing health promotion information at an appropriate level and in an accessible format is necessary. Alternative methods of providing health information are being developed by way of symbolized and pictorial health improvement material that can assist people with intellectual disabilities to quit.[62,63]

Smoking cessation clinics and self-help groups have been developed for the general population. People with intellectual disabilities who smoke should have the opportunity to attend and participate in these, with additional support where needed. Modified therapy and interventions counselling may be necessary as part of a treatment programme tailored to individual needs. Cognitive behavioural therapy (CBT) approaches have been developed to assist smokers to quit, and include preparation to quit, coping with the challenges after quitting, and becoming a long-term non-smoker.[61-63]

Health screening programmes targeted at people with intellectual disabilities need to include a specific focus on smoking and the possibility of associated respiratory problems. Primary care and specialist intellectual disabilities health services, as a result of health screening, have the opportunity to identify people who require education and support to enable them to stop smoking. Assisting people with intellectual disabilities to stop smoking will bring about wider improvements in their health and avoid complications associated with cardiovascular disease.[64,65]

Consideration and recognition need to be given to the possibility of weight gain in a population that faces challenges with their weight. It is appropriate therefore to consider support for stopping smoking, in the wider context of a plan aimed at supporting healthy lifestyles and choices for people with intellectual disabilities.[65]

Medication options to help people with intellectual disabilities to stop smoking need to be considered carefully, to ensure that they are appropriate to the individual and that any additional support needs are identified and clearly set out and agreed by them and their carers in the patient's care plan. Ongoing review and monitoring are necessary.

References

59 McGuire BE, Daly P, Smyth F (2007). Lifestyle and health behaviours of adults with an intellectual disability. *Journal of Intellectual Disability Research*. 51: 497–510.

60 Gale L, Naqvi H, Russ L (2009). Asthma, smoking and BMI in adults with intellectual disabilities: a community-based survey. *Journal of Intellectual Disability Research*. 53: 787–96.

61 Kerr S, Lawrence M, Darbyshire C, Middleton AR, Fitzsimmons L (2013). Tobacco and alcohol-related interventions for people with mild/moderate intellectual disabilities: a systematic review of the literature. *Journal of Intellectual Disability Research*. 57: 393–408.

62 Singh NN, Lancioni GE, Winton AS, *et al.* (2013). A mindfulness-based smoking cessation program for individuals with mild intellectual disability. *Mindfulness*. 4: 148–57.

63 Taggart L, Cousins W, eds. (2014). *Health Promotion for People with Intellectual and Developmental Disabilities*. Open University Press: London.

64 Cooper SA, Morrison J, Melville C, *et al.* (2006). Improving the health of people with learning disabilities: outcomes of a health screening programme after 1 year. *Journal of Intellectual Disability Research*. 50: 667–77.

65 De Winter CF, Bastiaanse LP, Hilgenkamp TIM, Evenhuis HM, Echteld MA (2012). Cardiovascular risk factors (diabetes, hypertension, hypercholesterolemia and metabolic syndrome) in older people with intellectual disability: results of the HA-ID study. *Research in Developmental Disabilities*. 33: 1722–31.

Accidents

People with intellectual disabilities frequently experience accidents, falls, fractures, and trauma.[66-68] Accidents and falls are associated with epilepsy, the side effects of medication, such as anticonvulsants, visual impairment, impulsivity, and epilepsy, and are multifactorial. People with profound and multiple intellectual disabilities are at significant risk for fractures.[69]

Epilepsy is common in people with intellectual disabilities and can be related to specific syndromes and conditions such as Angelman syndrome, tuberous sclerosis, fragile X, Rett syndrome, and Down syndrome. Epilepsy has been implicated in contributing to injuries and sudden unexplained death in people with intellectual disabilities.[70] Seizures can result in fractures, subluxation, joint dislocation, and soft tissue injury. Fractures to the skull may result from trauma to the head following a seizure.[71]

It is now recognized that people with intellectual disabilities are more at risk of developing osteoporosis due to vitamin D deficiency and lower bone density than does the general population.[72,73] Osteoporosis can go unrecognized and may contribute to bone fractures that result from falls, nutritional issues, and the menopause.[73-75] There is also the possibility that fractures can occur even with very minor injury, and this needs to be borne in mind if people with intellectual disabilities stumble, trip, or fall. Women with intellectual disabilities are at risk of fractures and should be recommended to have bone density tests and medication to improve the bone's density.[75]

Nurses working in unscheduled care services, such as accident and emergency departments, need to be aware of the possibility of fractures. Detection and treatment of fractures are important, as they eliminate pain and suffering, as well as the possibility of deformity and reduction in functioning. Exercise, good nutritional supplements, and medication for the treatment of osteoporosis can reduce the progress of this disorder.

People with intellectual disabilities can experience mobility problems due to conditions such as cerebral palsy and severe intellectual disabilities.[69] Mobility problems may also be associated with disorders of the foot, which, if not treated, can contribute to falls and associated trauma and injury in this population. Older people with intellectual disabilities, as with the general population, are at risk of falls.

Nurses have an important contribution to make in collaborating with dieticians, physiotherapists, primary care colleagues, carers, and people with intellectual disabilities to minimize the impact of health conditions and associated complications, thereby helping to reduce the possibility of accidents that, in some circumstances, may result in further disability and can contribute, in extreme cases, to premature death.

References

66 Hsih K, Rimmer J, Heller T (2012). Prevalence of falls and risk factors in adults with intellectual disability. *American Journal on Intellectual and Developmental Disabilities*. 117: 442–54.

67 Finlayson J, Jackson A, Mantry D, Morrison J, Cooper SA (2015). The provision of aids and adaptations, risk assessments, and incident reporting and recording procedures in relation to injury prevention for adults with intellectual disabilities: cohort study. *Journal of Intellectual Disability Research*. 59: 519–29.

68 Wagemans A, Cluitmans J (2006). Falls and fractures: a major health risk for adults with intellectual disability in residential settings. *Journal of Policy and Practice in Intellectual Disability*. 3: 136–8.

69 Glick N, Fischer M, Heisey D, Leverson G, Mann D (2005). Epidemiology of fractures in people with severe and profound developmental disabilities. *Osteoporosis International*. 16: 389–96.

70 Kiani R, Tyrer F, Jesu A, et al. (2014). Mortality from sudden unexpected death in epilepsy (SUDEP) in a cohort of adults with intellectual disability. *Journal of Intellectual Disability Research*. 58: 508–20.

71 Camfield C, Camfield P (2015). Injuries from seizures are a serious, persistent problem in childhood onset epilepsy: a population-based study. *Seizure*. 27: 80–3.

72 Burke EA, McCallion P, Carroll R, Walsh JB, McCarron M (2017). An exploration of the bone health of older adults with an intellectual disability in Ireland. *Journal of Intellectual Disability Research*. 61: 99–114.

73 Jaffe J, Timell A, Elolia R, Thatcher S (2005). Risk factors for low bone mineral density in individuals residing in a facility for the people with intellectual disability. *Journal of Intellectual Disability Research*. 49: 457–62.

74 Vanlint S, Nugent M (2006). Vitamin D and fractures in people with intellectual disability. *Journal of Intellectual Disability Research*. 50: 761–7.

75 Schrager S, Kloss C, Ju AW (2007). Prevalence of fractures in women with intellectual disability: a chart review. *Journal of Intellectual Disability Research*. 51: 253–9.

Sexual health and personal relationships

People with intellectual disabilities are unique individuals who have their own relationships and friendship needs.[76,77] They are also sexual beings and have the right to express their sexuality, in line with their peers and all other members of society, but their sexuality and sexual health needs have historically been ignored, and their rights not recognized or ignored.

Young people and their parents

There is a need to include young people with intellectual disabilities in sex education programmes within schools, and materials have been developed to assist in this regard. Regardless of age, they should have accessible sexual health information that enables and supports them to make informed choices within their relationships.[78] Nurses have an important role in supporting and facilitating them to form relationships and express their sexuality. By working with small groups, nurses can support and develop understanding of puberty menstruation, masturbation, and contraception. It is important to recognize the needs of parents and differences in views and opinions that may be expressed by them regarding relationships and friendships that their adult son or daughter may form. Parents may have anxieties regarding the ability of their son or daughter to enter into sexual relationships and may be concerned about abuse and exploitation.

Women with intellectual disabilities

Women with intellectual disabilities have sexual and reproductive health needs. Additional support and education may be required by some young women at the onset of menstruation to enable them to understand and meet their personal care needs. Contraception and additional information that may be required to enable choices to be made by these women offer opportunities for nurses in sexual health services, primary care teams, and specialist intellectual disabilities teams to support these women. Sexually active women should attend regular cervical screening; women with intellectual disabilities are sometimes not included because it can be distressing and embarrassing, so nurses working in specialist services should work collaboratively with colleagues in primary care and sexual health services to overcome this. Women should attend for breast screening, and as this group is now living longer, breast screening is indicated, because there is the possibility of an increase in cervical and breast cancers.[79] Nurses should ensure that health screening programmes take account of their sexual health and contraception needs, and that they are included in national screening programmes.[80] As women age, they will also experience the menopause. Literature highlights a delay or absence of puberty in some women with intellectual disabilities, whereas others, as a result of syndrome-based conditions, may fail to produce sex hormones.

Men with intellectual disabilities

Men with intellectual disabilities have their own distinct sexual health needs, and yet many are not included in well-men activities, and this is an issue that needs to be addressed. Testicular cancer can occur in young men, and it is important to ensure that men with intellectual disabilities have the necessary knowledge and support to examine their testicles and seek help if indicated. As men age, there is a need to recognize the possibility of prostate disease and prostate cancer; all social and healthcare workers must ensure that their care needs are addressed within screening and well-men programmes, and they are given information, advice, and support about relationships, sexuality, their sexual health, and options for them to make informed choices.[81]

Sexual health and abuse in intellectual disabilities

People with intellectual disabilities who are sexually active may be at risk of developing sexually transmitted infections (STIs), such as gonorrhoea, syphilis, and chlamydia, and the possibility of human immunodeficiency virus (HIV) infection and hepatitis. It is important to recognize that they may enter into same-sex relationships, and this may bring with it an increased risk of STI.[82] People with intellectual disabilities have been victims of a range of abuses, and this includes sexual abuse.[83] As a result of their cognitive impairment and communication difficulties, perpetrators may target such people, and all social and healthcare workers need to be mindful of this and implement safeguarding procedures where indicated.

References

76 Scottish Government (2013). *The Keys to Life: Improving Quality of Life of People with Learning Disabilities*. The Stationary Office: Edinburgh.

77 Department of Health (2009). *Valuing People Now: A New Three-year Strategy for Learning Disabilities*. HMSO: London.

78 Schaafsma D, Kok G, Stoffelen JM, Curfs LM (2015). Identifying effective methods for teaching sex education to individuals with intellectual disabilities: a systematic review. *Journal of Sex Research*. 52: 412–32.

79 Cobigo V, Ouellette-Kuntz H, Balogh R, Leung F, Lin E, Lunsky Y (2013). Are cervical and breast cancer screening programmes equitable? The case of women with intellectual and developmental disabilities. *Journal of Intellectual Disability Research*. 57: 478–88.

80 Swaine JG, Dababnah S, Parish SL, Luken K (2013). Family caregivers' perspectives on barriers and facilitators of cervical and breast cancer screening for women with intellectual disability. *Intellectual and Developmental Disabilities*. 51: 62–73.

81 Merrick J, Morad M (2016). Men and their health. In: IL Rubin, J Merrick, DE Greydanus, DR Patel, eds. *Health Care for People with Intellectual and Developmental Disabilities Across the Lifespan*. Springer International Publishing: New York, NY; pp. 1359–64.

82 Stoffelen J, Kok G, Hospers H, Curfs LMG (2013). Homosexuality among people with a mild intellectual disability: an explorative study on the lived experiences of homosexual people in the Netherlands with a mild intellectual disability. *Journal of Intellectual Disability Research*. 57: 257–67.

83 Cambridge P, Beadle-Brown J, Milne A, Mansell J, Whelton B (2011). Patterns of risk in adult protection referrals for sexual abuse and people with intellectual disability. *Journal of Applied Research in Intellectual Disabilities*. 24: 118–32.

Gastrointestinal disorders

Gastrointestinal disorders are common in people with intellectual disabilities and increase with the severity of their disability.[84] GORD is experienced by some 70% of people with intellectual disabilities.[84] Gastric aspiration is associated with swallowing, nutritional, and feeding issues experienced by this population. As a consequence of GORD, people with intellectual disabilities, particularly those with cerebral palsy, scoliosis, and severe and profound intellectual disabilities, may regurgitate the acidic gastric contents up the oesophagus, which is then inhaled into the lungs. Material inhaled results in inflammation of the respiratory tract, which, in turn, results in pneumonia, which, if not promptly and effectively treated and managed, results in potentially avoidable death.[85] Trial treatments with proton pump inhibitors, such as omeprazole and lansoprazole, are indicated and should be instigated without an endoscopy.

It is important to identify and treat gastric disorders in people with intellectual disabilities, because they cause pain and distress and have been linked to cancers.[86] Nurses have an important role in working with carers, dieticians, physiotherapists, SLTs, and colleagues in gastroenterology units in general hospital services, to ensure that risk assessments are undertaken, and plans of care developed and implemented, thereby ensuring that nutritional and care needs are met.

Some people with intellectual disabilities may require nasogastric nutrition or a percutaneous endoscopic gastrostomy (PEG) tube (see ➔ PEG and PEJ feeding, pp. 198–200). This requires the surgical insertion of a tube into the stomach where it remains *in situ* and is used to provide nutrition. Nurses need to be familiar with the care needs of people with intellectual disabilities who have additional nutritional needs, and the safe management of the equipment they require. They also have a key role in providing education and support for carers and family members, and in reassessing care needs.[87]

H. pylori is a Gram-negative bacterial infection of the stomach lining and small intestine that, if untreated, results in gastritis and ulceration of the mucosal lining. It is more common in people with intellectual disabilities than in the general population, and many do not present with symptoms.[88]

Diagnosis is made by breath, blood tests, or endoscopy and biopsy, and obtaining specimens can be challenging.[89] It is treated with antibiotics; the infection can recur and further treatment may be required. Side effects are common.[90] Evidence suggests a link with an increased risk of stomach, oesophageal, and gall bladder cancers within this population.[86] Nurses need to be aware of the possibility of *H. pylori* within the intellectual disabilities population and of the presence of symptoms such as vomiting, weight loss, haematemesis, and melaena, which may indicate infection.[89] Good infection control measures are required, such as scrupulous attention to hand hygiene, and particular attention is required when dealing with faeces and salivary secretions to minimize the spread of infection.

References

84 Galli-Carminati G, Chauvet I, Deriaz N (2006). Prevalence of gastrointestinal disorders in adult clients with pervasive developmental disorders. *Journal of Intellectual Disability Research*. 50: 711–18.

85 Haveman M, Heller T, Lee L, Maaskant M, Shooshtari S, Strydom A (2010). Major health risks in aging persons with intellectual disabilities: an overview of recent studies. *Journal of Policy and Practice in Intellectual Disabilities*. 7: 59–69.

86 Emerson E, Baines S (2011). Health inequalities and people with learning disabilities in the UK. *Tizard Learning Disability Review*. 16: 42–8.

87 Liley A, Manthorpe J (2003). The impact of home enteral tube feeding in everyday life: a qualitative study. *Health and Social Care in the Community*. 11: 415–22.

88 Clarke D, Vemuri M, Gunatilake D, Tewari S (2008). *Helicobacter pylori* infection in five inpatient units for people with intellectual disability and psychiatric disorder. *Journal of Applied Research in Intellectual Disabilities*. 21: 95–8.

89 Wallace R, Philip J, Schluter P, Forgan-Smith R, Wood R, Webb P (2003). Diagnosis of *Helicobacter pylori* infection in adults with intellectual disability. *Journal of Clinical Microbiology*. 41: 4700–4.

90 Wallace R, Schluter P, Webb P (2004). Recurrence of *Helicobacter pylori* infection in adults with intellectual disability. *Internal Medicine Journal*. 34: 131–3.

Constipation

Constipation is characterized by difficulty in passing faeces, or a change in the usual bowel pattern. Having a bowel movement is a routine activity of daily living, although not necessarily occurring every day. The 'usual' bowel pattern varies between individuals. People with intellectual disabilities are more likely to be constipated than those in the general population.[91,92] There are a range of preventable factors that contribute to constipation with the intellectually disabled population.[93]

What are the causes of constipation?
- Inadequate fluid intake;
- Inadequate fibre in the diet;
- Limited physical activity;
- Side effects of medications;
- Associated with stress.

Factors associated with constipation and people with intellectual disabilities
- Not eating a balanced diet;
- Inadequate fluid intake and limited food choices, particularly when dependent on others;
- Less physical activity than is recommended;
- Side effects from medications that contribute to constipation;
- Over-reliance on laxatives and/or as-necessary medications to try and prevent constipation;
- Inability to communicate the urge to defecate or being thirsty;
- Problems with sitting on the toilet in the right position or to use the toilet safely;
- Problems with eating and drinking (dysphagia);
- Lack of understanding in carers of the effects of food and fluid on the bowel.

Bristol stool chart

This is a recognized general measure of consistency and form that is understood by many.[94] This tool classifies faeces into seven types, according to their appearance. Type 1 has spent the longest in the colon and type 7 the least time, with type 4 being the easiest to pass with little discomfort (see Fig. 6.1).

Think about?
- Fluid intake—adults require on average 2L of fluid per day. For further details, seek advice from a dietician about the best options to suit an individual to ensure they are fully hydrated.
- Food intake—all people with intellectual disabilities need to eat regular balanced meals that contain both soluble fibre, such as porridge oats, fruit, beans, lentils, baked beans, and insoluble fibre, including wholemeal bread, pasta, wholegrain breakfast cereals, and brown rice. Any increase in dietary fibre should be done gradually to prevent any abdominal discomfort. A healthy, well-balanced diet can contribute to the prevention of constipation.[95] A food diary over a 7-day period to monitor fluid and food intake may help, and seek advice from a dietician.

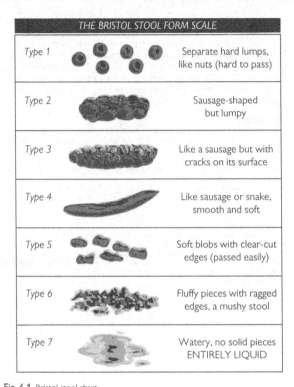

THE BRISTOL STOOL FORM SCALE	
Type 1	Separate hard lumps, like nuts (hard to pass)
Type 2	Sausage-shaped but lumpy
Type 3	Like a sausage but with cracks on its surface
Type 4	Like sausage or snake, smooth and soft
Type 5	Soft blobs with clear-cut edges (passed easily)
Type 6	Fluffy pieces with ragged edges, a mushy stool
Type 7	Watery, no solid pieces ENTIRELY LIQUID

Fig. 6.1 Bristol stool chart.
Reproduced by kind permission of Dr KW Heaton, Reader In Medicine at the University of Bristol.
© 2000 Norgine Pharmaceuticals Ltd.

- Position on the toilet—a person should be able to sit on the toilet comfortably, with their hips at right angle to the floor, and both feet on the floor or a firm base. See a physiotherapist or an occupational therapist for further advice.
- Increasing physical activity—increasing daily physical activity is a cost-effective way to help prevent constipation and improve overall health and well-being.[96] For those with profound and multiple intellectual disabilities, abdominal massage may be effective as part of a total bowel management programme.[94] Seek further advice from a qualified physiotherapist or a community nurse.
- Use of aperients—these can be prescribed, while dietary or other measures begin to take effect, for drug-induced constipation or when other measures fail. Aperients can be divided into four main groups; bulk-forming,

stimulant, faecal softeners, and osmotic laxatives. Discuss further with either a non-medical prescriber or a GP. It is important that these are reviewed once the food and fluids and physical activity have been increased.

- Privacy and dignity—recognizing the importance of privacy and the dignity of the individual needs to be considered when they are defecating. Consider how you might feel if defecating while someone was present and providing intimate personal care. What needs to be in place to ensure their privacy and dignity and protect their safety?

References

91 Carey IM, Shah SM, Hosking FJ, et al. (2016). Health characteristics and consultation patterns of people with intellectual disability: a cross-sectional database study in English general practice. British Journal of General Practice. 66: 264–70.

92 Cooper SA, Morrison J, Melville C, et al. (2006). Improving the health of people with intellectual disabilities: outcomes of a health screening programme after 1 year. Journal of Intellectual Disability Research. 50: 667–77.

93 Morad M, Nelson NP, Merrick J, Davidson PW, Carmeli E (2007). Prevalence and risk factors of constipation in adults with intellectual disability in residential care centers in Israel. Research in Developmental Disabilities. 28: 580–6.

94 Pawlyn J, Carnaby S, eds. (2009). Profound Intellectual and Multiple Disabilities: Nursing Complex Needs. Wiley: London.

95 Humphries K, Traci MA, Seekins T (2009). Nutrition and adults with intellectual or developmental disabilities: systematic literature review results. Intellectual and Developmental Disabilities. 47: 163–85.

96 Bartlo P, Klein PJ (2011). Physical activity benefits and needs in adults with intellectual disabilities: systematic review of the literature. American Journal of Intellectual and Developmental Disabilities. 116: 220–32.

Spirituality

Spirituality refers to those aspects of human experience that provide such things as meaning, hope, purpose, identity, value, love, and, for some people, a connection with the transcendent. Spirituality provides a way of looking at the world and of drawing attention to some important ways of being in the world that can easily be overlooked in our highly technologized society. Spirituality seeks to answer four key questions: Who am I? Where do I come from? Where am I going? Why? Some locate their spirituality within formal religion. For others, spirituality is found in such things as nature, friendship, work, community, and meaningful occupation. A person's spirituality is central for a healthy sense of wholeness, stability, wellness, security, hope, and peace. Spirituality comes sharply into focus at critical junctures in our lives, particularly when we face emotional stress, physical illness, or death.

Spiritual needs

Spiritual needs relate to the experiences that emerge from noticing the importance of spirituality in a person's life. These will include such things as the need for meaning and purpose, love, harmonious relationships, forgiveness, hope, trust, and the recognition of personal beliefs and values.

Spiritual care

At its simplest, spiritual care has to do with finding creative ways to meet the spiritual needs that are identified by patients in any given context. Spiritual care is not so much a set of competencies that a nurse has to learn. Rather it is the development of the kind of sensibilities that allow the nurse to be aware of the deeper dimensions that may be present in any caring encounter.

Narayanasamy (2001)[97] offers one way of formalizing spiritual care.

Assessment

Valuable information central to spiritual needs should be obtained from patients.

Planning

The information from a spiritual assessment may contribute to the formulation of spiritual care plans. When formulating the care plan, careful consideration should be given to the patient's individuality, the willingness of the nurse to get involved in the spirituality of the patient, the use of the therapeutic self, and the nurturing of the inner person (the spirit).

Implementation (giving spiritual care)

Implementation is about spiritual care intervention, based on an action plan that reflects caring for the individual. It is necessary to develop a caring relationship, which signifies to the person that he or she is significant. It requires an approach that combines support and assistance in growing spiritually.

Evaluation

As part of the evaluation, the following questions may be useful:
• Is the patient's belief system stronger?
• Do the patient's professed beliefs support and direct actions and words?
• Does the patient gain peace and strength from spiritual resources (such as prayer and minister's visits) to face the rigours of treatment, rehabilitation, or peaceful death?

- Does the patient seem more in control and have a clearer self-concept?
- Is the patient at ease in being alone? In having life plans changed?
- Is the patient's behaviour appropriate to the occasion?
- Has reconciliation of any differences taken place between the patient and others?
- Are mutual respect and love obvious in the patient's relationships with others?
- Are there any signs of physical improvement?
- Is there an improved rapport with other patients?[97]

Helpful as this framework may be, people should not think that once they have gone through this process, spiritual care has been done. Spiritual care is a way of being with people in deep and important ways, not a set of boxes to be ticked.

Further reading

Nonye Sango P, Forrester-Jones R (2014). Spirituality and learning disability: a review of UK government guidance. *Tizard Learning Disability Review*. **19**: 170–7.

Swinton J (2001). *Spirituality in Mental Health Care: Rediscovering a 'Forgotten' Dimension*. Jessica Kingsley Publishers: London.

References

97 Narayanasamy A (2001). *Spiritual Care: A Practical Guide for Nurses and Healthcare Practitioners*, 2nd edn. Quay Books: Wiltshire.

People with profound and multiple learning disabilities

Definition

The definition of adults with profound and multiple intellectual disabilities used in the Department of Health and Mencap in the UK[98,99] noted that people:

- Have a profound learning disability;
- Have more than one disability;
- Have great difficulty in communicating;
- Need high levels of support with most aspects of daily life and may have additional sensory and physical disabilities, complex health needs, or mental health difficulties and may have behaviours that challenge services.[98,99]

People with profound and multiple learning disabilities often face additional challenges in relation to aspects such as posture and mobility, dysphagia, respiration, epilepsy, hearing, vision, nutrition and hydration, continence, dental and oral hygiene, pain and discomfort, and access to health screening.[99] Mansell stated that good services for people with profound and multiple intellectual disabilities are individualized and person-centred, treat family carers as expert, focus on quality of staff relationships with the person with disability, are able to successfully sustain the package of care and are cost-effective.[98]

Assessment of abilities and needs

It is essential when undertaking a nursing assessment of a person with profound and multiple learning disabilities to pay careful attention to both their abilities and their needs. Assessment should be holistic, including physical, psychological, emotional, and spiritual needs. It should be particularly aware of the key areas noted above and ensure these are specifically addressed in any nursing assessment. Areas that may need to be addressed are the following:

- Firstly, seek to understand how the person communicates their wishes and needs. All people with profound and multiple learning disabilities are able to communicate in their own way, and family members will normally know this well. Learn how the person communicates emotions such as joy, interest, upset, distress, and worry in order to recognize these and act appropriately;
- Mobility—many people have difficulties with movement and control of posture. This can result in pain and breaks in the skin that need to be prevented or reduced. Specialized equipment may be required to aid mobility, support posture, and protect and restore body shape;
- Sensory disabilities—specialist assessment of how much a person can hear and see will be necessary;
- Respiratory system/breathing—often due to limited purposeful movement and physical disabilities of the chest or back, people will be at a greater risk of respiratory infections, and these can be very serious if not addressed promptly;

- Epilepsy—many people will have epilepsy, and therefore careful attention is needed to any clear triggers for seizures for that individual, an understanding of their 'normal' seizure type and pattern, and any medical or other intervention that may be required (see ➲ Epilepsy, pp. 160–1);
- Eating and drinking—some people are unable to take food by mouth and require gastrostomy feeding; others may experience severe swallowing difficulties, which must be assessed by an SLT. It is important to know what people's likes and dislikes in food are, as these are important factors to accommodate where possible. Oral and dental hygiene are also key aspects of nursing care;
- Continence and how this can be managed with most comfort and dignity for the person. Ensure any continence products are correctly measured for and comfortable for the person. These also need to provide proper protection for the person's skin.

Further detailed 'How to guides' covering 11 key areas directly related to working with people with profound and multiple learning disabilities are available at:[99] ℘ www.mencap.org.uk/advice-and-support/pmld

Learning

Despite having a profound intellectual disability, people can still learn throughout their lives, as long as appropriate and sustained efforts are made to provide individualized opportunities for learning. People may also be able to give consent for some decisions, and consent can be decision-specific. It is important to remember that staff are expected to start from a basis of presumed consent and seek to obtain this before moving to a position of taking best interests decisions.

References

98 Mansell J (2010). *Raising Our Sights: Services for Adults with Multiple and Profound Learning Disabilities.* Department of Health: London.
99 Mencap (2017). *Profound and Multiple Learning Disabilities.* ℘ www.mencap.org.uk/advice-and-support/pmld (accessed 30 October 2017).

Dysphagia

Dysphagia is a disorder of swallowing which may involve problems with any of the phases of a swallow, the reception and oral preparation of a bolus, the initiation of the reflexive swallow, and the pharyngeal phase, or the oe-sophageal phase.[100] Dysphagia can cause an increased risk of dehydration, malnutrition, respiratory tract infections, and aspiration and can lead to death. There is a significantly higher prevalence of dysphagia among people with intellectual disabilities, when compared to the general population, due to the impact of hypo-/hypertonia and poor coordination.[101]

The normal swallowing process

This involves three stages:
- Oral: food in the mouth is chewed, sucked, and mixed with saliva to create a bolus, to allow food to be swallowed;
- Pharyngeal: the swallowing reflex is triggered, allowing the bolus to be moved into the oesophagus. The epiglottis lowers to protect the airway and prevent aspiration of food;
- Oesophageal: the bolus is moved along the oesophagus towards the stomach by peristalsis.

Signs and symptoms of dysphagia

These include inability to recognize food and difficulty placing food in the mouth or controlling food or saliva and initiating a swallow.[101] Coughing, choking, frequent chest infections, unexplained weight loss, gurgly or wet voice after swallowing, regurgitation, and client complaining of swallowing difficulties can be indicative of dysphagia.[102] For those with communication difficulties, it is imperative that they are supported to communicate and discussion held with their carers. Dysphagia impacts in a variety of ways.[103]

Physical
- Inadequate nutrition, weight loss, dehydration, compromised skin;
- Integrity and oral health;
- Respiratory infections and physical exhaustion of the individual;
- Need for supplemental/enteral feeding;
- Parent/carer fatigue.

Social
- Diminished opportunity for social interaction;
- Social withdrawal by the individual and/or family;
- Unappealing presentation and choice of food;
- Support needs incompatible with specific environments, e.g. restaurants;
- Reduced time for social activities due to duration of meals;
- Restrictions on social activities of parents and siblings;
- Loss of social norms linked with milestones such as birthdays.

Psychological
- Anxiety and behavioural problems at mealtimes;
- Depression in the individual and/or the family/carers;
- Family stress, sibling conflict, and carer guilt;
- Embarrassment and loss of dignity;
- Emotional fatigue.

Management of dysphagia

For a further discussion, see Howseman (2013) and Dalton et al. (2011).[102,103]

- Where concerns exist, the individual should be referred to an SLT for full assessment.
- Dysphagia management procedures developed by the SLT should be strictly adhered to.
- Correct positioning in a chair, which provides head and trunk support, as required, assists in the oral preparation of a bolus and swallowing.
- The individual should be comfortable and free from distractions.
- Use verbal/non-verbal cues to direct the person's attention to eating.
- Use adaptive equipment and encourage independence during mealtimes using hand-over-hand techniques.
- Ensure food is presented in an appetizing manner, at an appropriate temperature; preparation of small amounts of food at a time may be advisable.
- Consistency of the food should be correct (pureed versus soft, thin versus thickened). If using commercial thickeners, follow manufacturers' directions. Observe for changes in food consistency; some foods become thicker/thinner as they heat up/cool down.
- Observe the person closely and allow time to eat; pace the intake of food to meet a person's needs. The person should remain upright for 30min after eating.
- Clear remaining food from a person's mouth when finished eating. Care of the oral mucosa is essential for people with dysphagia.
- Record dietary intake appropriately.
- Continuous assessment is required through direct observation and a diet history.
- Any deterioration, such as increase in incidences of aspiration, respiratory tract infections, and weight loss, may indicate the need for enteral feeding.
- Silent aspiration is difficult to detect; individuals present with recurrent respiratory tract infections, or pneumonia, which may be fatal. Video fluoroscopic swallow evaluation is required to identify silent aspiration.

References

100 Rubin L, Crocker A (2006). *Medical Care for Children and Adults with Developmental Disabilities.* Paul H Brookes Publishing Company: Baltimore, MD.
101 Howseman T (2013). Dysphagia in people with learning disabilities. *Learning Disability Practice.* 16: 14–22.
102 National Patient Safety Agency (2007). *Problems Swallowing Resources for Health Care Staff.* National Health Service: London.
103 Dalton C, Caples M, Marsh L (2011). Management of dysphagia. *Learning Disability Practice.* 14: 32–8.

PEG and PEJ feeding

Enteral tube feeding refers to delivery of a nutritionally complete feed into the intestinal tract through a tube. Enteral feeding is used when an individual is unable to meet their nutritional needs through oral intake alone and where the gastrointestinal tract is accessible and functioning and the intestinal absorptive function will meet all nutritional needs.[104] Enteral feeding requires insertion of a tube through a surgically created opening in the abdominal wall (see Tables 6.1 and 6.2 for further information on feeding methods and care of sites). A PEG involves the insertion of the tube directly into the stomach, whereas a percutaneous endoscopic jejunostomy (PEJ) involves the insertion of the tube directly into the jejunum.[104] A jejunostomy is preferable to a gastrostomy where a person has undergone upper gastrointestinal surgery or has severe delayed gastric emptying. [104] Issues and care of PEG/PEJ tubes and feeding regimens are similar.

Indicators for the use of PEG/PEJ feeding

- Aspiration, respiratory difficulties, dysphagia, limited gag reflex, poor appetite, cerebral palsy, presence of a cleft lip and palate, individual unable to meet nutritional requirements.

Advantages of PEG/PEJ feeding

- An effective means of long-term nutritional support. Ensures a person is adequately hydrated, enabling an individual to take in orally what they can, while ensuring adequate nutritional intake is achieved. It reduces the risk of aspiration and can be used during significant medical illness, and can be concealed by clothing; therefore, they are more cosmetically acceptable than nasogastric tubes.

Disadvantages of PEG/PEJ feeding

- Diarrhoea, constipation, nausea, vomiting, gastro-oesophageal reflux (associated more with PEG feeding);
- Invasive procedure, requires general anesthetic, wound infection, blockage, kinking or dislodgement of tube, can be difficult to relocate (associated more with PEJ feeding);
- Unnatural method of feeding, social element of mealtimes may be lost, loss of enjoyment and pleasurable experience of food;
- Rapid or excessive weight gain, continuous feeding (12–20h/day) may limit mobility and level of activity, care of oral mucosa may be overlooked.[105]

It is recommended that clinical monitoring of gastrostomy and jejunostomy be undertaken regularly[104] to assess for infection and to establish where in the gastrointestinal tract the tube tip lies. The tube size, type, insertion date, and method should be documented.

Methods of administering enteral feeds

• See Table 6.1 for a summary.[105]

Table 6.1 Methods of administering enteral feeds

Method of feeding	Advantages	Disadvantages
Bolus feeding	May reduce time connected to feed Very easy Minimum equipment required	May have increased risk of gastrointestinal symptoms May be time-consuming
Intermittent via gravity or a pump	Periods of time free of feeding Flexible feeding routine May be easier than managing a pump for some people	May have increased risk of gastrointestinal symptoms, e.g. early satiety Difficult if outside carers are involved with the feed
Continuous feeding via a pump	Easily controlled rate Reduction of gastrointestinal complications	Person connected to the feed for the majority of the day May limit the person's mobility

Administration of enteral feeds

• See Table 6.2 for a summary.[106]

Table 6.2 Gastrostomy or jejunostomy

Stoma site	Daily	To ensure site not infected/red, no signs of gastric leakage
Tube position (length at external fixation)	Daily	To ensure tube has not migrated from/into stomach and external over granulation
Tube insertion and rotation (gastrostomy without jejunal extension only)	Weekly	Prevention of internal overgranulation/prevention of buried bumper syndrome
Balloon water volume (balloon-retained gastrostomies only)	Weekly	To prevent tube from falling out
Jejunostomy tube position by noting position of external markers	Daily	Confirmation of position

Always confirm correct positioning of the tube for PEG using pH indicator strips; a pH of 5.5 or less indicates correct positioning of the tube. Before feeding, explain the procedure; gain consent and reassure the individual. Follow local policies and manufacturers' guidelines when administering the feed. The feeding regimen developed for the individual should be adhered to. After feeding, ensure the person remains seated in an upright position or with their head elevated for 30–40min to minimize the risk of aspiration. Assess skin integrity and report any signs of redness. Peristomal skin should be cleaned at least once a day with mild soap and water using a cotton swab or piece of gauze in a circular motion. The external fixation device should be rotated 390° and the skin underneath it should be cleaned; the skin should then be left to air-dry. Any indications of soreness, redness, swelling, or pain should be reported. Assessments and interventions should be documented.[106]

References

104 National Institute for Health and Care Excellence (2006). *Nutrition Support for Adults: Oral Nutrition Support, Enteral Tube Feeding and Parenteral Nutrition*. 🔗 www.nice.org.uk/guidance/cg32 (accessed 30 October 2017).

105 Dougherty L, Lister S (2015). *The Royal Marsden Hospital Manual Nursing Procedures*, 9th edn. Wiley-Blackwell Publishing: Oxford.

106 Kozier B, Erb G, Berman A, Snyder S, Harvey S, Morgan-Samuel H (2012). *Fundamentals of Nursing: Concepts, Process and Practice*. Pearson Education Ltd: London.

Nasogastric feeding

Nasogastric feeding is used to supplement feeding of individuals of all ages who have swallowing or feeding difficulties. It requires insertion of a disposable plastic feeding tube into the nose, extending into the stomach.[107] It is normally used on a short-term basis (2–4 weeks).[108]

Advantages

- Ensures adequate nutritional intake, allows individuals to take in orally what they can while ensuring adequate nutritional intake is achieved, ensures a person is adequately hydrated, reduces the risk of aspiration, less invasive procedure than gastrostomy, and can also be used as a trial prior to gastrostomy.

Disadvantages

- Diarrhoea or constipation, nausea, and vomiting;
- Erosion of nasal and oral mucosa, sinusitis, and/or nasal ulcers;
- Skin irritation from fixing the tube to the individual's cheek;
- Kinking/dislodgement, incorrect insertion of tube, aspiration;
- More 'visible' than gastrostomy, can cause distress when inserted, unnatural method of feeding, social element of mealtimes may be lost, long-term use can impact on swallowing and oral feeding.

Nasogastric care and feeding

Adhere to local health service and manufacturer's guidelines for use and disposal of nasogastric tubes.

Insertion of nasogastric tubes

- Explain the procedure to the person involved, and gain consent.
- Where possible, arrange a signal where the person can communicate discomfort to the nurse.
- Place the person in a semi-upright position, keeping the head well supported.
- Identify the length of tube required by measuring the distance on the tube itself to measure from the person's earlobe to the bridge of their nose plus the distance from the earlobe to the bottom of the xiphisternum.
- Wash your hands with bactericidal soap and water or bactericidal alcohol rub prior to gathering the required equipment, put on gloves, select the tube required.
- Follow manufacturer's guidelines when preparing the tube for insertion. For example, some indicate injecting sterile water down the tube or lubricating the proximal end of the tube with lubricating jelly.
- Check the nostrils are patent by asking the person to sniff with one nostril closed. Then repeat the procedure on the other nostril.
- Gently insert the rounded end of the tube into the nostril, and slide it backwards and inwards along the floor of the nose to the nasopharynx.
- If an obstruction is encountered, withdraw the tube and recommence in a slightly different direction. If the issue persists, use the other nostril.
- Unless swallowing is contraindicated, ask the person to swallow or to start sipping water as the tube travels into the nasopharynx.

- Continue to steadily pass the tube as the person swallows, until the desired length of tubing has been inserted. If the person shows signs of distress or cyanosis, immediately remove the tube.
- Then temporarily secure the tube to the person's cheek and behind the ear prior to checking that the tube is positioned correctly in the stomach.[108]

Confirming correct positioning of tube

- Either take an X-ray of the chest and upper abdomen; or
- Aspirate fluid from the tube (~0.5–1mL of aspirate will suffice). Place a few drops of the aspirate on a pH indicator strip, and allow 10–15s for any colour change to occur. Match the pH indicator strip with the colour code chart on the strip box. A pH of 5.5 or below indicates that the tube is correctly positioned, and feeding can start. A pH of 6 or above suggests that the tube may be incorrectly positioned. Recheck and the tube may need to be re-passed. Seek advice if the situation remains unchanged. Having confirmed the correct positioning of the tube, it must be attached securely with tape to either the left or right cheek. Observe the person for any adverse reaction to the insertion of the tube. It is essential to check the position of the tube before every feed. **If there is any query regarding the position and/or the clarity of the colour change on the pH strip, particularly between the range of 5 and 6, then feeding should not commence.**[108]

Feeding

Feeding via a nasogastric tube can take a variety of forms, including boluses and intermittent or continuous feeding (see ➔ PEG and PEJ feeding, pp. 198–200). If the person can take fluids and food orally, then feeding via a nasogastric tube should only be used to supplement oral intake. Particular attention should be given to oral hygiene, to alleviate mouth dryness. Care of the nasal mucosa is also important.

References

107 Batshaw ML, Pellegrino L, Roizen NJ (2007). *Children with Disabilities*. Paul H Brookes Publishing: Baltimore, MD.

108 Dougherty L, Lister S (2015). *The Royal Marsden Hospital Manual Nursing Procedures*, 9th edn. Wiley-Blackwell Publishing: Oxford.

Hearing

Feeling, emotions, knowledge, information, enthusiasm, and enjoyment can be established, strengthened, and developed through the medium of sound. Our hearing is used to gain large amounts of information about our environment and the people in it. If you close your eyes and listen, you will notice that there is a cascading stream of sounds around, all with something to offer. For this reason, it is very important to establish what a person can and cannot hear and how their hearing can be maximized. In developing and maintaining communication skills, information from all five senses is important. However, the main channels for communication are the distance senses of hearing and sight. Evidence suggests that up to 40% of people with intellectual disabilities have some level of hearing loss and that this often goes undiagnosed.[109] Hearing is vital for the development of spoken language. People with a pre-lingual profound hearing loss will not have access to speech sounds and therefore will not develop verbal communication.

Behaviours that may indicate hearing loss

- Watching the speaker's face and lips constantly.
- Tilting the head to one side towards the source of sound.
- Speaking loudly—this is typical of a sensorineural hearing loss where people raise their voice so that it is audible to themselves.
- Speaking softly—typical of conductive hearing loss where people match their own voices to the level at which they hear others.
- Appearing startled when someone approaches, particularly if they have not been seen approaching.
- Do not react to your requests or sounds in their environment.
- Need to have things repeated several times.
- Complain that they cannot hear as well as they used to.
- Dislike of loud sounds—people have a reduced range between the point where they can just hear sounds and the point where sound is perceived as unbearably loud.
- Complain about others mumbling.
- Pulling/poking the ears.
- Visible signs of discharge from the ears or excessive wax.

Causes of hearing impairment

- Conductive hearing loss—sounds have difficulty passing through the outer or middle ear; hearing loss is usually mild/moderate.
- Sensorineural hearing loss—the cause of the hearing loss is in the cochlea or auditory nerve; hearing loss is usually severe or profound.
- Mixed hearing loss—combination of both.
- Central: involves damage to the central nervous system.

Levels of hearing loss

The level of a person's hearing loss can vary considerably and is measured in relation to the hearing thresholds. There are four levels of hearing loss, ranging from mild hearing loss when it can be difficult for people to follow conversations in a noisy environment, through moderate (often need hearing aids) and severe hearing loss (difficulty in hearing continues even when using hearing aids, often needing to lip-read or using sign language), to profound hearing loss when a person needs to lip-read or use sign language.[110]

Communication

When communicating with someone with hearing loss, you need to be patient and take the time.[110] These are some of the things you can do to make communication straightforward for both of you.

- 'Even if someone is wearing hearing aids, it doesn't mean they can hear you perfectly. Ask if they need to lip-read.
- If you are using communication support, always talk directly to the person you are communicating with, not the interpreter.
- Make sure you have face-to-face contact with the person you are talking to.
- Get the listener's attention before you start speaking, maybe by waving or tapping them on the arm.
- Speak clearly but not too slowly, and don't exaggerate your lip movements—this can make it harder to lip-read.
- Use natural facial expressions and gestures.
- If you're talking to a group that includes deaf and hearing people, don't just focus on the hearing people.
- Do not shout. It can be uncomfortable for hearing aid users and it can be interpreted as aggressive.
- If someone doesn't understand what you've said, try saying it in a different way instead, don't keep repeating it.
- Find a suitable place to talk, with good lighting and away from noise and distractions.
- Check the person you're talking to is following you during the conversation. Use plain language, do not waffle, and avoid jargon and abbreviations.
- To make it easy to lip-read, don't cover your mouth with your hands or clothing.'

It should be remembered that hearing declines as we age, and this is equally so for those with intellectual disabilties.[111]

Further reading

Buskermolen WM, Hoekman J, Aldenkamp AP (2017). The nature and rate of behaviour that challenges in individuals with intellectual disabilities who have hearing impairments/deafness (a longitudinal prospective cohort survey). *British Journal of Learning Disabilities*. 45: 32–8.

McClimens A, Brennan S, Hargreaves P (2015). Hearing problems in the learning disability population: is anybody listening? *British Journal of Learning Disabilities*. 43: 153–60.

McShea L (2015). Managing hearing loss in primary care. *Learning Disability Practice*. 18: 18–23.

References

109 Action on Hearing Loss (2016). ℘ www.actiononhearingloss.org.uk (accessed 7 March 2018).

110 Action on Hearing Loss. *Glossary*. ℘ www.actiononhearingloss.org.uk/your-hearing/about-deafness-and-hearing-loss/glossary/levels-of-hearing-loss.aspx (accessed 30 October 2017).

111 Bent S, McShea L, Brennan S (2015). The importance of hearing: a review of the literature on hearing loss for older people with learning disabilities. *British Journal of Learning Disabilities*. 43: 277–84.

Integration of sensory experiences

There is an increased prevalence of sensory impairments within the population of people with intellectual disabilities, when compared with the general population.[112–114]

Hearing and visual impairments are common and may be apparent from birth. Others may be acquired in later life and may be associated with genetic conditions related to the cause of the intellectual disabilities, such as Down syndrome, where visual and hearing problems are common.[114,115] Some people with intellectual disabilities can experience congenital cataracts, retinal abnormalities, optic atrophy, or abnormalities of the eye structure that result in visual impairment.[116]

Access to assessment and remedial prosthesis and other treatments, such as cataract surgery, can be beneficial, and therefore early detection, treatment, and regular review are important and will contribute to reducing the possibility of accidents and injury resulting from visual impairments. Attention should also be paid to the sense of smell and touch, and there have been developments in the provision of therapies, such as reflexology and aromatherapy, provided for people with intellectual disabilities and cerebral palsy.

As people with intellectual disabilities are ageing and living longer, they will also experience visual changes and hearing loss associated with the ageing process.[114] The possible changing needs must be recognized, and routine health screening programmes provide an ideal opportunity for nurses to incorporate visual and hearing screening at the same time.

Effective screening and management can have positive benefits to the quality of life of the person with intellectual disabilities; barriers can exist, however, when undertaking assessment of vision and hearing.[117]

Nurses can play an important role in enabling access to visual and hearing assessments, and in ensuring there is support to adapt to their prosthesis, such as glasses and hearing aids, as well as educating carers of their importance.[114]

References

112 Robertson J, Hatton C, Emerson E, Baines S (2014). The impact of health checks for people with intellectual disabilities: an updated systematic review of evidence. *Research in Developmental Disabilities.* 35: 2450–60.

113 Meuwese-Jongejeugd A, Vink M, van Zanten B (2006). Prevalence of hearing loss in 1598 adults with an intellectual disability: cross-sectional population based study. *International Journal of Audiology.* 45: 660–9.

114 McCarron M, Swinburne J, Burke E, McGlinchey E, Carroll R, McCallion P (2013). Patterns of multimorbidity in an older population of persons with an intellectual disability: results from the intellectual disability supplement to the Irish longitudinal study on aging (IDS-TILDA). *Research in Developmental Disabilities.* 34: 521–7.

115 Määttä T, Määttä J, Tervo-Määttä T, Taanila A, Kaski M, Iivanainen M (2011). Healthcare and guidelines: a population-based survey of recorded medical problems and health surveillance for people with Down syndrome. *Journal of Intellectual and Developmental Disability.* 36: 118–26.

116 Evenhuis HM, Theunissen M, Denkers I, Verschuure H, Kemme H (2001). Prevalence of visual and hearing impairment in a Dutch institutionalized population with intellectual disability. *Journal of Intellectual Disability Research.* 45: 457–64.

117 Evenhuis H, van Splunder J, Vink M, Weerdenburg C, van Zanten B, Stilma J (2004). Obstacles in large-scale epidemiological assessment of sensory impairments in a Dutch population with intellectual disability. *Journal of Intellectual Disability Research.* 48: 708–18.

Oral health

Oral health refers to 'a standard of health of the oral and related tissues which enables an individual to eat, speak and socialize without active disease, discomfort and embarrassment and which contributes to general well-being'.[118]

People with intellectual disabilities experience poorer oral health than does the general population. In the past, oral disease was not given as much priority as other medical problems experienced by people with intellectual disabilities, despite the severity of the impact of oral disease on this population.[119]

Impact of oral disease

• Dental caries, coronal caries (of the crown part of the tooth);
• Root caries (of the root part of the tooth);
• Periodontal disease (of the gum and supporting bone);
• Lower number of natural teeth;
• Higher level of tooth extraction and lower levels of restorations;
• Significant pain;
• Inability to consume nutritious food;
• Poor quality of life (destruction of self-image, lack of confidence).

Oral disease has been linked to other systemic diseases such as:
• Cardiovascular disease;
• Cerebrovascular disease;
• Diabetes;
• Respiratory infection;
• Periodontal bone loss;
• Osteoporosis.

Specific factors such as bruxism (involuntary grinding of the teeth), altered salivary flow resulting in xerostomia (dry mouth), and hypertrophy or overgrowth of the gingival tissues, due to long-term use of certain medications, need to be addressed.[120]

Other factors such as congenital or developmental anomalies can impact on the ability of people with an intellectual disability to receive adequate personal and professional care.[121] Alongside these factors, other issues such as behaviours that challenge, mobility issues, neuromuscular issues affecting the oral cavity, gastro-oesophageal reflux, epilepsy, visual and hearing impairments, and latex allergies can further complicate oral health care for this population.[122]

Effective oral care

Oral assessment—simple oral assessment can be carried out by carers; healthy gums are firm in texture and do not bleed when brushed. Inflamed gums often bleed. Observe for changes in teeth such as cavities, trauma, or loose teeth. Observe the lips, gums, tongue, palate, and soft tissue of the oral cavity for damage and mouth ulcers. A full assessment by a dentist needs to be undertaken to identify signs and symptoms of oral disease, and they should undertake an annual review, whether or not they have teeth. People with intellectual disabilities may require an advocate or a HF to arrange dental visits and ensure an effective oral care plan is developed. A review of medical history should be undertaken prior to a dental appointment. Reasonable adjustments may be needed such as arranging an appointment to familiarize the individual with the dental surgery to reduce anxiety and stress. Keeping appointments short and only undertaking treatment that the person can tolerate at one visit may help promote cooperation.

An oral care plan should:[120,123]

- Ensure teeth are brushed effectively to ensure no part of the mouth is missed. If an individual has difficulty tolerating this, brush different parts of the mouth throughout the day;
- Record oral care appropriately, including any abnormalities noted;
- If a person can brush their teeth with assistance, this should be encouraged to promote independence;
- Skills training programmes can be developed to teach someone to brush their teeth;
- Adapt the toothbrush to make it easier to hold, e.g. buying a toothbrush with a bigger handle or attaching a foam handle to the brush may facilitate independence. An electric toothbrush may be of use in promoting independence;
- For those who cannot brush their teeth independently, when brushing teeth, always explain to them what is to happen, and gain consent;
- Brushing someone's teeth is an invasive procedure and can be frightening. Be aware of how long a person can tolerate having their teeth brushed; brush more frequently and for shorter lengths of time if required. Use pea-size amounts of toothpaste with fluoride. Be aware that some people may find toothpaste difficult to tolerate. If this is the case, brush with water instead;
- Stand behind and to one side of a person, gently drawing back the lips with the thumb and forefinger on one side of the mouth to gain access to teeth;
- Commence with the upper teeth; brush them with short back-and-forth motions, paying particular attention to the gum margins. Brush the inner and biting surfaces of all teeth as far as possible, and gently;
- Floss the teeth, or encourage the individuals to do this for themselves;
- Rinse the mouth, or clean with a damp swab. In some instances, a dentist may recommend a mouthwash to prevent cavities or manage gum disease;
- Good nutrition is required to ensure good oral health. No drinks (other than water) should be given after toothbrushing at night. It is important to remember that people with enteral feeding devices also require effective oral healthcare.

Medication can impact on oral health; over 400 medications cause xerostomia (dry mouth), and some antiepileptic therapy is linked to gingival overgrowth. Some medicines have high sugar content; 'sugar-free' options should be used.

References

118 Waldman B, Perlman S (2007). Oral health, nurses and patients with developmental disabilities. *International Journal of Nursing in Intellectual and Developmental Disabilities*. 3: 4.

119 Department of Health, Social Services and Public Safety (2005). *Survey of Dental Services to People with Learning Disabilities in Northern Ireland*. Department of Health, Social Services and Public Safety: Belfast.

120 Doyle S, Dalton C (2008). Developing clinical guidelines on promoting oral health: an action research approach. *Learning Disability Practice*. 11: 12–15.

121 Anders P, Davis E (2010). Oral health of patients with intellectual disabilities: a systematic review. *Special Care Dentist*. 30: 110–17.

122 National Institute of Dental and Craniofacial Research (2009). *Practical Oral Care for People with Developmental Disabilities*. National Institute of Dental and Craniofacial Research, National Oral Health Information Clearinghouse.

123 National Institute of Dental and Craniofacial Research (2012). *Dental Care Everyday. A Caregiver's Guide*. National Institute of Dental and Craniofacial Research, National Oral Health Information Clearinghouse.

Healthy skin

The skin is the largest organ of the body, covering 1.5–2.0m^2. It is made up of a number of layers and contains nerve endings, sweat glands, and blood capillaries.[124]

Functions of the skin

- Protects the body against noxious agents and infectious organisms;
- Helps to regulate the body temperature;
- Assists with the body's fluid and chemical balance;
- Sensitivity to pain, temperature, pressure, and touch;
- Production of vitamin D with exposure to sunlight;
- By being visible to the outside world, the skin is also integral to an individual's personal identification.

People with intellectual disabilities are at greater risk of suffering from skin complaints than the general population. For example, dryness and eczema is common in people with Down syndrome, and a variety of skin lesions and abnormalities are associated with phenylketonuria and tuberous sclerosis. An accurate nursing assessment and care are therefore essential to maintain good skin health for people with intellectual disabilities.

Nurses should remain very aware of the discomfort and annoyance dry or cracked skin can cause for people with intellectual disabilities. What appears to be a minor skin problem may cause itching, discomfort, and embarrassment, all of which may impact on a person's confidence, mood, enjoyment, and willingness to engage in social activities.

Assessment

Skin care is integral to person-centred health action planning. Assessment should be individualized and holistic and take account of personal preferences and cultural factors. Carers should be mindful of the impact of skin colour on the presentation of skin conditions. For example, lesions that appear red or brown in white skin may appear black or purple in pigmented skin, and mild degrees of redness (erythema) may be masked completely in black skin. Personal and intimate care can provide an opportunity for carers to assess the skin. People with intellectual disabilities who are able to carry out their intimate care independently should be educated to examine their skin and to report any worrying changes they notice to a carer or their GP. Assessment of the skin should include consideration of:

- Family history of skin disease;
- Medication and its side effects;
- Seasonal effects;
- Allergies and changes in the use of cleansing agents, washing liquid, and cosmetics.

Use of skin care products and cleansing agents

A balanced diet and drinking plenty of water are thought to be important for the health of the skin. Good personal and intimate care is also essential for maintaining the health of the skin, and the use of appropriate skin care products can promote healthy skin. Products should be chosen according to an individual's particular skin type and based on individual assessment and preference. Soap and perfumed products should be used with caution because they can cause dryness and irritation, and soap substitutes, known as emollients, are more suitable for many people. Dry skin can be itchy, sore, and unsightly. This can be reduced and prevented with the use of appropriate emollients and moisturizers. Excessive washing, use of detergents (such as soap), failing to remove soap from the skin, extensive soaking, and very hot bath water can cause dryness and lead to dermatitis.

Common skin conditions and their symptoms

- Eczema—dry, red, scaly skin that can be intensely itchy;
- Psoriasis—the most common forms appear as patches of silvery scales on top of areas of red skin;
- Leg ulcers—swelling, brown discoloration of white skin, presence of eczema;
- Pressure sores—initially appear as an area of red skin and feel warm and spongy or firm to the touch. In people with darker skin, the mark may appear to have a blue or purple cast, or look flaky or ashen. If pressure is not relieved, an open sore may develop that looks like a blister and, in advanced stages, can appear as a deep, crater-like wound;
- Herpes simplex—ulcers or sores, found particularly on the face, hands, and genitals;
- Dandruff—white, oily-looking flakes of dead skin appearing on the hair and shoulders, and an itchy, scaling scalp;
- Cellulitis—a bacterial infection resulting in redness, swelling, warmth, pain, and tenderness;
- A GP should be consulted for advice on specific skin complaints.[125]

Care of the skin in the sun

The risk of skin cancer as a result of over-exposure to the sun has been well documented and established. The risk can be greatly reduced by taking the following precautions:

- Stay out of the sun during the hottest part of the day. In the UK, this is usually 11 a.m. to 3 p.m. in the summer months. Never allow the skin to burn.
- Particular caution should be taken for people who are on psychotropics or any medication that can cause skin sensitivity to sunlight.
- Wear clothing made of cotton or natural fibres that are closely woven and offer good protection against the sun.
- Protect the face and neck by wearing a wide-brimmed hat.
- Use a high-factor sunscreen (SPF 30 or above) whenever you are exposed to the sun. Follow the instructions on the bottle, and reapply as recommended, particularly after swimming.
- Report changes to skin moles or unusual skin growths to the GP promptly.

References

124 Boore J, Cook N, Shepherd A (2016). *Essential of Anatomy and Physiology for Nursing Practice.* Sage Publications: London.
125 NHS Choices (2016). *Healthy Skin and Skin Conditions.* ℳ www.nhs.uk/Livewell/Skin/Pages/Skinhome.aspx (accessed 30 October 2017).

Personal and intimate care

Personal and intimate care includes a wide range of activities such as bathing and showering, dressing, changing continence pads, helping someone use the toilet, changing sanitary towels or tampons, shaving, skin care, hair care, and brushing teeth. Many people with intellectual disabilities are dependent on others for their personal and intimate care, which may be as a result of sensory disabilities or physical disabilities, which restrict movement and the ability to carry out fine and gross motor skills that are required for self-care. Good personal and intimate care is essential for health, hygiene, psychological well-being, and self-esteem. Personal and intimate care is carried out for hygiene, comfort, pleasure, and personal appearance.

Nurses may also find providing intimate care challenging[126] and must recognize and continue to remain sensitive to the intimate nature of much of the care they deliver and avoid seeing such care as routine because it may be undertaken frequently. They should also be very aware of the views and preferences[127] of the person with intellectual disabilities in relation to things such as how they would prefer to provide personal care, the gender of the staff involved, and which aspects of their personal care the person finds personally most intimate. Most services have local policies on personal and intimate care, and nurses should be aware of, and follow, these; there will also be clear guidance within the care standards set up by local care regulators[128] that must be followed.

Good hygiene

Ensuring the skin is kept clean will limit the amount of microorganisms present and reduce the risk of infections. It is important that hygiene of the genital and anal areas are given careful and sensitive attention, as the presence of bacteria and bodily fluids can increase the risk of infections and skin discomfort. Thorough hygiene is necessary to provide comfort and maintain dignity, as well as prevent infections in these areas.

Male hygiene

When attending to the hygiene of a person who is not circumcised, the foreskin needs to be pulled back in order to see the glans (or head of the penis). This should be washed carefully and then the foreskin extended again to cover the glans. There is a need to be careful to monitor any reaction to soap or other products used, as these may cause balanitis (inflammation and itchiness of the head of the penis), whereas poor hygiene can result in viral infections.

Female hygiene

Daily washing of the vulva and perineal area is important to reduce the risk of infections. When doing so, contact with soap and care need to be taken to avoid the internal mucous membranes, as these can be damaged by soap or other solutions for external only use, including deodorants. When selecting clothes for the person, ensure they have enough room to move comfortably and that their clothes are not too tight. Always observe the condition of the skin when the person is wearing synthetic material, as these can contribute to irritation and potentially vulvitis. When washing a person, in order to reduce the risk of movement of potentially harmful microorganisms, it is important to wash them from front to back. Carefully attention should also be given to skinfolds of the abdomen and underneath the breasts due to these being areas that can develop redness and other skins problems. These areas should be washed and then care taken to make sure these are dried.

Assessment and planning

Nursing care should be planned on the basis of a nursing assessment of a person's abilities and needs, with attention to their physical and cognitive abilities, as well as their personal preferences. Other issues that need to be considered when assessing and planning care are:

- Informed consent and capacity to consent;
- Maintaining and promoting privacy and dignity;
- Building and maintaining independence in personal care—consider possible aids, adaptations, and reasonable adjustments to assist;
- Particular needs around continence care;
- Choice of products after bathing to keep the skin supple and smooth).

Cultural and religious considerations

In Hindu, Muslim, and Sikh religions, physical cleanliness is extremely important. Many people who belong to these religions have a preference for washing under running water; for these people, showering is more appropriate than bathing. Modesty is important, particularly for women; legs and upper arms may need to be covered. The necessity for washing rituals prior to prayer time may need to be considered. In the Muslim faith, genitals are washed with the left hand, because the right hand is used for eating. In Sikhism, hair and beards may need to be kept uncut; men and women fix their hair on their head with a plastic comb known as a 'kangha'. Hair should not be cut without permission of the person or family.

Risk assessment, policies, and training

Areas that need to be addressed in risk assessments, policies, and training include:

- Prevention of abuse, and cross-gender care;
- Epilepsy and environmental safety (e.g. water temperature, need for slip mats);
- Moving and handling;
- Infection control (use of gloves, aprons, and good hand hygiene).

Good practice tips

- Be discrete when talking about incontinence to others and in front of others; prepare the environment and ensure all items are close to hand.
- Respect dignity at all times, e.g. do not undress the person until the last minute when they need to be undressed, and use appropriate communication strategies, use short sentences and objects of reference.
- Be aware that the person may have sexual wishes. If they indicate by touching themselves, they would like to be alone, and if it is safe to do so, provide the person with time alone in private.
- Intimate and personal care can be used as an opportunity for close observation of the health of the skin and may also provide opportunities for one-to-one communication.

References

126 Crossan M, Matthew TK (2013). Exploring sensitive boundaries in nursing education: attitudes of undergraduate student nurses providing intimate care to patients. Nurse Education in Practice. 13: 317–22.
127 O'Lynn C, Krautscheid L (2011). How should I touch you? A qualitative study of attitudes on intimate touch in nursing care. American Journal of Nursing. 111: 24–31.
128 Health Information and Quality Authority (2014). Guidance for Designated Centres: Intimate Care. Health Information and Quality Authority: Dublin.

Continence

Definition
Continence is the voluntary control over urinary and faecal discharge. Failure to achieve or maintain continence is referred to as 'incontinence' and is the involuntary loss of urine or faeces. Incontinence ranges from occasional leakage to an inability to control voiding; it may be a short-term or a longer-term issue, depending on the reason.

Prevalence
Prevalence of incontinence is difficult to determine because a variety of definitions have been used, and also because of the stigma associated with it. Incontinence can happen to anyone and occurs across all age groups. It is, however, more common in older age. People with intellectual disabilities are recognized as a group of people at greater risk of incontinence.[129] Among people with intellectual disabilities, continence is more likely to be delayed later into childhood, and some people remain incontinent throughout adulthood. Incontinence is more common in people with intellectual disabilities than in the general population, particularly among people with more severe intellectual and physical disabilities.

Causation
Continence is dependent on hormonal, muscular, and neurological control. Incontinence is therefore associated with a variety of conditions, and the primary cause for people with intellectual disabilities is likely to be related to the nature of their intellectual and/or physical disability. Neurological and physical disabilities can be the root causes of incontinence and UTIs, and renal abnormalities can exacerbate the problem. Many people with intellectual disabilities may have problems achieving continence if they are unable to understand the biological signals for urination and defecation. There may also be psychological and behavioural reasons for failing to urinate and defecate appropriately.

The cause of incontinence among people with intellectual disabilities should be investigated, consistent with national guidance.[129,130] It should not be considered inevitable or unresponsive to interventions at any age. Nurses need to provide opportunities for people to develop and maintain continence to whatever degree is possible. This may range from the person being able to signal the need to go to the bathroom or staff prompting people to use the toilet.

Assessment
Assessment should:
- Be individualized, dignified, and holistic and lead to a person-centred treatment package;
- Be made by an interdisciplinary team, which might involve a GP, a community nurse, a continence advisor, a physiotherapist, and carers;
- Identify underlying problems and the type of incontinence;
- Comply with national guidelines;[129,130]
- Include consideration of mobility and physical and mental health;
- Involve the measurement of fluid and dietary intake and output;
- Determine bladder and bowel habits and patterns.

Consider also the following factors, which may contribute to incontinence:
- Medication;
- Constipation/diarrhoea;
- Lack of access to toilet facilities and lack of privacy;
- Difficulties with psychomotor skills needed for undressing and using the toilet independently.

Treatment

Incontinence is often viewed as an inevitable consequence of having intellectual disabilities, and therefore treatment is not always prioritized or even considered. However, with assessment, planning, and appropriate support, many people with intellectual disabilities have a real chance of becoming continent. A training programme for incontinence might include:
- Positive reinforcement for appropriate voids;
- Teaching skills required for dressing and undressing;
- Regulating fluid and dietary intake;
- Making toilet facilities accessible;
- Training in pelvic floor exercises to increase muscle control for continence.

Management of incontinence

Good, person-centred, and intimate care is essential when caring for someone who has incontinence. This involves prompt skin care after defecation to reduce odour and skin problems. Brisk rubbing should be avoided to prevent damaging the skin, and moisturizing cream or ointment can be applied to protect the skin from future exposure to urine and stool. Appropriate use of continence aids, such as the correct size of pads, is important. Catheterization can be considered and may be successful for people with neurological conditions.

The impact of incontinence

Incontinence can have serious effects on physical, psychological, and emotional well-being, both for the person and their carers, including:
- Increased risk of skin infections and perineal dermatitis and discomfort;
- Reduced independence and problems with access to social opportunities, school, and work, and difficulties with accessing the community for extended periods of time due to limited changing facilities;
- The effects of stigma from a society that tends to undervalue people who have not mastered continence;
- Shame, embarrassment, depression and anxiety, lowered self-esteem, and negative body image;
- Barriers to sustaining relationships and leading a sexually fulfilling life;
- Physical, practical, emotional, and financial burden to carers and the family; dealing with incontinence can be unpleasant and is a factor that may lead to a request for residential care.

References

129 NHS England (2015). *Excellence in Continence Care*. NHS England: Reading. ℳ www.england.nhs.uk/commissioning/wp-content/uploads/sites/12/2015/11/EICC-guidance-final-document.pdf (accessed 30 October 2017).
130 National Institute for Health and Care Excellence (2015). *Urinary Continence in Women*. ℳ www.nice.org.uk/guidance/cg171/chapter/1-Recommendations#assessment-and-investigation (accessed 30 October 2017).

End-of-life care, preferred place of care

Planning for the future

On approaching the end of life, it is important to consider preferences regarding where people wish to be cared for. Most people would prefer to die at home, but many do not and are admitted to hospital in the last few days or hours of life.[131] Reasons for this in the general population are complex but are compounded in marginalized groups (such as people with intellectual disabilities) who may lack the ability to fully understand, make informed, personal choices, or articulate their own needs and wants at this difficult time.

End-of-Life Care Programme

Patients who are dying should have access to palliative care and opportunities for a good death in the place of their choosing. The Department of Health's End-of-Life Care Programme recognized the importance of patient involvement in aiming to reduce the number of unnecessary admissions to hospital. It supports nationally recognized tools for end-of-life care, including the five Key Priorities of care,[132] which remain important if death is likely to be imminent. The five Key Priorities include:

- A recognition and communication that death is imminent, with decisions made in accordance with the person's needs and wishes;
- The use of sensitive communication to the patient and family;
- Active involvement of the patient and those important to them in any decision-making process, as directed by the patient themselves;
- The needs of families and others important to the patient are explored, respected, and met wherever possible;
- An individual care plan is agreed, coordinated, and delivered, including the support of eating, drinking, symptom assessment and management, and psychological, social, and spiritual support.

Such Key Priorities should be '*relevant and accessible to everyone*' and are supported by NICE (2015) guidance.[133]

Advance care planning

The ACP is a tool to record patient preferences and priorities in relation to care and place of death. Belonging to the patient, the ACP recognizes that views are likely to change. The ACP is a generic tool and does not easily translate across to those who may have communication impairments such as people with intellectual disabilities. The ability of care staff involved to facilitate the ACP process and the person's ability to communicate clearly needs to be assessed. Patients should be supported to make informed (often difficult) choices about sensitive issues. Communication at this level should be facilitated in the most appropriate manner suitable for each person and their circumstances. Those closest to the person can be supported by palliative care professionals to sensitively record the needs of the individual at this time in the ACP or other appropriate document.

Issues for people with intellectual disabilities

Marginalized groups, such as people with intellectual disabilities, have an increased risk of disenfranchised death, resulting from a lack of autonomy and choice and social exclusion, particularly at the end of life.[134] Challenges to reciprocal communication and processing complex information and limited writing skills can make end-of-life choices around patient preferences difficult for both the staff and the patient. A multidisciplinary team using a person-centred approach[135] and supporting the carers will facilitate expression of options for that individual. In domiciliary settings, the team usually consists of community nurses, specialist nurses, matrons, and the patient's GP. People with intellectual disabilities may have already expressed their options to those closest to them or have been engaged in processes where they have reflected on their own losses and formed an opinion about their future care.

Person-centred approaches

Discussions with people with intellectual disabilities should not be left until death is imminent, but held as early as possible following a diagnosis or prognosis. Person-centred approaches to care planning promote inclusion, civil rights, and independence for people with intellectual disabilities. Person-centred planning and palliative care share similar philosophies—adopting a holistic approach, placing the person at the centre of the palliative care process, and incorporating active listening throughout. HAPs and essential lifestyle plans are well suited to providing holistic end-of-life care.[136]

Compassionately supporting people with intellectual disabilities to make choices at the end of life may not be easy. Shared values across different professional groups will promote collaborative working to support and help individuals to die in places of their own choosing. Further research around this topic should inform a sound evidence base for future development and support.

Further reading

European Association for Palliative Care (2015). *Consensus Norms for Palliative Care of People with Intellectual Disabilities in Europe (EAPC White Paper)*. European Association for Palliative Care: London. ℘ www.eapcnet.eu/LinkClick.aspx?fileticket=lym7SMB78cw%3D (accessed 30 October 2017).

NHS England. *End of Life Care*. ℘ www.england.nhs.uk/ourwork/ltc-op-eolc/improving-eolc/ (accessed 7 March 2018).

References

131 Higginson IJ (2003). *Priorities and Preferences for End of Life Care in England, Wales and Scotland*. National Council for Palliative Care: London.

132 Leadership Alliance for the Care of Dying People (2014). *One Chance to Get it Right*. ℘ wales. pallcare.info/files/One_chance_to_get_it_right.pdf (accessed 5 March 2018).

133 National Institute for Health and Care Excellence (2015). *Care of Dying Adults in the Last Days of Life*. ℘ www.nice.org.uk/guidance/ng31 (accessed 30 October 2017).

134 Read S (2006). Communication in the dying process. In: S Read, ed. *Palliative Care for People with Learning Disabilities*. Quay Books: London; pp. 93–106.

135 Department of Health (2001). *Valuing People: A New Strategy for Learning Disability for the 21st Century*. Department of Health: London.

136 Read S, Elliott D (2006). Care planning in palliative care for people with intellectual disabilities. In: B Gates, ed. *Care Planning and Delivery in Intellectual Disability*. Blackwell Publishing: Oxford; pp. 195–211.

Medicines management

Many people with intellectual disabilities may be prescribed medication for physical health conditions which they may need to take for the short or long term. These medications should be prescribed following an assessment of the person's abilities and needs and because it is believed that the medication will be of benefit to the person with intellectual disabilities. The medication will be prescribed by a suitably qualified person who has successful completed the necessary education and assessment for medical prescribing or independent and supplementary prescribing as required by their professional regulator. Prescribed medication can be an important aspect of the provision of effective healthcare within a wider bio-psycho-social model of care.

Nurses' overall responsibility in relation to medication

Both the NMC (UK) and the NMBI (Republic of Ireland) have published standards relating to the administration and management of medication. These standards are reviewed on an ongoing basis, and therefore nurses should be aware of the current guidelines from their professional regulator and ensure they are working within the most current document, which they should obtain directly from the professional regulator's website (ஃ www.nmc.org. uk/standards/additional-standards/standards-for-medicines-management/ and ஃ www.nmbi.ie/Standards-Guidance/Current-Projects/Medicines-Management). These standard documents are extensive and clearly state the expected level of practice of nurses across key areas such as: method of supplying and/or administration of medicines, dispensing, storage and transportation, standards for practice of administration of medicines, delegation, disposal of medicinal products, unlicensed medicines, complementary and alternative therapies, management of adverse events (errors or incidents) in the administration of medicines, and controlled drugs.[137]

Nurses' responsibility in relation to the administration of medication

This is largely consistent across professional regulators about the standards of administration of medication. These reflect ten key points that underpin the safe administration of medication in hospital, community settings, and residential and nursing homes. These include:[137,138]

- You must be certain of the identity of the person to whom the medicine is to be administered;
- You must check that the person is not allergic to the medicine before administering it;
- You must know the therapeutic uses of the medicine to be administered, and its normal dosage, side effects, precautions, and contraindications;
- You must be aware of the person's plan of care (care plan/pathway);
- You must check that the prescription or the label on the medicine dispensed is clearly written and unambiguous;
- You must check the expiry date (where it exists) of the medicine to be administered;

- You must consider the dosage, weight where appropriate, method of administration, route, and timing;
- You must administer or withhold in the context of the person's condition and coexisting therapies, e.g. physiotherapy;
- You must contact the prescriber or another authorized prescriber without delay where:
  - Contraindications to the prescribed medicine are discovered;
  - The person develops a reaction to the medicine;
  - Assessment of the person indicates that the medicine is no longer suitable;
- You must make a clear, accurate, and immediate record of all medicine administered, intentionally withheld, or refused by the person, ensuring the signature is clear and legible; it is also your responsibility to ensure that a record is made when delegating the task of administering medicine.

When working with people with intellectual disabilities, a challenge can at times occur when obtaining informed consent (see ➔ Consent to examination, treatment, and care, pp. 506–7) and ensuring reasonable adjustments and accessible resources are available to assist people in understanding the relevant information. When working with psychotropic medication, further attention is required due the potential added risks of these medicines (see ➔ The undesired or side effects of psychotropic medication, pp. 344–5).

References

137 Nursing and Midwifery Council (2008, updated 2015). *Standards for Medicines Management*. Nursing and Midwifery Council: London. (This document is being updated at the time of writing; please refer to the NMC website for the latest version.)

138 Health Improvement and Quality Authority (2015). *Medications Management Guidance*. Health Improvement and Quality Authority: Dublin.

Independent nurse prescribers in intellectual disability

Non-medical prescribing (NMP) is an area of advanced practice within nursing. It has seen extensive developments in primary care and is evolving within other areas of practice, including intellectual disability and mental health nursing. There is currently a small cohort of learning disability nurses in intellectual disability services working as NMPs across the UK. They are involved in prescribing a range of medications within their specialty to meet the individual's physical health needs such as epilepsy and mental health needs. Nurses within these areas have developed enhanced knowledge relating to the assessment and pharmacological interventions for the health needs in which they prescribe.

Becoming an NMP

In order to become an NMP prescriber, nurses must have 3yrs post-qualifying experience and complete an NMC-approved Independent and Supplementary Nurse Prescribing course.[140] The course is assessed both academically and through supervised clinical practice by a medical practitioner. On completion of the course, the nurses can work as independent or supplementary prescribers. It is common practice that the nurse will work as a supplementary prescriber for a period of time, prior to progressing to independent prescribing.

- **Supplementary prescribers** work in partnership with a medical practitioner through the use of a clinical management plan (shared care plan). This plan will provide information on conditions for treatment, medications that can be prescribed by the NMP, and any specific details regarding the name of the medication, reason for prescribing the medication, dose schedule, and specific indications for referral back to the medical practitioner.
- **Independent prescribers** hold all of the accountability for the assessment of the health needs of the individual and for the clinical decisions that they make relating to the individual's care, including prescribing practice. They are therefore prescribing independently of medical prescribers.

Prescribing in intellectual disability

People with an intellectual disability have a higher incidence of health needs and often experience multiple health needs, leading to an increased risk of polypharmacy.[141] NMPs in intellectual disability nursing must apply specialist knowledge and skills in evidence-based assessment of the individual's needs in order to ensure assessments are accurate. This can present as a significant challenge due diagnostic overshadowing, communication difficulties, and reliability on information from informants. Accurate diagnosis is the foundation for identifying the correct intervention. NMPs must be highly competent within their specialty and are accountable for maintaining and updating their knowledge and skills and prescribing practice. To do this, NMPs will develop their personal formulary of medications that they are competent to prescribe. Although NMPs may specialize in a particular health need and prescribe certain groups of medication to meet that health need (i.e. mental health or epilepsy), they must ensure that they have a good under-standing of other medications and how medications interact with one another.

It has been identified that people with an intellectual disability are being prescribed psychotropic medication without a clear diagnosis of mental illness.[141,142] This is often due to behaviours that are challenging. There is currently a strong move to reduce inappropriate or unnecessary prescribing of these powerful medications, unless there is a clear clinical indication for their use and a sound evidence base for prescribing.[142] Medical prescribers and NMPs must consider social and psychological interventions, to help reduce reliance on medication. There is a clear role for NMPs to work with psychiatrists and GPs, to ensure that regular medication reviews are undertaken, where appropriate medication is discontinued or reduced, and that there is an accurate assessment and diagnosis prior to introducing medication.

Advantages of NMP in intellectual disability nursing

There are a range of benefits of NMP in delivering care to people with an intellectual disability. These include:

- Increased knowledge of medication and how medication interacts with the physiological systems of the body.
- The intellectual disability nurse developing a therapeutic relationship with the individual and providing increased opportunities to review medication and to make clinical decisions relating to bio-psycho-social interventions and prescribing practice.
- Working in partnership with medical prescribers in assessing and titrating medication safely and effectively.
- Increased autonomy for the NMPs.

References

139 Bhaumik S, Gangadharan SK, Branford D, Barrett M (2016). *The Frith Prescribing Guidelines for People with Intellectual Disability*. Wiley-Blackwell: London.

140 Nursing and Midwifery Council (2015). *Standards of Proficiency for Nurse and Midwife Prescribers*. Nursing and Midwifery Council: London. (This document is being updated at the time of writing; please refer to the NMC website for the latest version.)

141 Public Health England (2015). *Prescribing of Psychotropic Drugs to People with Learning Disabilities and/or Autism by General Practitioners in England*. Public Health England. London. ℘ www.gov. uk/government/publications/people-with-learning-disabilities-in-england-2015 (accessed 30 October 2017).

142 Royal College of Psychiatrists (2016). *Psychotropic Drug Prescribing for People with Intellectual Disability, Mental Health Problems and/or Behaviours that Challenge: Practice Guidelines*. Royal College of Psychiatrists: London. ℘ www.rcpsych.ac.uk/pdf/FR_ID_09_for_website.pdf (accessed 30 October 2017).

Mental health and emotional well-being

Introduction

Mental health

Good mental health is integral to general health and well-being, which highlights the bio-psycho-social aspects to good health. Current mental health services are underpinned by a 'recovery'-based approach.[1,2]

Mental health relies on an individual's positive sense of self and is intertwined with our sense of self-purpose. Good mental health provides us with the ability to cope with both positive and negative life events. This includes our abilities to develop and sustain relationships, to learn and adjust to new environments and situations, and to interact with other people and the world around us.

Everyone has mental health needs. These needs and their causes are unique to each individual. When mental health needs go unmet, the individual is vulnerable to developing mental health problems.

Mental health problems

Mental health is concerned with self-concept, emotion, perception, and cognition. It frequently manifests in human behaviour, which can be difficult to measure because of its subjectivity and varying behavioural norms that occur across cultures and societies. The term 'mental health problems' implies a deterioration in an individual's functioning in areas such as cognition, emotions, thoughts, and behaviour, which has a negative impact on their overall functioning.

Classification of mental health problems

There are a range of symptoms that affect mental well-being. These can be clustered to form formal mental health diagnoses. The most widely recognized systems of classifying mental disorders, and guidelines for their diagnosis, are:

- International Classification of Diseases, 10th revision (ICD-10) classification of mental and behavioural disorders: clinical descriptions and diagnostic guidelines[3] (used in UK clinical practice—ICD-11 due for release in 2018);
- DSM-5: Diagnostic and Statistical Manual of Mental Disorders, 5th edition.[4]

These manuals, in turn, group the different types of diagnoses into related sections. The example below is from ICD-10:

- Organic disorders—dementias, delirium;
- Psychotic disorders—schizophrenia;
- Mood disorders—depression, bipolar disorder;
- Neurotic disorders—anxiety disorders, post-traumatic stress disorder;
- Behavioural syndromes— eating disorders;
- Personality disorders.

Both ICD-10 and DSM-5 are commonly used with people with intellectual disabilities, although problems have been noted in their application because of a number of reasons, including: atypical presentation, poverty of experience, and ability of, or opportunity for, an individual to express themselves.

This occurs across the range of abilities, but particularly in people with severe and profound intellectual disabilities. To address this, specialist diagnostic systems have been developed for this population:

- DC-LD: diagnostic criteria for psychiatric disorders for use with adults with learning disabilities.[5]
- DM-ID-2: a clinical guide for the diagnosis of mental disorders in persons with intellectual disabilities.[6]

These systems, however, continue to be noticeable by their absence in general mental health settings where most people referred may have mild intellectual disabilities, in which case ICD-10 or DSM-5 can be used.

Mental health and people with intellectual disabilities

Only over recent decades has it been accepted that people with intellectual disabilities can develop mental health problems just as the wider population. Studies have shown that people with intellectual disabilities are at increased risk of developing mental health problems. This vulnerability is thought to be due to the combination of developmental, biological, psychological, and social factors that people with intellectual disabilities are more likely to encounter in their lives. The impact of mental health problems on people with intellectual disabilities can significantly affect quality of life, as the individual may not detect or understand changes or indeed the significance of what is happening to them. It is vital that registered nurses in intellectual disability services have an understanding of what good mental health is and how to promote and maintain this, as well as an understanding of mental health issues affecting the people to whom they provide services. This will include the ability to recognize atypical presentations of mental health problems and will involve carers, family, and friends who know the individual well.

There is an increasing body of evidence showing the importance of early intervention in supporting people with mental health problems. Interventions need to be proactive and include interventions and/or support aimed at promoting mental well-being and detection and assessment of mental health problems. This requires nurses supporting individuals with intellectual disabilities to know the range of interventions and services available, as well as the relevant legislation.

References

1 Slade M, Longden E (2015). Empirical evidence about recovery and mental health. *BMC Psychiatry*. 515: 285.
2 Shepherd G, Boardman J, Slade M (2008). *Making Recovery a Reality*. Sainsbury Centre for Mental Health: London.
3 World Health Organization (1992). *ICD-10 Classification of Mental and Behavioural Disorders: Clinical Descriptions and Diagnostic Guidelines*. World Health Organization: Geneva. (Keep up-to-date on ICD-11 updates at: www.who.int/classifications/icd/revision/en/)
4 American Psychiatric Association (2013). *Diagnostic and Statistical Manual of Mental Disorders*, 5th edn. American Psychiatric Association: Arlington, VA.
5 Royal College of Psychiatrists (2001). *DC-LD: Diagnostic Criteria for Psychiatric Disorders for Use with Adults with Learning Disabilities/Mental Retardation*. Gaskell: London.
6 National Association for the Dually Diagnosed (2017). *DM-ID-2: Diagnostic Manual–Intellectual Disability*. National Association for the Dually Diagnosed: New York, NY.

Promoting emotional well-being

In contrast to the promotion of physical health, the promotion of emotional well-being of people with intellectual disabilities has been given much less coverage and priority. Promoting mental health and emotional well-being is recognized as very important for everyone, and NICE have used the following definitions:[7]

- Emotional well-being—this includes being happy and confident, and not anxious or depressed;
- Psychological well-being: this includes the ability to be autonomous, problem-solve, manage emotions, experience empathy, and be resilient and attentive;
- Social well-being: to have good relationships with others, and not having behavioural problems, i.e. not being disruptive, violent, or a bully.[7]

Many factors can impact on a person's ability to develop and maintain emotional well-being. ➔ Factors contributing to mental health problems, pp. 242–3 identifies the bio-psycho-social factors that contribute to this population developing high levels of psychiatric disorders. For many people, spiritual well-being is also an important aspect of their mental health (see ➔ Spirituality, pp. 192–3). In addition to these inter-related risk factors, there are further issues that need to be acknowledged:

- **Professional barriers**: primary healthcare professionals may have limited experience, less confidence, limited clear referral systems in working with people with intellectual disabilities. There may also be unlikely to utilize specific health screening tools and also may have difficulty in communicating with people with intellectual disabilities;
- **Societal barriers**: stereotypical views that people with intellectual disabilities inevitably develop mental health problems, and limited political willingness to provide supportive services that seek to promote and maintain recovery;
- **Individual barriers**: personal attributes, personality traits, strengths, and protective factors. People with intellectual disabilities may lack the knowledge required of what to do when feeling unwell and where to go and seek help;
- **Carer barriers**: many people with intellectual disabilities are dependent upon family and carers to identify the symptoms of when they are unwell and make a prompt referral to a GP. However, many of these carers may not recognize the early indications/triggers.

These professional, societal, individual, and carer barriers may prevent the person with intellectual disabilities from being proactive about accessing professional advice and receiving adequate levels of support, early screening, assessment, and treatment.

Models of promoting emotional well-being

Proactive measures are considered to have an important impact on preventing the onset of mental health problems, and where mental health problems do arise, proactive measures can help to reduce their severity and the potential need for crisis management. Nurses should have a clear awareness and understanding of the risk factors that may predispose the person to develop mental health problems and use this knowledge in the development of proactive and preventative individualized and group interventions

A plan for promoting emotional well-being

- Increased use and development of targeted group-based programmes to promote mental health that focus on:
  - Promoting positive self-esteem and empowerment;
  - Developing the person's ability to make informed choices, and promoting advocacy balanced with person-centred risk management;
  - Ensuring effective receptive and expressive communication with individuals and groups, so people can speak up for themselves;
  - Providing environments where individuals feel safe and secure;
  - Ensuring and enhancing feelings of achievement and success;
- Promotion of mental health should become a routine component of assessment and care planning for every person seen; identifying those most at risk by utilizing early screening tools such as the PAS-AAD Schedules (see ➲ Screening of mental health problems, pp. 96–7);
- Informal and formal carers receiving health promotion information and training to identify warning signs earlier; likewise people with intellectual disabilities having access to health promotion material in a format that they can understand;
- Ensuring optimal physical health, adequate leisure, exercise, and physical exercise by participation in more community and group activities;
- Developing and maintaining positive relationships and friendships with peers, including positive family connections;
- Improving and facilitating access to mainstream primary and mental health services;
- Education, awareness, and support from specialists within the intellectual disability field to primary care and mental health services;
- Effective management of transition and loss;
- Developing specific relapse prevention plans for individuals who are particularly vulnerable or in the stage of recovery from a specific mental health problem.

Further reading

Campbell MA, Gilmore L (2014). The importance of social support for students with intellectual disability: an intervention to promote mental health and well-being. *Cypriot Journal of Educational Sciences*. **9**: 21–8.

Taggart L, Cousins W (2014). *Health Promotion for People with Intellectual and Developmental Disabilities*. Open University Press: Maidenhead.

References

7 National Institute for Health and Care Excellence (2013). *Social and Emotional Wellbeing for Children and Young People. Local government briefing [LGB12]*. ℘ www.nice.org.uk/advice/lgb12/chapter/Introduction (accessed 30 October 2017).

Promoting assertiveness

Being able to assert oneself is a skill many take for granted. Assertion is the ability to communicate confidently in a socially appropriate manner, clearly making your points and respecting the rights of others, and being able to do so without becoming upset. Effective communication happens in a cycle; someone needs to be able to communicate their point of view and to have this responded to appropriately.[8] If someone feels that they are not being listened to, they might respond in a number of ways. They might simply give up, or they might compensate through other behaviours, e.g. withdrawal, aggression, or avoiding situations. Therefore, having the ability to assert oneself is integral to human communication in order to feel valued and to have one's needs met. The ability to assert oneself can fluctuate, depending on internal factors such as mood or level of health, and it is also context-specific. People may lack assertion in certain situations, such as at a medical appointment, but not in others, e.g. at home or with friends where assertion may not be an issue or a problem.

People with intellectual disabilities, like everyone else, will encounter difficult situations, and it is important they are able to communicate effectively. People may talk to their family and carers, rather than them, or they are treated as if they are a child, naïve, or incompetent, or they might find themselves in situations where they feel bullied and/or abused.

The individual's expectations in any given situation will be informed usually by their previous experience or preconceived ideas that may or may not be realistic and will be influenced by a number of factors, including thought disorder, limited previous experience, or difficulty in understanding the complexity of any given situation and following closely what is being said, verbally and non-verbally.

Developing assertiveness

Assertiveness training normally uses cognitive behavioural and self-help techniques. It will include techniques to address the overt behavioural components of assertion, including the content of the message, but also vocal characteristics, non-verbal behaviours, and social interaction skills.[9,10]

Assertiveness should facilitate and enable a person to
- Respond in difficult situations in an appropriate manner.
- Build confidence and self-esteem.
- Engage in longer-term treatment on a more equal footing.
- Replace verbal and physical maladaptive communication behaviours.

Assertiveness programmes use a number of techniques, including
- Structured role play, providing repeated opportunities to practise.
- Using their own experiences to re-enact and learn from positive feedback and the opportunity to rehearse future behaviours.
- Homework to set goals that recognize areas to improve and practise scenarios.

Assertiveness training can be facilitated in groups or individually, within a structured programme that will encompass educational issues around social skills, such as how people might conduct themselves, how to handle feelings, and coping with daily events, and then, within these scenarios, looking at more positive ways of expressing feelings, abilities, and needs. Other strategies that may be adopted include the individual having aids to complement the programme such as a prompt cards tailored to them. This might give guidance on how to cope in difficult situations, or it may be used to help the person practise difficult situations in a systematic manner. Using a solution-focused approach can allow the person to identify what they wish to achieve from an interaction and to identify the steps they need to take to reach this.

Assertiveness training is designed to help the individual through positive and social reinforcement, to enable them to learn new skills, and also to maintain these with the added bonus of increasing self-confidence, effectiveness, and self-esteem. It also develops self-awareness to enable the individual to recognize and manage, as much as possible, their own emotions within the scenario and to recognize behaviours that are not assertive or helpful.

In seeking to support and enhance the assertiveness of people with intellectual disabilities, nurses should encourage and provide opportunities to practise communication skills that reflect the following:

- A positive solution-focused orientation, and not presuming the outcome;
- Listening to the other person and following what is being said;
- Knowing what the individual wants to say and saying it;
- Focusing on the topic, and not what the individual thinks about the other person;
- Being direct but not rude; focus on the person's action, and not judging them as a person;
- Helping the individual to recognize if they are becoming upset and having a way to effectively manage this.

References

8 Hargie O (2017). *Skilled Interpersonal Communication: Research, Theory and Practice*, 6th edn. Routledge: London.

9 Rakos R (2006). Asserting and confronting. In: O Hargie, ed. *The Handbook of Communication Skills*, 3rd edn. Routledge: London; pp. 345–81.

10 SkillsYouNeed. *Assertiveness: An Introduction.* www.skillsyouneed.com/ps/assertiveness.html (accessed 30 October 2017).

Supporting people with intellectual disabilities in general mental health services

People with intellectual disabilities have the right to use the same mental health services as any other citizen, and this is reflected in policy across the UK, the Republic of Ireland, and internationally. This policy has not been met without apprehension, from professionals in both general mental health services and intellectual disability services. Current policy recognizes that some people will require specialist intellectual disability services for their mental health, though the majority of people will use general health services, with or without extra support. There is a changing role for intellectual disability services, moving towards a tertiary role, to offer expertise and support and facilitate movement within and between services by providing advice and support to general mental health services. There are still issues in accessing these services, as discussed in the following sections below, along with ideas on how they can be addressed.

Care pathways

Service boundaries and eligibility criteria have been problematic for people with intellectual disabilities and mental health problems trying to access services, with many ending up with no service, until they reach crisis point. Many services are addressing this issue by developing joint protocols. This is where both general mental health services and intellectual disability services develop a care pathway for people with intellectual disabilities to access general health services, when possible, with both parties offering advice and support where needed.

Vulnerability

Like anyone else, people with intellectual disabilities may be vulnerable at times within general mental health services, but this does not automatically indicate exclusion. It is expected within equality legislation that reasonable adjustments are made to support people access general service, and this would also involve any vulnerability being risk-assessed and managed. The risk to each person should be assessed and plans should be put in place to minimize the risk; if this cannot be achieved, then intellectual disability services should be available until general mental health services make the necessary provision.

Developing confidence, knowledge, and skills among staff

Staff in general mental health services often believe they lack the skills or knowledge to support people with intellectual disabilities. This can be due to a lack of confidence and experience and a perceived fear of the unknown, although it is likely that staff who have supported people with mild intellectual disabilities are often unaware of this, as the person may not have had a formal diagnosis or attended a special school.

The use of general mental health services has been stated policy in the UK for over a decade, and although some progress is being made, it is less than accessing primary care and general hospital services. Staff in intellectual disability services can support further developments by providing advice in some key areas and helping the transfer of skills:[11]

- Rights and values of people with intellectual disabilities to general mental health services;
- Recognizing the incidence of mental health problems and, at times, atypical presentation;
- Strategies for interviewing people and reducing the risk of suggestibility and acquiescence;
- Recognition of associated unmet physical health needs;
- Adapting therapeutic interventions, e.g. simplification of cognitive behavioural techniques;
- Being aware of unwanted effects of treatment, e.g. side effects such as susceptibility to seizures;
- Supporting people with ASC;
- Range of intellectual disability services available.

Communication

Many people with intellectual disabilities will have specific communication needs, some of which are very apparent and others which can be easily overlooked. Making sure that communication is pitched at the appropriate level is essential for ensuring an equal relationship between the person using the service and staff. Also, it is a requirement that any information provided about local services, the person's rights, and treatments available are produced in an accessible format.

An example in practice

One example of how the inclusion agenda is being driven forward is the Green Light Toolkit[11] in England. It is primarily an audit tool that examines how well services are working together to meet the mental health needs of people with intellectual disabilities. It is based on a traffic light scoring system and offers examples of how services can be improved. It is a tool that should be used in partnership with those using services, their carers, and other local services.

Further reading

Hardy S, Chaplin E, Woodward P (2010). *Mental Health Nursing of Adults with Learning Disabilities*. Royal College of Nursing: London.

References

11 National Development Team for Inclusion (2013). *Green Light Toolkit (2013): A Guide to Auditing and Improving Your Mental Health Services so that it is Effective in Supporting People with Autism and People with Learning Disabilities*. Department of Health: London.

Primary care

Primary care is defined by the WHO as the first-line intervention that is provided as an integral part of general healthcare and mental healthcare by primary care workers who are skilled, able, and supported to provide mental health services.[12] Primary care is usual the entry point to the healthcare system and is part of the stepped care model of assessment delivery and monitoring of treatments (see ➔ Primary Care, pp. 348–9), so in primary care services, the most effective, yet least, resource-intensive treatment is delivered to patients first, with referral on to intensive/specialist services if clinically required. There is no single primary care model, and how services are delivered is subject to wide variation within and across countries. This means access to evidence-based mental health assessment and treatment cannot be taken for granted. Primary care is responsible for referral to access to the wider range of specialist healthcare services, usually through the GP. An example of referral within primary care services for people with mental health problems might be referral to diabetes or cardiac services for those at risk from the side effects of psychotropic medications.

Primary care and mental health

For people with mental health problems, primary care should be the first point of call, this generally being their GP. It is estimated that, in the wider population, 20–25% of all appointments concern a mental health issue.[13] The focus on primary care is often on prevention and early intervention and can offer a wide range of services to people with mental health needs, including mental health promotion, advice, education and support, assessment, interventions such as low-level psychological interventions or medication, and referral to secondary mental health services. Prevention of mental health problems is divided into three levels:

- Primary—preventing illness, health promotion;
- Secondary—early identification and treatment;
- Tertiary—early intervention to promote recovery and prevent relapse.

Primary care is able to meet the needs of people presenting with a wide range of mental health problems, most commonly assessing and treating those with anxiety and depressive disorders. People with more acute and complex needs or presenting with severe/enduring mental health problems, such as chronic schizophrenia or bipolar disorder, are likely to be referred on to secondary mental healthcare services. However, many people do not access primary care services for their mental health issues, worried that they would be wasting their GP's time or due to a lack of confidence that the GP would be able to help. A good primary care mental health service[13] should be based on the underpinning principles of:

- The primary/secondary interface should not interrupt care, cause delays, or exclude people because of rigid access criteria;
- There should be a systematic process of organizing allocation to, and progress along, care pathways in primary care settings;
- All healthcare professionals should understand what collaborative care means;
- GPs must have the confidence and resources to treat people with mental disorders themselves.

Primary care, mental health, and people with intellectual disabilities

Part of the focus of primary care is to encourage self-management. However, it is known that people with intellectual disabilities[14] may be less likely to be offered health screening services (i.e. cancer) and access to health promotion services such as exercise and advice on smoking, alcohol, and mental and sexual health. Although there is inequality accessing health services, there are many examples of positive action such as the introduction of annual health checks, emotional well-being, and training programmes for primary care professionals, and the development of nurse liaison posts has gone some way to redress this balance. Another issue is that, in some services, some of the treatments offered may inadvertently exclude people with intellectual disabilities because of the assumed cognitive level required and lack of reasonable adjustment needed for them to take part. This is particularly true of low-level psychological interventions. People with intellectual disabilities have higher rates of mental health problems than the general population, often with complex physical health comorbidities, which may necessitate referral to secondary mental or physical health services for specific aspects of the individual's care and treatment, to improve overall management and prognosis. People with intellectual disabilities should be able to access primary care for their mental health, with or without the advice and support of learning disability services.

References

12 Funk M, Ivbijaro G (2008). *Integrating Mental Health into Primary Care: A Global Perspective*. World Health Organization/World Organization of Family Doctors: Geneva.

13 Joint Commissioning Panel for Mental Health (2012). *Guidance for Commissioners of Primary Mental Health Care Services*. ℘ www.jcpmh.info/good-services/primary-mental-health-services/ (accessed 30 October 2017).

14 Improving Health and Lives: Learning Disability Observatory, RCGP, and RCP (2012). *Improving the Health and Wellbeing of People with Learning Disabilities: An Evidence-Based Commissioning Guide for Clinical Commissioning Groups* (CCGs). Improving Health and Lives: Learning Disability Observatory: Durham. ℘ www.rcgp.org.uk/learningdisabilities/ (accessed 30 October 2017).

Secondary care

Access to secondary mental health services is initially via a primary care referral, though once known to services, often patients will access secondary service directly, with the person's GP being kept informed. There are a few services that are self-referrals such as walk-in or emergency clinics.

Examples of secondary mental healthcare services

Community mental health teams (CMHTs)

Throughout the UK and the Republic of Ireland, community services are delivered locally in most areas through interdisciplinary CMHTs. They can be accessed by any adult of working age, who has a severe and/or enduring mental health problem. CMHTs provide assessment, support, and a range of treatment options. In some rural areas, CMHTs may see people with a full range of mental health problems. However, many areas are now developing sub-specialty teams, which are described in the sections below. There are similar CMHTs for children and adults: child and adolescent mental health services (CAMHS) (<18yrs), and CMHT for older adults (>65yrs)

Assertive outreach teams (AOTs)

Some people with mental health problems present with complex needs, may be at a higher risk of relapse, or have a history of disengaging with services (e.g. substance misuse). AOTs are specifically designed to support these individuals, offering a more intense style of intervention.

Home treatment/crisis resolution teams

These teams offer an alternative to hospital admission for those who are in the acute phase of mental illness. Treatment and support are offered in the least restrictive environment, normally the individual's home. They respond rapidly to people in crisis and can offer a wide range of support and interventions. They also facilitate early discharge from hospital, offering a home-based support package.

Early-onset psychosis teams

Early-onset psychosis teams are designed for young adults (generally 18–35yrs) who are experiencing a first episode of psychosis. Their aim is to provide an individually tailored package of care that will facilitate access to services, promote recovery, support people to adapt to their mental health problems, and reduce the likelihood of relapse.

Inpatient services

Most people receive mental healthcare in the community. A small minority, such as those either in crisis or experiencing a severe/acute episode, may need hospital admission, particularly where there is a risk to self or others. Acute inpatient services are available throughout the country and can be based on a general hospital site. They are staffed by nurses, with input from psychiatry, occupational therapy, psychology, and other professionals. Admission is voluntary, wherever possible, but in some instances people may be detained under mental health legislation. Inpatient services work very closely with community services, trying to ensure a smooth transition home.

Secondary care intellectual disability services

Commissioners need to work in partnership with local authorities to ensure that vulnerable groups, including those with intellectual disabilities and autism, receive appropriate high-quality care.[15,16] In recent years, a lack of appropriate services have seen people receiving treatment outside of their local area, as they fall between gaps in local services. There is still a need to provide required reasonable adjustments within local mental health services; this is a legal obligation for health providers. To address this, clinical outcomes have also focused on the safety and acceptability of services and those who support them to provide person-centred care pathways tailored to the needs of the individual.

In terms of current provision, most areas will have some type of community team for people with intellectual disabilities (some may only work with adults) and many will offer inpatient admission, as required, to general mental health services. The extent to which mental health teams currently meet the needs of people with intellectual disabilities is variable, as many can lack awareness of the clinical presentation of mental disorders in people with intellectual disabilities. Some areas have a specialist CMHT for people with intellectual disabilities, which are attached to local mental health services.

These joint working models in secondary care can be positive in terms of more effective care and provision of reasonable adjustment and provide the following benefits:

- Identifying links between intellectual disability and secondary care services;
- Assisting with communication strategies;
- Supporting a person-centred planning approach;
- Working collaboratively to facilitate valid consent;
- Developing training programmes for secondary care staff on meeting the health needs of people with intellectual disabilities;
- Producing awareness and educational resource packs for secondary care services;
- Supporting the development of joint protocols and care pathways to ensure a smooth transition between services.

References

15 Department of Health (2012). *The Mandate: A Mandate from the Government to the NHS Commissioning Board: April 2013 to March 2015*. Department of Health: London. ℘ www.gov.uk/government/publications/the-nhs-mandate (accessed 30 October 2017).
16 Joint Commissioning Panel for Mental Health (2012). *Guidance for Commissioners of Primary Mental Health Care Services*. ℘ www.jcpmh.info/good-services/primary-mental-health-services/ (accessed 30 October 2017).

Tertiary care

Tertiary services are specialized health services that are provided by statutory or independent providers. These services tend to cover regional and/or national areas. They are for those people who need highly specialized care and, in regard of mental health, those with the most serious or complex needs that cannot be treated appropriately in local secondary services. The need for such services has been explored with service and policy reviews across the UK.[17,18]

As well as offering expert assessment and treatment, many tertiary services can fulfil wider functions that will support local services in their development and provide an evidence base that will influence practice across other services. This knowledge can be disseminated in a number of ways, including education and training, research, and consultancy.[19]

There is much debate as to when a service is classified as a tertiary specialist, rather than a sub-specialist linked to secondary care services; identifying characteristics would include a separate management structure. Such services are, to a greater or lesser degree, self-financing, generating income from external organizations, i.e. the commissioning or purchasing of beds. Some will provide secondary care services within their locality, while also providing similar care on a regional or national basis at a tertiary level, e.g. forensic, challenging behaviour, and autism services. Tertiary services are also referred to as level 4 services. Tertiary services may be defined by the client group they service or the condition that is their focus of the services such as autism, epilepsy or secure-services mental illness, behaviour problems, and offending behaviour. Tertiary services can be either inpatient or community-based. However, there should be effective pathways to ensure that the aim is to ensure once treatment is finished, the person accesses local secondary and primary care services.

Nursing roles within tertiary services

Nurses within tertiary services are employed increasingly in a variety of roles. These include working within specialist clinical inpatient settings, e.g. forensic, or clinics for people with specific conditions, such as autism or ADHD, and offer specialist assessment and/or treatment at a regional level in some areas. Some services will be used in other roles that promote collaboration through dissemination of specialist skills through training and consultancy, e.g. audit or service evaluation. They may also provide academic and skills-based training programmes to local services, including adult mental health and residential services in areas such as intellectual disability awareness, risk assessment, or assessment and treatment strategies. The aim is to support these services to develop their own skills and knowledge base on the way to providing greater collaboration and a more defined care pathway.

Specialist intellectual disability services

Specialist services are defined within the Specialized Services National Definitions Set; intellectual disability was removed from version 3 and is incorporated into a number of service types, including mental health and autism, as well as child and adolescent categories. As part of the Health and Social Care Act 2012, the responsibility for the commissioning of NHS services was charged to the CCGs.

Traditionally, tertiary services for people with intellectual disabilities were dominated by the treatment of severe mental health problems and people who are referred as a result of offending or offence-type behaviours that cannot be addressed by general mental health services. The provision of tertiary services for specific conditions such as autism or severe challenging behaviour is also increasing. The transforming care agenda, which came about following abuse of patients at Winterbourne View and the inappropriate admission of people to assessment and treatment units, has seen a shift away from tertiary inpatient services being a long-term option and the development of appropriate local crisis and community services.

For this to become a reality, there needs to be progress to reduce the health inequalities experienced by people with intellectual disabilities by minimizing the impact of:[20]

- 'Exposure to social determinants of poorer health such as poverty, lack of personalized, meaningful activity, poor housing, unemployment, and social isolation;
- Health problems—including those associated with specific genetic and biological conditions associated with learning disabilities;
- Personal health risks and behaviours such as self-harm, poor diet, and lack of exercise;
- Communication difficulties and reduced understanding of health issues (health literacy);
- Deficiencies related to access to healthcare provision.'*[20]

References

17 Department of Health (2001). *Valuing People: A New Strategy for Learning Disability for the 21st Century*. Cm 5086. HMSO: London.

18 Department of Health and Social Services and Public Safety (2005). *Equal Lives: Review of Policies and Services for People with Learning Disability in Northern Ireland*. Department of Health and Social Services and Public Safety: Belfast.

19 The Estia Centre. ♂ www.estiacentre.org (accessed 30 October 2017).

20 Improving Health and Lives: Learning Disability Observatory, RCGP, and RCP (2012). *Improving the Health and Wellbeing of People with Learning Disabilities: An Evidence-Based Commissioning Guide for Clinical Commissioning Groups (CCGs)*. Improving Health and Lives: Learning Disability Observatory: Durham. ♂ www.rcgp.org.uk/learningdisabilities/ (accessed 30 October 2017).

* Extracted from Improving Health and Lives: Learning Disability Observatory, RCGP and RCP (2012) with permission from the Royal College of General Practitioners.

Prevalence rates

There are three main groups of population-based studies (or epidemiological studies) into the prevalence of psychiatric disorders among people with intellectual disabilities:

- Studies that examined people with intellectual disabilities in hospitals—prevalence rates were found to vary between 60 and 100%;
- Studies that examined people referred to community psychiatric clinics—prevalence rates were again found to vary between 60 and 100%;
- Community samples of adults with intellectual disabilities were reported to be between 14 and 50%.

These studies clearly show that people with intellectual disabilities are significantly more likely to develop a psychiatric disorder, compared with the general population.[21]

Similar international studies have reported that children and adolescents with intellectual disabilities living with their natural families were also likely to have a psychiatric disorder, compared with their non disabled peers. Prevalence rates were 31–50%. These figures contrast sharply, compared with those reported for young people 10–15yrs without intellectual disabilities of 9%.[21]

Difficulties in obtaining accurate prevalence rates

Such discrepancies in obtaining accurate prevalence rates are a result of a combination of methodological difficulties and issues pertaining to people with intellectual disabilities and third-party informants:

- Depending on the level of intellectual disabilities (i.e. mild or severe/profound), diagnosis may or may not be achieved;
- For people with limited or no communication skills, accurate diagnosis becomes more difficult;
- How the information is gathered either from family/staff or from the person with intellectual disabilities;
- Methodological problems related to what is meant by a 'psychiatric disorder' or a 'mental health problem';
- The type of classification system used to diagnose a psychiatric disorder (i.e. ICD-11, DSM-V, or DC-LD).[22]
- The different assessment methods used to identify such clinical conditions (i.e. case records, screening tools, e.g. PAS-ADD, REISS, and structured interviews);
- The reliability and validity of the screening tools used by frontline staff to identify potential cases;
- Whether 'behavioural disorders' are included within the diagnosis.

Prevalence rates of specific psychiatric disorders

- *Affective disorder*—a number of studies report that people with intellectual disabilities are more likely to develop a depressive disorder, compared with their non-disabled peers. As within the general population, women with intellectual disabilities were more likely to develop depression than men with intellectual disabilities.[23]

- *Anxiety disorder*—people with intellectual disabilities have been reported as more likely to develop an anxiety disorder, adjustment disorder, and also post-traumatic stress disorder, compared with the general population.
- *Dementia*—5–8% of the general population will develop dementia, compared with 15.6% of people with intellectual disabilities of 65–75yrs, 23% in those of 75–84yrs, and 75% in those of ≥85yrs. For people who have Down syndrome, the prevalence rate of Alzheimer's disease is 8% in people of 35–49yrs, 55% in those of 50–59yrs, and 75% in those of ≥60 years.
- *Psychotic disorders*—a small number of studies have examined schizophrenia in people with mild/moderate intellectual disabilities and have reported that prevalence rates are four times higher than those reported in the general population.
- *Eating disorder*—there is clear evidence of higher obesity rates in people with intellectual disabilities, compared with the non-disabled population. In addition, other eating disorders are evident in this population: binge eating, pica, anorexia nervosa, bulimia nervosa, food refusal, and psychogenic vomiting. However, unlike the general population, no gender differences were found in these eating disorders.
- *Substance abuse*—alcohol and illicit drug misuse in people with intellectual disabilities has been reported to be lower, compared with the general population, although people with intellectual disabilities are at a higher risk to abuse such substances (see ➜ Substance misuse, pp. 258–9).[24]

Further reading

Jacobs M, Downie H, Kidd G, Fitzsimmons L, Gibbs S, Melville C (2016). Mental health services for children and adolescents with learning disabilities: a review of research on experiences of service users and providers. *British Journal of Learning Disabilities*. **44**: 225–32.

Mesa S, Tsakanikos E (2014). Attitudes and self-efficacy towards adults with mild intellectual disability among staff in acute psychiatric wards: an empirical investigation. *Advances in Mental Health and Intellectual Disabilities*. **8**: 79–90.

References

21 Bouras N (2013). Reviewing research of mental health problems for people with intellectual disabilities. *Journal of Mental Health Research in Intellectual Disabilities*. **6**: 71–3.

22 Royal College of Psychiatrists (2001). *DC-LD: Diagnostic Criteria for Psychiatric Disorders for Use with Adults with Learning Disabilities/Mental Retardation*. Gaskell: London.

23 Lunsky S, Canrinus M (2005). Gender issues, mental retardation and depression. In: P Sturmey, ed. *Mood Disorders in People with Mental Retardation*. NADD Press: New York, NY; pp. 56–68.

24 Tsakanikos E, McCarthy J (2014). *Handbook of Psychopathology in Intellectual Disability: Research, Practice and Policy*. Springer: New York, NY.

Factors contributing to mental health problems

Fig. 7.1 shows that a dynamic interaction of biological, psychological, developmental, and social factors may contribute to the development of mental health problems in people with intellectual disabilities.[25,26]

Biological (examples)

- Behavioural phenotypes such as fragile X, Lesch–Nyhan, and Prader–Willi, and a link with psychiatric conditions;
- Strong link between people with Down syndrome and Alzheimer's disease;
- Organic brain damage;
- People with intellectual disabilities have higher rates of psychotic disorders, possibly linked with brain abnormalities;
- People with temporal lobe epilepsy may also experience auditory hallucinations;
- Difficulties in personal development that may arise secondary to sensory and physical impairments, or undesired effects of antipsychotic medication may also contribute to the development of a psychiatric disorder.

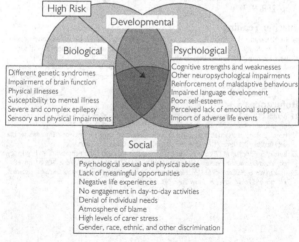

Fig. 7.1 Factors contributing to mental health problems in people with intellectual disabilities.

Reproduced from IASSIDD 2001, (2001) *Mental Health and Intellectual Disabilities: Addressing the mental health needs of people with intellectual disabilities*, Report by the Mental Health Special Interest Research Group of IASSID to the WHO.

Psychological (examples)

- Impaired intelligence, memory deficits, and limited coping behaviours;
- Poor communication and social skills;
- Poor problem-solving abilities and coping strategies;
- Wanting to appear normal;
- Low levels of self-esteem and disempowerment;
- Higher levels of frustration, loss of motivation, and greater vulnerability of stress.

Social (examples)

- Most people with intellectual disabilities will experience more negative life events than the non-disabled population;
- Higher levels of institutionalization, labelling, stigmatization, bullying;
- Lack of choice and control;
- Higher levels of separation and loss;
- Greater loss in keeping friends/peers;
- Limited social support networks;
- Lack of opportunities regarding employment, education, and recreational activities;
- Limited spiritual well-being;
- Many of the support services fail to fully understand the needs of people with intellectual disabilities and mental health problems, and have little training in this area.

Risk factors in young people with intellectual disabilities

Young people with intellectual disabilities are also more likely to develop a mental disorder, compared with other young people, as a result of a range of bio-psycho-social variables. Moreover, there are also a range of family and community variables that are also significant risk factors:[27]

- High levels of social deprivation/poverty;
- Family composition (i.e. being brought up by a single parent);
- Poor mental health of primary caregiver/family history of mental health;
- Presence of negative role models with less punitive child management practices/family in disharmony;
- Negative life events (i.e. accidents, abuse, domestic violence, bereavement);
- Lower opportunities for employment, education, and recreation;
- Excessive amounts of free time;
- Limited relationships/friends;
- Lack of meaning in life and routine/social exclusion.

References

25 International Association for the Scientific Study of Intellectual Disabilities (IASSID) (2001). *Mental Health and Intellectual Disabilities: Addressing the Mental Health Needs of People with Intellectual Disabilities*. Report by the Mental Health Special Interest Research Group of IASSID to the WHO.

26 Bouras N (2013). Reviewing research of mental health problems for people with intellectual disabilities. *Journal of Mental Health Research in Intellectual Disabilities*. 6: 71–3.

27 Hassiotis A, Barron DA (2007). Mental health, learning disabilities and adolescence: a developmental perspective. *Advances in Mental Health and Learning Disabilities*. 1: 32–9.

Anxiety disorders

People with intellectual disabilities are exposed to greater risks of developing psychiatric disorders as a result of a dynamic interaction of physical, psychological, and social factors (see ➜ Factors contributing to mental health problems, pp. 242–3). Cumulatively, these risk factors will make the person more vulnerable to anxiety disorders.

Definition

Anxiety disorder is characterized by excessive, exaggerated worry about everyday life events. People suffering from an anxiety disorder may anticipate the worst and cannot stop worrying about their health, relationships, family, work, or other specific concerns. These excessive anxieties and worries are often unrealistic or out of proportion to the situation. Daily life becomes a constant state of worry, fear and dread. Eventually, the anxiety controls the person's thinking and interferes with their daily functioning (social activities, relationships, family, work).

Symptoms of anxiety

According to ICD-11, the main symptoms reported are:
- Somatic—headaches, sweating, nausea, trembling, palpitations, muscle tension;
- Emotional—excessive ongoing worry, emotional tension, crying, irritability, being easily startled;
- Motivational—unrealistic view of problem, concentrating on difficulties;
- Thoughts—a restlessness or a feeling of being 'edgy';
- Behavioural—including reduced appetite and sleep problems.

Types of anxiety disorders

- Generalized anxiety disorder—the anxiety is not restricted to a specific event or situation, but generalized to everyday life (free-floating);
- Adjustment disorder—a mix of both depressive and anxiety symptoms that have resulted from a specific life event (bereavement, change in living circumstances);
- Post-traumatic stress disorder—a severe reaction to a specific life event (physical or sexual abuse, road traffic accident);
- Panic disorder—recurring attacks of severe anxiety that are not attached to a specific event or situation; normally associated with intense feelings of having a 'heart attack' and 'doom';
- Obsessive–compulsive disorder—characterized by recurrent obsessions and compulsions, causing severe anxiety and repulsive thoughts, leading the person to undertake certain behaviours repetitively;
- Phobia disorder—excessive anxiety is present whereby the person avoids the event or situation; even thinking about the event or situation can trigger intense worry and cause a panic attack. There are three types:
  - Agoraphobia—fear of being in crowds or public places;
  - Social phobia—fear of being noticed by other people;
  - Specific phobia—restricted to specific events or situations.

Prevalence

People with intellectual disabilities have higher levels of anxiety-related behaviour and also anxiety disorders, compared with the non-disabled population, and rates vary between 5 and 27%.[28] Stavrakaki and Lunsky reported
that people with intellectual disabilities were more likely to have a coexisting
diagnosis of a generalized anxiety disorder, an adjustment disorder, and a
depressive disorder than their non-disabled peers.[29] These authors also
report that people with intellectual disabilities can also experience post-
traumatic stress disorder.

Symptom presentation

For many people with mild intellectual disabilities, they will show similar
signs and symptoms of anxiety disorder as their non-disabled peers. In addition, other atypical symptoms may be displayed:
- Aggression/disruptive behaviours;
- Agitation, irritability;
- Obsessive–compulsive phenomena (self-injury, obsessive fears, ritualistic
  behaviours, and insomnia);
- Greater likelihood of displaying more somatic/physical symptoms, and
  also appetite and sleep disturbance.

Assessment

Self-rating scales are widely used in general psychiatric practice; however, there is no reliable and valid method for assessing anxiety in people
with intellectual disabilities. A number of specific screening tools have
been developed for nurses to use with this population and may be worth
considering:
- PAS-ADD schedules;[30]
- Glasgow Anxiety Scale;[31]
- Zung Anxiety Rating Scale: Adults Intellectual Disability Version.[32]

References

28 Hassiotis A, Stueber K, Thomas B, Charlot L (2014). Mood and anxiety disorders. In: E
Tsakanikos, J McCarthy, eds. *Handbook of Psychopathology in Intellectual Disability: Research,
Practice and Policy*. Springer: New York, NY: pp. 161–75.
29 Deb S, Mathews T, Holt G, Bouras N (2001). *Practice Guidelines for the Assessment and Diagnosis
of Mental Health Problems in Adults with Intellectual Disability*. Pavilion Publishing: Brighton.
30 Moss S (2002). *PAS-ADD Schedules*. Pavilion Publishing: Brighton.
31 Epsie CA, Mindham J (2003). Glasgow Anxiety Scale for people with intellectual disability (GAS-
ID): development and psychometric properties of a new measure for use with people with mild
intellectual disability. *Journal of Intellectual Disability Research*. 47: 22–30.
32 Lindsay WR, Michie AM (1988). Adaptation of the Zung self-rating anxiety scale for people with
a mental handicap. *Journal of Mental Deficiency Research*. 32: 485–90.

Psychotic disorders

Definition

This grouping of psychosis brings together schizophrenia, schizotypal, and delusional disorders. They are generally characterized by the following two groups of symptoms:

- Positive—distortion of thinking (i.e. thought interference, insertion, withdrawal, broadcasting), perception (hallucinations, delusions), mood (rapid changes of highs and lows, incongruous, flattened), and behaviour (i.e. bizarre, impaired social functioning);
- Negative—apathy, lack of communication, social withdrawal, mutism, blunted mood.

Types of disorders

According to ICD-11, there are several different types of disorders within this grouping:

- *Paranoid schizophrenia*—Dominated by relatively stable, often paranoid delusions, usually accompanied by hallucinations, particularly of the auditory variety, and perceptual disturbances;
- *Hebephrenic schizophrenia*—affective changes are prominent, delusions and hallucinations fleeting and fragmentary, behaviour irresponsible and unpredictable, and mannerisms common;
- *Catatonic schizophrenia*—dominated by prominent psychomotor disturbances that may alternate between extremes such as hyperkinesis and stupor, or automatic obedience and negativism;
- *Simple schizophrenia*—progressive development of oddities of conduct, inability to meet the demands of society, and decline in total performance.

Prevalence

A small number of studies have examined schizophrenia in people with mild/moderate intellectual disabilities and have reported that prevalence rates are at least three times higher than those reported in the non-disabled population (3–3.7%).[33]

Assessment

Diagnosis is based on the presence of a number of complex and subjective symptoms, and thus a certain level of communication is needed to describe such symptoms (i.e. voices). Therefore, for those people with severe/profound intellectual disabilities with very restricted communication, diagnosis will be more difficult to obtain.[34]

There are a number of screening tools designed specifically to aid nurses to assess a person's experiences of voices or disturbing thoughts; however, these will be helpful only for people with borderline/mild intellectual disabilities, with good communication skills:

- PAS-ADD;
- The Cognitive Assessment of Voices Schedule;
- The Hallucinations Rating Scale;
- The Delusions Rating Scale.[34,35]

Within the area of intellectual disabilities, there are no specifically developed rating scales for nurses to use in relation to psychosis; however, within the PAS-ADD Schedules, a number of questions are set to collate some information about the person's thinking, perception, mood, and behaviour.[36]

Difficulties in assessment

Deb et al. have offered nurses some advice in order to accurately assess psychosis in people with intellectual disabilities:[36]

- As sensory impairments are common in this population, these should be checked as they may aggravate symptoms.
- Some people may have 'imaginary friends', which may be observed as a positive symptom of schizophrenia.
- As many people may have limited communication, they may express themselves using behaviour that may appear odd or bizarre.
- People may have difficulty recognizing their own thoughts and therefore may attribute them to others.
- Some of the behaviours normally displayed by people (i.e. marked apathy, paucity of speech, underactivity, passivity) may represent negative symptoms of this condition.
- Negative symptoms may be a consequence of medication and/or unstimulating environments.
- For many people, they will have little control of their own lives, as carers and professionals supervise them.

Further reading

Hemmings C, Bouras N (2016). *Psychiatric and Behavioural Disorders in Intellectual and Developmental Disabilities*, 3rd edn. Cambridge University Press: Cambridge.

References

33 Tsakanikos E, McCarthy J, eds. (2014). *Handbook of Psychopathology in Intellectual Disability: Research, Practice and Policy*. Springer: New York, NY.

34 Clarke D (2007). Schizophrenia spectrum disorders in people with intellectual disabilities. In: N Bouras, G Holt, eds. *Psychiatric and Behavioural Disorders in Intellectual and Developmental Disabilities*, 2nd edn. Cambridge University Press: Cambridge: pp.131–42.

35 Moss S (2002). *PAS-ADD Schedules*. Pavilion Publishing: Brighton.

36 Deb S, Mathews T, Holt G, Bouras N (2001). *Practice Guidelines for the Assessment and Diagnosis of Mental Health Problems in Adults with Intellectual Disability*. Pavilion Publishers: Brighton.

Organic disorders

Both international classification systems (i.e. ICD-11 and DSM-V)[37,38] clearly distinguish between two groups of psychiatric disorders, based on a system of diagnosis:

- Organic disorders;
- Non-organic or functional disorders.

This distinction between organic disorders and non-organic disorders is important, as the causes for each of the two groups are different. The central clinical feature of most organic psychiatric disorders is impaired cognitive functioning. Cerebral dysfunction can, however, also cause organic mood states and personality change, as well as organic psychotic or neurotic states.

Organic disorders result from cerebral malfunction of the brain caused by certain metabolic, toxic, or other cerebral pathogens/dysfunctions of the brain. Examples include:

- Anoxia;
- Trauma;
- Degenerative disease.

System of classification

A practitioner undertaking an assessment/diagnosis using ICD-11 and DSM-V has to be fully aware of three facts when attempting to diagnose an organic or functional psychiatric disorder:

- A small number of psychiatric disorders are known to result from an organic cause such as brain injury.
- People suffering from any organic brain disorder can experience any psychiatric symptoms (i.e. hallucinations, delusions) as described by a person with a functional disorder.
- Many psychiatric symptoms can also be caused by ingestion of psychoactive substances.

In making a diagnosis, both classification systems highlight that organic disorders are examined first and, if appropriate, excluded before a non-organic functional psychiatric disorder can be clearly identified.

Organic disorders

Within the ICD-11 classification of psychiatric disorders, there are a wide range of organic conditions. The following are some of the main organic disorders.

- *Dementia*—there are a number of organic causes of dementia, which need to be identified clearly before a general diagnosis of dementia can be made. Some of these include cerebrovascular disease, Parkinson's disease, Huntington's disease, multiple sclerosis, epilepsy, hypothyroidism, vitamin B12 or folic acid deficiency, hypercalcaemia, and alcohol or drug misuse. Frontal lobe dementias can be caused by other brain diseases such as Pick's disease and Creutzfeldt–Jakob disease.

- *Delirium (acute and subacute confusional states)*—occurs more readily in older persons, acutely and chronically physically ill. Causes of delirium include septicaemia, urinary, chest, central nervous system, and other infections, cancer, and cardiopulmonary, liver, renal, metabolic, autoimmune, and other systemic physical health disorders. Delirium may also follow medication changes and include medication toxicity, especially during anticonvulsant/psychotropic polytherapy. Delirium can also result from substance intoxication, substance withdrawal, and multiple aetiologies.

Other organic disorders listed in different categories with ICD-11 include:
- Psychoactive substance use;
- Acute intoxication;
- Harmful use;
- Dependency syndrome;
- Withdrawal state with delirium;
- Organic affective disorder;
- Organic anxiety disorder;
- Organic delusional disorder: possible cause of epilepsy, amphetamine intoxication;
- Organic catatonic disorder;
- Organic sleep disorders.

Further reading

Tsakanikos E, McCarthy J (2014). *Handbook of Psychopathology in Intellectual Disability: Research, Practice and Policy*. Springer: New York, NY.

References

37 World Health Organization (2015). *ICD-11 Classification of Mental and Behavioural Disorders: Clinical descriptions and Diagnostic Guidelines*. World Health Organization: Geneva.
38 American Psychiatric Association (2015). *Diagnostic and Statistical Manual of Mental Disorders*, 5th edn. American Psychiatric Association: Arlington, VA.

Dementia (in people with intellectual disabilities)

While some studies report prevalence rates similar to those in the general population, it is generally accepted that people with intellectual disabilities are at increased risk of earlier-onset dementia. Compared with the general population, Cooper found that the prevalence rate of dementia in adults with intellectual disabilities other than Down syndrome is 15.6% in the 65–75yrs age group, 23.5% in the 65–84yrs age group, and 70% in the 85–94yrs age group.[39] People with Down syndrome are acknowledged to be at even greater risk (see ➔ Older people with Down syndrome, pp. 138–9). Of dementias among people with intellectual disabilities, 50–60% are of the Alzheimer's type. Alzheimer's disease is an irreversible, progressive brain disease that slowly destroys memory and thinking skills. It is characterized by impaired memory and judgement, disorientation, impaired ability to learn and reason, high levels of stress, and sensitivity to the local and social environment.

The diagnosis of dementia in persons with intellectual disabilities relies on evidence of change from the person's previous level of functioning and on meeting the following ICD-10 criteria:[40]

• Decline in memory;
• Decline in other cognitive skills—thinking, planning, and organizing;
• Clear consciousness;
• Decline in emotional control, motivation, or social behaviour;
• Six-month duration;
• Exclusion of other disorders.

The TSI, DSMSE, DMR, and DLSQ have proved to be effective instruments in the diagnosis of dementia in people with Down syndrome, with the DSMSE proving less sensitive than the other instruments.[41]

Changes in personality, behaviour, and global day-to-day function are often more relevant as warning signs than changes in cognition and memory. Identification of changes is more likely if there is frequent and early screening for such changes; recommendations are for annual baseline screening for people with Down syndrome >35yrs, a full diagnostic work-up, and a person-centred approach to care.[42] Each person is unique and will experience dementia differently, yet clients and the services they need tend to fall into three groupings:[42]

• *Group 1*—some people may experience a relatively slow progression of dementia over 5–8yrs. While these individuals will require increasing supports, particularly in terms of staffing and some relatively low-cost environmental modifications to their living spaces, they can often be maintained within their family unit, i.e. the home they have lived in throughout their decline. Retaining contact with familiar environments, family, and friends is the optimal approach to service delivery for this group.

• *Group 2*—for some people, while decline may not necessarily be compressed, they present, particularly at mid-stage dementia, with behavioural and psychotic features: night-time wakening, wandering, agitation, screaming, and visual and auditory hallucinations. Some behavioural issues may be addressed in existing settings with improved communication, programming, and environmental approaches. For others, dementia-specific environments with specialist-trained staff will better respond to their additional care needs.

• *Group 3*—for others, decline may be compressed and the person may progress to a stage of advanced dementia within a relatively short time, i.e. 1–2yrs. As dementia progresses, specialist nursing and palliative care will become increasingly important.

Intellectual disability services system has traditionally been focused on serving and maintaining people in the community for as long as possible and has been driven by a service philosophy that emphasizes positive approaches, skill acquisition, and increasing independence.

The inevitable decline associated with dementia challenges this philosophy, and there is a danger that, with changing needs when dementia presents, service providers will seek to transfer a person to other, often more expensive, alternatives. This often does not need to happen, as there are opportunities to support ageing in place and a growing interest in understanding the role of specialized services and dementia-specific homes for people with intellectual disabilities and dementia.[43,44]

References

39 Cooper SA (1997). High prevalence of dementia among people with learning disabilities not attributable to Down's syndrome. *Psychiatric Medicine*. **27**: 609–16.

40 Aylward E, Burt D, Thorpe L, Lai F, Dalton A (1997). Diagnosis of dementia in individuals with intellectual disability. *Journal of Intellectual Disability Research*. **41**: 152–64.

41 McCarron M, McCallion P, Reilly E, Mulryan N (2014). A prospective 14-year longitudinal follow-up of dementia in persons with Down syndrome. *Journal of Intellectual Disability Research*. **58**: 61–70.

42 Burt DB, Aylward EH (2000). Test battery for the diagnosis of dementia in individuals with intellectual disability. Working Group for the Establishment of Criteria for the Diagnosis of Dementia in Individuals with Intellectual Disability. *Journal of Intellectual Disability Research*. **44**: 175–80.

43 McCarron M, McCallion P, Reilly E, Mulryan N (2014). Responding to the challenges of service development to address dementia needs for people with an intellectual disability. In: K Watchman, ed. *Intellectual Disability and Dementia: Research into Practice*. Jessica Kingsley Publishers: London; pp. 241–69.

44 McCarron M, Reilly E, Dunne P (2013). *Achieving Quality Environments for Person Centred Dementia Care*. Daughters of Charity Service: Dublin.

Psychopathology

Psychopathology is a term that refers to the study of mental illness, mental distress, and behaviours which may be indicative of mental illness or psychological impairment. It examines the biological, psychological, and social causes, and is a synonym for mental illness, even if the symptoms do not constitute a formal diagnosis.

Psychopathology is not the same as psychopathy, which examines antisocial personality disorders and criminality.

Our earliest explanation, of what we now refer to as psychopathology, can be seen in the sixteenth and seventeenth centuries when bizarre behaviours were associated with evil spirits and demons. By the eighteenth century, recognition of psychopathology as a treatable condition, rather than the act of a demon, was being acknowledged. However, until the 1970s, it was widely believed that people with intellectual disabilities did not have the cognitive ability to experience mental illness. It is now recognized that psychopathology and intellectual disabilities coexist.

Psychopathology can also be defined using two related diagnostic protocols that contain these specific criteria: the DSM (American Psychiatric Association) and the ICD (WHO). For people with intellectual disabilities, the DC-LD can be used alongside the ICD-10.

Models of psychopathology can be divided into three main groups: medical, psychological, and social.

Medical/biological models of psychopathology

This model focuses on studying signs and symptoms of disease, neurochemical abnormalities, brain defects, and possible genetic factors. It classifies psychopathology into diagnostic groups. Evidence of this model is based on a scan of biological markers [(e.g. CT, positron emission tomography (PET)] and their response to medication and disease treatments. Depending on the aetiology, treatment regimens may involve medication, electroconvulsive therapy (ECT), and, to a very limited extent, neurosurgery. A variant of the medical model is the diathesis–stress model. This psychological theory explains behaviour as a result of biological and genetic factors and life experiences (nature and nurture). It suggests that a mental disorder is produced by the interaction of a predisposition to mental ill health and a precipitating event in the environment, with this example being used to explain schizophrenia and bipolar mood disorder.

Psychological models of psychopathology

This model examines psychological actions, e.g. early experiences, traumatic events, maladaptive learning experiences, and illogical thinking. Sigmund Freud was the first to formalize the psychoanalysis model, and this has influenced this approach ever since. In the psychoanalysis model, there is emphasis on the behaviour being seen as a result of an abnormal symptom; the importance of unconscious conflicts, early childhood experiences, and stages of psychosexual development are emphasized. The range of therapeutic treatments include cognitive therapy models. In cognitive therapy, the counsellor and the client work together to highlight, explore, and challenge inaccurate thoughts and then develop new ways of replacing these thoughts and beliefs with more effective thought processes. The emphasis is on the person's current situation and how their major problems may be resolved.

Sociocultural models of psychopathology

This model considers the social and cultural influences on behaviour, arguing that these forces exert important influences. It views biological and psychological models as incomplete because they do not consider societal norms and expectations, subgroup influences, and family dynamics. Suggested interventions include family therapy, couples therapy, group therapy, and community interventions. The family dynamics model embraces a view that families can be a source of stress, can discourage change, and can encourage a member to be sick, and therefore the family as a whole should be the target of intervention.

A combination of approaches

People with intellectual disabilities need to be able to access a combination of approaches, as more general mental and behavioural disorders are probably better understood within a more comprehensive biological-psychological-social-developmental framework.

Further reading

Bouras N, Hardy S, Holt G (2013). *Mental Health in Intellectual Disabilities: A Reader*, 4th edn. Pavilion Publishing: Brighton.

Hemmings C, Bouras N (2016). *Psychiatric and Behavioural Disorders in Intellectual and Developmental Disabilities*, 3rd edn. Cambridge University Press: Cambridge.

Matson J, Matson L, eds. (2015). *Comorbid Conditions in Individuals with Intellectual Disabilities* (Autism and Child Psychopathology Series). Springer: London.

Tsakanikos E, McCarthy J, eds. (2014). *Handbook of Psychopathology in Intellectual Disability Research, Practice and Policy*. Springer: London.

Autistic spectrum conditions

The term autism, as an umbrella term for all autistic conditions, including Asperger syndrome, was adopted by the Department of Health in 2011. Autism is a life-long neurodevelopmental condition, affecting around 1.1% of the population. Autism is a spectrum disorder, because of both the range of abilities and difficulties that may be present among adults with autism and the way that these present in different people. Autism is not an intellectual disability, but research suggests that around half of people with autism may also have an intellectual disability.

Autism is broadly defined with difficulties in three main areas, known as the triad of impairments, being **social communication**, **social interaction**, and **social imagination**. These are combined with restricted interests and rigid and repetitive behaviours.

In addition to these features, many people with autism have at least one other physical or mental health problem such as epilepsy, dyspraxia, sleep problems, and self injurious behaviours.

People with autism may display one or more of the following

- **Need for routine**: as the world can seem a very unpredictable and confusing place;
- **Adherence to rules**: with difficulty in taking a different approach once they have learnt one way of doing something;
- **Adapting to change**: change can be difficult and uncomfortable and may require advanced preparation;
- **Special interests**: some people with autism can have intense special interests;
- **Sensory processing issues**: hyper- or hyposensory sensitivity in one or more of their senses;
- **Mental health**: including anxiety, depression, bipolar disorder, and obsessive–compulsive disorder;
- **Catatonia**: catatonic and parkinsonian features;
- **ADHD**: should not be considered as an additional diagnosis until their needs relating to their autism are addressed first;
- **Tourette syndrome**: tics, stims, and stereotypies are common;
- **Eating disorders**: gastric disorders can result in restrictive diets. Individuals with autism are also known to be sensitive to foods such as wheat (gluten) and all dairy products (casein).

Reasonable adjustments that may support people with autism

- **Improving appointments**: think about the best time of the day and fitting in with their routines. Make a longer appointment.
- **Tell people what you are doing**: explain at every stage what you are about to do, what will happen next, and why.
- **Keep language straightforward**: avoid humour and double-meaning words, as these can be taken literally. Make sure facial expressions and the tone of voice match what is being said. Avoid complex social language. Using a variety of media may be helpful.

- **Helping people understand**: allow time for them to process what is being said (at least 6s). Check they have understood. Be prepared to repeat and rephrase.
- **Information from people**: ask direct questions. Questions about time and frequency are often difficult to understand. Check answers; ask in a different way. Be aware of acquiescence.
- **Good environments**: consider sensory processing difficulties. Keep the environment calm. Avoid busy areas. Familiarity is important.
- **Understanding behaviours**: behaviours may be a coping mechanism. Social difficulties may include lack of eye contact, unusual body language, or talking inappropriately.
- **The support people need**: ask the person and/or parent, carer, or advocate what support they might need. Respect confidentiality.
- **Social stories**: are short descriptions of a particular situation, event, or activity? Which include specific information about what to expect in that situation and why?

Examples of interventions and approaches

There is currently no cure and no specific treatment for autism. There are a variety of approaches, therapies, and interventions which can improve an individual's quality of life. These can include medication to alleviate anxiety and depression, diet, psychological interventions, psychoeducation, and standard therapies. Any treatment or intervention should be carefully tailored to suit the individual.

Further reading

Autism Act 2009. ℘ www.legislation.gov.uk/ukpga/2009/15/contents (accessed 30 October 2017).
Autism Act Northern Ireland (2011). ℘ www.niassembly.gov.uk/visit-and-learning/autism-and-the-assembly/autism-legislation/ (accessed 30 October 2017).
Autism (Scotland) Bill (2011). ℘ www.scotland.gov.uk (accessed 30 October 2017).
Autism NI. ℘ www.autismni.org (accessed 30 October 2017).
Department of Health (2014). Think Autism. Fulfilling and Rewarding Lives, the Strategy for Adults with Autism in England. Department of Health: London.
National Autistic Society. ℘ www.autism.org.uk/ (accessed 30 October 2017).
National Institute for Health and Care Excellence (2012). Autism in Adults: Diagnosis and Management. Clinical Guideline [CG142]. ℘ www.nice.org.uk/guidance/cg142 (accessed 30 October 2017).
National Institute for Health and Care Excellence (2014). Autism. Quality standards [QS51]. ℘ www.nice.org.uk/guidance/qs51 (accessed 30 October 2017).
Welsh Autism Strategy Action Plan (2008). ℘ www.asdinfowales.co.uk/strategic-action-plan (accessed 30 October 2017).

Self-harm

What is self-harm?

Self-harm is when an individual deliberately self-inflicts pain on themselves, causing physical harm, often to relieve emotional distress. Although self-harm is not a mental health diagnosis per se, it is associated with a range of mental disorders, including borderline personality disorder, depression, anxiety disorders, and bipolar disorder. There are various methods of self-harm which range in severity in terms of harm to the individual. The most common method is cutting, but other forms of self-harm include poisoning, burning, punching self, ingesting toxic substances, and throwing self into an object.

Self-harm is often used as a coping mechanism, a way to survive, and while a person who self-harms can be at risk of suicide, self-harm in itself does not imply a suicidal intent, which should be considered as part of the mental state examination. There are also less obvious ways of self-harming; these can be subtle and more difficult to detect, e.g. not taking care of physical and mental health, overeating, excessive exercise, and scratching the skin.

Although the intention may be to get some relief from emotional distress, for many, self-harm will bring feelings of guilt that others are judging you as not coping. Many people will try and keep any self-harming behaviour a secret from others. Whatever the reasons for self-harming, there is no single reason for the behaviour. It has been described as a way to:[45]

- Express something that is hard to put into words;
- Make painful thoughts or feelings into something visible;
- Change emotional pain into physical pain;
- Reduce overwhelming emotional feelings or thoughts;
- Have a sense of being in control/escape from traumatic memories;
- Stop feeling numb, disconnected, or dissociated;
- Create a reason to physically care for yourself;
- Express suicidal feelings/thoughts without taking your own life;
- Communicate to other people your severe distress.[45]

Self-harm and people with intellectual disabilities

Self-harm should be considered at all levels of intellectual functioning. The presentation and mode of self-harm may differ according to the level of ability. This has implications for assessing intent and understanding the individual's motivations to harm themselves. For example, a person with intellectual disabilities who walks out onto the road in front of traffic—staff may believe this is due to a lack of road safety and overlook any suggestion of self-harm or suicidal intent.

The assessment, management, and intervention of self-harm will differ from service to service. Although assessment is normally based on the biological-psychological-social model, interventions and management often adopt cognitive and/or behavioural approaches according to the level of ability (see ➡ Self-harm, pp. 256–7; ➡ Self-injury, pp. 592–3). Often treatment may be risk-averse and focus on reducing opportunities to self-harm by removing hazards from the environment. This can be accompanied by increased monitoring and observation levels. At the other end of the continuum is a harm minimization approach. Harm minimization approaches consider the actual harm that can occur from a person's current behaviour and then considers how the threat of harm to the individual can be minimized by altering the environment and reducing access to opportunities for the impact of self-harm. In addition, a range of psychological treatments, e.g. problem-solving therapy and dialectical behaviour therapy, may be provided. When self-harm occurs in the context of mental disorders, e.g. depression, treatment may also include the prescription of medication to bring about a reduction or discontinuation of the behaviour by treating the underlying condition. Addressing the individual's social and relationship needs are also pivotal for a successful approach.

Self-injurious behaviour and people with intellectual disabilities

The term 'self-injurious behaviour' is commonly used in services for people with intellectual disabilities. Its use can be confusing, as its meaning is somewhat different to that of self-harm. Self-injurious behaviour can include head banging and biting, or hitting oneself. Self-injurious behaviour is often associated with people with more severe intellectual disabilities and is used as an intentional (and non-intentional) form of communication. For example, it may be used to express feelings of pain or ill health, to avoid situations that the person does not understand or wish to be in, or to gain some form of interaction with those around them. Also, self-injury may be present as a form of sensory stimulation for people with sensory impairments. In these instances, self-injurious behaviour is referred to as a type of challenging behaviour. Interventions will differ and are based around supporting the person to engage in meaningful activities, developing relationships, and teaching the person new skills, e.g. alternative forms of communication.

Further reading

Dick K, Gleeson K, Johnson L, Weston C (2011). Staff beliefs about why people with learning disabilities self-harm: a Q-methodology study. *British Journal of Learning Disabilities*. 39: 233–42.

Fish R, Woodward S, Duperouzel H (2012). 'Change can only be a good thing:' staff views on the introduction of a harm minimisation policy in a Forensic Learning Disability service. *British Journal of Learning Disabilities*. 40: 37–45.

Heslop P (2011). Supporting people with learning disabilities who self-injure. *Tizard Learning Disability Review*. 16: 5–15.

Rees J, Langdon PE (2016). The relationship between problem-solving ability and self-harm amongst people with mild intellectual disabilities. *Journal of Applied Research in Intellectual Disabilities*. 29: 387–93.

The Mix. *Self-harm: Recovery, Advice, and Support.* ℘ www.selfharm.org.uk (accessed 30 October 2017).

References

45 Mind. *Self-harm.* ℘ www.mind.org.uk/information-support/types-of-mental-health-problems/self-harm/#.VzCuE9KDGkp (accessed 30 October 2017).

Substance misuse

There is debate regarding the prevalence of alcohol and illicit drug misuse in people with intellectual disabilities as a result of methodological problems. Nevertheless, lower prevalence rates of substance misuse are reported, compared with the general population; however, these figures may be underestimated, as they are based on only those people known to intellectual disability services.

Definition

According to ICD-11, three or more of the following must be present in the previous year to obtain a diagnosis of a 'dependence syndrome':
- A strong desire or sense of compulsion to use the substance;
- Difficulties in controlling substance-taking behaviour;
- A physiological withdrawal state;
- Evidence of tolerance;
- Progressive neglect of alternative pleasures;
- Persisting with substance use despite clear evidence of overtly harmful consequences.

Aetiology

People with intellectual disabilities are comparatively more likely to develop a substance abuse problem. A clearer picture is emerging of the characteristics that place individuals most at risk from misusing substances:[48]
- *Intrapersonal variables*—borderline/mild intellectual disabilities, young, ♂, mental health problems, low self-esteem, inadequate self-control, illiteracy, short attention span, poor problem-solving skills, and frustration;
- *Interpersonal variables*—living in the community, low levels of supervision, homelessness, parental alcohol-related mental health problems, negative role models, negative life events, limited employment, educational and recreational opportunities, excessive amounts of free time, restricted friendships/relationships, loneliness, desire for 'fitting in'.

Assessment

Difficulties exist in assessing this population as a result of staff issues (i.e. a lack of skills/knowledge) and complex issues presented by the person (i.e. aggression, mental and physical health problems, offending behaviour). Furthermore, people with intellectual disabilities who misuse substances sometimes can be 'unwilling' or 'uncooperative' to fully engage in the assessment process—or may be labelled as such. Areas that need to be assessed include:
- Substance use patterns and impact;
- Reasons for, and knowledge of, substance misuse;
- Mental health;
- Offending behaviour patterns;
- Motivation to fully want to change and engage in the process of helping.

There are a number of general addiction clinical screening tools that have been developed to assess substance abuse. Some are designed for self-administration and others for use in clinical interviews, although these have not been validated for use with people who have intellectual disabilities:

with some minor amendments to the wording and reading these aloud to the person, they could be easily used with this population. The Alcohol Use Disorder Identification Test (AUDIT) was developed by the WHO as a simple method of screening for excessive drinking and to assist in brief assessment.[47]

Biological-psychological-social interventions

- *Biological*—detoxification and psychopharmacological treatments;
- *Psychological*—individual education (anger management, relaxation training, challenging negative statements), modifications of AA & Twelve Step Programme, group therapy, assertiveness skills, motivational interviewing, and relapse prevention programmes;
- *Social*—develop coping and refusal skills, self-monitoring skills, promote interpersonal communication, role-plays, and staff education.

Kerr et al.[48] (2013) reported that there is little evidence of the effectiveness of these interventions to guide practice, and more robust research is needed.

Advice to help people diminish substance abuse

- Target the person's intrinsic motivation to want to change and engage in self-help using motivational interviewing.
- Offer education with more time flexibility, repetition, and greater use of role-play.
- Provide information leaflets about the harmful effects on people's bodies, minds, relationships, and lifestyle in a user-friendly format.
- Address unresolved problems (i.e. bereavement, abuse, loneliness).
- Target specific offending behaviours.
- Identify trigger factors of relapse.

References

46 Taggart L, Chaplin E (2014). Substance abuse disorder. In: E Tsakanikos, J McCarthy, eds. *Handbook of Psychopathology in Intellectual Disability*. Springer Publishing: New York, NY.

47 Taggart L, Temple B (2014). Substance abuse. In: L Taggart, W Cousins, eds. *Health Promotion for People with Intellectual Disabilities*. Open University Press/McGraw-Hill Publishers: Maidenhead; pp. 128–37.

48 Kerr M, Laurence C, Darbyshire C, Middleton AR, Fitzsimmons L (2013). Tobacco and alcohol related interventions for people with mild/moderate intellectual disabilities: a systematic review. *Journal of Intellectual Disability Research*. 57: 393–408.

Responding to bereavement

Reactions to loss

Loss is a universal experience, to which people respond in many different ways. Reactions to death as loss can affect people in an emotional way (e.g. feeling guilty, profoundly sad, or helpless), in a physical way (e.g. lacking energy, being lethargic, or having a hollowness in the stomach), and/or in a behavioural way (e.g. sleeplessness, crying, and restlessness). Most bereaved people seek the support they need from family and friends, but for a small percentage of people, the need for professional support (such as a bereavement counsellor or therapist) is required.

Intellectual disability and loss

The person with intellectual disabilities may experience many more losses than others, because of the nature of their disability and societal reactions to the person who may be perceived as being 'different' in some way. People with intellectual disabilities do experience death and grief but sometimes express it in ways that may be misinterpreted or express grief a long time after the death, which may mean it is overlooked. They may also be prone to multiple and successive losses as a result of the death of, for example, their main carer (mother or father), as illustrated in Fig. 7.2.

Often, when multiple losses are experienced, the raw realities of living (such as where the bereaved person will be sleeping that night) overtake the overwhelming sadness of death, and mourning the deceased may be delayed for weeks or months.

Factors affecting support

It seems that the more complex the nature of the intellectual disabilities, the less likelihood of being actively involved in loss and bereavement issues and associated mourning opportunities. Subsequently, many people with intellectual disabilities often do not get the support they need following the death of their loved ones, and some may not even be told of the death, because of:

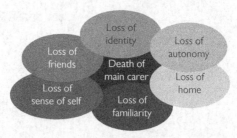

Fig. 7.2 Multiple and successive losses.

- Difficulties in communicating effectively, which precludes meaningful reciprocal information and explanations;
- Challenges associated with cognition, as some people may struggle to understand complex and abstract concepts (such as death);
- Limited attention span;
- An inability to articulate feelings in a socially acceptable and meaningful way;
- So much reliance placed on other people to help them to facilitate their loss;
- Carers not feeling comfortable talking about loss and bereavement;
- Carers wanting to protect them from the sad business of bereavement;
- Carers not knowing how to offer appropriate bereavement support.

Such compounding issues can make bereavement and grief work difficult for this client population.

Disenfranchised grief

When a loss such as death cannot be openly acknowledged, publicly mourned, or socially supported, it often results in disenfranchised grief,[49] and people with intellectual disabilities are at risk of this happening to them.

- The relationship to the deceased is not recognized.
- The loss is not recognized.
- The griever is not recognized.
- The circumstances around the death preclude involvement.
- The way people have learnt to grieve (or not) may influence involvement and coping styles.

These factors often result in the bereaved person being excluded from the rituals associated with death (such as attending the funeral or sending a wreath) and create additional problems for the bereaved by removing or minimizing sources of appropriate support.

The nurse should remain open and honest with the grieving person with intellectual disabilities. They should take every opportunity to actively include the person throughout the grief process and associated rituals. This helps to affirm the death and minimize the possibility of disenfranchised grief, which can lead to complex grief reactions and indicate the need for grief counselling or therapy.

Further reading

picTTalk. Communicating with People with Learning Disabilities about Loss and Ill Health (communication tool to support and facilitate conversations about ill health, loss, and bereavement, free to download from). 🔊 itunes.apple.com/gb/app/picttalk-communicating-people/id951053318?mt=8 (accessed 30 October 2017).

Read S, ed. (2014). Supporting People with Intellectual Disabilities Experiencing Loss and Bereavement: Theory and Compassionate Practice. Jessica Kingsley Publishers: London.

Stancliffe RJ, Wiese MY, Read S, Jeltes G, Clayton JM (2015). Knowing, planning for and fearing death: do adults with intellectual disability and disability staff differ? Research in Developmental Disabilities. 49–50: 47–59.

References

49 Doka K (2002). Disenfranchised Grief: New Directions, Challenges, and Strategies for Practice. Research Press: Champaign, IL.

Planning with people and their families

Undertaking a nursing assessment

In undertaking an assessment, nurses should select an appropriate structured nursing framework on the basis of the initial information provided in the referral to them. All nurses need to be careful to undertake a full nursing, and not to only use a broad interprofessional assessment or a specific secondary assessment, such as those that are psychology-based (behavioural) or medical-based (epilepsy), without a comprehensive nursing assessment having been completed first.

There is a range of person-centred planning frameworks for developing individualized plans for support with people with intellectual disabilities, such as those discussed in ➡ Life planning, pp. 302–3. Although such frameworks are not profession-specific, nurses have a unique contribution to make in providing a nursing perspective in these discussions through the completion of a structured nursing assessment.

Nursing assessment

A nursing assessment requires the systematic collection of information by a nurse, which is guided by a nursing framework and involves some or all of the following processes: observation of the individual, active listening, questioning, information gathering on physical/mental health, and physical examination.

The purpose of a nursing assessment is to gain comprehensive information on the person's current abilities and needs within a recognized nursing framework and to establish priorities for nursing intervention.

Preparing for an assessment
- Prior to commencing a nursing assessment, it is necessary to explain the process to the person (and their carers if present).
- Keep your focus on the person with intellectual disabilities and direct your questions to them.
- Provide opportunities for the person (and family members) to ask further questions they may have about what the process involves.
- Develop a rapport with the person, sufficient for them to feel comfortable during the assessment process.
- Obtain valid consent for the assessment to be undertaken and for information to be sought from other relevant professionals.
- The preparation for a nursing assessment often requires more than one meeting with the person, and family members if they are actively involved in their care.

Conducting a nursing assessment
- Focus on the person and their current situation (including family circumstances).
- Select a structured nursing framework that identifies the areas to be considered within the nursing assessment.
- Provide opportunities for the person to demonstrate their abilities through day-to-day activities and, where possible, in a range of settings.
- Undertake the assessment within an environment with which the person is familiar.

- Avoid undertaking nursing assessments when people are distressed, if at all possible.
- Provide positive feedback to the people involved during the process of the assessment.
- Undertake the nursing assessment in manageable chunks, so that the person can maintain their concentration.
- With the permission of the person, seek information from other professionals/carers involved in providing support, in so far as it assists in the completion of the nursing assessment.

Recording and reporting
- All nursing assessment documents and related care plans are legal documents and must be treated accordingly.
- Record objective information on what was observed, heard, and measured during the nursing assessment.
- Write clear statements about what the person can do, before listing areas of need.
- Avoid value judgements on behaviour observed, previous history, and value-laden words such as 'vulnerable', 'aggressive', and 'difficult'.
- When identifying the abilities and needs of a person, clearly state the abilities and needs as expressed by the person and those views expressed by other people.
- Comply with the professional nursing regulator's requirements for reporting and record-keeping.

Identifying priorities for nursing action
- In discussion with the person, review the information recorded and seek to identify their priorities, areas of strengths, and need.
- Decide if further detailed assessment is required in relation to specific aspects, e.g. physical mobility, epilepsy, mental health.
- Review the areas of need identified, and consider which of these may be responsive to nursing interventions (consistent with the nursing framework used for nursing assessment).
- Write a prioritized list of areas for nursing intervention, and share these with the person with intellectual disabilities. This will form the basis of the nursing care plans.

Further reading

McCormack B, McCance T, eds. (2016). *Person-Centred Practice in Nursing and Health Care: Theory and Practice*, 2nd edn. Wiley-Blackwell: Oxford.
Wilson B, Barrett D, Woollands A (2012). *Care Planning: A Guide for Nurses*, 2nd edn. Taylor Francis: London.

Writing nursing care plans

Documented 'plan' for nursing actions

Nursing care plans provide details of the prioritized area of need, the objective of nursing intervention, the nursing interventions to be undertaken, and the date for evaluation of the nursing care plan. Nursing care plans are central documents to the organization of nursing interventions, have an important legal status, and provide the record for what care was meant to be delivered. Nurses should start to plan interventions from the priorities identified by the nurse and the person with intellectual disabilities within the nursing assessment. The focus of nursing care plans must be consistent with the structured nursing framework used for assessment and should be written within the headings used within the nursing framework.

Nurses often work within a wider interdisciplinary context and may be contributing to an overall interdisciplinary person-centred plan. In such situations, they must remain cognisant of the fact that only a nurse can write a nursing care plan and they will remain personally accountable for the quality of the nursing care plan developed and delivered, and how this is documented, including any core care plan they sign without personalizing the content.[1,2] Therefore, an individual who has an overall person-centred plan should also have nursing care plans that link to that overall plan. Nursing care should not be delivered without a nursing care plan in place, except in emergencies, after which the care delivered and care plans should be documented as soon as possible.

Area of need

Nursing care plans arise from the results of a nursing assessment of a person's abilities and needs, so they must demonstrate a clear link to the priorities identified within a nursing assessment. Nurses should clearly state the area of nursing needs within the wider context as it relates to the individual, e.g. eating and drinking—'Mary is underweight (providing her weight and BMI) and is at risk of pressure sores'. Nurses should not use short phrases or single words in outlining the nursing needs, such as 'restricted mobility', without providing the wider context and contributing factors.

Person-centred objectives

It is essential that people with intellectual disabilities are enabled to be actively involved as much as possible, in developing their objectives within their nursing care plans. Objectives should start with the client's name and be written as a clear statement of:
• The skill/knowledge the person is seeking to achieve (self-administer their own medication/eat three meals a day);
• The support the person will need to do this (from pre-prepared blister packs/using adapted cutlery);
• The criteria that will be used to establish when the person's objectives have been achieved (for 5 consecutive days);

- A measure of success (without error/either by using a recognized instrument or self-reports from the person and/or family carers);
- A specific calendar date for evaluation, rather than 'in 4 weeks' or the date for evaluation being described as 'ongoing'.

Progress towards the person's objectives should be reviewed with them and their families (if relevant). When nursing care plan objectives have been agreed, nurses should ensure all necessary resources (staff, equipment) are in place before the care plan is commenced. Any delay in commencing the care plan should be recorded, and a rationale provided, as well as any unmet need, and the appropriate line manager/professional manager within the service provider notified.

Nursing interventions

These should be written as clear action statements, which fully describe any actions required, e.g. provide information explaining the components of healthy eating in a format that is accessible to (client's name), or provide three 15-min sessions of walking each week.

All nursing interventions to be undertaken should have the informed consent of the person and be based on best available evidence. Nursing interventions should be written in a format accessible to all staff who will need to read the care plan, and abbreviations should not be used in describing nursing interventions.

Recording amendments in nursing care plans

Nurses should keep an ongoing record of all nursing interventions provided and outcomes achieved by the person with intellectual disabilities. These notes should be cross-referenced by the number or title to the ongoing nursing care plans. This will provide the necessary information for ongoing and summative evaluations. When the objectives of the care plan have been achieved, the care plan should be discontinued and this recorded. Any amendment to nursing care plans or interventions within these should be signed and dated, and the time entered, together with a rationale for any change being recorded within the nursing notes.[3,4] Nursing interventions not written in the care plan should not be undertaken; if additional interventions are deemed necessary, these should be added to existing care plans, or a new care plan developed in which the new need is identified.

Further reading

Wilson B, Barrett D, Woollands A (2012). *Care Planning: A Guide for Nurses*, 2nd edn. Taylor Francis: London.

References

3 Nursing and Midwifery Council (2015). *The Code: Standards of Conduct, Performance and Ethics for Nurses and Midwives*. Nursing and Midwifery Council: London.

4 Nursing and Midwifery Board of Ireland (2014). *Code of Professional Conduct and Ethics for Registered Nurses and Registered Midwives*. Nursing and Midwifery Board of Ireland: Dublin.

Advocacy

Advocacy is fundamentally about promoting the voice, choices, and rights of individuals.[5] It is a process by which people, individually or in groups, make others aware of their views and interests.

It exists in various forms:

- For oneself, as in self-advocacy—for small personal decisions such as what to wear or larger ones such as with whom to live and healthcare decisions;
- With others in a group through collective advocacy—this could be about access to resources or to challenge political or service agendas;
- Through others in citizen, peer, family, professional, and independent advocacy.

Advocacy is used for micro-, mezzo-, and macro-level issues. Each person's ability to be involved in decision-making will vary over time and according to the issue being considered; however, the ultimate goal of all forms of advocacy should be to enable every individual to speak for themselves as much as possible. Advocacy can be instructed (following the clear directions and wishes of the person) or non-instructed (when the person is unable to communicate what they want and advocacy is necessary to secure their rights, best interests, and preferences). It is about people who use services setting the agenda and is not merely about being consulted by professionals or organizations.

Effective advocacy requires a relationship based on partnership, trust, and moral support. Key functions are undertaken without controlling or making choices for the person or the group, and include assisting with: finding accessible resources and information; generating ideas and possible courses of action; understanding options and their implications; expressing the needs and wishes of the person; upholding rights; and obtaining the appropriate support and care.

Statutory advocacy services

In some regions, local authorities are required to commission specific types of advocacy that are independent from service providers in the areas of: mental capacity; mental health; NHS complaints; and in relation to care and support for people who receive, or are eligible to receive, care and support, *regardless of who is providing that support*, who have 'substantial difficulty' being involved in the process of care and have no other suitable person to represent them. Each jurisdiction has different requirements for the provision of advocacy, and nurses must be familiar with what is available in their country of practice (and the country of origin of clients who are placed in a service that is not in their usual country of domicile). It is increasingly acknowledged that individuals often use a range of services across their lifetime, sometimes simultaneously. The *whole-systems* approach to advocacy that has one point of contact facilitates continuity in the advocacy relationship and works across services aimed to address this.[5]

Nurse advocacy/professional advocacy

Section 3.4 of the NMC Code (2015) requires all nurses to '*act as an advocate for the vulnerable, challenging poor practice and discriminatory attitudes and behaviour relating to their care*'.

While this rightly raises questions about who is considered vulnerable, it is probable that all clients supported by a registered nurse can reasonably expect advocacy support from the nurses who work with them. In the Republic of Ireland, the NMBI Code (2014) explicitly states that nurses respect each person's right to self-determination as a basic human right and requires nurses to advocate for patient's rights when necessary. Attributes of nurse advocacy include safeguarding, listening to the client's voice, promoting well-being, ethical decision-making, promoting client autonomy, representing clients, and championing social justice.[6,7]

In order to protect and secure rights, nurses must be familiar with the legislation (including mental health advocacy, ➔ www.scie.org.uk/independent-mental-health-advocacy/) that is pertinent to people with intellectual disabilities. This will include, but is not limited to, the law regarding: human rights; equality; disability discrimination; mental health; capacity; and health and social care (see ➔ The law, pp. 477–524; ➔ Independent Mental Capacity Advocates, pp. 274–5).

However, this advocacy role can pose particular challenges to nurses who are often not independent of the system providing services to the individual. Registered nurses must consider the impact of their advocacy actions upon other clients and may find it impossible to align themselves with one client to the exclusion of others. Inevitably, they will also deliberate its impact upon themselves and their relationships with colleagues, other professionals, and families. These dilemmas and conflicts of interest challenge the concept of a registered nurse as advocate and highlight the crucial significance of reflective practice.

It is vital that registered nurses recognize their role to create an organizational culture and service environment where advocacy can flourish. This could involve, but is not limited to, supporting individuals to build skills in decision-making and speaking up, training staff to create opportunities to promote choice and to actively listen to the people they support, enabling clients to access advocacy groups, welcoming friends and family members and recognizing their role as advocates, referring to independent advocacy services, and campaigning for them where they do not exist.

Further reading

Baker N, Wightman C (2015). *Same Difference? Advocacy for People who have a Learning Disability from Black and Minority Ethnic Groups.* British Institute of Learning Disabilities: Kidderminster.

Hafal (2012). *Care and Treatment Planning. A Step by Step Guide for Secondary Mental Health Service Users.* ➔ www.hafal.org/pdf/Care_and_Treatment_Planning_1.pdf (accessed 30 October 2017).

Mental Health (Wales). *Measure 2010.* ➔ www.legislation.gov.uk/mwa/2010/7/contents/enacted (accessed 30 October 2017).

References

5 Social Care Institute for Excellence (2014). *Commissioning Independent Advocacy.* Social Care Institute for Excellence: London.

6 Nursing and Midwifery Council (2015). *The Code: Professional Standards of Practice and Behaviour for Nurses and Midwives.* Nursing and Midwifery Council: London. ➔ www.nmc.org.uk/standards/code/ (accessed 7 March 2018).

7 Nursing and Midwifery Board of Ireland (2014). *Code of Professional Conduct and Ethics for Registered Nurses and Registered Midwives.* Nursing and Midwifery Board of Ireland: Dublin. ➔ www.nmbi.ie/Standards-Guidance/Code (accessed 7 March 2018).

Patient advice and liaison service

In 2002,[8] the then NHS Plan announced its commitment to setting up a patient advice and liaison service (PALS) in every Trust in England by April 2002. PALS are still to be found across England and aim to provide information, steer users towards appropriate service, and resolve problems. According to the Department of Health, their core functions were to:

- Be identifiable and accessible to patients, and their carers, friends, and family;
- Problem-solve promptly and efficiently;
- Signpost patients to independent advice and advocacy, both locally and nationally;
- Provide information about Trust services and health-related services;
- Initiate change and improvement via its feedback mechanisms;
- Link with other PALS;
- Support staff throughout the organization to respond to patients.[8]

For people with intellectual disabilities, PALS may be more difficult to access than for non-disabled people. Abbott et al. have pointed out that PALS may be underused by people who are already marginalized or demoralized.[9] Findings from the National Evaluation of PALS did not specifically mention access difficulties or adaptations, and reasonable adjustments that may need to be made for people with intellectual disabilities who intend or need to use PALS.[10]

The Department of Health's preliminary report described case studies whereby people felt enabled and empowered having used PALS.[10] Outcomes have been positive for people who have approached PALS with issues to address, such as with 'uncommunicative Trust systems' or complaints. It is believed that PALS effects and reduces the number of formal complaints, thus increasing public confidence, although the evidence has not been presented for this yet. Sometimes PALS is a last source of hope for some, yet people have still reported an improved experience of the Trust having accessed PALS. Abbott et al. suggested that people do need to go on to find independent advocates if inside problem-solving does not remedy their issue.[9]

Early findings of the Department of Health's National Evaluation revealed vast differences in staffing, establishments, and budgets, as well as differences in how PALS fed back within Trusts and at which level of seniority.[10]

One way of avoiding complaints in the first instance about NHS care is for providers of services to be aware of the particular communication needs that some people with intellectual disabilities may have. Another excellent resource is web-based and provided by University College Hospitals NHS Foundation Trust. They have a suite of videos that they have produced to help patients with intellectual disabilities better understand their visits to the hospitals within the Trust.[11]

A final example of how healthcare providers can support people with intellectual disabilities is Dartford and Gravesham NHS Trust.[12] At this Trust, in order to ensure that people with intellectual disabilities have equality of access and care, they have appointed a service lead. They have set up regular meetings between the Trust and members of the Social Services intellectual disabilities. The Trust has an excellent website, with numerous resources that include an easy-read complaints leaflet.

In the spirit of why PALS were first established in England, it is important to note that they were not simply to provide a mechanism for making complaints. It was always intended that they provide information, steering healthcare users towards appropriate services, and to this extent, this might prevent complaints. Notwithstanding this, some PALS have organically evolved beyond this to provide comprehensive and accessible information for people with intellectual disabilities. In doing so, they recognize the sometimes compromised nature of communication in people with intellectual disabilities, as well as a need to make reasonable adjustments to the services and care provided.

References

8 Department of Health (2000). *The NHS Plan. July 2000*. HMSO: London. ♒ webarchive. nationalarchives.gov.uk/20130123203805/http://www.dh.gov.uk/en/Publicationsandstatistics/Publications/PublicationsPolicyAndGuidance/DH_4002960 (accessed 30 October 2017).

9 Abbot S, Meyer J, Copperman J, Bentley J, Lanceley A (2005). Quality criteria for patient advice and liaison services: what do patients and the public want? *Health Expectations*. 8: 126–37.

10 Department of Health (2006). *Developing the Patient Advice and Liaison Service: Key Messages for NHS Organisations From the National Evaluation of PALS*. HMSO: London.

11 University College London Hospitals NHS Foundation Trust. *Learning Disabilities Videos*. ♒ www.uclh.nhs.uk/PandV/LD/Pages/Learningdisabilitiesvideos.aspx (accessed 30 October 2017).

12 Dartford and Gravesham NHS Trust. *Learning Disabilities*. ♒ www.dvh.nhs.uk/for-patients-and-visitors/learning-disabilities/ (accessed 30 October 2017).

Consent to examination, treatment, and care

At the most fundamental, 'consent to treatment' refers to the legal right that every single adult (and some children) has with regard to accepting or refusing care or intervention from a health or social care professional. People with capacity have the right to choose and to make decisions regarding care and interventions offered to them, even if that decision may appear unwise to the health or social care professional.

'Valid consent to care or treatment is therefore absolutely central in all forms of health and social care, from providing personal care to undertaking major surgery'[3] and applies as much to those receiving care and treatment in the community and residential care settings, as it does to those receiving surgery under anaesthesia in a general hospital.

What is legal and valid consent?

Three essential criteria are required to be met for consent to be regarded as legal and valid:

- The person must be deemed to have sufficient capacity to make the decision (see ⊃ Chapter 13);
- Their decision must be made voluntarily, with no evidence of coercion;
- The person must have sufficient knowledge about the care or intervention being offered.

It is important to understand that consent is a process and that simply obtaining a client's signature on a form does not equate to obtaining valid and legal consent. How the principles are applied, such as the amount of information provided and the degree of discussion needed to obtain valid consent, will vary depending on the nature and permanency of the decision. However, if any one of the above three criteria is shown or proved to be missing from the process of obtaining consent, in any setting, then valid consent cannot be said to have been achieved, leaving the health or social care professional liable to claims of assault, negligence, breach of human rights, or misconduct.

Legal and policy frameworks

The right to have a choice in the receipt of health and social care interventions is protected in a number of ways. These laws and policy differ across the UK and Republic of Ireland. For example, the Mental Capacity Act (2005)[14] provides the legal framework to protect people living in England and Wales who lack the capacity to consent, supporting and empowering people to make decisions for themselves.

The Adults with Incapacity Act (Scotland)[15] provides the legal framework in Scotland. At this point in time, Northern Ireland and the Republic of Ireland both have equivalent capacity legislation enacted and are awaiting implementation. Specifically, with regard to consent, practice in Northern Ireland is guided by Consent to Examination, Treatment and Care,[13] whereas practice in the Republic of Ireland is guided by the National Consent Policy.[16]

NBMI[17] and NMC[18] Codes of Practice make it explicit that nurses must ensure that proper and valid consent is obtained, that a person's right to accept or refuse treatment is respected, and that professionals need to understand and work to the relevant laws and policy about mental capacity and consent that apply in the country in which they are practising.

Is the right to consent absolute?

There are some exceptions and circumstances when the consent of the individual may not be necessary. For example, the law around consent in children and minors allows their consent to be overridden in some circumstances. This will, of course, be dependent on the age and maturity of the child, as well as the decision to be made. The law with regard to consent in children is complex and differs across UK jurisdictions. Therefore, to ensure legal and valid consent for those under 18, practitioners should refer to the law and policies in the country in which they practise. Treatment can also be provided without consent in emergency situations under the doctrine of necessity and, in some circumstances, when people are detained under mental health legislation. In all of the above circumstances and when adults lack capacity to consent to treatment or care, healthcare professionals can deliver interventions without consent but are required to do so in the person's best interests.

Best interests

Where an individual is found to lack capacity, it is lawful to proceed in their 'best interests'. The principles and legal frameworks that guide 'best interests' decision-making are addressed in ➜ Chapter 13.

References

13 Department of Health, Social Services and Public Safety (2003) *Good Practice in Consent: Consent for Examination, Treatment or Care: A Handbook for the HPSS*. Department of Health, Social Services and Public Safety: Belfast. ℘ www.health-ni.gov.uk/publications/consent-guides-healthcare-professionals (accessed 30 October 2017).

14 Department of Health (2005). *The Mental Capacity Act 2005*. HMSO: London. ℘ www.legislation.gov.uk/ukpga/2005/9/contents (accessed 30 October 2017).

15 The Scottish Government (2000). *Adults with Incapacity (Scotland) Act 2000*. HMSO: Edinburgh. ℘ www.legislation.gov.uk/asp/2000/4/contents (accessed 30 October 2017).

16 Health Service Executive (2014). *National Consent Policy*. Health Service Executive: Dublin. ℘ www.hse.ie/eng/services/list/3/nas/news/National_Consent_Policy.pdf (accessed 30 October 2017).

17 Nursing and Midwifery Board of Ireland (2014). *Code of Professional Conduct and Ethics for Registered Nurses and Registered Midwives*. Nursing and Midwifery Board of Ireland: Dublin.

18 Nursing and Midwifery Council (2015). *The Code: Professional Standards of Conduct and Behaviour for Nurses and Midwives*. Nursing and Midwifery Council: London.

Independent Mental Capacity Advocates

An Independent Mental Capacity Advocate (IMCA) is a statutory advocate that can be instructed to support the decision-making process for a person who lacks capacity under the Mental Capacity Act 2005. The role of the IMCA is established within the act to provide a legal safeguard for people who are unable to make a decision on their own upon a significant issue.

The role of the IMCA

An IMCA is appointed by local authorities or by NHS staff where a complex health or social care decision needs to be made. The IMCA is an independent professional advocate, employed within an advocacy organization which is separate to health and social care bodies. They are specially trained in issues concerning capacity and mental health legislation and in communicating with individuals who lack capacity.

An IMCA should be appointed to ensure that a decision is made under the principles of the MCA. They will ensure that the person's best interests are being considered, that the least restrictive options have been identified, and that the individual's personal beliefs and wishes are being taken into account.

The IMCA will meet with the person referred to establish their views and consult others involved in their care. They will gather other relevant information through the review of health and care records and other relevant documentation. The IMCA should be invited to all relevant meetings and they will ask questions pertinent to the situation. They will prepare a preliminary and final report, the recommendations of which must be considered by the decision-maker. The IMCA has the right to challenge the final decision.

The IMCA does not make the final decision or offer their opinion.

An IMCA must be appointed when the individual is over the age of 16 and has been formally assessed and deemed to lack capacity under the Mental Capacity Act 2005 **and**:

- Decision is to be made on a serious medical treatment or a long-term change of accommodation; and
- There are no family or friends willing to and/or able to be consulted (other than paid staff and professionals);
- Local authorities or the NHS may consider appointing an IMCA if they are undertaking complex care reviews and/or where incidents of safeguarding are an issue.

An IMCA does not need to be instructed when the:

- Decision can wait until the person regains capacity;
- Individual has family or friends that are willing to and able to represent them;
- Individual has a personal welfare attorney appointed to deal with the same issue;
- Court of protection has appointed a deputy to deal with the same issue.

Key principles

- An IMCA is independent.
- Local authorities and NHS staff have a duty to appoint IMCAs in decisions involving serious medical treatment and/or changes in accommodation.
- The IMCA does not offer their own opinion.
- The IMCA does not make the decision; their role is to support the decision-making process.
- An IMCA should not be appointed where the individual is receiving treatment under the Mental Health Act 1987; an Independent Mental Health Advocate (IMHA) should be appointed in these circumstances.
- Should disputes occur, referral to the court of protection should be considered.

Further reading

Department of Health (2005). *Mental Capacity Act 2005*. The Stationary Office: London. ℬ www. legislation.gov.uk/ukpga/2005/9/contents (accessed 30 October 2017).

Office of the Public Guardian (2007). *Making Decisions: The Independent Mental Capacity Advocate (IMCA) service*. Available to download from: ℬ www.publicguardian.gov.uk (accessed 30 October 2017).

Circles of support

> 'A circle is hard to describe; it's too simple.'
>
> (Regina DeMarasse, Circles Network, 2005).*[19]

A circle of support, sometimes called a circle of friends, is a group of people who meet on a regular basis, with the ultimate aim of helping the focus person reach their dreams and aspirations in life. A circle might be created for a number of reasons—some people may be at risk of, or experiencing, social isolation; for others, a circle may arise as a consequence of their person-centred plan.

The concept of circles of support was initiated in Canada, then spread through North America before arriving in the UK in the mid 1980s.[19] A circle of support is a markedly different idea to advocacy or befriending. An advocate or befriender may not naturally occur from the focus person's wider network, whereas one purpose of a circle is to 'draw together a group of people who are committed to helping someone they care about (or maybe love) to change his or her life.'[20]

Circles of support are not exclusively for people who have intellectual disabilities. They may be of benefit to any person who feels isolated, excluded, or in need of support to realize or achieve a better life. For example, these include children or adults who are living in deprived circumstances, disabled students in education, parents who themselves have intellectual disabilities, people receiving palliative care services, people who have committed sexual offences, or those who have mental health problems.

Circles of support derive from truly person-centred principles. To this end, the focus person is in charge, as they decide who can join the circle and which direction the energy of the circle is taken. Initially, a circle has a facilitator to get it started and to keep account of the action that is required to keep it working. Once formed, the circle meets regularly to assist the focus person to recognize their dreams and imagine their most desirable future. In order to help the dreams become reality, the members of the group 'realize their gifts and skills'. In addition, the circle helps to problem-solve and continues to build networks in order for the focus person to broaden their opportunities and achieve greater inclusion in their (chosen) community. Finally, a key ingredient is to have fun! It is expected that the facilitator withdraws once the circle is up and running, and fully operational for the focus person.

An important aim of a circle of support for a child or young person is to include at least one peer, often a peer who is non-disabled. Jay describes the merits of this to both the focus person and the non-disabled peers.[21] Jay recognizes that young people who have intellectual disabilities often miss out on the 'ordinariness' of growing up and that advocacy is usually provided through adults. By involving non-disabled peers in the circle who have got to know the focus person, Jay professes that they have a different slant on life and 'are bound to have a closer and more accurate view of what young people want from life than an adult'.[21]

---

* Circles Network (2005). Circles of Support. ℰ www.circlesnetwork.org.uk/index.asp?slevel=0z114z115&parent_id=115 [Accessed 30th October 2017]

A circle may start small, even only three members. The members comprise family, friends, and community members, usually people who are not paid to be there. There may be a role for paid professionals, but the aim and focus of the circle must remain. As time goes on, the whole circle may not meet in its entirety each time. As the circle builds momentum, and gifts and strengths are identified, certain members may meet (always with the focus person) with respect to specific goals.

A circle of support is not the end-result of a planning process; in fact, once a circle has been formed, further person-centred planning takes place. It is a planning style in itself, but it may also employ one or even a variety of planning tools such as PATH or McGill Action Planning System (MAPS). Circle meetings usually take place monthly, more often in a period of crisis, and may last <2h. As an important aim of a circle is to have fun, celebrate, and enjoy being together, the meetings may take place in a whole variety of settings such as the focus person's living room, a pub, or a café.

There is a limited evidence base for circles of support. This is partly due to the small number of services and the diversity of their focus. It is also linked to the paradox of trying to be a roots-led, values-based social movement for inclusive communities, while simultaneously needing to show effectiveness in service-defined outcomes that will bring resources for development.[22]

An expressed fear of a family carer might be that a circle is actually intended to replace or avoid paid support where it is needed. Circles Network (2007) insist that a circle of support is 'not a replacement for human services'.[23] Once a circle is formed, therefore, it must ensure that the focus person does not lose necessary paid support. One answer would be to ensure that a care/budget manager is involved where this fear is sensed, so plans can be made to develop or protect the focus person's paid support package. Also there might be concern that any efforts to befriend the focus person were tokenistic. However, the role of the facilitator is to ensure that everyone's gifts and skills are shared and used to work towards change.

References

19 Circles Network (2005). *Circles of Support*. ஃ www.circlesnetwork.org.uk/index.asp?slevel= 0z114z115&parent_id=115 (accessed 30 October 2017).

20 Circles Network (2007). *Circles of Support: An Introduction to Person Centred Planning and the Values of Inclusion*. Circles Network: Rugby.

21 Jay N (2007). Peer mentorship: promoting advocacy and friendship between young people. *Learning Disability Today*. 7: 18–21.

22 Elliot I, Zajac G (2015). The implementation of Circles of Support and accountability in the United States. *Aggression and Violent Behavior*. 25: 113–23.

23 Circles Network (2007). *Circles Network Impact Report*. Circles Network: Rugby.

Making best interests decisions

When are 'best interests' decisions required?

All national policies that underpin services for people with intellectual disabilities include clear principles about the need to involve people with intellectual disabilities in decisions that affect them. The consent policies in the respective jurisdictions highlight the right of people to be involved in decisions and the need for, and importance of, maximizing their opportunities to do so, through providing additional support and making reasonable adjustments such as providing information in an accessible manner and providing more time for decision-making (see ➔ Consent to examination, treatment, and care, pp. 506–7).

All countries in the UK and the Republic of Ireland also now have legislation in place or approved, and the process of being implemented (as in Republic of Ireland and Northern Ireland) relating to mental capacity for all people and people with intellectual disabilities are included within this. It is also clearly stated within the policy documents and legislative provision that when a person is over 18yrs old and is unable to give consent, no one, including family members, are able to give consent on their behalf and that decisions must be taken in their 'best interests'.

The Mental Capacity Act (2005) provides the legal framework to ensure that anything done for, or on behalf of, a person who lacks capacity to consent is done in the best interests of the person concerned.[24] The decision-maker is protected from liability if they ensure that the care/treatment is in the best interests of the person concerned. Currently, the legislation only covers England and Wales, and in Scotland, the Adults with Incapacity Act (2000) applies.[25] In Northern Ireland and Republic of Ireland, the separate guidance on *Consent to Examination, Treatment and Care* applies.[26,27]

What could I do to ensure that care and/or treatment is in the best interests of the person?

It is necessary to be clear about the process of making a 'best interests' decision, and this should be documented, very clearly showing what factors were considered in developing possible options for consideration, exactly what options were considered, together with the benefits and limitations of each option, and finally how the decision was made and who was involved.

A clear record of the process of making a best interest decision must be made on the appropriate forms within your service. In developing options for consideration, reviewing these, and the final decision-making process, the following points should underpin the 'best interests' decision-making process and be clearly documented:[24]

- Encourage participation of the person with intellectual disabilities and people involved in their care.
- Identify all relevant circumstances.
- Find out the person's views.
- Avoid discrimination.

- Assess whether the person might regain capacity.
- If the decision concerns life-sustaining treatment, it should not be motivated in any way by a desire to bring about the person's death.
- Do not make assumptions about the person's quality of life.
- Consult others; an independent advocate may be consulted in certain circumstances.
- When consulting, remember that the person who lacks capacity to make the decision or act for themselves still has a right to keep their affairs private.
- Avoid restricting the person's rights (least restrictive alternative).
- Take all of this into account and weigh up all of these factors in order to work out what is in the person's best interests.[24]

Best interests decisions must be made on the basis of weighing up the possible benefits against the possible disadvantages for the person (sometimes referred to as a 'balance sheet' approach). Medical, emotional, social, and welfare benefits and disadvantages should be considered. It is only if the benefits outweigh the disadvantages that the proposed action should be taken.

Who is the decision-maker?

The decision-maker can be a number of different people and is dependent on the decision in question, i.e. for day-to-day actions, the decision-maker would be the carer directly involved with the person. Where the decision involves medical or dental treatment, the decision-maker would be the doctor or dentist responsible for carrying out the treatment or procedure. It is the responsibility of the decision-maker always to ensure that the decision is in the best interests of the person concerned at that time.

Best interests meetings

For major decisions with regard to healthcare, if the person is found to lack capacity to consent, then a best interests meeting must be arranged and all relevant parties invited. These meetings may, at times, need to be arranged quickly, and it is therefore important to understand that only those people relevant to the specific decision in question need to be part of the best interests meeting. Clear consideration should be given to whether an independent advocate should be appointed to be part of these discussions.

References

24 Office of the Public Guardian (2014). *Mental Capacity Act 2005: Code of Practice*. The Stationery Office: London. ॐ www.gov.uk/government/publications/mental-capacity-act-code-of-practice (accessed 30 October 2017).

25 The Scottish Government (2000). *Adults with Incapacity (Scotland) 2000. A Short Guide to the Act*. ॐ www.gov.scot/Publications/2008/03/25120154/1 (accessed 30 October 2017).

26 Department of Health, Social Services and Public Safety (2003). *Consent to Examination, Treatment and Care*. Department of Health, Social Services and Public Safety: Belfast. ॐ www.health-ni.gov. uk/publications/consent-guides-healthcare-professionals (accessed 30 October 2017).

27 Health Service Executive. *Republic of Ireland National Consent Policy Documents*. ॐ www.hse.ie/eng/about/Who/qualityandpatientsafety/National_Consent_Policy/consent.html (accessed 30 October 2017).

Vulnerability

What is vulnerability?

Vulnerable—'Exposed to the possibility of being attacked or harmed, either physically or emotionally'.[28] Within the context of intellectual disability, some may argue this term is pejorative in leading people to assume that the whole of this population, when described as vulnerable, are in need of other people to take 'control' over their lives to varying degrees. While this is not the case (as people may not be vulnerable all of the time), it is important to examine some key issues.

Why may people with intellectual disability be vulnerable?

There are many reasons why people experience different levels of vulnerability when we consider the word exposure in the above definition. Exposure may be influenced and affected by personal circumstances and/or subsequent dependency on others and can change over time. For some people, this dependency may centre on complex physical needs, sensory impairment, expressive and receptive communication problems, social isolation and/or lack of supportive relationships, mental health problems, and behaviour that challenges others. Other influencing factors can include where people are cared for and institutional regimes and lack of recognition or disputes about whether that person has a learning disability or not. Most obviously, the presence of a cognitive impairment may prevent people from recognizing risk and danger and/or being able to take independent action to prevent it. More specifically, within care situations, the person's environment can increase their level of vulnerability and can include lack of care plans, rigid routines, poor staff morale, high levels of sickness, inadequate complaints systems, lack of advocacy, lack of community involvement, lack of client involvement in decision-making, lack of personal possessions, and a lack of privacy.[29]

There have been several recent serious case reviews concerning the abuse of people with intellectual disabilities where there have been inequalities in care relationships.[30] These care relationships have often been domineered by control and power imbalances. Vulnerability is not only symptomatic of such scenarios but is exacerbated by them. Also, for people with intellectual disabilities in general hospital settings, a lack of care giver's knowledge can be equally detrimental.[31] The effects of many of the above influences can lead to disempowerment.

Conversely, a move away from group care settings has changed the landscape regarding vulnerability patterns. Terms such as 'mate crime' have evolved to describe people with intellectual disabilities being befriended before being coerced and bullied into prostitution, selling drugs, and storing stolen goods.[32] Recent increases in social media and wider Internet use have varied the methods in which people may target vulnerable individuals, e.g. through online dating sites or email scams. These risks may be heightened when the social isolation that many people with intellectual disabilities experience is considered.

What can we do to help reduce a person's vulnerability?

- Help develop protective behaviours where people are comfortable talking about all areas of their life and experiences.
- Empower people to have as much control over their lives as possible.
- Assist people with intellectual disabilities to develop and maintain positive and supportive relationships with others.
- Identify actual and potential risks to people with intellectual disabilities and help plan strategies to minimize the risk of harm.
- Work closely with care staff and families to raise awareness of factors that may increase vulnerability of a person and important strategies to reduce the level of vulnerability.
- Understand that people have the right to make what others may consider a 'poor decision' as long as they have the capacity to do so.
- Where there are concerns regarding potential abuse, local safeguarding and policies for escalating concerns need to be followed.
- Lead by example to challenge inappropriate power imbalances and share information across services, as those most at risk are most commonly known to multiple agencies.[33]

References

28 *Oxford Dictionaries*. ℛ www.oxforddictionaries.com (accessed 4 July 2016).
29 Jenkins R, Davies R (2011). Safeguarding people with learning disabilities. *Learning Disability Practice*. **14**: 32–9.
30 Department of Health (2012). *Transforming Care: A National Response to Winterbourne View Hospital*. Department of Health Review: Final Report. Department of Health: London.
31 Heslop P, Blair P, Fleming M, Hoghton M, Marriott A, Russ L (2013). *Confidential Inquiry into Premature Deaths of People with Learning Disabilities (CIPOLD)*. Norah Fry Research Centre: Bristol. ℛ www.bris.ac.uk/cipold/ (accessed 30 October 2017).
32 Grundy (2011). Friend or fake? Mate crime and people with learning disability. *Journal of Learning Disability and Offending Behaviour*. **12**: 167–9.
33 Manthorpe J, Martineau S (2015). What can and cannot be learned from serious case reviews of the care and treatment of adults with learning disabilities in England? Messages for social workers. *British Journal of Social Work*. **45**: 331–48.

Child protection

Child protection is a term used to refer to activities undertaken to prevent or reduce the risk of children and young people experiencing significant harm. It is part of the wider process known as safeguarding which aims to promote the safety, well-being, and optimal development of all children up to the age of 18.

Each nation of the UK and the Republic of Ireland has its own policies and laws regarding safeguarding and child protection. It is important to be familiar with the laws and guidance that govern where you practise. However, the principles of child protection are generally relevant nationally and internationally.

Everyone who works with children or young people in any setting has a responsibility to safeguard and act to protect children and young people if they have concerns about their safety. Each agency should have its own guidelines and protocols, and all nurses must be familiar with these and know what to do in the event that they have concerns.

Children with intellectual disabilities may be particularly vulnerable to abuse because of their difficulties in communication, their need for intimate care, and the provision of such care by a number of carers in a range of locations.

What are the different types of abuse?

Perpetrators of abuse against children can be any age.[34] It can happen in any location, including online. All forms of abuse require a response from professionals and other adults around the child/young person.

Children and young people have the right to be protected from:

- Physical abuse—including hitting, slapping, shaking, burning, pinching, biting, throwing, and anything that causes physical injury, leaves a mark, and/or causes significant physical pain or induced illness;
- Emotional abuse—can be difficult to identify, as there may not be any physical signs. It includes situations when shouting and anger causes distress and when parents and/or others constantly criticize or threaten children so that their self-esteem and feelings of self-worth are damaged;
- Sexual abuse—any type of sexual activity that takes place between an adult and a person under 16yrs. Sexual abuse can also occur between children. Child sexual exploitation involves using a child sexually for money or power;
- Neglect occurs when a child or young person does not have adequate physical and emotional care to promote their well-being and development. This is a common form of child abuse;
- Bullying and cyberbullying can have physical and emotional effects;
- Child trafficking—involving the movement or recruitment of children who may be forced to work or be sold;
- Female genital mutilation (FGM)—the partial or complete removal of external ♀ genitalia for any non-medical reason;
- Grooming—when a person makes an emotional relationship with a child or young person with the intention of abusing or exploiting them. This could include radicalization;

- Sexually harmful behaviour—involving engaging in sexual language, activity, or observation of images that are the beyond the developmental stage of the child. This can harm the child engaging in the activity and with other children.

What do you need to know?

There is interprofessional agreement regarding the minimum standards of knowledge, skills, and values about safeguarding children/young people.[35] Nurses should be able to identify signs of abuse or neglect, make appropriate referrals, advocate for the child/young people, work effectively in an interdisciplinary context, be aware of how parents'/carers' mental and physical health may negatively affect a child, and know to whom to report and the processes to follow.

What should you do?

Always be ready to actively listen to children/young people (listening and observation). Reflect on how your own experiences and beliefs may impact on your work in this area. If you have concerns about a child, do something; do not ignore your suspicions. Talk to:

- A teacher, health visitor, community nurse, social worker, or GP;
- Your clinical supervisor;
- Your local safeguarding/child protection team.

It is particularly important to ensure that events are recorded accurately with dates and times.

What do professional codes say?

As a registered nurse, you must protect the rights and interests of individuals and act in such a way that justifies the trust and confidence the public holds of you, as required in your regulator's 'Code' of conduct.

Nurses must act immediately if concerned a child or young person is at risk of harm, neglect, or abuse. You need to follow professional guidelines in relation to escalating concerns.[36] You have a responsibility to share information about those concerns (with due regard to laws regarding disclosure of information) and must ensure your knowledge of safeguarding policy and legislation is current. You are also accountable for your actions and omissions, regardless of advice or directions from anyone.

References

34 NSPCC (2016). *Child Protection in the UK*. ℛ www.nspcc.org.uk/preventing-abuse/child-protection-system/ (accessed 30 October 2017).

35 Royal College of Paediatrics and Child Health (2014). *Safeguarding Children and Young People: Roles and Competences for Health Care Staff*. Royal College of Paediatrics and Child Health: London.

36 Nursing and Midwifery Council (2015). *Raising Concerns. Guidance for Nurses and Midwives*. Nursing and Midwifery Council: London.

Adult safeguarding

Adult safeguarding is a process to promote and protect the rights of adults to live a life free from abuse and neglect. Legislation and policy particularly focus on individuals who may need care or support to achieve this.[35–39] All staff are responsible for safeguarding. This requires partnership between individuals, professionals, communities, and organizations to be effective. The key duty for adult safeguarding rests with local authorities, the police, and the NHS. Every person who has concerns with regard to suspicion of abuse should follow the relevant local policies and procedures or directly contact the adult protection team.

Who is a vulnerable adult?

At different times in our lives, we are all vulnerable to harm. Different contexts, issues, and environments may all impact on whether, and to what extent, any individual may be at risk of some sort of physical or psychological danger; put another way, our 'vulnerability' can change with time and place. There is some disagreement about what vulnerability means and the concept itself can be challenged. Recognizing that some groups of people (e.g. those with dementia or intellectual disabilities) have historically been mistreated and may be more at risk of harm offers services the potential to afford them greater protection. However, it must also be acknowledged that being recognized as a 'vulnerable adult' may make an individual more at risk of being stigmatized, infantilized, and treated as part of a homogenous group, rather than a unique human being. We need to be alert to the idea that being labelled a vulnerable person may have the effect of making someone vulnerable; the emphasis should be on supporting people when they are vulnerable, rather than treating people as 'vulnerable' all the time. There is a need to approach safeguarding through a focus on being person-centred and guided by the wishes and needs of the individual. [35–39]

The six key principles of safeguarding

- Empowerment—led by the person with their informed consent;
- Prevention—act before harm happens;
- Proportional responses—is it an actual or a potential risk? Offer the least restrictive response;
- Protection—support and advocacy for those in greatest need;
- Partnerships—co-producing solutions with the individual, their networks, and relevant third-sector organizations;
- Accountability—effective and transparent.[35]

Working with 'vulnerability'

When working with individuals around their vulnerabilities, it can help to consider: for this individual, at this time, and in this context, what are they vulnerable to? Is the risk actual or potential? Who are the right people to work together on this? What does the individual want? It then becomes possible to consider what support can be put into place to manage those specific risks and who the right people to be involved are.

What is abuse?

Abuse covers a wide range of actions and could be:

- Financial, e.g. theft, fraud, misuse of property, possessions, or benefits;
- Physical, e.g. hitting, inappropriate use of punishments, misuse of medications that make a person drowsy;
- Sexual, e.g. rape, sexual assault, sexual acts without consent;
- Psychological, e.g. threats of harm, restraint, intimidation, threats to restrict a person's liberty;
- Neglect and acts of omission, e.g. ignoring a person's medical or physical care needs, failing to provide health or social care, or withholding a person's medication or basic care needs;
- Exploitation and coercion, including grooming to commit crime, acts of terrorism, or forced marriage.

What do professional codes say?

As a registered nurse, you must protect the rights and interests of individuals and act in such a way that justifies the trust and confidence the public holds of you, as required in your regulator's 'Code' of conduct.

Nurses must act immediately if concerned an adult is at risk of harm, neglect, or abuse. You also have a responsibility to share information about those concerns (with due regard to laws regarding disclosure of information) and must ensure your knowledge of safeguarding policy and legislation is current. You are also accountable for your actions and omissions, regardless of advice or directions from anyone.

What do people with intellectual disabilities say?

There has been a limited amount of research exploring what women and men with intellectual disabilities think about abuse. However, one mixed-method participatory study[40] established that people are clear that what they want from the people who support them is for them to actively *listen* to the person (what is said, how they act, and what is not said), to *believe* they are in distress and need support, and then to *do* something by acting upon this knowledge and following relevant procedures.

Further reading

Northway R, Jenkins R (2017). *Safeguarding Adults in Nursing Practice*, 2nd edn. Learning Matters: London.

References

35 Department of Health (2014). *The Care Act (2014)*. Department of Health: London.
36 Welsh Government (2014). *Social Services and Well-being (Wales) Act (2014)*. Welsh Government: Cardiff.
37 Scottish Government (2007). *The Adult Support and Protection (Scotland) Act (2007)*. Scottish Government: Edinburgh.
38 Department of Health, Social Services and Public Safety (2015). *Adult Safeguarding Protection and Prevention in Partnership*. Department of Health, Social Services and Public Safety: Belfast.
39 Health Service Executive (2014). *Safeguarding Vulnerable Persons at Risk of Abuse. National Policy and Procedures*. Health Service Executive: Dublin. ℘ www.hse.ie/eng/services/publications/corporate/personsatriskofabuse.pdf (accessed 30 October 2017). (This document is being updated; check ℘ HSE.ie for the most recent document.)
40 Northway R, Melsomme M, Flood S, Bennett D, Howarth J (2013). How do people with intellectual disabilities view abuse and abusers? *Journal of Intellectual Disabilities*. **17**: 361–75.

Care pathways

What is a care pathway?

A care pathway is an integrated and structured interdisciplinary care plan outlining the care to be undertaken and the order in which care should be delivered. A care pathway should be based on best evidence, standards, and protocols available in relation to a particular clinical condition. A care pathway lays out a framework as to how care should be delivered appropriately, in the right order, and at the right time, and with the correct outcome for the individual. It must be remembered, however, that nurses are required to consider how a care pathway relates to each individual in their care and will need to make professional decisions if there is a need to adapt this in the provision of individualized care.

Different terms for care pathways

It has been identified that a number of terms are used interchangeably to describe a care pathway.[1] All the following terms have been used within the literature to describe care pathways:

- Clinical pathways;
- Anticipated recovery pathways;
- Interdisciplinary pathways of care;
- Integrated care management;
- Collaborative care pathways;
- Care profiles;
- Coordinated care pathways.

Implementing care pathways

The stages in developing and then implementing a care pathway are as follows:

- Appointment of a credible facilitator;
- Identification of interdisciplinary team members;
- Selection of topic;
- Definition of problem or issue;
- Review of evidence base, guidelines, and protocols;
- Audit of current practice;
- Identification of users' views on current and future practice;
- Consideration of local abilities and constraints;
- Development of the actual pathway documentation:
  - Desired outcomes;
  - Decision points;
  - Procedures to follow;
  - Outcomes and milestones to achieve;
  - Detail of variance tracking;
  - Detail of review;
  - Detail of audit;
  - Staff education;
- Pilot of the pathway;
- Review of pilot;
- Amendment as required;
- Implement pathway.

Variance tracking and analysis
Variance in a care pathway is the difference between the predicted outcome and the actual outcome. Thus, if delivered care varies from the care pathway, this should be recorded as variance. It is important that unexpected outcomes can be tracked. It is also apparent that if these unexpected occurrences happen in a number of cases, analysis should be undertaken, which may lead to new and improved pathways.

Potential benefits of care pathways
Care pathways should:
• Enable research-based practice to underpin care;
• Provide a framework for interdisciplinary working;
• Aid the use of local protocols and guidelines;
• Aid the incorporation of national policies, protocols, and guidelines;
• Enhance communication between everyone involved;
• Reduce unnecessary variations in care;
• Ensure that people's care journeys are straightforward.

Barriers to developing care pathways
There are many barriers to developing pathways, including:
• Time;
• Increase in meetings;
• Education;
• Evaluation;
• True involvement.

Care pathways for people with intellectual disabilities
There are care pathways that are used within services for people with intellectual disabilities, but there appears to be only a small amount of literature available. Care pathways that are detailed in the literature include:
• Crisis in challenging behaviour;
• Oral healthcare;
• Access to general healthcare;
• Epilepsy;
• Hearing impairment.

Further reading
Rotter Y, Kinsman L, Jame EL, et al. (2010). Clinical pathways effects on professional practice, patient outcomes, length of stay and hospital costs. *Cochrane Database of Systematic Reviews*. 2010; 3: CD006632.
Van Gerven E et al. (2010). Management challenges in care pathways: conclusions of a qualitative study within 57 health care organisations. *International Journal of Care Pathways*. 14: 142–9.

References
41 Powell H, Kwiatek E (2006). Integrated care pathways in intellectual disability nursing. In: B Gates, ed. *Care Planning and Delivery in Intellectual Disability Nursing*. Blackwell Publishing: London; pp. 21–52.

Care Programme Approach

The CPA, first introduced in 1990, is a structured approach in which services are assessed, planned, coordinated, and reviewed for someone with mental health problems or a range of related complex needs. An individual might be offered CPA support if they:

- Are diagnosed as having a severe mental disorder;
- Are at risk of suicide, self-harm, or harm to others;
- Tend to neglect themselves and do not take treatment regularly;
- Are vulnerable; this could be for various reasons such as physical or emotional abuse, financial difficulties, because of mental illness or cognitive impairment;
- Have misused drugs or alcohol;
- Have learning disabilities;
- Rely significantly on the support of a carer or have their own caring responsibilities;
- Have recently been detained under the mental health legislation—this will depend on the jurisdiction;
- Have parenting responsibilities;
- Have a history of violence or self-harm.

Anyone experiencing mental health problems is entitled to an assessment of their abilities and needs from a mental healthcare professional. If required, a care plan will be constructed which will be regularly reviewed by that professional.

Involvement of people with intellectual disabilities and their carers

The importance of involving users and carers has been stressed in successive guidance on the implementation of the CPA. Users should be involved in discussions about their proposed care programmes so that they can discuss different treatment possibilities, agree with the programme, and identify the outcomes. It is also important to involve relevant others in the development of the care programme. Carers often know a great deal about a person's life, interests, and abilities, as well as having personal experience of the person's mental health problems.[42]

Key components

The four key components or stages of the CPA are:[43]

- Systematic assessment of both health and social care needs;
- Formation of a care plan, including identification of providers;
- Appointment of a key worker or care coordinator;
- Regular review.

As well as involving the person and their carers, the development and implementation of a care programme should be an interdisciplinary activity.

Levels of the care programme approach

It should be noted that the person may move up and down the levels detailed below, as the mental healthcare abilities and needs change.

Standard care programme approach
This approach is suitable for people who require minimal social support, are relatively stable, and have low healthcare needs.

Enhanced care programme approach
This level is suitable for people who require medium/high levels of support and are less likely to remain stable. The person may also require further assessment, and it is likely that they will receive support from more than one professional, and the actual care plan will be more complex. Alternatively, they may have a severe mental health problem or be unstable and volatile, posing a risk either to themselves or to others. It is likely that the person requiring this level of support would also be unable to function socially. In this case, the care plan will be detailed with arrangements for continual evaluation so that changes in the mental health status can be identified quickly. It is imperative that the role of the differing professionals is identified within the plan in detail and that the professionals communicate effectively.

Supervision register
This level of care programme is required for people who present a significant risk to themselves or others. The person is continually and actively followed up, and they may be placed on the supervision register.

Advantages of the care programme approach
The CPA:
- Supports multidisciplinary working;
- Supports 'joined-up' management;
- Encourages explicit roles;
- Enhances communication;
- Formalizes communication;
- Provides clarity for the person and their carers.

Disadvantages of the care programme approach
The CPA also has some disadvantages in that it may:
- Increase bureaucracy;
- Increase stress for the person and their carer.

Further reading
NHS Choices (2018). *Care Programme Approach.* (The mental health charity Rethink has produced a factsheet providing further information about the CPA.) ⌨ www.nhs.uk/conditions/social-care-and-support-guide/pages/care-programme-approach.aspx (accessed 30 October 2017).

References
42 Carpenter J, Sbarani S (2007). *Choice, Information and Dignity: Involving Users and Carers in Care Management in Mental Health.* The Policy Press: London.
43 Hepworth K, Wolverson M (2006). Care planning and delivery in forensic settings for people with intellectual disabilities. In: B Gates, ed. *Care Planning and Delivery in Intellectual Disability Nursing.* Blackwell Publishing: London; pp. 125–57.

Health action plans and health facilitation

The terms 'health action plan' (HAP) and 'health facilitation' originated from the Department of Health's White Paper *Valuing People*.[44] These terms have since been endorsed with similar documents and are recognized good practice elsewhere in the UK and Ireland. This initiative was needed because there was growing evidence that people with intellectual disabilities had greater health needs than the general population, yet accessed health services less often. It is expected that all people with intellectual disabilities will have the opportunity to have a personal HAP.[45] This should be developed in partnership with the person with intellectual disabilities, the nurses working them, and other relevant professionals such as primary healthcare providers and allied health professionals and GPs. Information that comes from these health checks can form the basis of the individual's HAP. In practice, a HAP forms part of an individual's person centred plan and will normally include details about the individual's health under various domains:

• Oral health and dental care;
• Fitness and mobility;
• Continence;
• Vision;
• Hearing;
• Nutrition;
• Mental health needs;
• Emotional, spiritual, and sexual needs;
• Medication taken—desired effects/side effects;
• Screening tests results.

A critical aspect and persistent challenge of health facilitation and health action planning is to demonstrate consistent positive outcomes and health improvement for people with intellectual disabilities. Following the health check, any interventions required can be put into action, e.g. a dental appointment could be made for a man with intellectual disabilities who complains of pain in his mouth or for someone who had not seen a dentist in the last 12 months. It is important that all HAPs consider the person's lifestyle choice, culture, and values. Actions arising from HAPs should be agreed with the individual, and choices offered (e.g. regarding treatment decisions). A copy of the HAP is held by the person with intellectual disabilities, so like all 'care plans', it should person-centred and outcomes-based and be written in an accessible format, according to the person's communication abilities and needs, in order that the individual can understand it. To ensure that health needs are closely monitored, it is recommended that a HAP is conducted at key points such as:

• Transition from education or young peoples' services;
• Leaving home/moving into residential services;
• Moving from one service provider to another;
• Moving to an out-of-area placement;
• If there has been a change in health status (e.g. following an illness);
• On retirement;
• When planning transition for those living with older family carers.

Health facilitator

One of the roles of the HF, where these roles have been appointed as separate from nursing roles, is to ensure that the actions arising from the HAP are followed up and that the person gets the medical or other attention they need. In doing so, they should liaise with other professionals involved, e.g. GPs, allied health professionals, staff in general hospitals, or other services when planning appointments for screening or conducting further assessments. Exactly who undertakes this role varies from area to area and depends on the nature of the service and the abilities and needs of the individual. It may be a professional carer or alternatively someone close to the person who is not paid to work with them (such as an advocate or friend). However, a registered nurse in intellectual disability with up-to-date knowledge and skills in health promotion and healthcare could undertake this role.

More recently, the Department of Health has endorsed the role of the 'strategic health facilitator'.[45] This is a broader role to be undertaken by a professional (e.g. registered nurse with specific education in working with people with intellectual disabilities). It concerns the need to overcome the barriers between primary and secondary healthcare and people with intellectual disabilities and to enable effective liaison with health staff in both these environments to improve the access to, and outcomes of, healthcare experience. One way this may be achieved is through proactive education of other professionals who have a responsibility for the care of people with intellectual disabilities. This role is considered critical to the effectiveness of local health and social care services for people with intellectual disabilities, as it aims to provide an interface between the strategic, the operational, and the individual.

Further reading

McConkey R, Taggart L, Kane M (2015). Optimizing the uptake of health checks for people with intellectual disabilities. *Journal of Intellectual Disabilities*. **19**: 205–14.

Robertson J, Hatton C, Baines S, Emerson E (2015). Systematic reviews of the health or health care of people with intellectual disabilities: a systematic review to identify gaps in the evidence base. *Journal of Applied Research in Intellectual Disabilities*. **28**: 455–523.

Royal College of General Practitioners. *Learning Disabilities*. www.rcgp.org.uk/learningdisabilities (accessed 30 October 2017). (See examples of HAP templates.)

References

44 Department of Health (2001). *Valuing People. A New Strategy for Learning Disability for 21st Century*. Department of Health: London.

45 Department of Health (2007). *Health Action Planning and Health Facilitation for People with Learning Disabilities: Good Practice Guide*. Department of Health: London.

Care management, case management, and continuing care

It is widely accepted that some people with intellectual disabilities will have some element of a 'looked-after life', and while not advocating that everyone needs professional intervention within their lives, it is necessary to acknowledge that lessons in support packages are learnt to ensure that individuals receive the care they need and deserve. While the notion of 'managing care' for people is not new, the concept of specific 'care management', as we know it today, was first introduced in the 1989 *Griffith Report*. This became the template for the White Paper *Caring For People* in England,[46] with related documents elsewhere in the UK. One of the key objectives of the White Paper challenged services 'to make proper assessment of need and good care management the cornerstone of high quality care; packages of care should then be designed in line with individual needs and preferences.'[46]

From this, it can be argued that a clear focus and definition of care management are to ensure that a specific, individualized package of resources is in place to ensure that the person's needs and wishes are met; it is not about fitting a person's service into a budget. Essentially, care management is a collaborative process—one which appropriately assesses, ethically plans, effectively implements, coordinates, and evaluates the holistic package of health and social care services required to meet an individual's needs.

However, since headline issues, such as Winterbourne View, the commissioning and provision of services for adults with intellectual disabilities has been in flux and under review. The government pledged in 2012 in the *Transforming Care*[47] report, 'By 1 June 2014 we expect to see a rapid reduction in the number of people with challenging behaviour in hospitals or in large scale residential care—particularly those away from their home area. By that date, no-one should be inappropriately living in a hospital setting.'

As with all systems of care, there are inherent difficulties, e.g. care managers are often placed in invidious positions, particularly in relation to rationing and resource allocation/management. They frequently find themselves aligned to both the purchaser (i.e. the person in receipt of care) and the provider, entering into deliberations of 'best practice'.

There is no doubt that the Transforming Care Programme has wide and much needed impact on care management; the Transforming Care Programme is focusing on addressing long-standing issues to ensure sustainable change that will see:

- More choice for people and their families, and more say in their care;
- Providing more care in the community, with personalized support provided by multidisciplinary health and care teams;
- More innovative services to give people a range of care options, with personal budgets, so that care meets individuals' needs;
- Providing early more intensive support for those who need it, so that people can stay in the community, close to home;
- But for those that do need inpatient care, ensuring it is only for as long as they need it (℘ www.england.nhs.uk/learning-disabilities/care/).

It is important to acknowledge within this section long-term conditions and NSFs, as both of these impact on a model of case management and lead into continuing care. It is interesting to note that there is a specific service framework for people with intellectual disabilities which has been developed in Northern Ireland, but as yet none exists in England, Wales, or Scotland dedicated to people with intellectual disabilities. Professionals often need reminding that all other NSF applies to all citizens.

Case management

Not all people with intellectual disabilities have a 'labelled' long-term condition or need intensive case management. However, this approach may have value as a method of coordinating services. It is recognized that for people who live with a long-term condition, their care becomes disproportionately complex and presents management problems for practitioners and the individual with the condition. Case management, as defined by the Department of Health, sets out to address this complexity: 'Case management is also the first step to creating an effective delivery system and implementing the wider NHS and Social Care Long Term Conditions Model'.

Continuing care is not solely about health needs, and there needs to be an acknowledgement that effective social care is a facet of holistic healthcare, and vice versa. It is well documented that people with intellectual disabilities have higher levels of unmet healthcare needs and therefore would benefit from such an approach, as outlined in continuing care strategies. There is no universally accepted definition—particularly where there has been concern that the term 'case' is derogatory—but there is some consensus about the main components of case management. These are: screening or case finding, assessment, care planning and implementation, monitoring, reassessment, or review. Challis describes case management itself as: 'a specific job, a task within an existing job role within a single agency, a job or task within a joint health and social work structure, an organizational process'.

Further reading

Department of Health (2012). *Transforming Care: A National Response to Winterbourne View Hospital.* ℰ www.gov.uk/government/uploads/system/uploads/attachment_data/file/213215/final-report.pdf (accessed 30 October 2017).
Department of Health, Social Services and Public Safety (2015). *Service Framework for Learning Disability.* ℰ www.health-ni.gov.uk/sites/default/files/publications/dhssps/service-framework-for-learning-disability-full-document.pdf (accessed 30 October 2017).
NHS England. *Homes Not Hospitals.* ℰ www.england.nhs.uk/learningdisabilities/care/ (accessed 30 October 2017).
NHS England (2015). *Building the Right Support.* ℰ www.england.nhs.uk/wp-content/uploads/2015/10/ld-nat-imp-plan-oct15.pdf (accessed 30 October 2017).

References

46 Department of Health (1989). *Caring For People.* Department of Health: London.
47 Department of Health (2012). *Transforming Care: A National Response to Winterbourne View Hospital.* Department of Health: London.

Direct care payments

Introduction

There is now a requirement on health and social care services across the UK to offer people who are in receipt of care the opportunity to receive and manage direct care payments. Direct care payments or personal budgets are aimed at providing more control and choice to people who are assessed by their local social services, department, or health and social care provider as requiring services. Through the use of direct care payments, it is anticipated that services a person feels best meet their needs can be arranged on a more individualized and person-focused manner. A direct care payment provides the opportunity for a person in receipt of care or a carer to receive a payment which they have more control over what it is spent on. The amount of money paid as a direct care payment is then deducted from the amount of money that has been allocated to your carer by the local services.

Direct care payments may be paid to people receiving care who have capacity, young people (16–17yrs), and carers in their own right. All of these can request a direct care payment if they have the capacity to do so and if the local authority (health or social care) is satisfied they are capable of managing the budget allocated to them. Direct care payments can also be requested by parents of younger children and an identified person acting on behalf of an adult without capacity if the local authority making the payment is satisfied that appropriate arrangements are in place to manage the budget. In all situations, the local authority making the payment must also agree that providing a direct care payment is an appropriate way to meet the needs of the person for whom the payment is being made.

What care direct care payments are used for?

Direct care payments are designed to enable people have more control and flexibility over how their care needs are met and how their care is provided in a way that works better for them. There is a need to agree what the money can be spent on with the service making the direct care payment, and it needs to be demonstrated that the proposed use of the money will meet an individual's assessed care needs. These payments may be used to employ their own care workers, purchase care services from an independent or private agency, buy equipment, or pay for home adaptations. These payments can also be used more flexibly to buy other types of support to meet the individual's assessed needs, such as planning leisure activities, or a more personalized way of meeting needs such as doing shopping or other necessary activities.

There are some limits as to what direct care payments can be used for, and it is important to remember these payments are designed to meet a person's care needs as assessed by the service providing the direct care payment. Direct care payments are not used to pay for support already available within the family (although there may be exceptions that can be agreed with your local service). Direct care payments would not normally be used to pay for care provided by a spouse, civil partner, live-in partner, or close relative who lives in the same household as the person requiring care, in order to provide care for them. These payments would be used to buy services from the local council or pay for permanent care in a care home, although it could be used to pay for a period of respite care within locally agreed guidelines.

People in receipt of direct care payments must be able to clearly account for how the budget is spent and need to be aware of potential employer responsibilities, pension, and tax matters if they employ someone directly. They may choose to pay for services from people who are self-employed or obtain the assistance of an agency or arrangements such as a 'microboard' to manage their direct care payments who will manage much of these aspects.

Supporting the use of direct care payments

Nurses working with people with intellectual disabilities and their supporters should ensure that they:

- Are familiar with national and local guidelines for direct payments within the jurisdictions in which they are working;
- Are able to explain the overall process to people with intellectual disabilities and their carers in order that they can consider the possible use of this approach;
- Are fair and transparent in all the information they provide and let people with intellectual disabilities and their carers know where they can seek independent advice;
- Are aware of the challenges of managing direct care payments and be sensitive to people if these challenges arise;
- Remain up-to-date with the information they need to know about a person's personal support plan;
- Are confident in raising any concerns about possible mistreatment or neglect with local safeguarding services.

Further reading

NHS Choices (2015). *Your Guide to Care and Support*. England and Wales. ℰ www.nhs.uk/ Conditions/social-care-and-support-guide/Pages/direct-payments-personal-budgets.aspx (accessed 30 October 2017).

Northern Ireland (2002). *Carers and Direct Payments Act (Northern Ireland) 2002*. ℰ www.legislation. gov.uk/nia/2002/6/section/8 (accessed 30 October 2017).

Scottish Executive (2003). *A Guide to Receiving Direct Payments in Scotland*. ℰ www.sehd.scot.nhs.uk/ publications/grdps/grdps-00.htm (accessed 30 October 2017).

Effective teamworking

The need for teamwork

Effective teamworking is necessary in order to respond to the fact that no one profession has all the knowledge, skills, and resources necessary to meet the increasingly complex and varied needs of all people with intellectual disabilities. Teams should always involve and focus on the abilities and needs of the person receiving care. They may involve a wide range of people from one professional group/agency or the team members may be from a range of backgrounds, usually referred to as an interdisciplinary team. Teams, whether uniprofessional or interdisciplinary, can provide a way for services to deliver effectively coordinated services that can be jointly planned and funded, which bring together people from a range of services and prevent fragmentation of care packages within services that are increasingly becoming narrowly focused 'specialist', with at times quite exclusive referral criteria.

Without effective interdisciplinary teamworking there is a real possibility that people with intellectual disabilities and their families will encounter fragmented, uncoordinated, and at times competing services, providing conflicting advice and support. Failure to work cooperatively and as an effective team is also a common finding in many inquiries into poor quality care[48] (see further reports on care regulators websites).

Effective teamwork

It is important to recognize that a group of people working in the one place is not necessarily a team and may be more accurately described as a group of people. To move from being a group of people to become a team, it is necessary for the people involved to:

• Agree to work together;
• Hold shared values;
• All work collaboratively to achieve agreed goals and objectives.

Effective teamwork also requires team members to recognize their interdependence on each other if the objectives of the team are to be achieved. This is why the term 'interdisciplinary', rather than 'multidisciplinary' (implies multi-, and perhaps separate, parts), is used. Team members need to work flexibly, challenging traditional divisions and stereotypes and allocating work on the basis of the ability of people to effectively undertake it, rather than only on the basis of previous practices or professional titles. Together the members of an effective team should be able to achieve more for people within intellectual disabilities than each of them working individually; put another way, 'the whole should be greater than the sum of its parts'.

The requirement for nurses to work as effective team members

All nurses are required to work as effective team members; it is not an optional extra for any nurse. This requirement and associated details are clearly stated within the codes of conduct from both the NMC (2015)[49] and the NMBI (2014).[50] The NMC Code highlighted this under the heading of 'Practise effectively' and notes the requirements to:

• Always practise in line with the best available evidence;
• Communicate clearly;
• Work cooperatively;
• Share your skills, knowledge, and experience for the benefit of people receiving care and your colleagues;
• Keep clear and accurate records relevant to your practice;
• Be accountable for your decision to delegate tasks and duties to others.

Similar requirements are also noted within the NMBI Code.

Supporting effective teamwork

It is recognized that at times effective teamwork is not easy and may involve trying to reach agreement among differing professional views of team members. These differing views may result in strong disagreements, and team members should have the confidence to address this openly and positively. Nurses are expected to respond to differences of professional opinion by discussion and informed debate in a timely and appropriate manner.[49,50]

There are a wide range of possible team structures and memberships; it is important therefore that decisions about team structures in services should be selected to match locally identified client abilities and needs. Effective teamwork does not just happen; it requires time and support to develop, with an investment of time and personal, as well as organizational, commitment.[51] Finally, it is important to evaluate the overall work of the team;[48,49] unfortunately, this is often not done and the focus remains on the performance of individuals within the team, which means that largely systemic problems are not acknowledged and addressed.

References

48 Raine R, Wallace I, Nic a' Bháird C, et al. (2014). Improving the effectiveness of multidisciplinary team meetings for patients with chronic diseases: a prospective observational study. *Health Services and Delivery Research.* 2(37):ISSN 2050-4349. ℛ www.ucl.ac.uk/dahr/pdf/study_documents/MDT_Study_Published_NIHR_Report_Oct_2014.pdf (accessed 30 October 2017).

49 Nursing and Midwifery Council (2015). *The Code: Standards of Conduct, Performance and Ethics for Nurses and Midwives.* Nursing and Midwifery Council: London.

50 Nursing and Midwifery Board of Ireland (2014). *Code of Professional Conduct and Ethics for Registered Nurses and Registered Midwives.* Nursing and Midwifery Board of Ireland: Dublin.

51 Reeves S (2010). *Interprofessional Teamwork for Health and Social Care.* Wiley-Blackwell: Oxford.

Interagency working

Defining interagency working

Interagency working refers to people working collaboratively who are employed by, or working in, voluntary capacity for a number of different agencies that have different organizational arrangements and separate management structures. It often results in new ideas emerging as each agency brings differing perspectives to the same situation and new insights can emerge. Interagency working may occur at a number of different levels, ranging from formal structures such as those with transition planning for teenagers with intellectual disabilities or those required for the care and support of people who are vulnerable or a risk to others. In such situations, the remit of the group is clearly defined, as is the purpose of the meeting which is formally chaired, with a record kept.

Often interagency working is in the form of a network-based approach in which people from a number of agencies are not within a formal team setting but working collaboratively, e.g. when people belonging to a number of other formal teams come together to plan leisure activities within a locality which could be made accessible to people with intellectual disabilities, or managing the support of a person with intellectual disabilities to access primary or secondary healthcare services, or developing new supported living options. At times, interagency working can focus on wider strategic decisions related to policy-making and setting agreed priorities across organizations, e.g. between health services, social services, housing, police and criminal justice services, focusing on a particular initiative such as support for the risk of crime of people with intellectual disabilities.

Potential challenges in interagency working

When it works effectively, people with intellectual disabilities could potentially receive a flexible, yet coordinated, service in which people are clear about their roles, the interface between these, and the lines of communication. However, interagency working is not without challenges, and the difficulties with making it work effectively have been reported and highlighted in inquiry documents and sadly bear witness to the fact that when it goes wrong, it can have catastrophic consequences often for people most in need of care.[52,53]

In particular, difficulties can arise when appropriate governance arrangements are not in place; the differing operational cultures (the tacit knowledge of how things are done in the team, 'practice wisdom', the unwritten rules and procedures) of agencies lead to events being viewed differently, e.g. a difference in opinion about the right of an individual to make their own decisions and concern over a potential risk of exploitation or child protection issues being underestimated.

There is a risk that the potential for interagency working can be restricted due to priorities or budgets of separate agencies involved becoming competing, and managers wishing to maintain autonomy, gain control, or retain perceived hierarchical position, or are reluctant to share information that may show their organization in a poor light and wishing to 'save face'.

In particular, the need for effective sharing of information and a clear audit trail on how this was shared has been highlighted in several major inquiries that investigated failures in interagency working.

Towards effective interagency working

Effective interagency working requires, among other things:
- The need for senior managers in each agency to be supportive of collaborative working between agencies;
- The active involvement of people with the necessary knowledge and autonomy to make the necessary decisions, rather than people who will always have to refer back to their managers for further discussion (although this may happen from time to time in major decisions);
- A willingness to seek new solutions and ways forward for people with intellectual disabilities and their families, as this is the primary purpose for entering into interagency working;
- Clear information on what each agency is prepared to bring to the joint venture in relation to time, people, budgets, and other resources;
- Agreed procedures for managerial and professional supervision (if appropriate) of all staff involved within their respective agencies which also consider their role in interagency working;
- Clear procedures for highlighting concerns and resolving any differences of opinions or disagreements around decisions made and conflicts of interest, potentially including 'whistle blowing arrangements'.
- A regular review of the arrangements for interagency working by the people involved and their respective managers.

References

52 Raine R, Wallace I, Nic a' Bháird C, et al. (2014). Improving the effectiveness of multidisciplinary team meetings for patients with chronic diseases: a prospective observational study. *Health Services and Delivery Research*. 2(37):ISSN 2050-4349. ℅ www.ucl.ac.uk/dahr/pdf/study_documents/MDT_Study_Published_NIHR_Report_Oct_2014.pdf (accessed 30 October 2017).
53 Department of Health (2012). *Transforming Care: A National Response to Winterbourne View Hospital*. Department of Health: London.

Commissioning services

Introduction

Health and social care services are in place because these have been identified as necessary, commissioned, and funded. The process of commissioning is often referred to as the 'commissioning cycle' and traditionally involves the stages of assessing need, reviewing current provision, deciding priorities, specifying services, deciding how services will be supplied, managing demand and ensuring appropriate access to services, ongoing clinical decision-making, and managing performance against criteria set for quality, performance, and outcomes.[54] It is now expected that there will be effective patient and public involvement at all stages in the commissioning process. Once services are being provided, these should be monitored on an ongoing basis to ensure the quality of the service provided and that the services are achieving the outcomes for which they were put in place. Increasing the achievement of outcomes, measured against agreed criteria, is an important aspect of commissioning services and the continuing funding of services.[55]

Most health and social services are commissioned for a defined locality, which could be a local Trust area or a defined area within a Trust where a specific need has been identified. Some services are commissioned on a larger regional level when these relate to specialist high-cost services or services for people with less frequent conditions and a local service is not practical due to the level of expertise required and/or the cost of setting up multiple services.

Services may be commissioned by a single agency, e.g. a health commissioner, by more than one health commissioner, or increasing by more than one agency such as health services and local authorities as the number of 'integrated' commissioning arrangements grow.[56] The principles of effective commissioning apply, irrespective of who is commissioning services. Each country with the UK and the Republic of Ireland has its one specific arrangements for commissioning services and in order to be able to input into, and understand commissioning, processes, it is important that you are aware of who commissions which services within your country.

Commissioning services for people with intellectual disabilities

The commissioning and delivery of services for people with intellectual disabilities should be underpinned by the values stated within national policy documents. The effectiveness of services commissioned to support people with intellectual disabilities continues to be a major area of concern. Recent years have continued to show limitations of poorly commissioned services and the massive negative impact this can have on the lives of people with intellectual disabilities. Two major examples are the services provided at Winterbourne View[57] and Aras Attracta.[58] It is not always clear from the subsequent inquiries why such poor services were delivered, but it does appear a major aspect is the lack of clear and robust monitoring by the commissioner of the services and perhaps an overreliance on inspections by health and social care regulators.

Nurses working with people with intellectual disabilities and their supporters should ensure that:

- They are familiar with national guidelines for the commissioning of services for people with intellectual disabilities overall and for specific services in which you may be working, such as mental health, complex disability, or behavioural services, e.g. ℘ www.jcpmh.info/good-services/learning-disabilities-services/ and ℘ www.rcgp.org.uk/learningdisabilities/;
- They are aware and have discussed local commissioning plans at a level appropriate to their role;
- They are aware of the principles of effective service commissioning and contribute to interagency working, regional commissioning, and local plans;
- People with intellectual disabilities and their supporters have information about local commissioning strategies and that there are ways for people to influence these at all levels;
- There are fair and transparent commissioning processes and that providers of services have regular opportunities to share information with commissioners, e.g. at providers' forums;
- They take every opportunity to talk to commissioners and provide opportunities for them to talk to people receiving services and to frontline workers.

References

54 Royal College of Nursing (2011). *Commissioning Health Services: A Guide for RCN Activists and Nurses*. Royal College of Nursing: London.

55 Humphries R, Wenzel L (2015). *Options for Integrated Commissioning*. Kings Fund: London.

56 Local Government Association (2015). *Commissioning for Better Outcomes; A Route Map*. Local Government Association: London.

57 Bubb S (2014). *Winterbourne View – Time for Change. Transforming the Commissioning of Services for People with Learning Disabilities and /or Autism.* ℘ www.england.nhs.uk/wp-content/uploads/2014/11/transforming-commissioning-services.pdf (accessed 30 October 2017).

58 Health Service Executive (2016). *What Matters Most. Report of the Aras Attracta Review Group.* Health Service Executive: Dublin. ℘ www.hse.ie/eng/services/publications/Disability/AASRGwhatmattersmost.pdf (accessed 30 October 2017).

Life planning

All of these approaches have been developed for use with people with intellectual disabilities and give the opportunity to take control and make decisions about their future. Planning gives individuals a choice and the opportunity to voice their views on their care and support as they age.

Essential life planning (ELP)

ELP was developed by Michael Smull and Susan Burke Harrison, and is a very detailed planning tool that helps people to find out what is important to the person and what support they need to get a good quality of life. Helpfully, it also identifies what is working well and what is not working well for the focus person. Unlike other planning tools, it does not make provision for the individual's desired future, dreams, or aspirations, although a section could be added. ELP is an excellent tool for getting to know someone and developing a service or team around them, especially when they do not use words to communicate. An ELP forms a useful support plan for an individual, but as with all planning tools, it must be implemented with consistency and regularly maintained as a live document.[59]

Planning Alternative Tomorrows with Hope (PATH)

PATH was developed by Pearpoint, Forest, and O'Brien, and it has the benefit of being suitable as a planning tool for both individuals and organizations. It is strongly focused and starts by setting out the person's dream, then builds momentum, with timescales and action plans towards it. PATH enables the capturing of outcomes (aspirations), as well as establishing outputs (goals), baseline data, capability and capacity (identifying additional support needed), and measurable indicators (action planning). However, the success of the PATH is heavily dependent on the commitment of the people who help to bring it together. A PATH does not result in a daily support plan for the person, as it specifically addresses their dreams, aspirations, and desires for a better future.[60]

Personal futures planning (PFP)

PFP, or life building, was developed by Mount and O'Brien, and enables a committed group of people to look at the focus person's life now and what they would like in the future. PFP encompasses eight steps, including:
• Bringing caring people together;
• Looking at the person's gifts and capacities;
• Finding new directions for change;
• Identifying the obstacles;
• Generating strategies and creating the vision;
• Making commitment;
• Taking action;
• Reflecting on what has been learnt.

It is geared at getting to learn more about the person's life (whereas PATH assumes this knowledge). The tool itself is designed to build on what is working well now and help the person move towards a desirable future. It does not create the support detail, which an ELP does.[60]

McGill Action Planning System (MAPS)

MAPS is a planning tool developed by Snow, Pearpoint, and Forest (with support from others). It works on the basis that there are important lessons to be learnt from looking at someone's past. It asks a series of questions about the person, their gifts, and their strengths but also allows time to explore their fears and 'nightmares'. It is pictorial in design, which can make it a very accessible tool for people who do not read or who do not use words to communicate. It is less focused than a PATH, and less detailed than an ELP. It requires careful and sensitive facilitation. Within MAPs, relationships are seen as a fundamental element, and one of the goals of MAPS is to 'continuously increase the focus of an individual's social connections'.[60]

The largest scale and most comprehensive review of person-centred planning found that the most significant benefits for people who have intellectual disabilities were improved community involvement, contact with friends and family, and increased choice.[61] This report goes on to explain that the key determinants of success are committed facilitators, the personal involvement of the service user, and a person-centred, supportive environment being in place at the time of planning.

It is important when commencing person-centred planning that the people involved remain aware of the possible challenges in service provision at that time. This does not mean that one should not elicit people's dreams and aspirations. However, when dreams become goals, reality must be sensed and facilitators must be open and honest about the seemingly difficult or impossible. The study by Robertson et al. claims that by clarifying the role of care managers and specialist practitioners in the policy and practice of life planning, access will be more equitable.[61]

Good-quality and person-centred life planning is about selecting planning tools appropriately and, in some situations, combining tools. It is important to understand that life planning is a continuous process and should be reviewed and updated. Planning is a process, not a single activity (see ➔ Person-centred planning, pp. 26–7)

Further reading

Sanderson H (2016). *Person Centred Practices*. ℠ www.helensandersonassociates.co.uk/person-centred-practice/maps/ (accessed 30 October 2017).

References

59 The Learning Community website (2016). ℠ www.learningcommunity.us/about.html (accessed 30 October 2017).
60 O'Brien J, Pearpoint J, Kahn L (2010). *The PATH & MAPS Handbook. Person-Centered Ways to Build Community*. Inclusion Press: Toronto.
61 Robertson J, Emerson E (2005). *The Impact of Person Centred Planning*. Institute for Health Research, Lancaster University: Lancaster.

Client-held records

These are documents that are held by the person with intellectual disabilities and aim to express the individual and important aspects of daily living in a way that is understood by the person. They are informative and helpful to others involved in the person's care.

Types of client-held records

There are a number of different client-held records relevant to the person with intellectual disabilities that may be in use within services. Basically, they are documents that help the person with intellectual disabilities and/or their carers to communicate with others across the range of services with which a person may come into contact, e.g. staff working within the person's home, within assessment and treatment services, or within general health services. Documents may vary in size and design, depending on the individual needs of the person. Some people use photographs or symbols to articulate their needs, while others may use audiovisual material. An accessible record may contain a mixture of photos, symbols, and text.

Health action plans

A HAP holds information about the person's health needs, the professionals who support those needs, and a record of various appointments and treatment interventions. The plan is constructed following an annual health check. A person can get assistance from a HF to develop a HAP or other member of staff/family member, act on it, and keep it under review. The HAP should indicate a range of services and supports the person might need. A HAP is particularly helpful when transitioning from child to adult services or when a person is growing older and their abilities and needs are changing.

Person-centred profiles (PCPs)

A profile captures all the important information about a person, sometimes on a single sheet of paper, under three clear headings: what people appreciate about me, what is important to me, and how best to support me.[62] Person-centred approaches support people to make informed decisions about, and to successfully manage, their own health and care. A PCP should challenge all to think about what they and/or society need to do differently to maximize the abilities and meet this person's needs and ensure the person is at the centre of care delivery.

Patient/client passport

These documents are sometimes referred to as health or hospital passports. These are an individualized document that highlights the abilities and specific health and social care needs of a person who has difficulty communicating those needs. It should be concise and adaptable, and be reviewed regularly. It should assist those who do not know the client well to make reasonable adjustments to their care. By doing so, this could decrease the incidence of diagnostic overshadowing, a term used to describe the tendency for clinicians to overlook symptoms of mental and physical health problems and wrongly attribute the symptom to being part of having an intellectual disability.

Communication passport

'A communication passport is a way of supporting a vulnerable person with communication difficulties across transitions, drawing together complex information (including the person's own views, as much as possible) and distilling it into a clear, positive and accessible format'.[63] It details how an individual communicates, together with information about the person's life and likes and needs in particular situations.

What client-held records seek to do

- Empower the individual, ensuring their own views are to the fore.
- Illustrate good practice.
- Highlight reasonable adjustments that may be required.
- Useful for new staff, helping them quickly to acquire key up-to-date information.
- Assist access to services, ensuring a seamless journey through the health and social care system.
- Promote partnership and joined-up interagency working.

Challenges

- Some people have a number of accessible records/documents, some people do not.
- The diversity and design of documents may be confusing.
- Promoting awareness of the value of client-held records.
- Training and development of staff.
- Avoiding duplication of information.

References

62 Sanderson H. *Person-centred Practices*. ℘ www.helensandersonassociates.co.uk/person-centred-practice (accessed 30 October 2017).
63 Communication Matters. ℘ www.communicationmatters.org.uk (accessed 30 October 2017).

Person-centred practice

What is person-centred practice?

'Person-centredness' is a term that is becoming increasingly familiar within healthcare globally and is being used to describe a standard of care that ensures people as individuals, communities, and populations are at the heart of planning and policy-making.[64,65] Person-centred practice challenges healthcare practitioners to think of the person first and then the disease or disability. It requires practitioners to work in a way that ensures people have access to healthcare services that reflect their needs, manage disease, and support self-management of long-term conditions, while at the same time promoting health in order to maximize well-being. It is an approach that is underpinned by values of respect for persons and individual right to self-determination, mutual respect, and understanding.

Who is the person in person-centred practice?

The word 'person' captures those attributes that represent our humanness and the way in which we construct our life. How we think about moral values, how we express political, spiritual, or religious beliefs, how we engage emotionally and in our relationships, and the kind of life we want to live are all shaped by our attributes as persons. The *person* in person-centred practice refers to 'all those involved in a caring interaction and therefore encompasses patients, clients, families/carers, nursing colleagues, and other members of the interdisciplinary team'. The 'person' is at the heart of care decision-making, and person-centredness is an approach to practice that focuses on the formation and fostering of healthful relationships between all those involved in care delivery.

How can person-centredness be promoted in practice?

As nurses, we have an expectation that people should receive a standard of care that reflect the person-centred principles. Translating the core concepts into everyday practice, however, is challenging.[65] The reasons for this come in many forms and are often indicative of the context in which care is being delivered and the fact that we are living in times of constant change particularly within healthcare.

The Person-centred Practice Framework has been developed over more than a decade, as a means of enhancing the understanding of person-centred practice and to provide insights that challenge accepted norms and ways of working.[65] It has been described as a tool that can illuminate practice and provides a language that can operationalize person-centredness within inter-disciplinary teams. The framework essentially comprises four domains:

* *prerequisites*, which focus on the attributes of the staff;
* *care environment*, which focuses on the context in which care is delivered;
* *person-centred processes*, which focus on delivering care to the patient through a range of activities;
* *person-centred outcomes*, which are the results of effective person-centred practice.

The relationship between the constructs of the framework proposes that to reach its centre, the attributes of staff must first be considered, as a prerequisite to managing the care environment, in order to provide effective person-centred processes, which leads to the achievement of person-centred outcomes.

What are the benefits of person-centred practice?

Our work to date would suggest that developing effective person-centred cultures has benefits for all, in terms of the care experience, feeling of well-being, involvement in care, and creating healthful cultures. The focus on healthfulness is consistent with contemporary theories of well-being and wellness as health goals and reflects the diversity of relationships that people experience. Furthermore, effective cultures have clearly articulated and shared values that are important in developing person-centred cultures.

References

64 McCormack B, McCance T, eds. (2010). *Person-Centred Nursing: Theory and Practice.* Wiley-Blackwell: Oxford.
65 McCormack B, McCance T. (2016). *Person-Centred Practice in Nursing and Healthcare: Theory and Practice.* Wiley-Blackwell: Oxford.

Chapter 9

Therapeutic interventions

Inclusive communication

As discussed in → Chapter 3, inclusive communication (sometimes also called total communication) is achieved when we provide information to others and demonstrate active listening to what they are telling us, through whatever means they may require/use to do so (see Fig 9.1 for a summary). Inclusive communication incorporates augmentative and alternative communication and simplifying language, using easier words and slowing down. It starts from the premise that everyone communicates and seeks to support people with communication difficulties both in understanding us and in telling us things. As such, it is fundamental to the delivery of person-centred services and should form the foundation of all professional relationships with people with intellectual disabilities. You need to know what inclusive communication is and how you can make reasonable adjustments in your communication style to meet the needs of people with intellectual disabilities.

So how do you do it?

Promoting understanding

- Do not make assumptions about a person's level of verbal understanding or about their ability to hear what you say/see what you are showing them—check it out (ask others if necessary).
- Consider how you are speaking, which words you are using, and how much information you are presenting at any one time.
- Simplify your language (short sentences, easy words).
- Aim to use words the person is likely to know.
- Present information in bite-sized chunks.
- Repeat and rephrase as necessary.
- Support your speech with gestures, signs, written words, symbols, drawings, photographs, video, gestures, facial expressions, actions/ mimes, vocalizations, and objects, as appropriate.

Individualized assessment is essential in order to get this right every time. An SLT can advise you on how to communicate with any particular individual, if referred for communication assessment. However, it is worth considering what you can do yourself by emphasizing non-verbal signals, learning signs and modifying the language used, and stockpiling a set of photographs and other resources that are likely to be useful time and time again. See → Principles in using augmentative and alternative communication (AAC), pp. 68–9.

Promoting expression

People with intellectual disabilities may need support to use these same methods of inclusive communication when interacting with you, especially where they have no speech and where their speech is limited or not always easy to understand. Even where people with expressive communication difficulties have their own AAC systems, they may require your help to initiate using them. People who know signs are unlikely to use these with you, unless you use signs with them. It is a good idea to learn at least a basic vocabulary (e.g. 'hello', 'yes', 'no', 'pain', 'nurse', 'doctor', 'medicine', 'injection', 'hospital', 'ill', 'happy', and 'sad', and to be able to sign the first letter of your name) and to practise using signs; otherwise, you will not retain your confidence in using them.

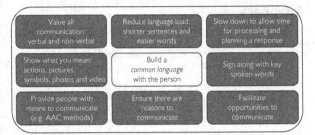

Fig. 9.1 Inclusive communication = good communication.

Inclusive means everyone

It could be assumed that people who have profound and multiple intellectual disabilities are not able to tell us anything. They may not have developed much (or even any) language but will use non-verbal means of communication (e.g. vocalizations, laughing, crying, looking, posture, actions, or objects) to express themselves. These signals may not be intended to deliberately signal a message, but people who know them well will often be able to interpret the meaning. You should make note of how a person indicates their 'like' and 'dislike' of something; you can also ask the family or key support staff. Gathering examples like this allows us to draw out themes that can be used to measure responses by that person to situations, thus helping us take their reactions into account regarding what happens to them.

Strategic considerations

In line with the Royal College of Speech and Language Therapists' (RCSLT) *Five Good Communication Standards*, professionals working within intellectual disabilities services should aim to apply inclusive communication methods meaningfully across a variety of service areas. To this end, a resource base of inclusive communication materials should be tailored for each service. In particular, any information provided to people with intellectual disabilities should be 'easier read' (i.e. with photos, drawings, or symbols to back up words). Each person with communication difficulties should have a clearly presented, individualized summary of communication needs (e.g. a communication profile) and/or a communication passport, as well as access to appropriate AAC systems. This should be supported by a systematic approach to inclusive communication training and linked to the supervision and management of continuing professional development.

Further reading

For links to examples of health-related Easy Read documents and brief Inclusive (Total) Communication training videos, see ℛ totalcommunicationnow.org/ (accessed 30 October 2017).

Advocacy

In the context of intellectual disability, and to all practical purposes, advocacy is mostly associated with four types of representation: self, an unpaid person, a paid person, or an organization (also see ⊃ Independent Mental Capacity Advocates, pp. 274–5).

Self-advocacy

Self-advocacy is practised by many of us as individuals, but groups can provide a good setting for developing self-advocacy skills, particularly for people who are at risk of being devalued in society. Self-advocacy has great potential to enhance the lives of people with intellectual disabilities, as they become more aware of their rights, express needs and concerns, and assert their interests. Self-advocacy is often described as the ultimate goal of all other forms of advocacy. Self-advocacy is concerned with speaking up for oneself, making one's own decisions, and taking action, as well as changing things with which one is not happy. Generally speaking, self-advocacy involves being:

• Able to express thoughts and feelings with assertiveness if necessary;
• Able to make choices and decisions;
• Clear on knowledge of rights and being able to make changes.

Other important components include: being independent, taking responsibility for oneself, getting things going, and being concerned for other people. Self-advocacy can permeate and influence a person's whole life.

Citizen advocacy

Citizen advocacy refers to a supportive partnership that results when a volunteer develops a relationship with a person who is vulnerable to being disadvantaged through illness, age, or disability. It is important that advocates are 'valued people' (i.e. not themselves disadvantaged). Advocates form a close personal relationship with their partners, helping them to make choices and decisions. They work independently of services to uphold the rights of their partners as citizens. Citizen advocacy refers to the persuasive and supportive activities of trained, selected volunteers and coordinating staff working on behalf of those who are disabled/disadvantaged and not in a strong position to exercise or defend their rights as citizens. Working on a one-to-one basis, they attempt to foster respect for the rights and dignity of those they represent. This may involve helping to express the individual's needs and wishes, helping them to access services, and providing practical and emotional support. The benefits of a partnership with a citizen advocate fall into two broad categories, according to the nature of the needs met: expressive (human, emotional, and social needs) and instrumental (material needs).

Peer advocacy

Peer advocacy refers to individual support provided by someone who is also a member of a section of society that is in danger of being devalued or stigmatized. Thus, a person with intellectual disabilities could be assisted to articulate their needs and wishes by a peer who also has intellectual disabilities. This is based on an assumption that the peer advocate is likely to have more insight into the experience of their partner than a non-disabled advocate would. This approach is now being used as a means of achieving co-production in designing services for people with intellectual disabilities.

Professional advocacy

Professional advocacy has an important role to play in supporting the empowerment of people with intellectual disabilities. This might involve introduction to a self-advocacy group or to an independent advocacy service. Whereas the UK's professional body the NMC[1] and the UK Chief Nurses[2] continue to endorse nurses taking on an advocacy role, it has been stressed that nurses should only advocate on a client's behalf after '*careful consideration of the issues involved*'.[3]

Collective advocacy

Collective advocacy is concerned with user representation. There is an important nuance here between advocacy and user representation. Self-advocates represent their own interests; citizen advocates uphold the rights of their partners. User organizations cannot represent each individual's views, but they can promote the 'cause' of minority groups, and this includes people with intellectual disabilities, by raising public awareness and lobbying policy-makers on their behalf. Key organizations that help to further the cause include: Mencap, People First, British Institute of Learning Disabilities (BILD), and Scope.

Further reading

Brolan CE, Boyle FM, Dean JH, Taylor Gomez M, Ware RS, Lennox NG (2012). Health advocacy: a vital step in attaining human rights for adults with intellectual disability. *Journal of Intellectual Disability Research*. 56: 1087–97.

Chapman M, Bannister S, Davies J, et al. (2012). Speaking up about advocacy: findings from a partnership research project. *British Journal of Learning Disabilities*. 40: 71–80.

Zisser AR, van Stone M (2015). Health, education, advocacy, and law: an innovative approach to improving outcomes for low-income children with intellectual and developmental disabilities. *Journal of Policy and Practice in Intellectual Disabilities*. 12: 132–7.

References

1 Nursing and Midwifery Council (2015). *The Code: Standards of Conduct, Performance and Ethics for Nurses and Midwives*. Nursing and Midwifery Council: London.

2 UK Chief Nursing Officers (2012). *Strengthening the Commitment: The Report of the UK Modernising Learning Disabilities Nursing Review*. Scottish Government: Edinburgh.

3 Jenkins R, Northway R (2002). Advocacy and the learning disability nurse. *British Journal of Learning Disabilities*. 30: 8–12.

Multisensory environments

The concept of multisensory rooms began in De Hartenberg, Holland in 1975. The idea of providing a specialized sensory environment in which the person could be actively or passively involved grew because of a positive response to an initial introduction to the approach. The Dutch term for this form of sensory intervention is Snoezelen (pronounced *snooze len*), a contraction of two words meaning 'to sniff' and 'to doze'. The term Snoezelen is used today only as a trade name for a company supplying sensory equipment in the UK and the term 'multisensory environment' or 'multisensory studio' is used.

A multisensory environment (MSE) provides an area within which, by using a range of equipment and materials, the stimulation of the primary senses—touch, taste, smell, see, sound—and proprioception (body parts in relation to each other) and vestibular stimulation can be catered for. This dynamic environment allows the user to choose the stimulation which they wish to use or a staff member may select this, based on an individual's assessment (see Fig. 9.2).

Many people with autism are unable to properly process sensory stimulation, being hyper-responsive or hyposensitive to incoming stimuli, and may become excited or heightened by self-produced stimulation. Without appropriate stimulation, individuals may resort to self-injury or repetitive behaviour as a substitute. This type of behaviour interferes with completion of activities of daily living.

A form of intervention, designed to reduce or avoid these traits, is an MSE. An MSE provides an area that offers individuals an opportunity to control, manipulate, intensify, or reduce stimulation within a safe environment.

The reported benefits of an MSE include:[1]
- 'Opportunity for affective/emotional development;
- Stimulation for all senses;
- Relaxation;
- Facilitation of therapy;
- Enhancement of communication;
- Minimization of challenging behaviour;
- Development of self-determination;
- Opportunity for social interaction with non-disabled children/families'.[1]

MSEs are used with individuals who have difficulties in sensory modulation, such as intellectual disabilities and people with autism, and can also be used to support people with profound and multiple disabilities. MSEs can provide people with opportunities to undertake self-stimulating activities which, in turn, may help them enhance the regulation of their nervous system. The potential benefits of MSEs for other groups of children and adults, in particular in relation to facilitating learning, is also being explored.[1]

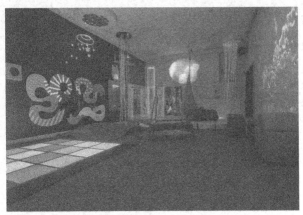

Fig. 9.2 Example of a multisensory environment.

Assessment and training

Multisensory studios are now included in many care environments, ordinary schools, as well as schools for pupils with special needs, day centres, residential units, and private homes. They have been developed to meet the need for more flexible spaces which enable people with intellectual disabilities to create whatever type of environment or mood they wish, either temporary or permanent. It is important that people who are using MSEs have their likes and dislikes carefully assessed and that the activities undertaken in the room have a positive benefit to the people with intellectual disabilities. It is not acceptable practice for people to be taken into MSEs and not be supported to engage in the environment. The equipment should have clear instructions, and staff training should be provided to ensure that they are confident to apply the technology and to ensure that the equipment is used in a safe and appropriate manner.

Further reading

van der Putten A, Vlaskamp C, Schuivens E (2011). The use of a multisensory environment for assessment of sensory abilities and preferences in children with profound intellectual and multiple disabilities: a pilot study. *Journal of Applied Research in Intellectual Disabilities.* 24: 280–4.

References

4 Pagliano P (2013). *Using a Multi-sensory Environment: A Practical Guide for Teachers.* David Fulton Books: Abingdon.

Sensory integration

What is sensory integration?

Through our senses, we are aware of where we are in relation to our surroundings, and it is through our senses of hearing, sight, touch, smell, and taste that we are kept informed about our movements. Our nervous system receives, filters, organizes, and uses motor and sensory information to provide information to our brains to make sense of all of this stimuli. This neurobiological process is known as sensory integration (SI) and is essential for us to make sense of, and respond to, our surroundings. Alongside our five senses, three other major systems provide us with information. These are: the vestibular system that responds to gravity and movement; the proprioceptive system that receives input from muscles and joints; and the interoception system which involves the internal sensation that our body uses to tell our brain what is happening inside our body, e.g. how our body tells our brain what is going on inside our body, e.g. hunger, 'butterflies in the stomach'.[3]

SI involves all of these systems and their interaction with our senses. From childhood, we learn how to make sense of, and integrate, information through our senses and sensations. This is learnt through day-to-day activities from infancy, and we continue to integrate this information throughout our lives, as this is necessary for the development of motor coordination and control.

Dysfunction in sensory processing

SI protects us from overstimulation and helps us to interact with, and learn from, our environment. Problems with SI have been grouped under four main headings,[5] which are:

- Problems with sensory modulation which normally involves an exaggerated or reduced response to sensory information;
- Sensory discrimination and perceptual problems which involve difficulties in discrimination between different types of touch;
- Vestibular bilateral functional problems largely relating to poor balance and coordinating body movements;
- Praxis problems relating to difficulties in planning and undertaking new body movements.

The presence of SI difficulties in children can be indicated by:

- Being oversensitive to touch, movement, sights, or sounds—may draw away if touched, dislikes specific textures, feeling of some clothes, or the sensation of certain foods;
- Under-reactive to sensory stimulation—seeks out intense sensory experiences such as body spinning or falling into objects; may appear oblivious to pain or body position;
- Unusually high/low activity levels—constantly on the move or may be slow to get going and tires easily;
- Difficulties with coordination—indicated by poor balance, reduced motor coordination which can make learning new actions challenging, at times people may appear to have clumsy, stiff, or other awkward movements;

- Slower progress than peers in learning new skills and/or activities of daily living, including activities associated with getting dressed, using various types of fasteners in clothing, or the development of handwriting;
- Behavioural issues that can be seen as challenges in integrating the sensations of new environments, which may result in the person withdrawing or reacting impulsively.

Through structured assessments and careful observation of the person in their environment, it is possible to highlight a person's abilities and needs in the area of SI.

Sensory integration therapy

Jean Ayres's work from the 1950s onwards laid the foundations for the development of SI. This is aimed at helping people develop more effective ways and pathways of sensory processing. Professionals, usually occupational therapists, following an assessment, can design a 'sensory diet' to help make life manageable for individuals with sensory dysfunction. This involves observation of an individual's developmental levels to establish how effectively their sensory–motor processing has developed.

Appropriately educated professionals can provide SI therapy for children, working alongside family members, by building important activities into their daily environment. SI therapy may be presented as play, as this is traditionally how children learn and develop. Activities are carefully chosen to stimulate development in specific areas. Although parents and carers can perform many of these activities at home with the child, professionals are trained to identify and address areas of specific need.

Further reading

Case-Smith J, Weaver LL, Fristad MA (2014). A systematic review of sensory processing interventions for children with autism spectrum disorders. *Autism.* **19**: 133–48.

Schaaf R, Mailloux Z (2015). *Clinician's Guide to Implementing Ayres Sensory Integration®: Promoting Participation for Children with Autism.* American Occupational Therapy Association: Bethesda, MD.

References

1 Sensory Integration Education. *What is Sensory Integration?* ℳ www.sensoryintegration.org.uk/What-is-SI (accessed 30 October 2017).

Behavioural interventions

Behavioural interventions originate from learning theories which are commonly referred to as a 'behavioural approach'.

The principles of a behavioural approach

- Behaviour is anything a person does or says that can be observed.
- Behaviour is learnt and can be shaped by the person's experiences and how reinforcement and punishment are provided.
- Both appropriate and inappropriate behaviours can be learnt, depending on experiences.
- Everyone has the ability to learn new behaviours.

The behavioural approach explains human behaviour as something that is functional and adaptive to the environment. Any behaviour may be under the 'influence' of external and/or internal events and can serve the following functions:

- *Sensory*—'I'm bored and have nothing else to stimulate me';
- *Escape*—'I don't like/understand what you're asking me to do';
- *Social attention*—'I want you to spend some time with me';
- *Tangible*—'I want that food/drink/ball.'

Assessment

Any behavioural intervention needs to commence with a baseline measurement to determine the functions of the behaviour/s under consideration. A functional assessment and analysis of behaviour using the ABC (Antecedents – Behaviour – Consequences) framework is helpful:

- *Antecedents* are observable events, stimuli, or occurrences that happen before a behaviour. Antecedents are usually triggers/prompts that lead to, or cause, the behaviour to occur.
- *Behaviour* measured in terms of frequency, intensity, and duration.
- *Consequences* are events/outcomes that immediately follow a behaviour. Consequences play a part in maintaining (reinforcing) or decreasing the occurrence of behaviours.

Assessment process

- Agree an *accurate description* of the problem/target behaviour.
- Investigate and rule out any underlying *physical and mental health issues*.
- Examine any *historical factors* relating to the behaviour.
- Assess the *functions* of the behaviour using ABC.
- Assess the person's *level of skills* and *opportunities* available to him/her.
- Assess the *environments* the person uses and the *activities* in which they take part.
- Assess the *motivators/reinforcers* for positive behaviour.
- Examine the *knowledge and skills* of carers who support the person.
- Obtain information from the *person, carers, families, friends and professionals*.
- *Analyse* all assessment information gathered.
- Summarize the *person's strengths*.
- Make a *formulation* of the most appropriate behavioural intervention/s.

Behavioural interventions

Behavioural interventions involve learning to repeat or stop behaviours because of the consequences they bring about. There are two main consequences:

- **Reinforcement (positive or negative)** is anything that follows a behaviour and causes it to be repeated. The use of positive reinforcement is by far the most frequently used behavioural interventions to support people with intellectual disabilities.
- **Punishment** is anything following behaviour that causes it to stop. Use of this intervention has serious professional, legal, and ethical implications and is no longer supported (see ➔ Positive behaviour support, pp. 336–7).

The provision of positive reinforcement can result in the 'shaping' of behaviours through the reinforcement of intermediate steps towards the learning of a complex behaviour. Conversely, the lack of reinforcement may result in the 'extinction' of a behaviour, i.e. the gradual elimination of an unwanted behaviour through repeated non-reinforcement. However, learning does not necessarily always require reinforcement. Learning can also occur as a result of simply watching someone else's performance or action. This type of learning is referred to as observational referred learning/modelling.

Use of behavioural interventions

Within the field of intellectual disabilities, behavioural interventions are used to support people to:

- Develop new skills—to facilitate their learning and to promote development and social functioning;
- Understand how people develop behaviours that may be inappropriate and is likely to put the person or others at risk of a reduced quality of life and may lead to inappropriate interventions that can be harmful to people. These types of behaviours are often referred to as challenging behaviours, as they present a challenge for services in terms of support and management.

Types of behavioural interventions

Behavioural interventions are likely to include one or more of the following:

- **Environmental interventions**—the environment can trigger/cause/ affect an individual's behaviour, and behaviours that challenge services are often caused by the interaction between the individual's needs and their environment.
- **Communication**—people with intellectual disabilities may not have the communication skills necessary to communicate their needs, choices, and feelings or explain that they have not understood what is expected of them. This can lead to anxiety, frustration, and, in some cases, increase the likelihood of challenging behaviour.
- **Positive programming/developing skills**—people with intellectual disabilities may lack skills in areas ranging from basic skills of daily living activities to complex skills of being in employment or in a relationship; this can lead to lack of participation, withdrawal, boredom, depression, and social isolation/exclusion.

- **Reactive strategies**—these can help carers to respond to violent or self-injurious behaviours quickly in a planned and safe way that will not make behaviour worse, and ensuring the safety of the person and that of others. Examples of reactive strategies include ignoring, redirecting, reducing demands, stimulus change, proximity control, relaxation, breakaway techniques/physical intervention, and chemical intervention. An example of working with people with intellectual disabilities and stereotyped behaviour is given in the references.[6]
- **Focused support strategies**—these are proactive strategies intended to establish rapid control over a behaviour to reduce associated risks, as well as minimizing the use of reactive strategies. Focused support comprises three main strategies, namely:
  - Differential reinforcement of other behaviour (DRO);
  - Differential reinforcement of low-rates behaviour (DRL);
  - Differential reinforcement of alternate responses (DRA).
- **CBT**—this is based on the idea that how one thinks and feels affects how one behaves, and if you can change how one thinks about a situation/event, then you can change how the person feels and behaves towards that situation/event.
- **Positive behaviour support (PBS)**—current evidence suggests that PBS is the most effective means of the behavioural interventions. PBS has evolved by integrating three major intervention strategies:
  - Applied behaviour analysis;
  - Normalization/social role valorization/inclusion movement;
  - Person-centred values.

For more information on PBS, please see ➔ Positive behaviour support, pp. 336–7.

Further reading

Emerson E, Einfeld SL (2011). *Challenging Behaviour*, 3rd edn. Cambridge University Press: Cambridge.

Hardy S, Joyce T (2011). *Challenging Behaviour: A Handbook: Practical Resource Addressing Ways of Providing Positive Behavioural Support to People with Learning Disabilities Whose Behaviour Is Described as Challenging*. Pavilion Publishing: Brighton.

Lloyd P, Kennedy H (2014). Assessment and treatment of challenging behaviour for individuals with intellectual disability: a research review. *Journal of Applied Research in Intellectual Disabilities*. 27: 187–99.

Medeiros K (2015). *Behavioral Interventions for Individuals with Intellectual Disabilities Exhibiting Automatically Reinforced Challenging Behavior: Stereotypy and Self-Injury*. ✍ www.omicsonline. org/open-access/behavioral-interventions-for-individuals-with-intellectual-disabilitiesexhibiting- automaticallyreinforced-challenging-behavior-stereotypy-andselfinjury-.pdf (accessed 30 October 2017).

National Institute for Health and Care Excellence (2015). *Challenging Behaviour and Learning Disabilities: Prevention and Interventions for People with Learning Disabilities whose Behaviour Challenges*. ✍ www. nice.org.uk/guidance/ng11 (accessed 30 October 2017).

References

6 Hill L, Trusler K, Furniss F, Lancioni G (2012). Behaviours assessed as maintained by automatic reinforcement. *Journal of Applied Research in Intellectual Disabilities*. 25: 509–21.

Family therapy

Family therapy offers conceptual frameworks and clinical approaches for understanding psychological problems. The focus is on the family system, rather than the individual. A consistent view is that difficulties do not arise within individuals but in the relationships, interactions, and the language that develop between individuals. There are many different models and theories of family therapy; however, all family therapists should be focused on the role of the family in problem resolution.

First phase

Family therapy developed as a distinct field during the 1950s. This was prompted by dissatisfaction with the effectiveness of psychoanalytical therapies, recognition of the significance of communication in the development of severe clinical problems, and the evolving practice of child guidance which involved working with families together. The first phase was exemplified by the structural model[7] and the strategic model.[8] Structural family therapy focuses on the hierarchical organization of the family—who makes decisions, who is in charge—and the effect on the family if the power balance becomes skewed, e.g. if a child is placed in a parental position. Structural ideas can be identified in the contemporary practice of multi-systemic family therapy. Strategic family therapy rests on the premise that family problems serve a function for some members of the family and that attempts to resolve problems only maintain them. Similarities between behavioural approaches and solution-focused therapy are evident.

Second phase

The mid-1970s to 1980s was dominated by Milan Systemic.[9] Early work saw a focus on communication, the use of a team of family therapists, and the key principles of hypothesizing, neutrality, and circularity. Hypothesizing (a collection of ideas about the causes of problems) remains relevant to contemporary practice.

Third phase

The third phase of family therapy, which spanned the mid-1980s to 2000 saw the development of narrative[10] and solution-focused[11] approaches. These models occurred against a backdrop of social constructionism which emphasizes the importance of social context in the development of knowledge and beliefs. This influenced family therapists to examine how language and culture shape problem perception and definition. Narrative therapy focuses on helping families generate new stories about their experiences, while solution-focused therapy focuses less on the problem and more on attempted solutions and exceptions.

Contemporary family therapy

Increasingly, the term family therapy has been replaced by systemic therapy to reflect the move to working with a range of organizations, in addition to families. There is a move away from adopting particular models to using frameworks which may involve a range of techniques. Emphasis is placed upon collaborative conversations with the family. The importance of context and relationships endures.

Family therapy and people with intellectual disabilities

Despite a growing interest in family therapy to problems encountered by individuals with intellectual disabilities and their families, literature remains sparse. Cognitive and behavioural approaches dominate the field. Fidell[12] identified four themes experienced by families that may benefit from family therapy:

- Loss—both in terms of grief following the birth of a disabled child and loss of an ordinary life for the disabled individual and his/her family;
- Transitional issues—these will often be out of sync with children without disabilities. There is evidence that the launching of children with a disability is often the most stressful time for parents;
- Involvement of professional systems—the break from child to adult services can be hard to negotiate;
- The dilemmas associated with achieving a balance between autonomy and dependence.

Purdy[13] highlighted the impact of contextual stressors and socio-economic inequalities on families. He suggested ways of adapting family therapy to include individuals with disabilities such as using simplified language, a slower pace, and the use of other forms of communication such as behaviour, drawing, and photos. Hutchison et al.,[14] in a recent paper on experience of family therapy for adults with intellectual disabilities, point out that health staff need clarity as to which families would benefit most from behavioural family therapy, that interventions will need to be adapted for people with intellectual disabilities, and that intellectual disability nurses, along with other health professionals, will need support from their managers to deliver such interventions.

Further reading

Association of Family Therapy (2009). *Current Practice, Future Possibilities. Association for Family Therapy and Systemic Practice in the UK.* ℘ www.aft.org.uk/SpringboardWebApp/userfiles/aft/file/Members/CurrentPracticeFuturePossibilities.pdf (accessed 30 October 2017).

References

7 Minuchin S (1974). *Families and Family Therapy.* Tavistock: London.

8 Haley J (1963). *Strategies of Psychotherapy.* Grune and Stratton: New York, NY.

9 Selvini Palazzoli M, Boscolo L, Cecchin G, Prata G (1980). Hypothesizing-circularity-neutrality. *Family Process.* 6: 3–9.

10 White M, Epston D (1990). *Narrative Means to Therapeutic Ends.* WW Norton: New York, NY.

11 De Shazer S (1985). *Keys to Solutions in Brief Therapy.* WW Norton: New York, NY.

12 Fidell B (2000). Exploring the use of family therapy with adults with a learning disability. *Journal of Family Therapy.* 22: 308–23.

13 Purdy L (2012). How to fail with people with learning disabilities. *Journal of Family Therapy.* 34: 419–30.

14 Hutchison J, Lang K, Anderson G, MacMahon K (2017). Health professionals' experiences of behavioural family therapy for adults with intellectual disabilities: a thematic analysis. *Journal of Psychiatric and Mental Health Nursing.* 24: 272–81.

Touch

Nurses frequently touch people for whom they are caring and supporting, and the positive and effective use of touch is an important set of skills that nurses need to become proficient in. The use of touch may involve the physical care of a person such as supporting or delivering intimate care. It may also be used to communicate empathy and understanding of a person's distress or happiness such as a comforting and welcome touch to a person's arm or shoulder. Nurses may also use touch in the purposive application of creams and massage of different parts of the body. There are also a number of therapies that rely on the use of touch such as massage.

People using nursing services are aware of the need for nurses to touch them and will normally permit a nurse to do so, as part of their role, but expect the use of touch to be respectful and appropriate. Therefore, prior to any nursing intervention or therapeutic practice, the nurse must gain the person's consent. Consent should be obtained through a local consent policy and documented accordingly (see → Consent to examination, treatment, and care, pp. 506–7).

People who are being touched will quickly be able to distinguish between a touch that they feel to be caring and supportive and a touch that they feel is unhelpful and unwelcome or intrusive. It is therefore very important that a nurse should be able to evaluate the person's response towards the touch interaction and to be aware of what touch could convey. Nurses need to develop a clear understanding of the use of touch and what is acceptable to an individual, as well as an awareness of cultural considerations. Touch can provide the nurse with a potent therapeutic tool with unexplored potential.

Touch as a communication tool

Aromatherapy and multisensory massage

Touch is key to the use of aromatherapy and is one approach that is often provided for people with intellectual disabilities. It is defined as the use of essential oils, obtained from plants, to promote health and well-being. Aromatherapy is mainly used to help people relax; however, aromatherapy is also used for stimulation, to promote concentration, and to build communication. Massage can be used purely for relaxation and to improve health, with the introduction of massage tools, e.g. electric massager. The activity can be identified as sensory stimulation, accompanied by oil, lotion, or cream.

Deep touch pressure

Deep touch pressure (DTP) involves hugging and stroking the skin, whereas light touch pressure (LTP) involves superficial stimulation, e.g. tickling or stroking. LTP arouses the sympathetic nervous system, leading to increased pulse rate and respiration, whereas DTP can be calming and leads to a reduction in pulse rate and respiration. DTP may be beneficial for people with ASC who are oversensitive to sensory stimulation or for people with acute anxiety.

Use of touch in multisensory environments

Tactile experiences can sometimes not be adequately explored in MSEs. We use our sense of touch all the time, and through doing so, we keep it focused and responsive. It is very important to our safety and can be a very important way of communicating to other people, e.g. caring, compassion, safety, or fear. The MSE provides an excellent place to stimulate the sense of touch by using tactile objects and panels. The sense and use of touch can be further highlighted with projectors, fibre optics, and other lighting equipment.

Tactile defensiveness

Some people with intellectual disabilities may have tactile defensiveness and find touch an uncomfortable and difficult experience and respond in a more defensive way. The cause of tactile defensiveness is neurological that can result in the person with intellectual disabilities perceiving tactile sensory input as extreme and uncomfortable; they have an ineffective ability to process touch sensations, which can result in them feeling very uncomfortable and, at times, distressed. SI techniques may be valuable in the process of attempting desensitization (see ➓ Sensory integration, p. 206).

A note on evidence

While the perceived benefits of effective touch is widely written about in nursing and healthcare, there continues to be debate about the robust research evidence base for the effectiveness of some interventions, and this is continuing to be developed. Like all interventions that nurses deliver, they need to be aware and be up-to-date with the current evidence base and, where possible, contribute in developing this.

Further reading

Buckle J (2014). *Clinical Aromatherapy: Essential Oils in Healthcare*, 3rd edn. Churchill Livingstone: London.

Burt J (2011). Delivering aromatherapy and massage in a day centre. *Learning Disability Practice*. 14: 25–9.

Chan SJ, Tse SH (2011). Massage as therapy for persons with intellectual disabilities. A review of literature. *Journal of Intellectual Disabilities*. 15: 47–52.

Complementary, integrated, and alternative therapies

Introduction

The term complementary, integrated, and alternative therapies refers to a range of therapies that are not usually considered to be part of western medical practice. There are distinctions between the words, and it is largely accepted that 'complementary' and 'integrated' therapies are used alongside more traditional medical interventions and recognize the value of these, as well as the added valued that may be brought by the use of additional therapies. 'Alternative' therapies are viewed as therapies that are used instead of more traditional medical approaches and are not used alongside these.[15] It appears that the use of complementary or integrated therapies is the most common arrangement.

Range of possible therapies

There is a wide and growing range of possible therapies, and these have been used across a large number of care settings, including maternity services, people with long-term conditions, palliative care, and people with intellectual disabilities. The provision of services may be limited by the availability of practitioners, as well as by local interest in, and funding for, the use of these therapies. Some of the most common therapies include:[16] homeopathy, acupuncture, osteopathy, chiropractic, and herbal medicines (further details of each of these is provided at ℘ www.nhs.uk/Livewell/ complementary-alternative-medicine/Pages/complementary-alternative-medicines.aspx). Aromatherapy is another approach that has been widely used among people with intellectual disabilities, both with and without the use of massage. Animal therapy has also been reported to have some benefits to people, including people with intellectual disabilities.[17]

Assessment and planning

Like all interventions, the use of complementary, integrative, or alternative therapies should be based on a careful assessment of a person's abilities and needs. The introduction of therapies should also be considered to be of benefit to the person receiving it. The need for the provision of adequate information to enable the person to understand what is being proposed and obtaining an informed consent are a requirement for all services that may be considered to involve examination, treatment, and/or care.

Potential benefits?

Many people have reported benefits to them from complementary, integrated, and alternative therapies. It has been reported that such approaches can contribute to an enhanced feeling of well-being, increased relaxation, and mobility.

A continuing challenge remains to develop a robust evidence base for many of these approaches when used with people who have intellectual disabilities. Much of the research that has been undertaken has provided limited evidence of effectiveness over a longer-term period and has often been questioned in relation to the adequacy of the methodology used in the studies.[17]

When considering the provision of complementary, integrated, or alternative therapies, NHS Choices[15] identify some helpful questions (particularly if intervention is being provided by a privately contracted therapist) you should consider asking any therapist. These are:

- 'The cost of treatment?
- How long the treatment will last?
- Are there any people who should not use this treatment?
- What side effects might the treatment cause?
- Is there anything you should do to prepare for treatment?
- What system does the practitioner have for dealing with complaints about their treatment or service?
- Documentary proof of their qualifications?
- Documentary proof that they are a member of their professional body?
- Association or voluntary register?
- Documentary proof that they are insured?
- Written references?'[15]

When providing these therapies for people with intellectual disabilities, it would also be useful to know what experience individual therapies have in doing so. Nurses in intellectual disabilities could become trained as therapists or work to support other therapists in providing these therapies.

References

15 NHS Choices (2016). *Complementary and Alternative Medicine.* ℜ www.nhs.uk/Livewell/complementary-alternative-medicine/Pages/complementary-alternative-medicines.aspx (accessed 30 October 2017) (Quotation reprinted under the Open Government License 3.0).
16 Maber-Aleksandrowicz S, Avent C, Hassiotis A (2016). A systematic review of animal-assisted therapy on psychosocial outcomes in people with intellectual disability. *Research in Developmental Disabilities.* **49**: 322–38.
17 Gartlehner G, Gaynes BN, Amick HR, et al. (2016). Comparative benefits and harms of antidepressant, psychological, complementary, and exercise treatments for major depression: an evidence report for a clinical practice guideline from the American College of Physicians. *Annals of Internal Medicine.* **164**: 323–30.

Art, drama, and music

Art opportunities can enable a person with intellectual disabilities to develop a wider range of methods of expressing thoughts and feelings and communicating with people around them. This can involve the use of images, music, language, gesture, and movement. Art, music, and drama can assist people to be more creative in their actions and communication. It encourages ideas that are personal and creative. A robust arts programme in the care setting can be exciting and a very positive experience for many of the people engaging in it. To be effective, people need to feel safe to express themselves, feel valued as people, and have their differences respected by others, be present and prepared to be spontaneous, and take some risks in their expressions. Art opportunities encompass a range of activities in the visual arts, music, and drama. These activities and experiences help the people with intellectual disabilities to make sense of, and engage more creatively in, the world.

Sensory art

Art in healthcare may take the form of sensory art where the medium used is carefully selected to stimulate the senses (touch, smell, hearing, sight) of the artist, while producing a valued and valid art piece. It is vitally important to recognize the contribution of the artist at their cognitive ability level, as therapeutic benefit could be compromised by the over-enthusiasm of a dedicated enabler.

Arts and crafts

Arts and crafts can provide an important part of leisure or day activities for people with intellectual disabilities. A fairly sophisticated arts programme can be observed in many modern day facilities. Silk painting, weaving, card making, pottery, and scrap booking are some of the current art activities on offer, with artists often progressing to exhibiting their work in local art galleries. Art pieces are often used to contribute to the cosmetic and therapeutic living and the working environment of people with intellectual disabilities.

Art therapy

Art therapy focuses on how the person is thinking and feeling. The therapist and the person with intellectual disabilities then explore the feelings and thoughts together by either talking and/or by enhancing further what has been developed during the course of the session. It is hoped that through this process, the person with intellectual disabilities will come to understand and better articulate personal emotional issues that they are having difficulty in expressing or coming to terms with.

Drama

Drama offers an integrating approach for people with intellectual disabilities that holistically addresses their learning needs—it can increase their ability to relate to others more effectively.

The appeal of drama to people with intellectual disabilities is that they can be caught up in situations that are both fun and intriguing. People are involved in their learning in a changing and real-time way which can learn strong memories. Drama can be used as a tool to help people recollect past experiences and anticipate new ones. There are many local successful drama groups for people with intellectual disabilities within voluntary and statutory services.

Drama therapy

Drama therapy is the purposeful use of drama with one person or a group of people, with the agreement that a therapist is using drama to primarily achieve therapeutic goals through these activities.

Music

Music is a highly motivating activity for many people with intellectual disabilities. It can help to elicit responses from individuals whose interest is often quite difficult to arouse. The elements of music sessions are usually made up of listening, observing, and singing, performing, and composing.

Music therapy

Music therapy is the use of sound and music within an evolving relationship between a person and a therapist to support and encourage well-being. In a typical session, the music therapist and the person with intellectual disabilities create music together. They establish a relationship through which the individual can communicate their thoughts and feelings in a safe and supported environment.

Further reading

Booker M (2011). *Drama Therapy Approaches for People with Profound or Severe Multiple Disabilities, Including Sensory Impairment*. Jessica Kingsley Publisher: London.

Clarkson AR, Killick M (2016). A bigger picture: community groups in residential settings for people with learning disabilities. *Voices: A World Forum for Music Therapy*. **16**: September 2016. doi: 10.15845/voices.v16i3.845. ♫ voices.no/index.php/voices/article/view/845 (accessed 8 March 2018).

Edwards J (2016). *The Oxford Handbook of Music Therapy*. Oxford University Press: Oxford.

Intensive interaction

Intensive interaction[18] is a research-based approach and draws heavily on parent–infant interaction. It is based on how babies first learn how to interact with others in usual development and adapts this teaching-learning approach in order to teach the fundamentals of communication (FOCs) to people with profound or multiple intellectual disabilities or severe and complex intellectual disabilities, additional multiple sensory impairment, dementia, developmental delay, and ASC. The FOCs include:[18]

- 'Enjoying being with another person;
- Developing the ability to attend to that person;
- Concentration and attention span;
- Learning to do sequences of activity with a person;
- Taking turns in exchange of behaviour;
- Sharing personal space;
- Learning to regulate and control arousal levels;
- Using and understanding eye contacts and facial expressions;
- Using and understanding other non-verbal communications;
- Using and understanding physical contacts;
- Vocalising and using vocalisations in a meaningful way.'*[1]

Learning the FOCs forms the foundation for more advanced communication and contributes to learning, development, and overall well-being. Activities are relaxed, enjoyable, and free-flowing and are led by the learner. The basic techniques are:

- **Tuning-in**—reading the person to understand their emotional, psychological, cognitive, and physical state, moment by moment;
- **Enjoyment**;
- **Holding back**—observing and waiting;
- **Allowing the person to lead, 'go first', or take the first turn**—allowing learners to initiate communication will raise their self-esteem and self-worth;
- **Responding in a variety of ways, including imitation and joining in**—imitation needs to be used carefully and thoughtfully; not everything is imitated, and practitioners need to think about, and understand, why they are imitating;
- **Being relaxed and unhurried**—interactions can last for seconds or many minutes, so be aware of time constraints;
- **Pausing**—when necessary;
- **Timing responses**—so that the pace of the interaction is right for the learner;
- **Positioning and available look**.

The only rule *is that the interaction stops when the person has had enough.*

Learners with whom we interact need our full attention; follow their actions and messages, and use these in play. This will allow them to learn skills needed for interactive communication and perhaps transfer these skills to other areas of their lives.

---

* Extracted from Nind, M and Hewett, D. (2001) *A Practical to Intensive Interaction.* Birmingham: British Institute of Learning Disabilitieso, with kind permission from BILD.

Useful and practical tips for successful interaction are:
- Be accurate and objective in your observations—learn their language; pay close attention to what they are doing; focus on even the smallest stimuli (e.g. changes in breathing, gentle teeth grinding, nails digging, and eye gaze);
- Learn their way of communication before choosing the appropriate way to interact (tune in and be responsive);
- Make sure you are aware of all their impairments. Sensory difficulties, problems with vision, hearing, or fine motor skills may be undiagnosed, and learners might have difficulty processing received signs. Take this into consideration during interactive activities;
- Always wait for a response or their initial signal that they are ready to interact—to allow the person to learn to initiate and that other people are interested in what they have to 'say'; overloading may cause a negative effect;
- Develop a good rapport—mutual trust and attention are always important for a successful interaction;
- Use their signals and ways of communicating, and try to expand on them during sessions;
- Listen to them and copy their behaviour closely, but not exactly. The object of this exercise is to initiate conversation;
- Make sure the environment is appropriate to the situation, whether that means finding a quiet place to keep distractions to a minimum or finding somewhere loud where the learner feels comfortable making a noise;
- Use minimal language, rather vocalize or imitate noises;
- Document and video-record sessions, and record progress and reflect on practice.

Further reading

Firth G, Elford H, Crabbe M, Leeming C (2007). Intensive interaction as a novel approach in social care: Care staff's views on the practice change process. *Journal of Applied Research in Intellectual Disabilities*. 21: 58–69.

Intensive Interaction. ℘ www.intensiveinteraction.org (accessed 30 October 2017).

References

18 Nind M, Hewett D (2001). *A Practical Guide to Intensive Interaction*. British Institute of Learning Disabilities: Kidderminster.

Hydrotherapy

Hydrotherapy has many benefits for people with a variety of disabilities and impairments or those recovering from surgery and injury, long-term and short-term conditions, pains in the joints and back, and other problems. Hydrotherapy pools are shallow with warm water and are used for any type of physiotherapy or gentle exercise, or for those who cannot access public swimming pools for a number of reasons. Physiotherapists usually create an exercise plan based on an individual's assessments and type of difficulties and should be carried out by people who have had special training.

The benefits of hydrotherapy may include

- Pain reduction—a warm and 'weightless' atmosphere can have a positive effect on a person's overall physique;
- A pleasurable and calm environment—this may reduce anxiety levels, relieve stress, and encourage relaxation;
- Improvement of overall physical and health well-being—e.g. improvement of skin conditions, development of the swallow reflex, relaxation and/or strengthening of muscles, reducing load on the joints and spine, improvement of circulation, posture, and balance, reducing muscle spasm and weight, increasing mobility, relieving strain on internal organs that could be caused by the person's limited mobility (e.g. people in a wheelchair), and improving breathing;
- Improvement of mental health well-being—enjoyable and fun; may help gain body control, increase self-confidence, and provide a secure and safe environment;
- Multisensory experience—e.g. water temperature, visual effects, sounds, feel of water on the skin, different types and textures of equipment, floating sensation of water, and smells.

The equipment used, specialist or otherwise, may include

- Specialist hydrotherapy chairs, hoists, and slings;
- Soft or specialist tubes/noodles with or without handles and Velcro™ and of different lengths and thickness;
- Arm bands, swim rings, swim vests, swim floats, loungers, boards, goggles, and swimming caps;
- Agua body belts, wrist bands, and specialist support braces;
- Specialist exercise kits (e.g. hydrotherapy hand bar weights and flotation devices);
- Toys, soft play balls, inflatable animals, and beach balls;
- Music and/or special effects (e.g. light displays and bubbles).

Before taking people for hydrotherapy

- Understand that some people may feel emotionally drained after hydrotherapy—offer emotional support and understanding, as well as be aware of their limits; negative behaviours may be displayed.
- Always take drinks and snacks with you.
- Have enough staff with you, usually a 1:1 ratio is optimal. This depends on the individual's disability, risk assessment, and behaviours.
- Be aware that hydrotherapy is relatively expensive.

- Be aware that there is no physiotherapist available, only a pool supervisor for health and safety purposes when hiring the pool privately.
- Do not perform any exercises with the individuals if you are untrained in their safe practising.
- Do not rush people to enter the pool. Rather offer alternatives (e.g. bring the water to them in a bucket and play with it, ask them to sit by the pool and dip their hands or feet into the pool).
- Contact the hydrotherapy pool before visiting, and let them know if you require any specialist equipment.
- Make sure that all the individuals going to the hydrotherapy pool have risk assessments, including manual handling.
- Bring people's favourite toys and/or equipment with you, if possible.
- Some people may need goggles, as the chemicals in the water may be irritating and cause distress.

Examples of different types and techniques of hydrotherapy include

- Balneotherapy and thalassotherapy;
- Kneipp system;
- Comprehensive aquatic therapies (the bad Ragaz ring method, clinical Aichi, and Halliwick concept);
- Thermal or mineral spas;
- Cryotherapy;
- Scotch hose;
- Foot spas and wraps.

Further reading

Eidson R (2008). *Hydrotherapy*. Delmar Cengage Learning: Ontario.

Ewac Medical (2016). *Methods of Hydrotherapy* [online]. ℘ www.ewacmedical.com/knowledge/articles-hydrotherapy/methods-of-hydrotherapy/ (accessed 30 October 2017).

Garcia MK, Joares EC, Silva MA, Bissolotti RR, Oliveira S, Battistella LR (2012). The Halliwick concept, inclusion and participation through aquatic functional activities. *Acta Fisiatr.* **19**: 142–50.

Kellogg JH (2007). *Outlines of Practical Hydrotherapy*. Kessinger Publishing: Whitefish, MT.

Mooventhan A, Nivethitha L (2014). Scientific evidence-based effects of hydrotherapy on various systems of the body. *North American Journal of Medical Sciences.* **6**: 199–209.

Conductive education

Conductive education (CE), developed in Hungary by Professor Peto in 1952, is an intensive, holistic approach to education, development, and training, concentrating on improvement of both gross and fine motor and cognitive skills through physical activities in a group environment. CE is for people with cerebral palsy, spina bifida, and other neuromotor-related *disabilities*. The purpose of CE is to provide support and instruction to gain or regain body control using minimal adaptive equipment in order to become independent and to raise their self-esteem.

The benefits of CE include

- Helping to regain lost skills; reinstating independence and improving their quality of life;
- Building confidence and the ability to problem-solve;
- Overcoming difficulties with fine motor skills;
- Reducing dependence on equipment; increasing mobility;
- Helping improve coordination, communication, and attention;
- Developing appropriate strategies to function in various environments;
- Focusing on building up personalities (e.g. determination, initiation, self-sufficiency, autonomy);
- Actively participating in the learning process.

Programmes are developed and implemented by specifically trained conductors and their assistants. Care providers and family members are involved in this intervention in order to support people in their care with acquired skills successfully. Every programme is condition- and age-specific and based on an individual assessment done by the conductor. When supporting people in this programme, never:

- Set people up to fail or de-motivate them;
- Set tasks that cannot be achieved or do them too fast;
- Reward only the results (reward the effort as well);
- Leave a person unsupervised for an extended period of time;
- Perform tasks without being specifically trained.

CE is an intensive life-long day-to-day learning process, so it is important for people to be kept motivated through visual representation of their achievements. A person (other than the conductor) assisting a client with CE needs to be aware of the key points of CE that includes:

- Developing a good rapport and trust among all involved;
- Creating a good learning environment;
- Working in groups as people learn and support each other with problem-solving in achieving day-to-day tasks (groups are usually condition-, age-, and skills-matched) and everyone in the group is involved;
- Providing a structured programme (including play to make it more interesting and creative) and timescale;
- Offering guidance to perform the task, rather than doing it for them;
- Each task needs to be tailored and made to suit the individual's needs;

- Linking together movement, speech, and thought (e.g. I roll from the left to the right side—the whole group has to repeat this and then perform the task using a count);
- Understanding people's conditions and how these can have an impact on their learning and lives;
- Planning support and identifying any required equipment;
- Emotional security.

The skills learnt through conductive education include

- Development of daily living skills (dressing, drinking, and potty/toilet training);
- Coordination and improving posture and weight-bearing;
- Eye and breathing exercises;
- Academic and social interaction skills;
- Facial expressions;
- Playing with others or peers, including play strategies.

Elements of conductive education

- The conductor—designs and delivers a programme to grow an orthofunctioning personality;
- Group dynamics—structured group activities that are broken down into a series of steps representing real-life settings. Goals include social skills development, friendship, encouragement, modification of behaviour, and acceptance;
- Daily routine—broken down into sequences of actions that are consistent. Goals include enhancement in cognitive, psychosocial, physical, and communication abilities;
- Rhythmic intention—by using the rhythm of language and music to pace movements to learn alternative ways to complete tasks;
- Task series—to function physically and mentally, participants learn to gain control of movements to increase cognitive functioning through tasking.

Further reading

Conductive Education. ♪ www.conductive-ed.org.uk (accessed on 30 October 2017) (information on CE).

National Institute of Conductive Education, Birmingham. ♪ www.conductive-education.org.uk/ (accessed on 30 October 2017).

TEACCH (Treatment and Education of Autistic and related Communication-handicapped Children)

TEACCH is a structured teaching approach with clear boundaries using an adapted learning environment that uses evidence-based practices and reflects an understanding of the learning and cognitive needs, characteristics, and challenges associated with autistic spectrum conditions (ASCs). The primary aim is to prepare people with ASCs for independent living (school, work, community) through skills development in order to reach their potential. A further goal is to encourage flexibility, self-efficiency, and meaningful engagement in activities.

Before an individualized programme is developed, it is important for the person developing it to:
- Understand the 'culture of ASC' (e.g. manifestations, impairments, strengths, and characteristics) to understand behaviours and learning styles;
- Assess the person's abilities—their skills, needs, and interests in order to make the programme effective;
- Involve people in their lives (parents, cares, siblings, teachers, assistance, professionals), as they help to maintain and develop it further (individualized person–family-centred plan);
- Consider the learning environment, the task/s to be taught, and how these will be achieved (e.g. task organization, physical organization, structured environment, teaching methods, reinforcements, cues, rewards), as consistency and clear instructions are important;
- Discuss all plans with the person at whom the programme is aimed (a communication aid might be needed);
- Attend TEACCH training to learn the principles, aims, skills, and strategies needed for successful delivery.

Difficulties and strengths presented by individuals with ASCs may be demonstrated by changes in behaviour and include:
- Communication—impairment in social use of language (e.g. non-verbal and verbal expressions, and difficulties in receptive language);
- Organization of oneself, ideas, materials, and activities (being easily distracted, difficulties with transition and concept of time);
- Processing of information (auditory difficulties);
- Having difficulties in understanding the bigger picture (frequent attention to details);
- Sequencing—not understanding what follows or what happens next; this may occur due to poor memory;
- Transfer of skills from one situation/environment/task to another—difficulties in generalizing;
- Resistance to change in routines and going back to familiar things, activities, or behaviours, therefore seek to motivate;
- A lack of understanding of social rules, visual learners, special interests, sensory preferences, dislikes, and unique skills.

When teaching people with ASCs using the TEACCH framework, always consider the following.[19]

Organization

- Appropriate environment (e.g. lighting, space, noise levels, organization, exits, distractions, colour of walls, use of dividers, smells, materials);
- Visual cues—for associating the activity/task to a place (e.g. a picture of handwashing on the wall above the sink, a toilet picture on the toilet door);
- Clear organization and structure of the tasks/activities;
- Identifying specific areas for specific tasks (e.g. playground—time-out area, kitchen—cooking);
- Accessible teaching materials (e.g. in a tray with their name and a photo);
- Clear boundaries and transition area identified (where the schedules are placed).

Schedules

- A sequenced visual timetable making clear the beginning and end of activities to be clearly visible;
- Tailor-made to a person's cognitive ability and experiences;
- Use—objects of reference, pictures, photos, symbols, numbers, words, diaries, own writing, ticking technique, magazine pictures;
- Presentation—a key ring (to take out), vertical or horizontal (with a person's photo or name);
- Time—beginning and end to be clear, e.g. use an egg timer, a clock (digital), colour coding (on the paper clock), hourglass.

Teaching approach

- Use verbal prompts (clear, consistent, key words only, sequenced—first do this, and then do that).
- Use gestures—e.g. pointing while talking to enhance the understanding, make sure the person follows what is being shown to them.
- Use non-verbal prompts—visual cues, written instruction, schedules.
- Use physical prompts—hand-over-hand approach, guide their hand, let them to model you, demonstrate first and let them to copy you.
- Use prompts for certain situations—what to say in certain situations (e.g. goodbye when leaving), provide reassurance.
- Use rewards and find motivators—always address behaviour at the time.

Further reading

Practical Autism Resources. ℘ www.practicalautismresources.com/printables (accessed on 30 October 2017).

The National Autistic Society. ℘ www.nas.org.uk (information about TEACCH) (accessed on 30 October 2017).

University of North Caroline at Chapel Hill School of Medicine. *TEACCH Autism Program*. ℘ www. teacch.com (accessed on 30 October 2017).

References

19 Schopler E, Mesibov G (1995). *Learning and Cognition in Autism*. Plenum Press: New York, NY.

Positive behaviour support

Introduction

Positive behaviour support (PBS) emerged in the USA in the late 1980s in response to increased awareness and public opposition to the use of aversive techniques to manage challenging behaviours.[20] It brings the science of applied behaviour analysis (ABA) together with the values of intellectual disability practice of inclusion and person-centred approaches.[21]

PBS is a constructive and normally an interdisciplinary approach that understands that all behaviours have a function, even those that are challenging.[22] It is a preventative approach which starts with where the person with intellectual disability is and is focused on enriching the environment, so that the person can get what they like without needing to use behaviours that are challenging in order to get the things that are important to them. Consider how many different ways you know to get the attention of another person. A person with intellectual disabilities may only have learnt one way. Is it right to take that 'one' way away from the person because we consider it challenging? PBS seeks to '*add*' behaviours with support, so the person has better, more efficient ways of meeting this function. This should make challenging behaviours redundant and reduce as a consequence of increasing their skills.

Key terms

Some of the terms used in ABA are used differently as to how they are used in everyday language, and understanding the use of these terms is an important starting point.
• Positive = adding;
• Negative = taking away;
• Reinforcement = making a behaviour more likely to happen in the future;
• Punishment = making a behaviour less likely to happen in the future.

There are no values added to these terms. Positive and negative do not mean good or bad. Punishment does not mean the use of abusive or aversive practices, only that the behaviour is likely to reduce.[23]

Importance of function

Understanding the function of behaviour is central to PBS. A functional assessment is completed to understand the function of the behaviour. This will usually include a semi structured interview and an analysis of event recordings (e.g. ABC charts), along with direct observations (see Fig. 9.3).

Functions are usually grouped into four areas, noting that a behaviour may serve more than one function:
• Sensory—a behaviour that meets an internal need such as expressing frustration;
• Escape—avoiding a task, area, or person;
• Attention—gaining attention from others;
• Tangibles—getting things such as food, activities, or preferred items.

When a functional assessment is completed, a function-based plan needs to be developed. Part of the plan should address the behaviour, and another part needs to focus on meeting the function.

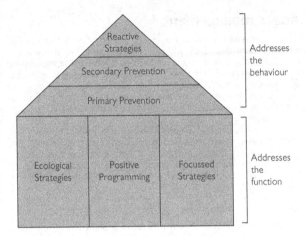

Fig. 9.3 A model for PBS.

Preventative approaches

Preventative approaches aim to prevent or respond to behaviours. Primary approaches aim to avoid the undesirable behaviours happening, e.g. by avoiding known antecedents. Secondary approaches aim to de-escalate a situation when there are early warning signs of undesirable behaviours, e.g. distraction and diversion strategies. Reactive strategies aim to safely and quickly bring an incident to an end when it occurs.

Proactive approaches

Proactive approaches aim to enable the person to meet the function in more effective ways. Positive programming focuses on teaching strategies that will be used for the development of a new skill. Ecological strategies describe how the environment and preceding factors will be adjusted to support the new behaviour. Focused strategies detail how reinforcement will be used for the new behaviours.

Further reading

Royal College of Nursing (2017). *Three Steps to Positive Practice*. Royal College of Nursing: London. ℳ www.rcn.org.uk/professional-development/publications/pub-006075 (accessed 30 October 2017).

References

20 LaVigna GW, Willis TJ (2012). The efficacy of positive behavioural support with the most challenging behaviour: the evidence and its implications. *Journal of Intellectual and Developmental Disability*. 37: 185–95.
21 Gore NJ, McGill P, Toogood S, et al. (2013). Definition and scope for positive behavioural support. *International Journal of Positive Behavioural Support*. 3: 14–23.
22 Carr EG, Dunlap G, Horner RH, et al. (2002). Positive behavior support: evolution of an applied science. *Journal of Positive Behavior Interventions*. 4: 4–16.
23 Cooper JO, Heron TE, Heward WL (2007). *Applied Behaviour Analysis*, 2nd edn. Pearson: Upper Saddle River, NJ.

Anger management

Anger management applied to people with intellectual disabilities draws on a range of techniques. These techniques are designed to enable people to cope better with their anger and the potential aggression that may develop from it. The techniques are generally of a cognitive behavioural nature (see → Cognitive behaviour therapies, p. 340), although some techniques are not. The techniques applied should be based on the cognitive ability of the person or people who could benefit from the technique(s), and the nature of their anger.

It is generally accepted that cognitive behavioural methods of anger management are best suited for use with people with a mild to moderate degree of intellectual disabilities, as the success of these approaches is underpinned by the ability to communicate and reason at a relatively high level. Taylor and Novaco[24] have proposed that anger is an emotion that has three components:

• Physiological;
• Behavioural;
• Cognitive.

Taylor and Novaco,[24] together with more recent theorists, have advocated that anger management plans should be built around these three areas. In very broad terms, the techniques recommended for each component of aggression are:

• Physiological—involving environmental management and relaxation techniques;
• Behavioural—involving the person recognizing how anger causes them to behave aggressively or inappropriately and to develop more acceptable coping skills;
• Cognitive—involving restructuring of distorted thinking that leads to anger.

Readers are advised to consult further reading for more detail. In order for anger management to work, preparatory measures should be undertaken:

• Thorough assessment of the anger and its consequences for the individual and others;
• Self-report questionnaires and interviews;
• A thorough exploration of the individual's history, to include the carer's views, triggers of anger, and environmental issues;
• Functional analysis and communicative function of the anger;
• The level of communication of the individual and their methods of communication.

Anger management techniques are normally developed during a series of structured facilitated sessions with individuals or within groups, the aims and methods of which are:

• To develop an understanding of anger and aggression;
• Individual and group reflections on the development of anger and its consequences;
• To develop coping skills that can help manage situations that have previously caused anger, and to generalize these to other anger-provoking contexts;
• To teach relaxation techniques.

Participants are encouraged to reflect on the sessions and their developing anger management skills by use of a reflective diary/self-report, which can be discussed in the sessions. Depending on the cognitive and communication level of participants, pictures, charts, pictorial rating scales, role-play, and 'traffic light' systems can be used.

For people with more severe intellectual disabilities and sensory impairments, it is recognized that the cognitive and some of the behavioural aspects may not be useful, and therefore physiological techniques should be encouraged, including:

- Aromatherapy;
- Reflexology;
- Hand massage;
- Multisensory rooms;
- Music therapy;
- Hydrotherapy;
- Art therapy.

The role of the registered nurse for people with intellectual disabilities

The cognitive aspects and anger management programmes are often facilitated by clinical psychologists; however, nurses are often involved with such groups. More specifically, nurses are likely to be involved with the assessment process and supporting individuals with behavioural and physiological aspects of anger management.

Further reading

Hamelin J, Travis RP, Sturmey P (2013). Anger management and intellectual disabilities: a systematic review. *Journal of Mental Health Research in Intellectual Disabilities*. 6: 60–70.

Wilner P, Rose J, Jahoda A, et al. (2013). Group-based cognitive—behavioural anger management for people with mild to moderate intellectual disabilities: cluster randomized controlled trial. *British Journal of Psychiatry*. 203: 288–96.

References

24 Taylor JL, Novaco RW (2005). *Anger Treatment for People with Developmental Disabilities: A Theory, Evidence, and Manual Based Approach*. John Wiley & Sons: London.

Cognitive behaviour therapies

CBTs are based on an assumption that individuals construct a world view that may be at variance from reality. These personal constructs, which are also known as schemata, are developed and maintained through everyday experiences, and they are used as coping mechanisms, which help people understand their own behaviour and that of others. If events and behaviours are consistently negative and emotionally damaging, then the individual can develop profoundly negative constructs and resulting behaviours such as self-injury. These constructs are called self-defeating beliefs and errors in thinking. These distorted errors in thinking and behaviour are often subconscious over which individuals have little control. CBT allows for individuals, through skilled therapeutic interventions,[25] to bring previously subconscious thought processes to a conscious level of self-awareness. This can then lead to an exploration of these thought processes and the development of a more accurate and healthy world view. Given that subconscious negative self constructs can develop due to persistently negative life experiences, it is suggested that some people with intellectual disabilities are likely to have developed negative self-views as a result from damaging ways in which they may have been treated. Some people benefit from CBT which can:

- Provide an opportunity to deconstruct negative self-views;
- Be a humanistic, person-centred intervention;
- Be a holistic approach that pursues personal growth;
- Offer opportunities for partnership working and the development of therapeutic relationships;
- Develop an understanding of seemingly irrational behaviours.

Using this approach shifts the focus from an emphasis on behaviours and symptomology to an understanding of the damaging nature of causative factors. CBT is less commonly used with people with intellectual disabilities at times because it:

- Requires and presupposes that an individual has the cognitive ability to do so;
- Demands compliance with what the therapist and others may agree to be an acceptable world view, rather than a real understanding of how a person with cognitive impairments makes sense of the world;
- Necessitates the individual being actively engaged in the process;
- Requires the person with intellectual disabilities to be able to use expressive language and have the ability to recognize and understand emotions.

Further reading

Jahoda A, Dagnan D, Stenfert Kroese B, Pert C, Trower P (2009). Cognitive behavioural therapy: from face to face interaction to a broader contextual understanding of change. *Journal of Intellectual Disability Research*. 53: 759–71.

References

25 Hassiotis A, Serfaty MK, Martin SAS, King M (2012). *A Manual of Cognitive Behaviour Therapy for People with Mild Learning Disabilities and Common Mental Disorders*. Camden & Islington NHS Foundation Trust and University College London: London.

Support associated with loss and bereavement

Supporting the person with intellectual disabilities

Just because a person has intellectual disabilities, it should never be assumed that they cannot grieve. Nurses should recognize the need to give them extra consideration because of their disability. Death never occurs in a vacuum, but within a social context, and that social context in which they are being supported may be crucial in helping a person with intellectual disabilities to deal with their grief in a constructive way.[26]

Facilitating grief

Nurses need to educate people about the impact of loss and its potential effects, using naturalistic opportunities such as events happening in the media or portrayed on the television. Nurses need to help people with intellectual disabilities to learn about loss and bereavement, actively participate in the grief process, and facilitate grief in a constructive way. Health and social care professionals need to remember that:

- Everyone has a right to know when someone close to them dies;
- Introducing and talking about difficult news need to be undertaken in conjunction with a familiar carer whenever possible;
- Nurses need to find out what the person knows (or indeed does not know) about the loss;
- Accurate information needs to be conveyed in a clear, consistent way, with active listening as key to personal support;
- Information may need to be clarified in a way that the person understands, repeated often, and reassurances regularly offered;
- Grieving individuals need an invitation to talk, which includes acknowledging the pain they may be feeling, recognizing the need for a safe, quiet space and privacy, ongoing constructive support;
- Individuals may find it difficult to articulate their feelings in a coherent manner. Picture and storybooks might help them to recognize and explore their feelings with support;
- It may take time for the grieving person to accept the reality and finality of the loss; accurate record-keeping is essential for ongoing support;
- Grief work takes time, and everyone grieves in their own unique way.

Creative approaches

Some people with intellectual disabilities may have communication challenges and may feel uncomfortable with support that relies on dialogue alone. Therefore, the nurse needs to be creative in the bereavement support process, using pictures, photographs, or artwork as a means of facilitating expression. Many people lack personal heritage and history, and the development of a life storybook is an excellent way of recording events in a tangible, accessible, and meaningful way. Similarly, the creation of a memory book around a particular person who has perhaps died captures vital information in an accessible format.

Responding to disenfranchised grief

Disenfranchised grief is described in ➔ Responding to bereavement, pp. 260–1, and according to Doka, ways of minimizing the chance of this occurring with people with intellectual disabilities include:[27]

- Acknowledging and legitimizing the loss, actively listening to the bereaved person, being empathic, trying to imagine how the person may be feeling, and helping the person to make sense of what has happened;
- Encouraging the constructive use of ritual (such as visiting the grave or memorial), sharing fears and anxieties, exploring spiritual needs and support, offering options for mutual support (such as group work), and bereavement counselling.

Those who may need therapeutic interventions

Although most people generally deal with their grief in their own way, without the need for therapeutic interventions, some people with intellectual disabilities may need to be referred for specific bereavement support from a counsellor or psychologist. People who may need additional help include those individuals who:

- Are unusually angry or who profoundly miss the deceased;
- Have a restricted social support network;[26]
- Are assessed as not coping;[27]
- Are excluded from the funeral or who have not been told about the death for some considerable time after the event.[27]

Impact of offering support

Working with loss and bereavement can affect health and social care professionals in different ways. It may make them recall friends and family who have died; it may make them think about current losses or even dwell on the potential for loss and death in the future. Professionals should remember to look after themselves. Clinical supervision is one way of accessing support during such difficult times, as is peer support and counselling.

Further reading

Read S (2007). *Bereavement Counselling for People with Learning Disabilities: A Manual to Develop Practice.* Quay Books: London.

Read S, ed. (2014). *Supporting People with Intellectual Disabilities Experiencing Loss and Bereavement: Theory and Compassionate Practice.* Jessica Kingsley Publishers: London.

Wiese M, Stancliffe RJ, Read S, Jeltes G, Clayton J (2015). Learning about dying, death and end-of-life planning: current issues informing future actions. *Journal of Intellectual and Developmental Disability.* 40: 230–5.

References

26 Read S (2008). Loss, bereavement, counselling and support: an intellectual disability perspective. *Grief Matters.* 11: 54–9.

27 Elliott D (1995). Helping people with learning disabilities to handle grief. *Nursing Times.* 9: 209–13.

Appropriate use of medication

Psychopharmacology

Psychopharmacology refers to the effects of medication on mental function and mental illness, and medication which can have these effects is referred to as psychotropic (medication that affects the mind). It is important to recognize that medication can have an important and, at times, a vital role to play in the therapeutic treatment of many people with intellectual disabilities with mental illness and can be very beneficial for some people at different times when their mental health is deteriorated. It is also important to understand that this is only one component of a holistic therapeutic plan, alongside possible psychological, educational, and social interventions in the pursuit of remission and recovery.

However, the inappropriate use of such medication is also a contentious issue, particularly concerning the use of such medications to manage behaviour, rather than for the purposes of therapeutic intervention in relation to a diagnosed mental illness. Equally, the long-term prescribing of such medication without effective monitoring of its continuing beneficial effects (rather than focusing on the absence of side effects) for the person taking the medication is not acceptable practice. This can also result in polypharmacy, when people are administered multiple medications, sometimes long after these continue to the needed, which can be further complicated by interactions between medications.

Types of psychotropic medication

Different medications are prescribed and used by people with intellectual disabilities who have mental health problems, including:
• Antipsychotics—used to treat psychosis; they may also be used to reduce the level of agitation, distress, and the risk of violence, as they can have a sedative effect;
• Antidepressants and mood stabilizers—can be used in the treatment of mood disorders such as depression or bipolar disorder;
• Anxiolytic medications—can be used to treat anxiety disorders or reduce symptoms of anxiety.

The undesired or side effects of psychotropic medication

The use of psychotropic medication can induce a number of severe and irreversible side effects, and it is essential that nurses have adequate knowledge and systems in place to identify such adverse effects early. Nurses should be up-to-date with the desired and undesired effects of all medication they are involved in prescribing and/or administering. This means nurses should read the product information leaflets that come along with the medication when these are supplied and also use a current and credible reference document (such as the current *British National Formulary*) to remain up-to-date on the desired and undesired effects of medication. This is particularly important when being involved in the use of medication with which they are unfamiliar or is new to the person with intellectual disabilities. There are some recognized longer-term undesired side effects that nurses should also be vigilant for, including:

- Memory impairment;
- Anticholinergic effects (including dry mouth, constipation, urinary retention, and confusion);
- Dyskinetic movement disorders (including involuntary repetitive writhing or jerking movements);
- Pseudo-Parkinsonian symptoms (including unsteady gait, bent posture, expressionless face, and tremors);
- Neuroleptic malignant syndrome is an uncommon undesired effect, but potentially very serious (including fever, severe muscle rigidity, altered consciousness, automatic arousal, potential death).

Good practice in the use of psychotropic medication

It is important that nurses carefully observe the effectiveness and undesired effects of the use of the medication. It is crucial that all staff follow good practice when involved in the prescribing or administration of medication. These are outlined below.

- Ensure adequate education and training of all staff involved in the administration of psychotropic medication.
- Ensure reasonable adjustments are in place and each person is given adequate and accessible information to enable to them to understand and to give or withhold an informed consent.
- If it has been established, through attempting to obtain informed consent, that the person does not have capacity at that time to make an informed decision, a 'best interests' decision should be considered and documented appropriately (see ➋ Consent to examination, treatment, and care, pp. 486–7).
- All staff involved in the administration of medication must have up-to-date knowledge of the expected desired and undesired effects and potential interactions of each medication administered.
- Side effect rating scales should be used to systematically identify the onset of side effects for psychotropic medication [e.g. Liverpool University Neuroleptic Side Effect Rating Scale (LUNSERS)].
- Close monitoring is necessary when reducing or stopping medication, particularly if medication is stopped abruptly.
- Ensure that there are clear parameters specified around the use of PRN (as necessary) medication, and when this is used, the reason for its administration and the effect of this should be clearly recorded.
- Ensure ongoing monitoring and review of treatment efficacy and the need for continued use, as part of the wider bio-psycho-social model of intervention.
- All prescribing medication has set review dates as actual calendar dates, not vaguely as in '3 months', to reduce the risk of people remaining on medication longer than is therapeutically useful.

Further reading

Royal College of Psychiatrists (2016). *Psychotropic Drug Prescribing for People with Intellectual Disability, Mental Health Problems and/or Behaviours that Challenge: Practice Guidelines*. Royal College of Psychiatrists: London. ⌘ www.rcpsych.ac.uk/pdf/FR_ID_09_for_website.pdf (accessed 30 October 2017).

Accessing general health services

Primary care

Primary care services are often the first point of contact for anyone wanting to access health services. The main route of access to primary care is through registration with a GP. Health and primary care commissioning is provided and managed separately within each of the four countries of the UK and in the Republic of Ireland. Within England, primary care is the responsibility of NHS England but, from 2015, increasing responsibility has been given to local clinical commissioning groups (CCGs).

Primary care settings

Historically, primary care has relied almost completely on GP services, predominantly doctors and nurses, based in local practices, offering face-to-face consultations, in the expert treatment of illness, between the hours of 9 a.m. to 5 p.m. With growing challenges, including an increasing and older population with complex medical conditions, combined with limited access to significant numbers of qualified GPs and an ageing population of nurses with problems in recruitment and retention, primary care is being forced to change.

The current focus of primary care is in prevention, working in partnership with individuals and communities to help them live a healthy life, detect any health challenges, and understand, maintain, and manage control of their health and any health conditions. This is requiring access to 24-hour services, a more diverse interdisciplinary workforce, different approaches, and new technology in the delivery of care offered in a range of different, expanded, and upgraded settings. There are a wide range of staff groups that work within primary care settings. These may include:

- GPs;
- Physician associates;
- Practice nurses;
- District/community nurses;
- Nurse practitioners;
- Mental health nurses;
- Prescribing pharmacists;
- Clinical pharmacists;
- Community pharmacists;
- Healthcare assistants;
- Paramedics;
- Practice managers;
- Receptionists;
- Administrative staff;
- Health visitors;
- Intellectual disability nurses;
- Optometrists;
- Podiatrists;
- Community dentists;
- Dental hygienists;
- Social workers;
- Community matrons;
- Occupational therapists;
- Physiotherapists;
- Dieticians;
- Psychology/CBT practitioners;
- Midwives;
- Phlebotomists.

Within the UK, primary care funding is largely based on meeting national and local contracts with commissioners. Additional voluntary contracts, called QOFs (quality outcome frameworks), offer financial incentives, associated with indicators that change annually. The QOFs include one to deliver an annual health check for people with intellectual disabilities aged above 16, introduced to try to standardize improvements in care delivery to this population. Confidential record-keeping is one important aspect of primary care, and to ensure integrated interagency care needs to be easily accessible. Most patient details are now recorded electronically and kept on electronic systems. Many areas now also have summary care records in place, which are stored electronically, at a central site and allow any health professional seeing the person, such as an out-of-hours GP, or an emergency department gain fast access to clinical information. Use of electronic systems allows easy access to anonymized data, which allow national data sets to be developed that record the numbers of people with specific health conditions, although this can be compromised when staff do not have adequate access to computer terminals.

Common chronic health conditions managed in primary care settings may include hypertension, diabetes, asthma, anxiety and depression, skin conditions, back pain, and arthritis. Home births, child development checks, vaccinations, and family planning may also be offered by primary care. When possible, care at the end of life will be managed at home, rather than in secondary care settings such as hospitals. Management of these conditions will require close working relationships and good communication between primary and secondary care.

Primary care and people with intellectual disabilities

The GP with whom a person is registered is responsible for the medical care of anyone living at home. People with intellectual disabilities should be able to access primary care in the same way as other members of the population. Local commissioning agreements may also be in place and audited to identify any reasonable adjustments that may be required to ensure that the person receives equal care to that of anyone else. All members of the extended primary care team should have access to this information; it should be documented in the summary care records and in any referral for secondary care services. Community nurses (learning disability) may occasionally work as members of primary care teams but are more likely to be based in community learning disability teams and work in close partnership with primary care staff. Often primary care staff lack confidence or experience in working with people with intellectual disabilities and may require support in this area. Community nurses in learning disabilities can improve access and understanding on their roles by developing close links and working in partnership with primary care staff. Delivering learning disability awareness training to the extended team, conducting joint home visits, and jointly assessing health needs in long-term conditions are examples of joint working in practice. Reasonable adjustments may include longer health appointments, access to easy-read information, and facilitating best interests decision-making meetings when informed consent is not given. Primary care staff may need help in both the identification and implementation of reasonable adjustments.

Further reading

Royal College of General Practitioners. *Learning Disabilities*. ℘ www.rcgp.org.uk/learningdisabilities (accessed 30 October 2017).

Secondary care

People with intellectual disabilities experience the same range of health problems as the general population, though their experience of ill health associated with both acute and chronic illness is greater than that of the general population.[1,2] Heslop et al. (2013) reports that both men and women with intellectual disabilities die much younger than the general population, with men dying 13 years younger and women dying 20 years younger.[3]

Access to secondary care

Given their increased acute and chronic healthcare needs, it is therefore understandable that people with intellectual disabilities attend and are admitted to secondary healthcare services more often that the general population, and their need for these services will continue to increase in the years to come. However, this group of people continue to experience inequity and barriers accessing all aspects of healthcare, including secondary care. Some of these barriers are associated with their difficulties with learning and communicating. Nevertheless, most of the barriers are associated with factors associated with healthcare professionals and the environment. Included in these is a lack of knowledge of healthcare professionals on the nature of intellectual disabilities and their health needs, negative or inappropriate attitudes and preconceptions about people with intellectual disabilities, diagnostic overshadowing (see ➔ Diagnostic overshadowing, pp. 110–1), inflexibility within appointment systems, too much use of written communication which is often not understood by people with intellectual disabilities and poor signage within departments, and poor transfer of information from intellectual disabilities services.[1,2]

Risks to safety

Although care for people with intellectual disabilities is improving, there is growing evidence that the barriers identified above can, in fact, increase risks to the safety of people with intellectual disabilities within secondary care. Equity of access to safe quality care is a right of us all; however, people continue to experience discrimination when in receipt of secondary healthcare. Examples of abuse and neglect and poor health outcomes, including premature avoidable deaths, have recently been reported.[3] Health is a right for all people, and there is emphasis on the need for general secondary health services to be accessible and non-discriminatory, with both treatment and polices being established within the context of the equality legislation across the UK and the Republic of Ireland.

Enhancing support in secondary care

Supporting people with intellectual disabilities within secondary care is the responsibility of all staff, and although it may seem challenging at times, some solid progress has been made. 1000 Lives Improvement and Abertawe Bro Morgannwg University Health Board[4] (ABMUHB) devised a 'care bundle' to support those working in general hospitals to be aware

of the needs of people with intellectual disabilities and to be able to respond to them and their families effectively, through:

- 'Early recognition of patients with learning disabilities;
- Effective communication with patients, carers, family members, and
  clinicians;
- Dignified, person-centred care and treatment;
- Effective review and discharge planning'.[4]

This 'care bundle' provides guidance for the several stages of the patient's
stay within hospital. However, all parts of the care bundle need to be
delivered for it to be effective.

View the associated Driver Diagram (access this document at
ℜ www.1000livesplus.wales.nhs.uk).

The National Public Health Service (NPHS) (2009) identified that safe
quality care for people with intellectual disabilities must ensure that 'reasonable adjustments' are in place. That requires health services to respect
the rights of people with intellectual disabilities, to provide a service that is
person-centred, to recognize individual needs, to anticipate these, and to be
flexible and responsive to these needs. This includes:

- The identification/removal of physical barriers to enhance access;
- Awareness by all staff of the distinct needs of this population;
- Ensuring frequent and timely communication occurs with people with
  intellectual disabilities and their families/carers in a format that is
  understood, to plan flexible appointments, admissions, and support
  while in hospital, and safe discharge;
- Ensure a request is made for any hospital passport;
- The use of straightforward signs to direct people where to go;
- The development of information in a format that is easily understood,
  with additions of pictures and signs which would enhance understanding
  and reduce anxieties;
- Respecting the right of the individual (adult) with intellectual disabilities
  to be involved in, and be adequately informed to support, their
  healthcare decisions;
- An appreciation of the role of the families/carers in supporting the care
  of the patient while in hospital, so that they are not expected to be the
  principal care givers;
- Introducing those concerned to the liaison nurse (if any);
- Having an awareness and record of support services that are available
  within or outside the hospital.

References

1 Parliamentary and Health Service Ombudsman (2009). *Six Lives: The Provision of Public Services
to People with Learning Difficulties 2008–2009*. The Stationary Office: London. ℜ www.gov.uk/
government/publications/six-lives-the-provision-of-public-services-to-people-with-learning-
difficulties-2008-to-2009 (accessed 31 October 2016).
2 Emerson E, Baines S (2012). *Health Inequalities and People with Learning Disabilities in the UK*.
Learning Disabilities Observatory/Department of Health: London.
3 Heslop P, Blair P, Fleming P, Hoghton M, Marriott A, Russ L (2013). *Confidential Inquiry into
Premature Deaths of People with Learning Disabilities (CIPOLD) Final Report*. Norah Fry Research
Centre: Bristol.
4 Browness B (2014). *Improving General Hospital Care of Patients who Have a Learning Disability*. NHS
Wales. ℜ www.1000livesplus.wales.nhs.uk (accessed 30 October 2017).

Tertiary care

Defining tertiary care

From a medical or nursing perspective, tertiary healthcare is specialized consultative care provided by professionals who have the appropriate resources, facilities, and expertise to provide specialist investigations or treatment usually for long-term or chronic conditions. Specialist cancer care, incontinence advisors, and epilepsy and dementia care specialists are common tertiary services required by people with intellectual disabilities. Referrals are usually made from primary or secondary care professionals.

Difficulties in accessing tertiary care

People with intellectual disabilities may have difficulties in accessing specialist care because:

- They may not be able to articulate their specific health needs;
- Their health needs may be overlooked and thus remain unrecognized;
- Interdisciplinary agency services do not talk to each other enough;
- There is a lack of clear information;
- There is little or no support for family carers;
- There is a lack of confidence, knowledge, and understanding of intellectual disabilities by general hospital staff;
- Hospital staff do not know about consent to treatment, the mental capacity legislation, and related consent policies.[5]

Although it is recognized that people with intellectual disabilities experience worse health than others, they also receive poorer healthcare.[6] Practical, administrative, communication, attitudinal, and knowledge barriers may make access to good healthcare difficult.[6,7] Nurses need to address these issues in a proactive way to facilitate appropriate healthcare at all levels.

Facilitating tertiary healthcare

To support nurses in accessing appropriate tertiary healthcare for people with intellectual disabilities, and to help support the person themselves in preparation for hospital appointments, tests, and investigations, roles, such as the HF and acute liaison nurses, have been developed in some places. The HF role includes working alongside other professionals in primary, secondary, and tertiary care teams to ensure that individuals with intellectual disabilities gain full access to the healthcare they require when they require it. Their role is to facilitate, advocate for, and support individuals (and their carers) to efficiently navigate their way around healthcare services.

Many people with intellectual disabilities have a variety of tertiary health needs which, if remain untreated, may at best be uncomfortable and at worse become life-changing or indeed life-threatening. Since some individuals may not be aware of their own health needs or are not able to articulate personal concerns, nurses need to remain vigilant in spotting any changes in the person that may indicate changes in potential health status. Nurses who care for people with intellectual disabilities may be among those best placed to encourage healthier lifestyles, and key issues for the nurse around accessing tertiary care include working proactively to ensure the following.

Adequate preparation prior to hospital appointments

Some individuals with intellectual disabilities will not be familiar with (and/ or may be fearful of) healthcare facilities, e.g. outpatient departments or clinics. Familiar carers can plan for the visit—perhaps take photographs of any diagnostic instruments or equipment that is likely to be used, to explain to the patient beforehand and arrange a visit to the clinic prior to the appointment to promote familiarity. Contact the clinic to arrange extra appointment time for the person in case the person needs more time to be guided through the anticipated procedure, and provide time to have complex terms translated and explained in a language that they are more likely to understand.

Accurate assessment

Communication can be the biggest barrier to accurate and appropriate assessment, and some health professionals may not be familiar with how to communicate effectively with people with intellectual disabilities. A familiar carer can support the individual by alleviating fears and anxieties during diagnostic consultations, by enhancing reciprocal communication and by supplementing information with personal knowledge where appropriate. Assessments are crucial to establishing specific health needs and subsequently identifying appropriate treatment options.

Developing links with health professionals

Collaborative working is key to effective support and includes establishing and maintaining up-to-date links with local health professionals, being aware of local and regional resources, and knowing when, where, and how to refer for specialist care and intervention.

Health action plans

HAPs can also help to identify and monitor health needs from a holistic perspective, incorporating details of health needs and interventions, oral care, dental care, fitness and mobility, continence, vision, hearing, nutrition, and emotional needs, in addition to details of current medications, side effects, and screening tests records. Such a plan seeks to ensure that health needs are not overlooked and can be monitored.

References

5 Michael J (2008). *Healthcare for All: Report of the Independent Inquiry into Access to Healthcare for People with Learning Disabilities*. Department of Health: London.

6 Emerson E, Baines S (2010). *Health Inequalities and People with Learning Disabilities in the UK: 2010*. Improving Health and Lives, Learning Disabilities Observatory: London.

7 Heslop P, Blair P, Fleming P, Hoghton M, Marriott A, Russ L (2013). *Confidential Inquiry into Premature Deaths of People with Learning Disabilities (CIPOLD) Final Report*. Norah Fry Research Centre: Bristol. ℐ www.bris.ac.uk/cipold/fullfinalreport.pdf (accessed 30 October 2017).

General practitioners

General practitioners, or GPs as they are generally known, are considered to be gatekeepers to health services. Across the UK, all British citizens are entitled to the services of a GP. People can register as patients with any local NHS surgery, providing they live in the practice catchment area and the practice has vacancies. It is through registering with a GP that people can access the full range of NHS services.

Education and employment status

GPs are qualified medical doctors, having completed at least 4yrs postgraduate experience and postgraduate training in general medicine. Some GPs specialize in particular aspects of medicine, within surgery settings. Most GPs work as independent contractors to the NHS, being responsible for providing adequate buildings and teams of staff to deliver a wide range of healthcare. They may do this individually or, increasingly, as shared partners in bigger practices. These teams may also include salaried GPs, working on a sessional or temporary basis.

Role in practice

In England, from 2013, GP commissioning became the responsibility of NHS England. Additionally, GPs started having responsibility for commissioning of other local health services, through sitting as members of CCGs. From 2015, however, co-commissioning was introduced, which gave CCGs more responsibility in also commissioning local GP services. There is a mixed picture on how co-commissioning is delivered across the country. GPs work to local health boards in Wales, regional health boards in Scotland, and local commissioning groups in Northern Ireland which are responsible for the commissioning, planning, and delivery of high-quality primary healthcare services to the local population. In order to treat NHS patients, GPs must have their name and details registered on a primary medical performers list. Every commissioning organization must ensure quality and governance checking that GPs have the right qualifications, skills, and experience to work in the NHS and that any services delivered are safe and of high quality.

On average, a GP has about 1800 patients registered with their practice; however, this number is extremely variable, depending on a number of factors. These include the size of the practice, the number of full-time GPs, and local area characteristics. GP practice numbers and demands associated with changing demographics are constantly increasing. In a practice of 1800, about 36 can be expected to have intellectual disabilities. Most patient consultations take place at the surgery and, less frequently, during home visits. Telephone triage is also increasingly available which enables initial consultations by telephone. GP practices can choose whether to provide 24-hour care or transfer it to an out-of-hours service. Out-of-hours care is often variable across the country and may be delivered at home or in local hospital settings. Other support services, including NHS walk-in centres or the NHS 111 service, will help signpost patients to GP services, when required.

GPs and other practice staff record their patient consultations on electronic clinical systems, using read codes. At present, electronic recording systems vary from practice to practice across the countries. Current negotiations are exploring the possibility of standardizing these. In England, since 2015, a summary electronic care record may be in place to enable key patient information to be shared with other medical staff or out-of-hours health services, as and when required.

GPs are paid under a UK-wide GP contract. Within this contract is a QOF. The aim of the QOF is to provide additional financial rewards, based on a points system, for offering GPs better management of chronic disease. The QOF is voluntary, although most practices choose to take part. The QOF is subject to an annual review. Since 2006/2007, QOF points have been in place for the development of a practice register of people with intellectual disabilities. Further standards were set within the specifications for annual health checks direct-enhanced services in 2007.

GPs and people with intellectual disabilities

GPs are responsible for the day-to-day medical care of people with intellectual disabilities who live in the community. GPs can experience a number of challenges in seeking to deliver an effective service for people with intellectual disabilities including:

- A lack of basic and postgraduate training in the skills of working with people with intellectual disabilities, resulting in reduced confidence;
- Limited skills in communicating directly with people with intellectual disabilities;
- Limited knowledge on the specific health needs of people with intellectual disabilities;
- Constraints associated with limited time for appointments;
- Difficulties in physical examination;
- Diagnostic overshadowing (reports of physical illness being viewed as part of the intellectual disabilities, and not investigated or treated).

A number of solutions have been proposed to address these barriers:

- Compulsory training for GPs in intellectual disabilities issues at undergraduate level, and availability of postgraduate refresher courses. This should be delivered by community intellectual disabilities staff, in collaboration with self-advocacy organizations;
- A coordinated approach to sharing information and closer working relationships between community intellectual disabilities teams and primary care services;
- Having a named GP within each practice to take the lead on the health issues of people with intellectual disabilities.

Further reading

Royal College of General Practitioners (curriculum statement 14). *Care of People with Learning Disabilities*. ℘ www.gmc-uk.org/14_Learning_disabilities_01.pdf_30450949.pdf (accessed 14 March 2018).

Royal College of General Practitioners. *Health Checks for People with Learning Disabilities Toolkit*. ℘ www.rcgp.org.uk/clinical-and-research/toolkits/health-check-toolkit.aspx (accessed 30 October 2017).

Health visitors

A health visitor (HV) is a qualified nurse or midwife, with post-registration experience and a further qualification in child health, public health, health promotion, and education [specialist community public health nurse (SCPHN)]. They are found and work across the UK; however, they have different priorities and models of working, based on the local evidence and actions identified within each country. HVs are considered to be SCPHNs, striving to meet specific outcomes identified and measured by country-specific health outcomes frameworks.

Working as members of multi-skill mix teams, and in close partnership with others, including GPs, school nurses, and midwives, HVs provide expert information assessments and interventions to babies, children, and families, including those with complex needs. They help to empower parents by providing expert information to help them make informed decisions on issues that affect their whole family health and well-being. Their role is central in achieving and improving the health outcomes of all children and offering additional support to populations experiencing the greatest health inequalities.

Health visiting role

HVs can be found working from different bases, including GP practices, children's centres, and community teams, supporting children, parents, and families within their own homes and communities. They provide expert advice, support, and interventions to all families with children in the first years of life. This is known as a universal service—through five key visits, a Healthy Child Programme delivers core elements, including health and development reviews, screening, immunizations, parenting support, and effective promotion of parenting health and behaviour change. Because it is a service accepted and valued by parents, it is known to promote positive parenting, emotional attachment, and bonding and to highlight potential safeguarding concerns at an early stage. If families are considered to be vulnerable and there is a risk of poorer outcomes, then increased support need can be provided. This is known as Universal plus and Universal partnership plus. In some areas, a family nurse partnership service may also be available. This is an intensive home visiting programme aimed at supporting families in which the mother is aged 19yrs or younger. Additional specialist health visiting roles may include working with older people or with children with special needs.

Since 2015, within England, the commissioning of all services for children aged 0–5yrs, including health visiting, has been transferred from NHS England to local authorities. This transfer facilitates a more coordinated, joined-up approach to working with young children between all local authority services, including public health, early years services, education, and housing.

Areas in which HVs may support families with young children

- Child growth, social and emotional development;
- Recognition and management of common infections;
- Managing teething, sleeping, eating, toilet training, anger, or other behaviour that parents find challenging;
- Breastfeeding, weaning, healthy eating;
- Safeguarding children, including looked-after children;
- Home safety;
- Postnatal depression;
- Child or family bereavement;
- Domestic violence.

HVs support families with young children by:
- Home visiting;
- Coordinating local child immunization programmes;
- Organizing and running baby clinics;
- Deliver, in some areas, portage (child development) programmes in partnership with families;
- Running health promotion groups, e.g. breastfeeding, parent support, parenting courses, home safety courses;
- Non-medical prescribing.

Health visiting and people with intellectual disabilities

HVs work with and support all families with children, including those with intellectual disabilities, based on their assessed individual needs. The HV is often the professional that detects an early delay in child development, referring the child on for specialist assessment and support. In these situations, child and family support is usually offered by the HV, in partnership with interdisciplinary children's disability teams, and they often work closely with school nurses, social workers, and community paediatricians. This support may continue after the child reaches school age but has usually finished by the time the child is 14yrs, the age when planning for child transition to adult services usually starts. For many families, the child will become the responsibility of the school nursing services by their fifth birthday.

People with intellectual disabilities are increasingly becoming parents themselves. The need for HVs to develop expertise in working with parents with intellectual disabilities has been highlighted.[8] The need for HV training in this area has been requested, along with the need to develop policies across community care services to define the parenting support role to this population.

Further reading

Scottish Consortium for Learning Disability (2015). *Supported Parenting: Scottish Good Practice Guidelines for Supporting Parents with a Learning Disability*. The Scottish Government: Edinburgh. ℅ www.scld.org.uk/publications/scottish-good-practice-guidelines-for-supporting-parents-with-learning-disabilities/ (accessed 30 October 2017).

Sines D, Aldridge-Bent S, Fanning A, Farrelly P, Potter K, Wright J (2013). *Community and Public Health Nursing*, 5th edn. Wiley-Blackwell Science: London.

References

8 Baum S, Gray G, Stevens S (2011). *Good Practice Guidance for Clinical Psychologists when Assessing Parents with Learning Disabilities*. The British Psychological Society: Leicester.

District nurses

District nurses, also known as community nurses, are a UK-wide resource. Working predominantly with people outside of hospital settings, they are central to keeping people with acute, chronic, and palliative care conditions at home, in residential care homes, and in other community settings. District nurses usually work within geographical boundaries, are often based in GP practices or health centres, and have a key role in integrated delivery of care, working in partnership with a range of different people and services. These may include family carers, primary and acute services, social care, hospices, and nursing and residential care providers. Some have specialist areas of expertise.

Education

District nurses are qualified nurses (registered nurse/registered general nurse), usually with graduate-level education and specialist qualification recordable with the NMC. In addition, they may have attended many other condition-specific courses, equipping them with the skills to manage a wide variety of different nursing needs. Specific additional training courses may include care assessment and coordination, nurse prescribing, chronic disease management [e.g. chronic obstructive airways disease (COAD), asthma, diabetes, stroke care], palliative care, and Doppler training (assessment and training of leg ulcer care).

> **What are the key principles of district nursing?**
> * Delivering high-quality care to people out of hospital, measuring practice outcomes.
> * Maximizing health and well-being, promoting independence.
> * Health protection and improvement, operating a public health, preventative, and healthy lifestyle approach.
> * Delivering a coordinated approach to hospital discharge and subsequent care in the community.
> * Prevention of hospital admission and readmission rates by support at an early stage of ill health.
> * Embracing new technology to enhance care.
> * Operating an evidence-based approach to clinical practice.
> * Promoting user involvement in service planning and evaluation.

Delivering services

District nurses visit people within their own homes, including residential care homes, or, along with treatment nurses and practice nurses, deliver services in health centres. In their nursing role, they provide direct care to patients, as well as supporting family members or paid staff in their caring roles.

Most district nurses work as members of a district nursing team. These comprise a number of qualified nurses/nursing assistants that work over a range of different hours, covering a 24-hr period. Many localities also have district nurses working within more acute services such as intermediate care teams and 'hospital from home'-type services that seek to prevent hospital admission or support earlier discharge.

District nursing teams are also often members of wider integrated care teams. These teams work across professional boundaries, preventing duplication of roles and promoting the need for good communication and partnership working. Membership of integrated teams is wide and may include:
- GPs;
- HVs;
- Practice nurses;
- Care home staff;
- Allied health professionals (e.g. physiotherapists, occupational therapists, podiatrists);
- Social workers;
- Community nurses in mental health;
- Community nurses in intellectual disabilities.

District nurses and people with intellectual disabilities

District nurses will meet people with intellectual disabilities in their working roles, but they may not have training in the specific health needs of the population or have knowledge of local intellectual disabilities service provision. This is an area of work in which nurses in intellectual disabilities teams should use their knowledge and skills to both offer awareness training and work collaboratively with district nurses to meet the healthcare needs of people with intellectual disabilities. Local agreements may be in place to define different roles and responsibilities.

District nurses may develop and support healthcare for people with intellectual disabilities in the following ways:
- Identify patients with intellectual disabilities on home visits to other family members. Check and ensure they are included on practice registers and are included in disease management or annual health checks.
- Offer and deliver health screening/health checks for patients with intellectual disabilities who will not attend GP visits.
- Identify unmet needs of patients with intellectual disabilities and refer to specialist services for intervention.
- Identify older family carers. Refer on to social services for carer's assessment or to access carer's support.
- Assist people with intellectual disabilities to understand and take control of their healthcare, by teaching them about their physical condition or disease management using accessible information.

Further reading

Sines D, Aldridge-Bent S, Fanning A, Farrelly P, Potter K, Wright J (2013). *Community and Public Health Nursing*, 5th edn. Wiley-Blackwell Science: London.

Community children's nurses

Community children's nurses (CCNs), also known as community paediatric nurses, work with babies, children, and young people up to the age of 18yrs. They work with children that have a wide range of complex health conditions and who are living at home. Their main role is to enable sick children with acute and chronic illnesses or disabilities to be cared for, in partnership with their parents, in their home or living environment. The aim, where possible, is to avoid admission to hospital. The delivery of nursing care to children at home, or in nurseries and schools, often enables children to remain within their families, to continue to attend normal daytime activities and reduce the disruption to routine of everyday family life. CCNs are employed and funded by a range of different organizations, including children's integrated trusts, charitable trusts, and primary and acute NHS trusts. CCNs often specialize in a particular aspect of nursing care. This may include chronic conditions, including asthma, cystic fibrosis, diabetes, or cancer or children with disabilities living with a life-limiting illness.

The Department of Health suggests a CCN service should provide care for the following groups:
- 'Children with acute and short-term conditions;
- Children with long-term conditions;
- Children with disabilities and complex conditions, including those requiring continuing care and neonates;
- Children with life-limiting and life-threatening illness, including those requiring palliative and end-of-life care'.[9]

There is considerable geographical variation in the role and services provided by CCNs. These may be influenced by factors, including:
- The extent and quality of evidence in the JSNA that clearly defines the medical, social, and cultural needs of children and families in the local area;
- Local commissioning priorities and levels of available funding;
- Numbers of qualified, skilled children's nurses available and the quality of local nursing leadership;
- Local commitment and access to high-quality postgraduate nurse training to develop additional knowledge, skills, competence, capability, and confidence to undertake new roles;
- Range of local resources, including children's hospital care, children's and young adult hospice provision, charitable services, and other community teams;
- Quality of local partnerships with children, families, and stakeholders in planning integrated services, monitoring design, and delivery.

Education

CCNs are generally qualified at degree level having the RN (children's) or former qualifications such as RSCN (registered sick children's nurse) qualification, with an additional community nursing qualification. All nurses must be registered to practise with the NMC. Children's nurses may also have qualifications in other branches of nursing, health visiting, or midwifery, as well as clinical skills or specific condition management training.

Role in practice

Qualified CCNs often work in skills mix teams, working from either hospitals or community office bases. Teams may include CCN assistants or home support workers who require support and supervision by CCNs. Effective collaborative working within a wider team is essential in order to provide integrated services and coordinated support and advice to children and their families.

Teams may include
- GPs, paediatricians, consultants, and other doctors;
- HVs, school nurses, community nurses (intellectual disabilities), and community nurses (mental health);
- Dieticians, physiotherapists, and occupational therapists;
- Social workers and home care staff;
- Specialist hospital and hospices, including any outreach workers;
- Specialist wheelchair, seating, or orthotics technicians.

In addition, they work in close partnership with parents and siblings in the provision of education, information, and support.

CCNs and children with intellectual disabilities

CCNs are often directly involved in the care of children with intellectual disabilities, who may also have complex physical healthcare needs. To deliver a coordinated approach to treatment and prevent duplication, CCNs often work in close partnership with nurses in services for people with intellectual disabilities, school nurses, and other paid carers. A strong focus of their joint role is on promoting and supporting independence and, where possible, providing accessible information to inform health decision-making. They may visit the child in their home, school, or respite care environment. All work is done in partnership with parents and families.

Further reading

Carter B, Coad J, Goodenough T, Anderson C, Bray L (2009). *Community Children's Nursing in England: An Appreciative Review of CCNs.* Department of Health: London (in collaboration with the University of Lancashire and the University of the West of England).

Royal College of Nursing (2014). *The Future for Children's Community Nursing: Challenges and Opportunities.* Royal College of Nursing: London.

References

9 Department of Health (2011). *NHS at Home: Community Children's Nursing Service.* Department of Health: London.

School nurses

The health of children in schools is a high government priority in all countries of the UK, with the focus of all school healthcare being to improve the health of all school-aged children (5–19yrs). School nurses are the single biggest workforce specially trained and skilled to deliver public health interventions to schools and to support school-aged children. Within England, since 2013, school nurses have been commissioned by directors of public health and are funded by the local authorities public health grant.

The key public health issues for school-aged children

• Exercise;
• Obesity;
• Healthy eating;
• Emotional health and mental well-being;
• Sexual health;
• Smoking;
• Drugs and alcohol;
• Vaccination and immunization;
• Home and community safety;
• Safeguarding;
• Defined support for children with additional and complex needs.

Education

School nurses are registered nurses, most of whom are qualified at degree level, who hold an additional specialist public health qualification, which is registered with the NMC.

School nursing role

Since the development of the school nursing service in 1908, the role has changed considerably. Periodic medical inspections have mostly been replaced by a public health and well-being focus to the role, with less emphasis on routine medical examination, although medical support is often still provided for children with complex health needs and for children at risk. All schools have a named school nurse and a medical officer linked with every school or a group of schools.

A number of different approaches exist to address school healthcare. Central to these is the role of the school nurse and the wider school healthcare team. This team may include community medical officers and community dental services. The school nurse's role is gradually changing from that of individual child screening and child health monitoring to that of a school public health practitioner. The focus of the role, however, can vary considerably to meet the above priorities across different countries. School nurses may also have a clinical role to meet the different and enhanced needs of children with physical impairments, long-term conditions, and emotional and mental ill health.

What are the key roles of a school nurse?

- Leading on the delivery of the Healthy Child Programme for children aged 5–19.
- Having a named nurse role for each school providing an integrated and joined-up link to all other key services, including GPs, social services, and hospitals.
- Delivering health promotion advice, screening and surveillance, and health education.
- Supporting in the management of long-term conditions.
- Delivering public health interventions to keep children safe and mentally resilient.
- Visiting and supporting parents and families.
- Working with schools to identify population health needs.
- Referring children, following local care pathways.
- Measuring and publishing service outcomes.
- Highlighting and addressing health inequalities and the health needs of vulnerable and priority groups.
- Safeguarding children.

In addition to school nursing, there are a number of whole-school approaches to health that also fall under the remit of local authorities. These include the national healthy schools programmes in England, and the healthy schools programme in Wales and Northern Ireland.

The key aims of healthy schools programmes

- To support children in developing health-promoting behaviours.
- To help raise pupil achievement.
- To help reduce health inequalities.
- To help promote social inclusion.

School healthcare and children and young people with intellectual disabilities

School nurses and community nurses for people with intellectual disabilities should work in partnership when planning the children's transition to adult services. There will need to be proactive planning, with clear communication between children and adult services. Planning for adult services, which are significantly different to children's services, may commence any time after the age of 14yrs, depending on local area commissioning protocols. GPs may now add children with intellectual disabilities to their practice register at age 14, and the young person may be eligible for an annual health check. A good HAP developed with the young person may help the person understand and take greater control of their health needs and help direct adult services to meet their identified needs.

Further reading

Public Health England (2014). *Maximising the School Nursing Team Contribution to the Public Health of School-aged Children.* Department of Health: London.

Midwives

Midwives' role is providing care to women who are pregnant and their baby during pregnancy and for up to 28 days after the baby is born. Midwives work in hospital and the community, meeting the individual needs of women, their partners, and babies.

Education

Qualified midwives are educated to degree level, when they are then eligible to register as a midwife with the NMC. Within their training, midwives have to work with, and support, women throughout the process of pregnancy, working in a number of different hospitals and community placements. Training includes caring for newly pregnant women, monitoring the woman and her baby throughout pregnancy, preparing them for child-birth, delivering babies, and caring for mothers and their babies in the new-born stage known as the postnatal period. Both men and women practise as registered midwives. Some older midwives may have initially trained as a registered nurse before retraining as a midwife

The rising birth rate within the UK is compromised by a shortage of midwives. In spite of there being an increasing number of spaces for training available, it is a very popular profession, and training places are often oversubscribed. There are a number of incentives to try to encourage non-practising midwives to return to the role.

Role in practice

Midwives are, in general, employed by NHS Trusts; however, small numbers of midwives practise independently. NHS midwives offer free maternity care. Independent midwives usually charge for their services. Midwives work across hospital and community settings.

Midwifery services are accessed by registration with a GP. Midwives are generally hospital- or GP-attached; therefore, as with other GP-attached staff, they cover a geographical locality. Midwives frequently work across a number of different GP practices; therefore, they may work from a central health base, a children's centre, or a hospital. There is no national uniformity of base. Midwives are, however, expected to work across professional boundaries and in partnership with other staff working with the woman. Other staff may include social workers, physiotherapists, HVs, GPs, children's centre staff, or specialist nurses, including community nurses (intellectual disabilities). A teamworking approach is provided to ensure women, their partners, and babies, receive care based on individual needs.

Where possible, midwives offer a named midwifery service to help promote consistency of care. Midwives meet with women, and their partners, at regular intervals throughout pregnancy. Women carry and look after their own maternity records, to aid accurate communication, for all working with the woman.

Midwives visit women and babies within a range of environments. All new mothers and babies are visited by midwives in their own homes, on the day after discharge from hospital, or after birth. Regular home visits will continue by the midwife, where necessary, for up to 28 days after birth, or until discharged by the midwife to the care of a HV.

Midwives and people with intellectual disabilities

Midwives may need to address issues relating to intellectual disabilities, in a number of significant areas.

What issues may midwives encounter relating to intellectual disabilities?

- Discussion and support regarding prenatal antenatal screening or testing scanning that might identify a baby with a condition associated with intellectual disabilities.
- Breaking the news and helping parents interpret and come to terms with the result that their newborn baby has a condition associated with intellectual disabilities.
- Supporting a woman with intellectual disabilities, and her partner, throughout the pregnancy, labour, and early postnatal period.

The manner and skill in which news regarding intellectual disabilities is shared with parents is crucial. In addressing the above issues, midwives require a good understanding of a number of issues. These include the ethics of scanning, knowledge on the range of scanning methods available, and the efficacy of the results. In addition, they need to know where to access current knowledge on a range of conditions associated with intellectual disabilities and contact details of parental support services for particular conditions. Effective counselling skills are also required.

Government strategies promote the requirement that all parents should access locally primary and acute service provision. Parents with intellectual disabilities may require the same, different, or increased service provision, to get their needs met. A number of issues have been identified to help midwives meet the needs of parents with intellectual disabilities.[10] These include:

- To have local policies, protocols, and guidelines in place for working with parents with intellectual disabilities;
- To identify the intellectual disabilities at an early stage;
- To refer to, and work in partnership with, staff in the local community learning disability team (CLDT);
- To complete an early and thorough assessment;
- To ensure all information is clear and is in an accessible format;
- To use models, videos, and pictures when available;
- To make reasonable adjustments, including longer appointments;
- To offer consistency of midwife and other support personnel.

Further reading

Harrison R, Willis S (2015). Antenatal support for parents with a learning disability. *British Journal of Midwifery.* 23: 344–8.

Royal College of Nursing (2008). *Pregnancy and Disability. A Guide for Nurses and Midwives.* Royal College of Nursing: London.

Scottish Consortium for Learning Disability (2015). *Supported Parenting: Scottish Good Practice Guidelines for Supporting Parents with a Learning Disability.* The Scottish Government: Edinburgh. ℛ www.scld.org.uk/publications/scottish-good-practice-guidelines-for-supporting-parents-with-learning-disabilities/ (accessed 30 October 2017).

References

10 Wilson S, McKenzie K, Quayle E, Murray G (2013). The postnatal support needs of mothers with an intellectual disability. *Midwifery.* 29: 592–8.

Parenting groups

Irrespective of an individual's level of cognitive ability, becoming and being a parent can, without doubt, be a struggle. When a parent has intellectual disabilities, they often require more support, accessible information, and communication about what is available to them in terms of supporting their child, particularly in the early years. With the right support. They are as capable of being great parents, as their peers in the general population. However, while attitudes have become more positive, there still exists negative societal assumptions which question their right to be a parent. That being said, people with intellectual disabilities are more likely to be parenting with limited support from family and friends, but with extensive involvement from statutory services. Without consistent and sustained support, particularly over the early days and years, it is less likely that their child will be able to remain with a parent who has intellectual disabilities. Therefore, in terms of support, healthcare professionals, in particular, need to learn how to support, advocate, lobby, and work with and for parents with intellectual disabilities. Equally, organizations and support groups which support parents with intellectual disabilities can be immensely beneficial. Research shows that families need support from the time the baby is born for a number of years, with extra support again at specific times, e.g. during toddler years, going to school, puberty, and adolescence. Parenting groups are one such way of support for parents with intellectual disabilities.

What can help parents with intellectual disabilities?
- Parenting groups (where available);
- Easy-read information;
- Support from peers;
- Information on rights and entitlements;
- Advocacy training for parents with intellectual disabilities and their support networks (family, friends, healthcare professionals);
- Professional advocates;
- Initiatives such as Sure Start and Best Beginnings (Baby Buddy app).

Parenting groups

Parenting groups across the UK and Ireland are varied, and it is difficult to find parent groups which specifically support parents with intellectual disabilities. Some groups, however, have been set up to support new mums and dads with all aspects of parenting. Sometimes these can be led by HVs or by working in partnership with intellectual disabilities services. Nurses in services for people with intellectual disabilities could be best placed to develop this supportive role and expertise. As facilitator of the groups, the framework of support would include discussion groups with a focus on education, advocacy, support, and keeping the family intact.

What will the groups talk about?
- What is it like to be a parent?
- How to keep your child healthy?
- What to do if your child becomes ill?
- How to keep your child safe?

- Helping your child develop.
- Managing difficult behaviours.
- Other issues initiated from concerns raised by parents.

The groups will also provide the opportunity for parents to talk and learn from each other and make friendships. These groups can provide ongoing support to people to review skills learnt and to support the maintenance of skills in the longer term.

Evidence from research shows that parenting is more successful using a combination of methods—group work alongside individual work within people's homes, showing people how to perform tasks with time to practise new skills in a supportive environment.[11]

The groups can support parents to learn together from each other, as well as from the HV or registered nurse in services for people with intellectual disabilities. It is vital that the facilitators of the parenting group are skilled and experienced in supporting people with intellectual disabilities, and are able to adapt to the person with intellectual disabilities within the group. It is important that the facilitators of the group are able to develop a trusting relationship, whereby parents feel safe to ask questions and seek support when they need it, without fear of reprisals, e.g. their children being taken into care.

Further reading

Best Beginnings. ℘ www.bestbeginnings.org.uk/parents-with-learning-disabilities (accessed 30 October 2017).

Inclusion Ireland. *Supporting Parents with Learning Disabilities: Good Practice Guidance*. ℘ www. inclusionireland.ie/sites/default/files/attach/basic-page/818/supportingparentsguidelineseasyt oread.pdf (accessed 30 October 2017).

Leaviss J, Ewins W, Kitson D, Watling E (2010). *Inclusive Support for Parents with a Learning Disability*. Mencap: London.

Scottish Consortium for Learning Disability (2015). *Supported Parenting: Scottish Good Practice Guidelines for Supporting Parents with a Learning Disability*. The Scottish Government: Edinburgh. ℘ www.scld.org.uk/publications/scottish-good-practice-guidelines-for-supporting-parents-with-learning-disabilities/ (accessed 30 October 2017).

References

11 Tarleton B, Ward L (2007). Parenting with support: the views and experiences of parents with intellectual disabilities. *Journal of Policy and Practice in Intellectual Disabilities*. 4: 194–202.

Dentists

Good oral and dental health is an important aspect of general health. The knowledge that your teeth look good and are straight and functional, and that one is able to smile, chew, and talk, without pain, all contribute greatly to feelings of well-being. Dentists are health professionals specializing in the care, diagnosis, and treatment of a range of problems that affect the mouth and teeth. Good oral health can contribute to good general health, confidence, dignity, self-esteem, social integration, and increased quality of life.

Education

The preparation of dentists is spread over 5yrs and results in BDS or BChD. The training process consists of academic, theoretical, and practical training in all aspects of dental care. A wide range of postgraduate courses in specialist areas are also available. Dentists have to register with their professional body (in the UK, this is the General Dental Council) before commencing practice.

Role of the dentist

A substantial focus of the dentist's role is on oral health promotion of the general public, in addition to dental treatment and surgery. A significant element of their role is preventing and treating dental and oral disease, correcting dental irregularities, and treating dental and facial injuries. People with intellectual disabilities are most likely to see dentists in NHS services, including family practices, community dental services, and hospital departments.

Oral health and people with intellectual disabilities

People with intellectual disabilities experience higher rates of dental disease than does the general population.[12] Good oral care is generally based on an individual's physical, mental, and cognitive ability to carry out effective oral hygiene, make informed choices about healthy eating, and seek and comply with dental treatment. They are seriously disadvantaged in some, or all, of these areas, with multiple barriers in their access to oral care.

Potential barriers in access to good oral care for people with intellectual disabilities

- A lack of perceived need for good oral care or an inability to express the need for treatment;
- A lack of awareness or ability in self-care with a poorly developed cleaning technique;
- An increased range of oral and facial development abnormalities;
- Increased drooling, tooth grinding, and dry mouth; dry mouth is sometimes linked to the side effects of medication;
- An increased need for high-energy food supplements and sugar-based liquid medication, leading to oral erosion;
- Reduced access to oral health education and dietary advice;
- Established fear and anxiety of health services, including dentists;
- Reduced physical access to dental clinics;
- Reduced choice in the range of dental services;
- Lack of dental staff training in intellectual disabilities.

Recommendations for improving oral care for people with intellectual disabilities

A number of recommendations have been made in response to meeting the oral health needs of people with intellectual disabilities.[12] These include the need for reasonable adjustments to be made and for dentists and other dental team members, specialist health professionals, carers, and people with intellectual disabilities to share the responsibility for improving oral healthcare.

- Dentists need to identify and assess the needs of their patients. Patients at high risk, or with active dental disease, should be seen at 3-monthly intervals. Persons with low risk should be seen every 6 months.
- Education and behavioural interventions that ensure appropriate diet and daily routines of good oral hygiene should be promoted and taught to people, including carers, when necessary. Meeting oral healthcare needs should be addressed at home, in school, and with adults in health checks and in HAPs.
- Preventative therapies, including use of fluoride toothpaste or antimicrobial agents, should be implemented, when indicated.
- NHS organizations, including dental commissioners, working with interdisciplinary intellectual disabilities staff teams, should facilitate training for all dental staff on working with people with intellectual disabilities, and placements for dental students within these community settings should be developed.
- General oral advice sheets, covering a healthy diet, oral hygiene, and visiting the dentist, should be given in an accessible format.
- When non-attendance at dental appointments is due to anxiety, referrals for support in desensitization should be made to the local intellectual disabilities service.

Good oral healthcare needs to be made everyone's business. Working with the local dental officer for public health, a local strategy should be developed, agreed across organizations, and included and monitored through commissioned providers on how good oral healthcare will be promoted actively and disseminated to all high-risk groups.

Further reading

Department of Health (2007). *Valuing People's Oral Health: A Good Practice Guide for Improving the Oral Health of Disabled Children and Adults.* Department of Health: London.

Oral Health Foundation. *Dental Care for People with Special Needs.* ℘ www.dentalhealth.org/tell-me-about/topic/caring-for-teeth/dental-care-for-people-with-special-needs (accessed 30 October 2017).

References

12 Royal College of Surgeons (2012). *Clinical Guidelines and Integrated Care Pathways for the Oral Health Care of People with Learning Disabilities.* Royal College of Surgeons: London.

Podiatrists

Registered podiatrists are also known in some services as chiropodists. Podiatrists are trained in the assessment, diagnosis, and treatment of the feet and lower limbs. They offer advice on the prevention of foot problems and the management of sports injuries. They perform nail surgery and teach people how to care for feet. Podiatrists work from a number of different resource bases, including local health centres, general hospitals, health clubs, shops, and private hospitals. They also visit patients in a range of different environments, including day centres, special schools, and residential, nursing, and family homes, and they sometimes work on their own, as members of interdisciplinary health teams, or as members of skill-mixed foot care teams. Other team members include podiatry assistants and orthotic technicians. Podiatry chiropody services delivered through the NHS are free of charge and are targeted at people with the perceived greatest risk of foot health problems. The general population, without high-risk health conditions, may access podiatry through private foot care services.

Education

Podiatry is concerned with the assessment and treatment of a person's foot, lower limb, and musculoskeletal function. Podiatrists are educated at university and are qualified at degree level. To practise as a podiatrist, they must be registered with the Health and Care Professions Council (HCPC).

Key health priorities in foot care for podiatry services

- Treatment for older people with deteriorating health;
- People with diabetes;
- People with osteoarthritis;
- People with rheumatoid arthritis;
- Post-surgical care;
- Neurological conditions;
- Immune deficiency;
- Terminal illness;
- Septic lesions and cellulitis;
- Vascular conditions/heart disease;
- Severe foot deformities;
- Ingrowing toenails;
- People with severe physical or intellectual disabilities.

Podiatry and people with intellectual disabilities

Little research has been completed on foot health and people with intellectual disabilities. People with intellectual disabilities are known, however, to experience increased foot risks affecting their health and mobility that may require particular care of their feet.[13] The number of people with intellectual disabilities with these conditions that receive chiropody support will be variable across the country. The fear of having a person work on one's feet and not fully understanding the rationale, particularly if discomfort is involved (even to reduce longer-term pain), may be an additional challenge in providing foot care and may need to be actively addressed within HAPs. Some areas across the UK do provide a specialist podiatry service to meet these enhanced needs.

There are a number of factors that may warrant additional monitoring and care in relation to foot care, including:

• Limited ability in foot self-care, including the cutting of toenails;
• Limited ability of older family carers in providing foot care;
• Difficulties in self-disclosing or communicating foot pain, other foot abnormalities, or infection;
• Increased risk and missed diagnosis of long-term health conditions, associated with a need for foot care;
• Fear and anxiety related to medical appointments;
• Non-attendance at medical appointments due to barriers to access;
• Challenging behaviour or limited ability to comply with foot care or medical appointments;
• The wearing of poorly fitting shoes;
• Changes in mobility may relate to foot problems, rather than injury.

Nurses working with people with intellectual disabilities have a part to play in monitoring foot care. As a number of people have difficulties in self-reporting of foot problems, early signs may be seen to indicate a need for support. Regular preventative foot care should be promoted, where available, with a podiatrist. Local protocols on the cutting of toenails, including the care of people with diabetes, should be developed and implemented at a local level.

Further reading

Your Health Matters. Leeds *Learning Disability Podiatry*. ℘ www.easyonthei.nhs.uk/learning-disability-podiatry-service (accessed 30 October 2017).

References

13 Courtenay K, Murray A (2015). Foot health and mobility in people with intellectual disabilities. *Journal of Policy and Practice in Intellectual Disabilities.* 12: 42–6.

Audiologists

National studies suggest that 16% of the general population experience significant hearing loss, but people with intellectual disabilities have been found to have a hearing loss of between 30% and 40%, over twice that of the general population. Much hearing loss in this population goes unrecognized. This may be masked by self-injurious and other problematic behaviours, which arise from pain in the ear or difficulties in hearing. An audiologist's role is to assess and treat problems with hearing or balance disorders, ensuring the necessary immediate and ongoing care is provided.

Education

There are currently three ways to become an audiologist. These are to complete a BSc, an MSc, or a Postgraduate Diploma. A BSc in audiology, the most common route into the profession, has been in existence since 2002 and is 3yrs in length. Training is shared between university learning and clinical placements. Qualified audiologists are eligible to apply for registration to practice with the Registration Council for Clinical Physiologists. Audiologists with a master's degree and specific higher clinical training may be known as audiology clinical scientists.

Roles in practice

Audiologists work predominantly in hospital settings, with adults and children. They generally work as members of interdisciplinary audiology teams. Referrals for assessment are usually made by GPs or SLTs. Audiology services vary in role and distribution across the country.

Key roles of audiologists

- Newborn and school hearing programmes.
- Screening for speech, cognitive communication, or other related disorders that may impact on education or communication.
- Identification and assessment of activities that identify hearing or balance problems.
- Assessment and interpretation of auditory problems, including non-medical management of tinnitus (ringing in the ear).
- Assessment and provision of balance rehabilitation therapy.
- Preventative strategies, including prevention of hearing loss and protection of hearing function.
- Assessment, selection, fitting, and dispensing of hearing assistive technology, including hearing aids.
- Identification and work with populations at high risk of hearing loss or other auditory dysfunction, e.g. people with intellectual disabilities.
- Conducting clinical examinations of the ear, using an auroscope.
- Assessment regarding potential surgery.
- Partnership working with SLTs, school staff, parents, and carers.
- Participation in noise measurements of the acoustic environment.
- Evaluation and management of children and adults with auditory-related processing disorders.
- Development of culturally appropriate hearing programme-based interventions, including hearing aids, counselling, and referral for speech and language therapy.
- Advocacy for the communication needs of all individuals.

Audiologists and people with intellectual disabilities

The provision of audiology services is gaining in importance, due to increasing evidence recognizing the unmet hearing needs of the population. Reflecting this, Hearing and Learning Disabilities (HaLD), a specialist interest group, has recently been set up to improve the quality of care in audiology clinics and to improve the support to people with hearing loss and their carers. Audiologists are often a limited resource, and some areas have difficulty in accessing their local service.

Specific roles of an audiologist in working with people with intellectual disabilities may include:
• Early detection of hearing loss;
• Developing approaches for the collection of baseline hearing measurements;
• Supporting young children and adults in the introduction wearing, and regular evaluation and maintenance of hearing appliances, based on individual needs;
• Supporting paid and family carers in the wearing of hearing appliances;
• Working in partnership with hearing and SLTs in relation to managing and responding to the hearing needs of individuals;
• Conducting otoscopy (clinical examination of the ear, using an auroscope) to detect impacted ear wax or other conditions that may be contributing to the cause of hearing loss;
• Educating staff on the specific factors that might indicate hearing loss in people with intellectual disabilities, e.g. ear poking, head banging, behaviour change, or discharge from the ear.

Significant hearing loss can be due to impacted ear wax. Any nurse or supporter that has concern about hearing loss should primarily book an appointment with a GP to check if this is the case. This can then be treated easily by softening the wax with oil, which allows the wax to be broken down and expelled.

Further reading

Hearing and Learning Disabilities Special Interest Group (HaLD). ℘ www.hald.org.uk/ (accessed 30 October 2017).

McClimens A, Brennan S, Hargreaves P (2015). Hearing problems in the learning disability population: is anybody listening? *British Journal of Learning Disabilities.* **43**: 153–60.

McShea L (2014). Hearing loss in people with learning disabilities. *British Journal of Healthcare Assistants.* **7**: 601–5.

Dieticians

Healthy eating and drinking have an important role to play for general health and quality of life. Registered dieticians are qualified experts in diet and nutrition. They give advice on all aspects of eating and diet, including diets associated with different long-term or medical health conditions. Dieticians are qualified professionals, having completed either a BSc in Dietetics, or a similar postgraduate qualification. Dieticians translate scientific information about food into dietary advice, to enable people to make informed and practical choices about managing food and lifestyle, in managing both health and disease. All qualified dieticians are registered with the HCPC.

Dietitians work in a variety of ways. Within the NHS, they work in both hospital and community settings, directly with the general public, in health promotion, in public health, and in acute and chronic disease management. They influence food and health policy across the spectrum, from government to local communities and individuals. Different to nutritionists who provide information on food and healthy eating in the well, within the UK, the title dietician can only be used by those who are registered with the HCPC.

Dieticians and people with intellectual disabilities

Dietetic provision varies across the country. In a few areas, there are specialist dieticians. More commonly, people will meet a dietician from within a wider community primary care or hospital service. Further information on what is available can be obtained from the local healthcare provider, GP, or dietetic department.

Recent documents have highlighted the importance of good dietary support for this population and their carers. As a result of awareness of the nutritional problems found in people with intellectual disabilities, there has recently been a call for an increased number of dieticians working directly with this population. Nutrition-related health problems are more common than in the general population, and those people who require enteral feeding or adapted diets require the support of a dietician.

> **Most common nutrition-related causes of ill health in people with intellectual disabilities**
> - Malnutrition: underweight and overweight;
> - Swallowing difficulties;
> - Gastro-oesophageal reflux;
> - Long-term conditions, including diabetes and heart disease;
> - Bowel disorders, including constipation;
> - Dental disease;
> - Mental health conditions;
> - Other long-term conditions, e.g. dementia, epilepsy.

Dieticians working with people with intellectual disabilities focus their work in a number of different ways, including:
- Nutritional assessment and support of the malnourished;
- Specialist support to people with chronic disease;
- Facilitating access to mainstream dietetic services;
- Keeping people who are well healthy;

- Training family and paid staff in healthy food preparation;
- Provision of accessible information, games, and resources to help in educating people with intellectual disabilities on heathy eating.

Conditions that should trigger a referral to a dietician working with people with intellectual disabilities

- Persistent underweight;
- Persistent overweight;
- Eating and drinking problems;
- Specific medical conditions requiring complex nutritional intervention, e.g. phenylketonuria, coeliac disease, diabetes;
- Chronic constipation;
- Use of enteral feeding.

A significant focus of the role of all dieticians is to promote guidelines on healthy eating. Healthy eating, however, is not only the responsibility of dieticians. Everybody working with people with intellectual disabilities should promote the following key messages and tips for a healthy diet, as advised by the Food Standards Agency (FSA). The two keys to a healthy diet are eating the right amount of food for how active you are and eating a range of foods to make sure you are getting a balanced diet.

FSA (2008): eight tips for eating well

- 'Base your meals on starchy foods.
- Eat lots of fruit and vegetables.
- Eat more fish.
- Cut down on saturated fat and sugar.
- Try to eat less salt.
- Get active and try to be a healthy weight.
- Drink plenty of water.
- Don't skip breakfast.'[14]

Further reading

British Dietetic Association. ℘ www.bda.uk.com (accessed 30 October 2017).
British Dietetic Association. *Nutrition and Dietetics, Delivered as Part of Multidisciplinary Approach, is Clinically and Cost Effective in the Management of Learning Disabilities (LD).* ℘ www.bda.uk.com/professional/iap/learning_disability_kf_sheet (accessed 30 October 2017).
NHS Choices (2017). *Managing Weight with a Learning Disability.* ℘ www.nhs.uk/Livewell/Disability/Pages/weight-management-learning-disabilities.aspx (accessed 30 October 2017).

References

14 NHS Choices (2017). *Eight Tips for Healthy Eating.* ℘ www.nhs.uk/Livewell/Goodfood/Pages/eight-tips-healthy-eating.aspx (accessed 30 October 2017).

Physiotherapists

Physiotherapists work with people of all ages, helping them manage physical problems caused by illness, accident, impairment, and ageing. At the core of their work is the belief that body movement is central to the health and well-being of all. A physiotherapist's role is focused on preventing loss of movement and optimizing the functional potential of individuals.

Training

Physiotherapy is a popular healthcare profession. Training programmes are available at a number of different universities across the country. Physiotherapy is a science-based degree, leading to a BSc, which takes either 3 or 4yrs to complete. In order to practise as a physiotherapist, all qualified staff must register with the HCPC.

Over the course of their training, all physiotherapists will have gained experience in a wide and diverse range of adult hospital settings. These may include orthopaedics, general medicine, surgery, neurology, cardiology, and respiratory care. Other placements available include paediatrics, maternity and women's health, mental health, or a variety of community settings, including primary care. In many courses, during their training, physiotherapists will seldom have had a placement focused specifically on working with people with intellectual disabilities. Many will graduate, having had little information and knowledge of the needs and skills of working with this population.

After qualification, physiotherapists may rotate through different hospital or community placements, until choosing to work in a specialist area. Further training may be available to them relevant to this specialism. In this role, physiotherapists are likely to work as members of profession-specific teams; this may include colleagues with different skills and levels of experience, including physiotherapy assistants. Physiotherapists also often work in wider multidisciplinary teams.

The core skills of a physiotherapist

- Holistic movement assessment, incorporating psychological, cultural, and social influences;
- Analysis of movement and function;
- Manual therapies, e.g. movement, massage, manipulation, electrical stimulation;
- Therapeutic exercise, e.g. hydrotherapy, group activities;
- Assessment for aids and appliances;
- Educating carers and staff in the techniques of moving and handling.

Physiotherapists are increasingly found working in primary care settings. This is due to the current focus in the provision of care outside hospital and the flexible role of the GP in the commissioning and provision of services to meet the needs of local communities.

How do physiotherapists work?
- Health promotion activities, e.g. sports groups;
- Preventative approaches, e.g. postural care, falls prevention;
- Individual treatment;
- Rehabilitation.

There is no common national model as to how physiotherapists are employed. They may be employed by GPs, primary care trusts, acute trusts, or charities, or they may be independent contractors. They may be based in any range of primary health, acute hospital, and social care settings. These include:
- GP surgeries;
- Private medical practice;
- Community hospitals;
- Special schools;
- Leisure and sports;
- Industry.

They may treat people in any of these environments or, where indicated, in the family home.

Physiotherapists in primary care and people with intellectual disabilities

People with intellectual disabilities experience many of the same conditions requiring physiotherapy as the general population. They use the same hospitals, hospital discharge teams, and health centres, and therefore they may have access to the same hospital and community healthcare services. When physiotherapy is required, people with intellectual disabilities are frequently, and successfully, treated by the generic teams.

Specialist physiotherapists are a limited resource and may not always be available within specialist services. They work closely with their physiotherapy colleagues in other services. They may refer people to generic services, helping the person access generic services and then help to support the staff in knowing the best ways to communicate and treat the person, in relation to their intellectual disabilities. Referral from the generic service to the intellectual disabilities service should be needed only where there are specific indications for a specialist service, such as communication difficulties, complex physical impairment, behaviour that challenges generic service delivery, and specialist individual needs, such as seating or postural care.

Specialist physiotherapists may make use of mainstream or specialist resources, including hydrotherapy pools, for individual treatment or prevention. In addition, they may run groups, such as for falls prevention, an area of risk known to be significantly higher in this population.

Further reading

Association of Chartered Physiotherapists for People with Learning Disabilities. ℰ acppld.csp.org. uk/about-acppld (accessed 30 October 2017).

Hodges C (2005). Getting to grips with learning disabilities. *Physiotherapy Frontline*. June 15, 21–3.

Occupational therapists

Occupational therapists (OTs) recognize that being independent and able to perform everyday activities is crucial to good health and wellbeing. OTs work with all age groups of people, in hospitals and across community settings. Their clinical role is based on the assessment and treatment of physical and mental health. Through the use of specific purposeful activity, they work to prevent disability and promote independent function, by addressing work and other aspects of daily life. Some OTs may also undertake a close partnership with housing departments and social services in the provision of aids and adaptations to houses where changes, such as a downstairs bathroom, are required, as a result of changes to a person's health and their ability to use household facilities.

In what areas do OTs work?
- Mental health services;
- Intellectual disabilities services;
- Physical disability services;
- Primary care;
- Children's services;
- Older peoples services;
- Rheumatology;
- Care management;
- Environmental adaptation;
- Equipment for daily living.

Education

OTs now undertake a 3-yr (or 4-yr in Scotland) degree. It can also be completed in 2yrs as a postgraduate qualification. All OTs must register with the HCPC prior to practice. Throughout their education, OTs complete a number of different placements, in a range of specialist areas. This might include intellectual disabilities; however, many OTs complete their education without having the opportunity to work in this area, and start to specialize after they qualify.

Role in practice

OTs in primary care often work as members of the primary care team. In some areas, primary care OTs are an integral part of joint rehabilitation teams. These are joint teams set up to coordinate work between primary care trusts and local authorities. These teams, led by the local authority, are usually responsible for providing the equipment, or any adaptations required, to enable someone to live at home. They also work increasingly in teams that focus on community care or care provision outside of hospital. OTs work with people who have injuries, illness, or disabilities on programmes of treatment based on an individual's lifestyle, environment, and personal choices. An assessment of needs may be done in the home, a community setting, or in hospital before discharge.

OTs may work with individuals for variable periods of time, depending on the needs identified. Referrals to the service are usually made by other medical professionals. As of 1 August 2016, there were 36 844 UK-registered OTs working across the UK.

What is the role of an OT working in primary care?
- Rehabilitation after amputation injury or illness, e.g. after a stroke or accident;
- Rheumatology, e.g. management of joint care in arthritis;
- Falls prevention in vulnerable older people, promoting home safety;
- Assessment and provision of aids and equipment, to facilitate independence or to support carers in their caring role;
- Assessment of the home, developing designs for housing adaptation;
- Provision of treatment, e.g. in running limb rehabilitation clinics after injury, offering hand exercises, splinting, pain management;
- Maintaining activities of daily living skills when living with a debilitating health condition, e.g. multiple sclerosis;
- Assessment of a person's work environment, to assess any aids required to facilitate return to work;
- Referrals for people who will need to use a wheelchair;
- At times, involvement in interventions related to behaviour management.

Occupational therapists and people with intellectual disabilities

OTs in primary care do not always have the communication skills or training in working with people with intellectual disabilities. Likewise, OTs in intellectual disabilities services may not have the specialist skills required in primary care. Within adult services, it is common practice for OTs in community intellectual disability teams to support primary care OTs in any rehabilitation work. This enables the sharing of skills to enable the individual to receive the best service. An OT in intellectual disabilities services will work with individuals to assess and develop daily patterns of self-care, leisure and productivity, motivation, and the impact of the environment on functional ability. They may also complete sensory processing assessments and develop sensory profiles for people with intellectual disabilities and associated conditions, including ASC or ADHD.

Further reading
Duncan EA (2012). *Foundations for Practice in Occupational Therapy*, 5th edn. Churchill Livingstone: Edinburgh.
Lillywhite A, Haines D (2010). *Occupational Therapy and People with Learning Disabilities. Findings from a Research Study*. College of Occupational Therapists: London.
Mountain G (1998). *Occupational Therapy for People with Learning Disabilities Living in the Community: A Review of the Literature*. College of Occupational Therapists: London.

Optical care

Regular assessment of vision and good care of the eyes is essential for good health and well-being. Having a regular eye test does not just tell you how short- or long-sighted you are. It can also reveal eye conditions that might lead to loss of vision (e.g. glaucoma). In addition, an eye test can detect evidence of general poor health or the existence of a previously undiagnosed health condition (e.g. diabetes).

The regularity of eye tests varies with age. Children are recommended to attend for an eye test 2-yearly, or more frequently as recommended by an optometrist. Adults are recommended to have regular eye tests from the age of 40yrs, the age when eyesight often starts to deteriorate and the risk of cataracts and glaucoma is increased. Follow-up examinations should take place every 2yrs, or more frequently, as advised. People with intellectual disabilities should follow the same recommendations. If detected early, the progress of some eye diseases can be stopped or slowed down.

Eye tests are conducted by ophthalmologists, optometrists, and opticians. Ophthalmologists are specialists in eye diseases, treatment, and surgery. As trained doctors, they are registered with, and regulated by, the General Medical Council (GMC) and mainly work in eye hospitals and hospital eye departments. They rarely work in high-street optical premises. High-street dispensing opticians advise on, fit, and supply spectacle frames and contact lenses after assessing a person's lifestyle and occupational needs.

> ### What is the role of optometrists?
> - Conduct eye examinations to detect injury, disease, abnormality, or defects.
> - Conduct eyesight tests.
> - Advise on eye care or visual problems.
> - Recognize abnormal eye conditions, e.g. squints.
> - Prescribe corrective lenses.
> - Fit spectacles and contact lenses.

Education

A qualified optometrist has completed a 3-yr training (4yrs in Scotland) and has obtained a university degree. On gaining the degree, an optometrist has to complete a year of salaried clinical experience with the NHS, and then pass a qualifying examination, before they can register with the General Optical Council. They are permitted to practise independently.

Role in practice

Optometrists work in private practice, or for the NHS, in both hospital departments and primary care. Optometrists work as members of eye care teams; other members include opticians, orthoptists, and ophthalmologists. Opticians are qualified to fit and adjust spectacles, some having an additional qualification to fit contact lenses and low vision appliances. Orthoptists are qualified to diagnose and work non-surgically, with people with eye problems. Based predominantly in hospital departments, orthoptists respond to GP or other medical referrals, to carry out visual screening after stroke or head injury. Ophthalmologists provide services in hospitals and community settings and are specialists in diseases of the eye.

Optical care for people with intellectual disabilities

People with intellectual disabilities experience significant impairments of sight, much of it undetected, such as premature cataracts.[15] In addition, high levels of eye problems have been found in people with specific conditions, such as Down syndrome, progressive visual failure associated with Prader–Willi syndrome and people born prematurely, who may have received oxygen therapy, and in association with cerebral palsy.

In the planning and provision of optical care to people with intellectual disabilities, a proactive approach often needs to be taken. Only a small number of optometrists may have the knowledge and skills of working with the population.

What issues need to be considered in optical care for people with intellectual disabilities?

- An inability to communicate eye pain or a change in visual function.
- A range of behaviours considered challenging, e.g. eye poking, head banging, may indicate a visual problem.
- Regular stumbling or falls may indicate a visual problem.
- A lack of knowledge in the need for regular eye checks or where to go to get them carried out.
- A fear of medical appointments and the use of unfamiliar optical procedures.
- An inability to provide medical information, to support optical assessments.
- Fear or behaviours that make the wearing of glasses difficult for individuals.

Best practice suggests that people with intellectual disabilities should be well prepared when going for optical assessment or treatment. A list of accessible resources and a preparation assessment form called *Telling the optometrist about me* are available from ℰ www.gmpec.co.uk/service/patients_with_learning_disabilities

Further reading

Emerson E, Robertson J (2011). *The Estimated Prevalence of Visual Impairment among People with Learning Disabilities in England.* Improving Health and Lives: Learning Disabilities Observatory: London. ℰ www.rnib.org.uk/sites/default/files/Emerson%20report.pdf (accessed 30 October 2017).

Pilling R (2011). *Ophthalmic Services Guideline. The Management of Visual Problems in Adult Patients who have Learning Disabilities.* Royal College of Ophthalmologists: London.

Royal College of Ophthalmologists, Vision 2020, See Ability (2015). *Eye Care for People with Learning Disabilities.* ℰ www.rcophth.ac.uk/wp-content/uploads/2015/09/Eye-Care-Services-for-Adults-with-Learning-Disabilities.pdf (accessed 30 October 2017).

References

15 Royal College of Ophthalmologists (2011). *The Management of Visual Problems in Adult Patients who have Learning Disabilities.* ℰ www.rcophth.ac.uk/wp-content/uploads/2014/12/2011_PROF_128_The-management-of-visual-problems-in-people-with-learning-disabilities.pdf (accessed 14 March 2018).

Community nurses mental health

Community nurses mental health (CNMHs), previously known as community psychiatric nurses (CPNs), play a significant role in the delivery of services to people with mental health problems living in the community. Working as members of primary care, community mental health teams, and hospital outreach teams, they have a number of different skills in order to treat, assess, and provide specific intervention to support people living with mental health conditions, either at home or other community settings. They may also work as mental health liaison nurses in accident and emergency departments, or in conjunction with other mental health outpatient services such as memory clinics.

Education

CNMHs have widely differing areas of skill and qualification. Most qualified nurses hold a registered nurse qualification in mental health, taken at either diploma or degree level. In addition, some nurses hold other nursing qualifications, e.g. in intellectual disabilities or adult nursing. After qualification, mental health nurses may work in hospital or residential settings where they gain a range of skills and experience, before moving into a community setting. Some undertake a post-basic qualification in community nursing. The skills of a CNMH may include:
• CBT;
• Substance misuse;
• Forensic psychiatry;
• Psychotherapy;
• Counselling;
• Family therapy;
• Nurse prescribing;
• Group therapy;
• Child and adolescent psychiatry;
• Mental health and learning disabilities.

What support does a CNMH offer primary care teams?
• Working with the team to help in the provision of care of people with mental health problems in the community;
• Developing realistic health promotion approaches;
• Facilitating link between the community mental health team and the primary care team;
• Updating the team on changes in mental health treatments and strategy.

CNMHs work across services and are required to have a number of key skills that are essential for both clinical patient care and teamworking. Community-orientated primary care, including the role of CNMHs, is the main driver for improvement of mental health services.

Key organizational skills of CNMHs

- Communication;
- Self-management;
- Teamworking;
- Leadership;
- Professional support and clinical supervision;
- Accountability at professional, managerial, and clinical levels;
- Referrals and caseload management;
- Management of resources;
- Evidence-based practice;
- Risk assessment.

Key clinical skills of CNMHs

- Assessment of physical and mental health;
- Development of therapeutic relationships;
- Treatment, e.g. medication, psychological interventions;
- Formulation of treatment plans;
- Re-enablement and relapse prevention;
- Clinical monitoring of health status;
- Carer support;
- Research and audit;
- Health promotion;
- CPA;
- Key worker responsibilities—case management and coordination.

CNMHs and people with intellectual disabilities

People with intellectual disabilities experience increased rates of long-term mental health conditions to that of the general population. Current UK policies promote the need for mental health services for the general population to be accessible to adults with intellectual disabilities. In some areas, this approach is well supported, with good joint working between services, enabling this to happen. Best practice is considered to be where there is clear local agreement between mental health and intellectual disabilities services at a local level about the commissioning and provision of services.

Further reading

Jacobs M, Downie H, Kidd G, Fitzsimmons L, Gibbs S, Melville C (2016). Mental health services for children and adolescents with learning disabilities: a review of research on experiences of service users and providers. *British Journal of Learning Disabilities.* **44**: 225–32.

Thornicroft G (2011). *Community Mental Health: Putting Policy into Practice Globally.* John Wiley & Sons: Chichester.

Yeager K, Cutler DL, Svendsen D, Sills GM (2013). *Modern Community Mental Health: An Interdisciplinary Approach.* Oxford University Press: Oxford.

General hospital services

General hospitals are an integral part of the structure of health service for all members of the population, including people with intellectual disabilities. These hospitals are required to provide equity of access to all people in the areas they serve. Contact with general hospitals can range from outpatient appointments and day procedures for investigations, review, or minor procedures, through to contact with accident and emergency departments, the need for major surgical intervention, and repeated lengthy admissions because of complex health needs.

Unfortunately, despite some innovative services to promote access to acute general hospitals, the consistent findings of inquiries and research projects over the past 20yrs have been that people with intellectual disabilities experience major difficulties in accessing and receiving high-quality services within many general hospitals, at times resulting in avoidable and premature death.[16,17] The failure of general hospitals to make 'reasonable adjustment' to meet the needs of people with intellectual disabilities continues to be highlighted as a major problem.

Challenges in achieving equity of access and outcome

Challenges, although often presented as difficulties arising from the presence of intellectual disabilities, can arise from three major areas:
- The presence of intellectual disabilities and the associated difficulties that may result in communicating directly with the patient for staff who are unfamiliar with the person;
- Difficulties in providing information about procedures;
- Confirming consent and gaining cooperation.

However, difficulties in communication cannot solely relate to the presence of intellectual disabilities and are also influenced by the lack of skills among staff in communicating non-verbally, lack of confidence in working with people with intellectual disabilities, and stereotypical attitudes which presuppose people will not be able to understand, give consent, or will be difficult to manage.

The risk of 'diagnostic overshadowing' has been highlighted as a potential major factor in failing to recognize the need to treat physical health conditions. This occurs when changes in physical (or mental) health are considered to be part of the presence of intellectual disabilities, even though the signs and symptoms are not associated with intellectual disabilities. As a result of this error in judgement, the necessary investigations are not undertaken, the appropriate diagnosis not made, or the necessary treatment not commenced. In addition, appointment systems, as well as inflexible policy-driven systems and procedures that are unable or unwilling to adjust to meet individual needs, can result in difficulties when seeking to plan for, or respond to, the differing abilities and needs of a person with intellectual disabilities.

Promoting access to a quality service within general hospitals

See ➔ Secondary care, pp. 350–1.

- Listen to people who know the person with intellectual disabilities; if they say something is wrong, investigate the possibility seriously.
- Ensure that all people with intellectual disabilities who have a planned contact with/admission to the general hospital should have the opportunity to have an assessment of their abilities and any additional support they may need to ensure their appointment/admission is a success.
- Clarify how the person with intellectual disabilities communicates, and ensure the necessary arrangements are in place to promote effective communication (including staff training).
- Provide information to people with intellectual disabilities and parents/carers about what they can expect when in contact with general hospital services. This should include contact details for key staff in both services that may be able to organize additional support, if required.
- In the first instance, information should be provided directly to people with intellectual disabilities in a format accessible to them, and they should be given the necessary time to comprehend as much of this as is possible for them to promote informed decision-making.
- When information needs to be shared, the permission of the person with intellectual disabilities should be sought and their right to confidentiality should be respected.
- Maintain frequent contact with the person with intellectual disabilities to monitor for any improvement or potential deterioration of their health.
- At all times, see the person first (not the intellectual disabilities), and remain alert to the possibility of physical health problems, and actively guard against diagnostic overshadowing. If you use the presence of intellectual disabilities to explain changes in behaviour, physical signs, symptoms, or overall health changes, you are probably making a mistake.

Further reading

Iacono T, Bigby C, Carolyn U, Douglas J, Fitzpatrick P (2014). A systematic review of hospital experiences of people with intellectual disability. *BMC Health Services Research*. **14**: 505.

MacArthur J, Brown M, McKechanie A, Mack S, Hayes M, Fletcher MA (2015). Making reasonable and achievable adjustments: the contributions of learning disability liaison nurses in 'Getting it right' for people with learning disabilities receiving general hospitals care. *Journal of Advanced Nursing*. **71**: 1552–63.

NHS Health Education England. *Learning Disabilities Made Clear Toolkit*. ℘ hee.nhs.uk/our-work/person-centred-care/learning-disability/workforce-development/learning-disabilities-made-clear-toolkit (accessed 30 October 2017).

References

16 Heslop P, Blair P, Fleming P, Hoghton M, Marriott A, Russ L (2013). *Confidential Inquiry into Premature Deaths of People with Learning Disabilities (CIPOLD). Final Report*. Noray Fry Research Centre: Bristol. ℘ www.bris.ac.uk/cipold/ (accessed 30 October 2017).

17 Department of Health (2013). *Six Lives: Progress Report on Healthcare for People with Learning Disabilities*. Department of Health: London. ℘ www.gov.uk/government/publications/six-lives-department-of-health-second-progress-report (accessed 30 October 2017).

Practice nurses

NHS policy changes have encouraged a shift from hospital-based care to community-based care, with procedures that were once only undertaken as an admission into hospital now being undertaken within the primary healthcare team (PHCT). Practice nurses work in a GP surgery as part of a PHCT, supporting the local people with their healthcare. The PHCT consists of a range of professionals such as doctors, practice nurses, HVs, dieticians, and counsellors.

What do practice nurses do?

- Offer health screening and health promotion.
- Undertake annual health checks.
- Offer family planning advice.
- Run nurse-led clinics, often for people with long-term conditions.
- Offer immunizations.
- Offer cervical smear tests.
- Take bloods for investigations.
- Treat minor injuries.
- Dress and re-dress minor wounds.
- Help with minor procedures under local anaesthesia.

What does this mean for people with intellectual disabilities?

We know that the life expectancy of people with intellectual disabilities has increased considerably over the past 20 years, which, in part, has been due to an increase in health promotion, a reduction in preventable illnesses, and more effective treatment of existing mental and physical health conditions. However, health inequalities and avoidable and preventable death encountered by people with intellectual disabilities continue to be an area of major concern.[18] It is increasingly important that community- and primary care-based services and agencies work together to improve the health of people with intellectual disabilities and, when necessary, to effectively meet a person's healthcare needs. As services continue to become more community-based, it will increasingly be staff in primary care settings that will support and meet the health needs of people with intellectual disabilities. People with intellectual disabilities will be seen more often in primary care across the full range of services the practice nurses provide.

As a registered nurse in intellectual disabilities, you should work closely with the practice nurse to ensure that the person with intellectual disabilities is able to receive high-quality care, treatments, and/or advice offered to the general population. This will mean getting to know who the practice nurses in your geographical are, providing them information that may be relevant to them about the mental and physical health of people with intellectual disabilities and, where necessary, working alongside them to help them design and implement reasonable adjustments to increase the accessibility of primary care services to people with intellectual disabilities.

Who is responsible for the health of people with intellectual disabilities?

It is everyone's responsibility. It is important that all services work together to address the person's healthcare needs. This should be written into a person's HAP or nursing care plan. The registered nurse in intellectual disabilities should work together with the practice nurse, supporting the person to access primary care and the practice nurse where possible; this may involve desensitization work and working to make information accessible in order for the person to understand the information (see ➔ Developing accessible information, pp. 70–1).

Developing collaborative working with practice nurses

- Taking opportunities to shadow each other in roles.
- Exchanging contact details with each other.
- Making presentations to practice nurses about the role of the registered nurses in services for people with intellectual disabilities.
- Attending events held by practice nurses to learn about developments in their role.
- Keeping in ongoing formal and more informal contact (perhaps for coffee occasionally) with staff in GP practices.
- Undertaking joint clinics to respond to local needs.
- Providing opportunities for practice nurses to visit people with intellectual disabilities who are well in range of settings to highlight the abilities of people with intellectual disabilities.
- Providing information to practice nurses on accessible resources for working with people with intellectual disabilities and meeting their key health needs.

Further reading

Royal College of General Practitioners. *Learning Disabilities*. ☞ www.rcgp.org.uk/learningdisabilities/ (accessed 30 October 2017).

Vanderbilt Kennedy Center. *Health Care for Adults with Intellectual and Developmental Disabilities: Toolkit for Primary Care Providers*. ☞ vkc.mc.vanderbilt.edu/etoolkit (accessed 30 October 2017).

References

18 Heslop P, Blair P, Fleming P, Hoghton M, Marriott A, Russ L (2013). *Confidential Inquiry into Premature Deaths of People with Learning Disabilities (CIPOLD). Final Report*. Noray Fry Research Centre: Bristol. ☞ www.bris.ac.uk/cipold/ (accessed 30 October 2017).

Outpatient clinics

People with intellectual disabilities are living longer, and by 2020, the UK will see a 10% increase in the number of people with intellectual disabilities and, in addition, the complexities of intellectual disabilities will also increase.[19] While this group of people are living longer, they have greater health needs than the general population and, as such, have the need to attend health services more often.[20] Outpatient clinics see more patients each year than any other hospital department, and many people with intellectual disabilities, due to their health profile, are high users of this service throughout their lifespan.

For many people, including people with intellectual disabilities, the experience of outpatient clinics is either the beginning of a period of investigations and treatment, or they are at the end-stage of their healthcare for a specific problem. Regardless of the reason for the outpatient appointment, people need to perceive that their needs are recognized, understood, and addressed. Unfortunately, this is too often not so for people with intellectual disabilities, as they continue to experience difficulties accessing healthcare services for various reasons.[21]

Within outpatient clinics, the professional barriers associated with access are inflexible appointments, long waiting times, overcrowded waiting areas, a lack of resources such as lifting equipment, a lack of knowledge and understanding of intellectual disabilities, poor staff attitudes, and a lack of effective communication.[22] Hospital services do rely heavily on written communication, which is often inaccessible for many people with intellectual disabilities, despite the legal requirement to provide information in a format that is understood. Any one of the conditions above can increase the individual's experience of distress and is a contributory factor in reducing patient safety. Regardless of the length of time or purpose of stay, hospitalization can be very distressing for a person with intellectual disabilities, but there are ways in which healthcare professionals can reduce the impact on the person and/or their family or carer.

Supporting people in outpatients

'Reasonable adjustment' in health services is key to ensuring that all people, including people with intellectual disabilities, have equity in accessing and availing of healthcare; this supports the principle of person-centredness, reflecting equality in health outcomes.[23] Various measures that can be viewed as reasonable adjustments in outpatient clinics have been identified, including:

- Preparation for the appointment should begin before the patient arrives at the outpatient clinic;
- The referral letter should indicate any special requirements such as difficulties waiting in crowded areas or lifting equipment. In addition, the appointment letter could ask for confirmation of any requirements;
- The hospital should identify people with intellectual disabilities on their records system in support of patient safety;
- Flexible appointments, either the first or last appointments of the individual clinic, or the day when it is least busy;
- If clinics are overrunning, there should be an opportunity for individuals and their families to leave the outpatient department for some time and a new time to return provided;

- Extra time should be given during the appointment to facilitate effective communication;
- Where appropriate, notify the person's advocate/carer/liaison nurse/ intellectual disabilities services;
- Check whether the patient has a hospital passport;
- Provision of sufficient space to facilitate wheelchair access and to maintain privacy and dignity;
- Where possible, there should be an option of the use of a separate waiting room for people who may be distressed on the day;
- Ongoing education of healthcare professionals on intellectual disabilities and on ways to enhance communication;
- Any journeys to another area of the hospital may need to be escorted and access to the area facilitated;
- Special requirements should be communicated to other healthcare professionals, e.g. by the nurse in outpatients to the radiographer in the X-ray department, so that they are ready for the patient's arrival;
- All communication to the individual needs to be in a format that is understood, and any further investigations, treatment, and care explained fully in order to support decision-making;
- Healthcare professionals need to have a clear understanding of the current legislation and guidelines on consent to examination, treatment, and care, to support decision-making.

There are many ongoing initiatives and good practice to improving access and streamlining patient pathways within outpatient clinics. Teams should seek an understanding of these to support their efforts in ensuring equity and safety in healthcare for people with intellectual disabilities.

References

19 Michael J (2008). *Healthcare for All: A Report of the Independent Inquiry into Access to Healthcare for People with Learning Disabilities.* HMSO: London.
20 Emerson E, Baines S (2012). *Health Inequalities and People with Learning Disabilities in the UK.* Learning Disabilities Observatory/Department of Health: London.
21 Department of Health (2013). *Government Response to the Confidential Inquiry into Premature Deaths of People with Learning Disability (CIPOLD).* Department of Health: London.
22 Bowness B (2014). *Improving General Hospital Care of Patients who have a Learning Disability. 1000 Lives Improvement.* ℘ www.1000livesplus.wales.nhs.uk/sitesplus/documents/1011/How%20 to%20%2822%29%20Learning%20Disabilites%20Care%20Bundle%20web.pdf (accessed 30 October 2017).
23 MacArthur J, Brown M, McKechanie A, Mack S, Hayes M, Fletcher J (2015). Making reasonable and achievable adjustments: the contributions of learning disability liaison nurses in 'getting it right' for people with learning disabilities receiving general hospitals care. *Journal of Advanced Nursing.* 71: 1552–63.

Radiology departments

Radiology departments are usually located within district and major secondary hospitals. These departments can vary considerably in size and the services they provide. While all offer X-ray investigations, and this equipment may also be seen within some dental surgeries and larger health centres, some radiology departments also provide more detailed scanning investigations in the screening, diagnosis, or interventions to treat health conditions.

Radiography departments use X-rays or other scanning equipment to check on bony injuries, soft tissues, the presence of thrombosis (clots), the condition of internal organs and new growths (tumours), and foreign bodies (e.g. pica, coins). It is also possible to use X-rays to view other body organs by introducing a medium that is visible on the X-ray. Radiology equipment may also be used to provide a 'picture' to guide and check the successful location of delicate internal procedures, e.g. the insertion of central venous lines. Some treatments for cancer involve the use of radiotherapy where the area of the body in which a tumour is present receives a targeted exposure to radiation.

Reason why people with intellectual disabilities may use radiology departments

People may have contact with staff in a radiology department for any of the reasons outlined above, in order to check for an injury or the functioning of body organs or to receive treatment. This is often a key step within the process of diagnosis, and therefore any difficulty in gaining cooperation for such procedures may delay the diagnosis, often resulting in prolonged discomfort and reducing the chances of success in any treatments. At times, practising to sit or lie still in advance may be useful, as this will be required during many investigations.

Some people with intellectual disabilities, including people with epilepsy, people with complex physical health needs, and older people, may be more likely to have contact with X-ray departments as a result of accidents, ill health (in particular chest infections), or as part of on-going monitoring of their health status.

Preparing for contact with radiology departments

In emergencies, it is not always possible to undertake detailed preparation for contact with a radiology department; however, patients with scheduled appointments known about in advance can be prepared. In seeking to support a person with intellectual disabilities who may have contact with a radiology department, the following actions may be helpful:

- With the agreement of the person with intellectual disabilities (or their parents, if a child), contact the radiology department to establish the reason for the visit and the nature of the procedure to be undertaken.
- Inform staff in the radiology department of any additional information they may need in relation to communication abilities, the ability to wait, and additional physical mobility issues. This information could be summarized and presented in a health/hospital passport document.
- Clarify with the person with intellectual disabilities what they understand about their forthcoming appointment/investigation.

- Provide information on the steps involved in using the department, including the possible need to change clothing, lying still, use of a scanner, and using accessible information, including photographs and videos if necessary (see Easyhealth link under ➲ Further reading). A pre-appointment visit to see the staff and equipment may be helpful if the department is nearby.
- Bear in mind that radiology departments are unfamiliar places for people not used to them. Investigations may include the use of equipment that is overhead or a large scanner; people are often required to lie still; staff may wear protective clothing and stand behind screens; lights may be dimmed; and sudden noises may come from the equipment. People may also be asked to move or allow a painful body part to be examined.
- Confirm if any pre-appointment preparation is required such as increasing/restricting fluid/food intake or taking premedication.

Support during contact with staff in radiology departments

Arrival at the department should be well planned—parents or carers accompanying a person should make available to radiology staff additional information using health passports and confirm ongoing consent to investigation/treatment. Provide ongoing information during the appointment, particularly if the person is to be left alone, and involve an acute liaison nurse if available. Give positive encouragement and feedback when things are going well.

Post-appointment

It is important to clarify if there are any restrictions of contact with other people, and explain any alterations from normal such as discoloured bowel motions. Before leaving, confirm whether a review appointment is required and the arrangements for this.

Further reading

Easyhealth. *X-rays and Scans (leaflets).* ✎ www.easyhealth.org.uk/categories/x-rays-and-scans-(leaflets) (accessed 30 October 2017).

Children's health services

The number of children with complex physical, mental, and behavioural healthcare needs has increased, as children and intellectual disabilities services have been able to support an increasing number of children with high level of complexity. Many of these children require intensive support throughout their childhood, at times being dependent on technology to receive adequate nutrition and at times for breathing.[24]

Children's services should be characterized by effective interdisciplinary and interagency communication in community/hospital-based provision, and integrated working that focuses on the needs of the child and family, rather than the needs of the service or professionals within the services. Nurses, whether nurses in intellectual disabilities services or children's services, need to consider their role in developing supporting services that recognize the abilities and needs of the child as an individual in a wider family context and working across interdisciplinary service structures, including being employed in services other than intellectual disabilities services.

All children with intellectual disabilities and their carers may have contact with general children's health services in both primary and secondary care. Some children with complex healthcare needs may have more frequent contact with general children's services or specific services for children with intellectual disabilities, which will be involved in promoting their overall physical, mental, and social health, reviewing and monitoring their development, responding to acute episodes of ill health, and, when necessary, seeking to provide palliative care.

Promoting collaborative working with children's services

The development of more inclusive children's services supports children to have equity of access to children's services and seeks to ensure that their general health needs should be met within children's services available to all children, rather than within a separate, and possibly parallel, intellectual disabilities services. While this may work for a large number of children, those children with complex healthcare needs will often require support from secondary specialist children's nursing teams in community and hospital settings. Many of these services have developed in response to the growing number of children with complex healthcare needs. Such services have a valuable contribution to make, as do intellectual disabilities nursing services, particularly when children and teenagers also have difficulties arising from behaviour that presents challenges or when more time is required to teach new skills that cannot be provided by general children's services.

Collaborative working is also very important to facilitate a smooth transition of care from children's to adult services. Through this, it is possible to provide the combined knowledge, skills, and commitment to support children and their families, resulting in a smooth and effective transition that provides children and parents with essential confidence in adult services to continue to support the development of young adults, to maximize their achievements, and to meet their needs. It is accepted that collaborative working can bring its own challenges and requires investment in time and personal commitment if it is to be successful (see ➜ Principles of working collaboratively with families, pp. 42–3, ➜ Effective teamworking, pp. 296–7, and ➲ Community children's nurses, pp. 360–1). Nurses within intellectual disabilities services should develop contact with their nursing colleagues within children's hospital and community services, sharing information on the possible contributions to care of a child, expressing willingness to work in partnership, and exchanging knowledge, skills, and contact details. There should be opportunities to meet regularly.

Many of these children are a 'new generation' of children with complex needs who would have been unlikely to survive into adulthood only 15yrs ago. Therefore, new service arrangements are required to effectively support children and their families. These should not be negatively impacted on by either intellectual disability or children's services claiming 'professional territory'. Such a position seeks to advantage one service but does little to enhance services for children.

Services for children with complex health needs that appear to be most successful are characterized by having committed staff who work as effective team members and listen carefully to children and young people. They give timely and appropriate information in a format that is understandable for the specific child. These services recognize the differing circumstances of families and respond to their changing abilities and needs, maintaining a focus on the human rights of all children.

Further reading

Department of Health (2010). *National Framework for Children and Young People's Continuing Care.* Department of Health: London.
Department of Children and Youth Affairs (2014). *Better Outcomes Brighter Futures: The National Policy Framework for Children and Young People 2014–2020.* Department of Children and Youth Affairs: Dublin.

References

24 Smith J, Cheater F, Bekker H (2014). Parents' experiences of living with a child with a long-term condition: a rapid structured review of the literature. *Health Expectations.* **18**: 452–74.

Emergency departments

The most common reason why people with intellectual disabilities in England attend emergency departments are epileptic seizures. Other reasons include constipation, diabetes, influenza/pneumonia, and mental health problems.[25,26] Fifty per cent of people with intellectual disabilities who present to the emergency care environment are admitted, compared to 31% who do not have intellectual disabilities.[27]

Barriers within the emergency care environment

Often nurses in emergency care experience challenges in ensuring equity of access to people with intellectual disabilities within this environment. These challenges are particularly associated with a lack of knowledge of intellectual disabilities, communication difficulties, and misunderstandings regarding the individual's right and ability to consent to healthcare and best interests decision-making.[28] Consequently, this reduces the nurse's confidence to assess needs to plan, provide, and evaluate care, and to arrange discharge and referrals where appropriate.

For many people, the emergency department is a fast-moving, noisy, bizarre, and unfamiliar environment. For a person with intellectual disabilities, a lack of understanding of what is happening can increase their levels of anxiety and distress, which may be demonstrated in challenging behaviours. Subsequently, there is a risk that these behaviours may be misinterpreted, being linked to the disability, and not seen as an indicator of distress (diagnostic overshadowing).

Additionally, assessment of patients in emergency care is conducted using the process of triage, a rapid assessment to prioritize the patient's needs. Triage assessments with people with learning disabilities will often need to be allocated more time to ensure people are able to understand and respond to the information provided to them and be actively involved in decision-making.

Enhancing support

It is important that healthcare professionals within emergency care have an awareness of the challenges encountered by people with intellectual disabilities and their families or carers when accessing this service. Patient safety in healthcare is a priority and is related to quality care. In order to support patient safety and increase equity to people with intellectual disabilities within the emergency department, 'reasonable adjustments' are required (Equality Act 2010).

These tend to fall within three broad categories.

Communication

Nurses within emergency care can improve communication with people with intellectual disabilities by:

- Seeking to understand how the individual communicates and employ various communication strategies to enhance safe assessment of needs (e.g. the Hospital Communication Book);
- Checking to see if they have a hospital passport that generally contains a range of key information about the patient and their health;
- Recognizing that behaviour is a means of communicating, not a symptom of intellectual disabilities;

- Providing regular information to them in a format that best suits them regarding their journey through the emergency care department and potential waiting times to reduce fears and anxieties;
- Providing discharge/referral letters in a format that is understood.

Organization
- Identify and address any lack of knowledge of the nature of intellectual disabilities.
- Understand that the health needs of this population are high, and that these needs may present and be communicated differently.
- Afford the extra time required to inform decision-making, assess needs, investigate, and provide treatment.
- Where possible, one nurse should remain with the person throughout the patient's journey for continuity.
- Respect the right of adults to consent to their healthcare, and apply the local guidelines on consent.

Collaboration
- Support the patient's autonomy; speak to the individual in the first instance, and see them as a person first, before seeing the disability.
- Appreciate the need to seek support from family/carers to aid assessment; often they use their intuition gained from experience of caring from the individual; listen to them, and respect their knowledge.
- Know who the liaison nurse (intellectual disability) is, their role, and how to contact them.
- Liaise with the community intellectual disability team.
- Sharing best practice between the team within emergency care and within intellectual disabilities services would enhance safe care through best practice.
- Monitor attendance; people who present repeatedly with seizures, hyperglycaemia, or hypoglycaemia may need the management of their condition reviewed by the primary care team.

References

25 Glover G, Evision F (2013). *Hospital Admissions that Should not Happen: Admissions for Ambulatory Care Sensitive Conditions for People with Learning Disabilities in England*. Improving Health and Lives: Department of Health: London.
26 Royal College of Nursing (2013). *Meeting the Health Needs of People with Learning Disabilities*. Royal College of Nursing: London. ℘ www.rcn.org.uk/professional-development/publications/pub-003024 (accessed 30 October 2017).
27 Emerson E, Copeland A, Glover G (2011). *The Uptake of Health Checks for Adults with Learning Disabilities: 2008/9 to 2010/11*. Improving Health and Lives: Learning Disabilities Observatory: London.
28 Cummings S (2012). How to tell whether patients can make decisions about their care. *Emergency Nurse*. 20: 22–6.

Dental services

Oral health, including dental health, is important in a number of ways, e.g. the presence of well-developed teeth in making it possible for people to eat a well-balanced diet, for clear speech, and confidence in one's appearance and smile. Good oral health is also important in preventing gum disease, halitosis (foul-smelling breath), dental pain, and mouth ulcers. Proactive steps to maintaining good dental and oral health include the eating of a well-balanced diet, an adequate intake of fluids, brushing teeth after meals, and regular check-ups by a dentist, in which they can examine the development and soundness of teeth and gums (see ➲ Dentists, pp. 368–9).

However, for many people with intellectual disabilities, achieving the above activities is difficult without practical support. The challenge to maintaining healthy teeth and gums can arise when some people may find it difficult to brush their teeth effectively, are unable to eat orally, have irregularly placed teeth that need specific dental interventions, or find it difficult to cooperate with dental examination or treatment.[29]

While most dental surgeries are based within community settings, it can be difficult to have people with intellectual disabilities who require dental treatment to be seen in a community-based dentist, if they or the dentist have any concerns about their own ability to manage or about other difficulties that may arise during examination or treatments. There can be long delays for people with intellectual disabilities in accessing dental services for major dental work, and often these are provided within hospital dental departments and involve the use of a general anaesthetic. In order to minimize the need for such a service and the associated risks, it is important that carers for people with intellectual disabilities encourage effective dental and oral health from a young age.

Preparing for an appointment

It is helpful for people with intellectual disabilities to have accessible information about services[30] and to meet a dentist and surgery staff before intervention is required as an emergency when they are in pain. Pre-appointment visits/pre-assessment at the dental surgery to meet the staff, sit in the dentist chair, experience some of the smells and noises of the dental surgery, and let the dentist look in their mouth and touch their gums (as well as applying a local anaesthetic) can be a worthwhile investment of time and should provide an opportunity to develop cooperative relationships and to reinforce positive behaviour for the person with intellectual disabilities, their carers, and staff within the dental surgery. The use of a 'health passport' may also be helpful in sharing important information about the person's abilities and needs with staff in the dental surgery.

If a visit to the surgery is not possible due to distance, time, or other issues, then a 'photographic tour' of the dental surgery may be possible. This could involve using a series of photographs of staff or a video tour of waiting rooms, chairs, some equipment, e.g. overhead examination light, and toothbrushes, as well as explaining that dentists may wear gloves and eye protectors, and nearby locations to familiarize the person with staff and location before they attend (see Easyhealth link under ➲ Further reading).

Support during contact

The requirements for valid consent apply to examination and treatment, and therefore it is important that this has been obtained prior to attending the dental surgery and confirmed when there. While parents may give consent for children under 18yrs (see ➜ Consent to examination, treatment, and care, pp. 506–7, and ➜ Vulnerability, pp. 280–1), good practice would seek to have all children involved in this process, because in reality, parental consent will be of little practical use if the person will not cooperate with the dentist.

People with intellectual disabilities do not seek to be difficult patients; therefore, a lack of cooperation should be explored and actively responded to. Carers should explain to the dentist how the person receiving treatment shows signs of distress and to monitor carefully for these, responding promptly with ongoing encouragement, an explanation of what is required, break in treatment, and, if necessary, further anaesthesia/analgesia. Active cooperation while in the dentist chair will also increase the prospects of establishing a pattern of regular visits and opportunities for proactive treatment and good dental and oral health.

Support after an appointment

Many visits to the dentist will not result in post-appointment pain, indeed it may relieve pain. However, care is needed in supporting people who have received anaesthesia, which will have numbed part of their mouth or cheek, to ensure they do not injure this. It is also important to assist the person with intellectual disabilities to follow the instructions they have received about eating and drinking hot and cold foods, care of the teeth that have been treated and dental sockets after treatment, and the use of pain relief. Opportunities should also be used for reinforcing success with the person with intellectual disabilities and the dental surgery staff.

Further reading

Oral Health Foundation. *Dental Care for People with Special Needs.* ℘ www.dentalhealth.org/tell-me-about/topic/caring-for-teeth/dental-care-for-people-with-special-needs (accessed 30 October 2017).

Turner S, Emerson E, Glover G (2012). *Making Reasonable Adjustments to Dentistry Services for People with Learning Disabilities.* ℘ webarchive.nationalarchives.gov.uk/20160704162752/http://www.improvinghealthandlives.org.uk/securefiles/160704_1732//IHaL-RA-2012-02.pdf (accessed 30 October 2017).

References

29 British Society for Disability and Oral Health/Faculty of Dental Surgery (2012). *Clinical Guidelines and Integrated Care Pathways for the Oral Health Care of People with Learning Disabilities.* British Society for Disability and Oral Health/Faculty of Dental Surgery: London. ℘ www.rcseng.ac.uk/library-and-publications/college-publications/docs/oral-health-care/ (accessed 30 October 2017).

30 Easyhealth. *Going to the Dentist (leaflets).* ℘ www.easyhealth.org.uk/listing/going-to-the-dentist-(leaflets) (accessed 30 October 2017).

Mental health services

Introduction

Although people with intellectual disability have higher rates of mental disorders, they still find difficulty in accessing mental healthcare, with many only being picked up or coming to the attention of services during a crisis, leading to a negative experience. National policies across the UK and the Republic of Ireland have stated for over a decade that people with intellectual disabilities have the right and should access general mental health services in line with the wider population. This policy is not without apprehension, from professionals in both general mental health and intellectual disabilities services, and joint work is required to enable general mental health achieved through this policy requirement.

Current policy also recognizes that some people will require specialist intellectual disabilities services for their mental health, although most people could and will use general mental health services with or without extra support.

There is a changing role for intellectual disabilities services, moving towards a tertiary role, in that they will offer expertise, support, and facilitate movement within and between services by providing advice and support to general mental health services.[31] There are still issues in accessing general mental health services, and the main ones are discussed below, along with ideas on how they can be addressed.

Supporting people with intellectual disabilities to access mental healthcare

Regardless of the care setting, there are a number of things that can be done to improve access to services. Table 10.1 offers practical advice on reasonable adjustments. Although this is for a community or out-patient setting, these measures can also be adapted to inpatient services.[32]

Table 10.1 Supporting access in mental healthcare

Reasonable adjustment	Rationale
Longer appointment times	To facilitate improved communication and comprehension
Appointment times at the beginning or end of the day	To avoid long waiting times or busy waiting rooms which can increase anxiety
Accessible information	To aid comprehension
Preparedness of person with intellectual disabilities and staff supporting them. Understand what the appointment is for, bring all relevant information and any communication aids or accessible information that could assist the consultation	To improve quality of consultation and enable comprehensive exchange of information to inform diagnosis, care, and treatment
Talking directly to the person with intellectual disabilities and only later clarifying with carers or family	To value and involve the person with intellectual disabilities and provide person-centred care

Table 10.1 (Contd.)

Reasonable adjustment	Rationale
Anchoring events, i.e. take your medicine after the late night news or 'remember when we did X ... ', rather than saying '4 weeks ago ... '	To enable improved communication
Environment—free from background noise, flicking lights, and medical equipment that is not required	To reduce anxiety and improve receptive communication
Check that the person has understood what you have said by asking them to explain it back to you	To check comprehension and avoid acquiescence
If using complex or technical words, check that you both have the same understanding of what is meant by that word	To avoid misdiagnosis or diagnostic overshadowing and to facilitate communication
Consider using pictures or symbols to augment verbal communication	To aid comprehension
Make the environment as friendly and predictable as possible, or complete the assessment at a venue in which person feels most comfortable	To reduce anxiety and increase rapport
Ask the same questions in different ways at different times during the appointment	To check comprehension and avoid acquiescence
Ensure that you fully understand what the concerns or difficulties are and that you fully understand what is normal for the person with intellectual disabilities Act on any changes that are reported, and consider possible physical or mental health diagnoses	To avoid diagnostic overshadowing and ensure timely access to appropriate healthcare
Conduct a thorough assessment of mental and physical health, which could include: • Physical examination and appropriate investigations • Medication history (neuroleptics, antihypertensives, steroids, etc.) • adverse effects of drugs (including antidepressants) • assessment to exclude other differential diagnoses Risk assessment (for both self-harm, self-neglect, harm to others, and adult safeguarding) is important	Differential diagnosis and diagnostic overshadowing Sometimes people with intellectual disabilities can experience different or 'atypical' signs and symptoms of illnesses or they seek help at a late stage of an illness which makes it appear different to what it might usually This can mean that serious illness is not diagnosed or incorrectly diagnosed, leading to delays in treatment

References

31 Chaplin E, Paschos D, O'Hara J, *et al.* (2010). Mental ill-health and care pathways in adults with intellectual disability across different residential types. *Research in Developmental Disabilities.* 31: 458–63.

32 Chaplin E, Marshall-Tate K, Hardy S (2016). *A Mental Health Guide for Those Supporting People with Intellectual Disabilities.* Pavilion Publishing: Brighton.

Maternity services

Maternity services are an important part of the range of health services available to members of the general public and are located within primary care, in health centres and GP services, and within maternity units linked to general hospitals. Maternity services are provided by GPs, midwives, and obstetricians and may also include ultrasonographers (who undertake ultrasound scans).

In a small number of services, the care of mothers and their partners may be provided by midwives, when it is anticipated that the pregnancy and birth will be uncomplicated; these units are sometimes referred to as 'midwifery-led units'. HVs often have a role to play in supporting new parents and usually meet with prospective parents during antenatal preparation.

Supporting inclusive maternity care

Recognizing the desire for parenthood

It is now recognized that some people with intellectual disabilities wish to be parents and therefore will require access to maternity services. People with intellectual disabilities, as prospective mothers and fathers, should have equity of access to maternity services.

Supporting consent to examination, treatment, and care

During contact with maternity services, prospective parents will be provided with a lot of new and unfamiliar information and choices on things ranging from choices of antenatal screening, various examinations that may be necessary, and their plans for the birth of the child.

Nurses within intellectual disabilities services would work collaboratively with their colleagues in maternity services to facilitate informed decision-making and to ensure that the requirements for consent to examination, treatment, and care are fulfilled (see ➔ Consent to examination, treatment, and care, pp. 506–7, and ➔ Vulnerability, pp. 280–1). There are a range of accessible resources that can support reasonable adjustments in how the service is delivered (See Easyhealth link under ➔ Further reading).

Developing agreed communication links

Nurses within intellectual disabilities services can have an integral role in supporting people in accessing services, through providing information about local services and encouraging people to consider their needs for antenatal care and education (see ➔ Parenting groups, pp. 366–7). They should also develop clear communication links with midwives in their local services and work collaboratively with them to support people with intellectual disabilities in making effective use of local maternity services, including antenatal and postnatal services.

Within each locality, identified nurses from within intellectual disabilities services could become the link to a designated midwife within maternity services. Staff could meet on a regular basis, once every 2–3 months, to discuss the strengths of each of the services and what their respective colleagues could bring to supporting women and men using maternity services.

Developing accessible information

Nurses and midwives could share examples of good practice such as accessible information, and revised protocols that are effective in making services accessible for people with intellectual disabilities can be identified and shared across intellectual disability and maternity services (see ➡ Providing information, pp. 64–5). It is important to remember when developing accessible information that this may also be useful with other people who have difficulty in understanding written English.

Establishing recognized links between local intellectual disability and maternity services will also provide a clear point of contact if any concerns or emergencies involving people with intellectual disabilities arise within maternity services. The suggestion of links between designated people within both services is to support the development of nurses and midwives who could be resource people for other professionals within the services which are seeking to support people with intellectual disabilities, rather than to support a designated midwife for people within intellectual disabilities who are expecting a baby, as this may place unnecessary restrictions on the parents' choice of midwife.

A balanced approach

It is important that a person's choice to have a baby is respected; however, if there are any indications that an assault, abuse, or exploitation has occurred, these should be discussed openly with the person and considered within local policy guidelines under the protection of vulnerable adults.

While some people seek to become pregnant, nurses within intellectual disabilities services, as well as midwives and HVs, should also be alert to the risk of exploitation and abuse of women with intellectual disabilities that would result in a pregnancy. Staff should also remain alert to the possibility of the exploitation or abuse of men. Irrespective of the origins of the pregnancy, if the woman's decision with capacity is to continue with the pregnancy, they will need to have supported access to maternity services.

Further reading

Best Beginnings. ℘ www.bestbeginnings.org.uk/parents-with-learning-disabilities (accessed 30 October 2017).

Evans R (2015). *Hidden Voices of Maternity. Parents with Learning Disabilities Speak Out.* Kings Fund: London. ℘ www.kingsfund.org.uk/sites/files/kf/media/Ruth_Evans.pdf (accessed 30 October 2017).

Porter P, Kidd G, Murray N, Uytman C, Spink A, Anderson A (2012). Developing the pregnancy support pack for people who have a learning disability. *British Journal of Learning Disabilities.* **40**: 310–17.

Planning for contact with general health services

As noted in the earlier sections of this chapter, people with intellectual disabilities may seek access to a range of services from primary care, secondary care, and specialist services. As citizens of the country, they should have equity of access to all health services (including mental health services; see ➋ Mental health services, pp. 398–9). There is a legal requirement on services to make 'reasonable adjustments' when people are unable to access services in the usual way. Failure to do so may result in a legal challenge of unlawful discrimination against health services.

Persistent challenges

It has been found that access to healthcare for people with intellectual disabilities can be much harder due to factors such as;
- Failure to make reasonable adjustments to support people with intellectual disabilities in accessing and using services;
- The views of parents and carers of people with intellectual disabilities are often ignored by healthcare professionals;
- Staff in general healthcare have limited knowledge about people with intellectual disabilities and often hold negative stereotypical attitudes about the limited abilities of people with intellectual disabilities;
- Staff in general healthcare services are not familiar with what help they should provide or from whom to get expert advice;
- Limited collaborative working occurs between staff in intellectual disabilities services and general healthcare services.[33,34]

Planning for contact

Most contact between people with intellectual and general healthcare services is known about in advance by staff and family carers. This contact is often in the context of appointments within primary care services, out-patient appointments, planned day-case admissions for minor procedures (e.g. dental treatment), or planned admission to a ward. In contrast, while people within intellectual disabilities may present specific challenges when admitted as an emergency,[34] such contact is less frequent.

Therefore, on most occasions, opportunities exist to plan more effectively for contact in advance. Practical steps that can be taken to increase the likelihood of a successful outcome are as follows:
- Staff in health services should ask if a 'health passport' exists and make use of the information contained within it.
- Staff in intellectual disabilities services should exchange names, address, telephone, email details, and emergency contact arrangements with key colleagues in primary care, mental health, or general hospitals services.
- The person requesting the appointment/admission should identify that this individual may have additional needs and what these may include.
- Information should be provided to people with intellectual disabilities and parents/carers about what they can expect when in contact with general health services.

- The above information should be presented in accessible formats and provide contact details for key staff in both intellectual and general health services who may be able to organize support.
- The procedures for making appointments should take account of the extra time that may be needed to complete the necessary examination and treatment.
- Consideration should be given to the need to reduce the usual level of examination/treatment and to plan this over subsequent contacts, rather than trying to complete it all in one session.
- Appointments should be provided at the start of a clinic session where this is convenient to people with intellectual disabilities, to increase the likelihood that the person is seen promptly.
- Staff in intellectual disabilities services should work collaboratively with their colleagues in general healthcare to assess additional support needed to ensure an appointment or admission is successful.
- Attention should be given to the practicalities of transport to and from the health service, parking, access to the building/room, and any toilet/ changing facilities that may be required. Reasonable adjustments should be identified in advance and the necessary arrangements put in place.
- At the end of the contact, the success of the arrangements should be reviewed and arrangements built upon for any subsequent contact.
- Feedback should be provided to staff, highlighting and reinforcing areas of good practice.

Further reading

Iacono T, Bigby C, Carolyn U, Douglas J, Fitzpatrick P (2014). A systematic review of hospital experiences of people with intellectual disability. BMC Health Services Research. 14: 505.

MacArthur J, Brown M, McKechanie A, Mack S, Hayes M, Fletcher MA (2015). Making reasonable and achievable adjustments: the contributions of learning disability liaison nurses in 'getting it right' for people with learning disabilities receiving general hospitals care. Journal of Advanced Nursing. 71: 1552–63.

Regulation and Quality Improvement Authority (2014). Review of Implementation of GAIN Guidelines on Caring for People with a Learning Disability in General Hospital Settings. Regulation and Quality Improvement Authority: Belfast. rqia.org.uk/RQIA/files/69/6992f0a9-b602-4832-ace7-e505d6dc1125.pdf (accessed 30 October 2017).

References

33 Michael J (2008). Healthcare for All: Report of the Independent Inquiry into Access to Healthcare for People with Learning Disabilities. Department of Health: London.

34 Heslop P, Blair P, Fleming P, Houghton M, Marriott A, Russ L (2013). Confidential Inquiry into Premature Deaths of People with Learning Disabilities (CIPOLD). Norah Fry Research Centre: Bristol. www.bris.ac.uk/cipold/fullfinalreport.pdf (accessed 30 October 2017).

Discharge planning

People with intellectual disabilities have greater health needs in relation to both acute and chronic illness, in comparison to the general population and, as such, are higher users of healthcare. Although they are admitted to general hospitals more often than the wider population, they actually spend less time within general hospitals and are discharged relatively quickly, though not necessarily appropriately.[35]

If an individual's care is complete, then delaying discharge poses a risk to the individual's safety, including the risk of infection, pressure ulcers, reduced independence, and depression.[36] Delayed discharge (also known as delayed transfer or bed blocking) is the term used to describe the fact that a person remains within the general hospital, even though they are medically fit for discharge, and this is often associated with incomplete plans for continuing care arrangements.[37] Conversely, if they are discharged too early in their care, there is a significant risk to their health and safety such as inappropriate preparation for home and early readmission.[35,36]

Discharge from hospital should be seen as a process, and not an end in itself, where discharge planning is ongoing, involving the individual, their family, and the interdisciplinary team. Although most people will be involved in their planned discharge, people with intellectual disabilities and their families/carers often experience problems with the discharge process.

The key principle underpinning an effective discharge is the partnership approach with patients and families, to plan discharge.[36] Many people with intellectual disabilities will be supported within the community by their families or paid carers, so advanced information is needed to prepare for the discharge. If the environment to which the person is transferred is unprepared, it may be an unsafe environment.

Preparing for discharge

Ten steps in effective discharge planning which can be adapted to any hospital setting are:[36]

- Start planning for discharge or transfer before or on admission. This is often supported through communications with the liaison nurse (if there is one in the hospital);
- The recognition of the role of the family/carers is key to effective discharge. Information should be gained from them about the best way to support the patient through their hospital journey, including their discharge. Identify whether the patient has simple or complex discharge and transfer planning needs, involving the patient and carer in your decision;
- The use of the HAP or hospital passport is critical to this understanding and person-centred approach. If the individual is in receipt of a care package, then the appropriate community support needs to be involved regarding admission and discharge;
- Develop a clinical management plan for every patient within 24 hours of admission. This should be in collaboration with the person with intellectual disabilities and family/carers and the multidisciplinary team;
- Coordination of the discharge or transfer of care process through effective leadership and handover of responsibilities at ward level;

- Set an expected date of discharge or transfer within 24–48 hours of admission, and discuss this with the patient and carer. The adult patient needs to be seen as an individual, with the right to be autonomous in decisions about his/her healthcare;
- Review the clinical management plan with the patient each day; take any necessary action, and update progress towards the discharge or transfer date;
- Involve patients and carers, so that they can make informed decisions and choices that deliver a personalized care pathway and maximize their independence;
- Discharges and transfers should take place over 7 days to deliver continuity of care for the patient;
- Use a discharge checklist 24–48 hours prior to transfer to identify any issues /concerns.

Information to support discharge should be provided in a timely fashion and in a format that the individual understands. People with intellectual disabilities and their families should, on discharge, have:

- Information on their diagnosis and any treatment given in a format that is understood by them;
- Clear advice on any treatment regime they need to follow at home;
- A contact number, should they require further advice or support;
- An evaluation of their understanding prior to discharge;
- An awareness of, and links with, the CLDT and, where possible, the liaison nurse.

Planning for discharge should be an integral aspect of care planning, and it is important for nurses within the clinical environment to ensure that good discharge plans are put in place. This can be facilitated through good working relations with the patient, carer, and multidisciplinary team, to promote good clinical outcomes and a safe discharge.[36]

Further reading

Pellett C (2016). *Discharge Planning: Best Practice in Transitions of Care*. The Queens Nursing Institute: London. ℘ www.qni.org.uk/wp-content/uploads/2016/09/discharge_planning_report_2015.pdf (accessed 30 October 2017).

References

35 Michael J (2008). *Healthcare for All: A report of the Independent Inquiry into Access to Healthcare for People with Learning Disabilities*. HMSO: London.
36 Department of Health (2010). *Ready to Go? Planning the Discharge and the Transfer of Patients from Hospital and Intermediate Care*. Department of Health: London.
37 Devapriam J, Gangadharan S, Pither J, Critchfield M (2014). Delayed discharge from intellectual disability in-patient units. *Psychiatric Bulletin*. 38: 211–15.

Palliative care

Noticing that someone is ill

People with intellectual disabilities may not recognize changes in their bodies that are indicators of potential palliative conditions. Additionally, some may lack the verbal repertoire to explain any associated discomfort and to identify changes in usual habits (such as eating, elimination, and/or weight loss), and thus some conditions may go unrecognized. Carers need to remain watchful in anticipation of such changes, which otherwise might go unnoticed in people with intellectual disabilities. Timely reporting of any suspicious changes to the person with intellectual disabilities must be reported promptly to their GP to reduce such late diagnosis and a poorer prognosis.

End of life

When disease is deemed to be advanced, progressive, and life-limiting, the focus of care should be on comfort and quality of life. End-of-life care supports people with an advanced, progressive, incurable illness to live as well as possible until they die. It 'enables the supportive and palliative care needs of both patient and family to be identified and met throughout the last phase of life and into bereavement'.[38]

Palliative care

Palliative care is described as active, holistic care, in which management of pain and other symptoms and provision of psychological, social, and spiritual support are paramount. It aims to affirm life and regards dying as a normal process—offering a support system to help patients and their families live as actively as possible until death—and, as such, is an important part of the nursing care of all those involved with the patient who has been diagnosed with a life-limiting condition. Such care can be delivered to patients in their own homes, in hospitals, and in hospice settings, supported by those healthcare professionals who specialize in palliative care.

Specialist palliative care

Specialist palliative care nurses provide advice, alongside the patient's own clinical team. They work in community, hospital, hospice, or care home settings, providing specialist advice in order to prevent or relieve suffering associated with a life-limiting illness. This may include advice regarding pain and symptom control or other problems relating to the patient's physical, psychosocial, or spiritual needs. However, studies indicate that healthcare professionals who specialize in palliative care may have little experience in caring for people with intellectual disabilities and will require advice, education, and support from the family and nurses for people with intellectual disabilities.[39]

Palliative care for people with intellectual disabilities

At the heart of good palliative care is a holistic assessment, which may prove difficult when the patient has intellectual disabilities. The DisDAT tool uses behavioural observations to assess distress in individuals who have limited verbal communication skills.[40] Similarly, the checklist 'Planning ahead to manage pain and distress confidently' helps carers to be proactive in identifying care strategies.[41] Nurses may be reliant on familiar carers to interpret symptoms and recognize indicators of distress and promote reciprocal communication, thus enhancing high-standard, individualized palliative care and support. Living with a life-limiting condition will bring a number of issues and problems, both for the patient and their family, which may change over time as the illness progresses and death approaches. It is important that the nurse identifies and anticipates any changes and is able to:

- Recognize and assess the holistic needs of the patient and the family in relation to their physical, psychological, social, spiritual, and informational needs;
- Provide the appropriate care and support to meet those needs within the limits of their own knowledge, skills, and competence in palliative care;
- Understand when they need to seek advice or refer to the specialist palliative care service;
- Collaborate with specialist palliative care services, families, and other health and social care professionals, in order to meet all of the needs of the patient with intellectual disabilities who has a life-limiting condition;
- Promote the concepts inherent in ACP;
- Apply the principles of the five key priorities for care.[42]

End-of-life care must be relevant to the patient's normal way of life, with an emphasis on quality of life. For the patient with intellectual disabilities, this will require a careful and collaborative approach by those healthcare professionals involved in the patient's care. See also ➲ Support associated with loss and bereavement, pp. 140–2.

Further reading

NHS England, PCPLD Network. *Delivering High Quality End of Life Care for People who have a Learning Disability*. ℰ www.england.nhs.uk/wp-content/uploads/2017/08/delivering-end-of-life-care-for-people-with-learning-disability.pdf (accessed 14 March 2018).

Tuffrey-Wijne I, McLaughlin D, Curfs L, et al. (2015). Defining consensus norms for palliative care of people with intellectual disabilities in Europe, using Delphi methods: a White Paper from the European Association of Palliative Care. *Palliative Medicine*. 30: 446–55. ℰ www.eapcnet.eu/LinkClick.aspx?fileticket=lym7SMB78cw%3D (accessed 30 October 2017).

References

38 National Council for Palliative Care (2007). *Palliative Care Explained*. ℰ www.ncpc.org.uk (accessed 30 October 2017).

39 Tuffrey-Wijne I, McEnhill L, Curfs L, et al. (2007). Palliative care provision for people with intellectual disabilities: interviews with specialist palliative care professionals in London. *Journal of Palliative Medicine*. 21: 493–9.

40 Regnard C, Mathews D, Gibson L (2003). Difficulties in identifying distress and its causes in people with severe communication problems. *Journal of Palliative Nursing*. 9: 173–6.

41 Brown H, Burns S, Flynn M (2005). *Dying Matters: A Workbook on Caring for People with Learning Disabilities who are Dying*. Mental Health Foundation: London.

42 Department of Health and Social Care (2014). *Liverpool Care Pathway Review: Response to Recommendations. One Chance to Get it Right*. ℰ www.gov.uk/government/publications/liverpool-care-pathway-review-response-to-recommendations (accessed 30 October 2017).

Continence advisors

Continence advisors are qualified nurses who have undertaken further education in the area of continence and are available within local health services. Their primary role is to support people with bladder and bowel problems, promoting continence and the management of incontinence. The continence advisor works together with the person with continence problems, their carers, and other health professionals, providing education and specific advice and equipment to enable the person and relevant others to effectively manage the problem. Continence advisors will normally offer services such as continence clinics, community prostate assessment, continence product advice, and education programmes. They will also be able to assist with aspects of continence such as pelvic floor exercises, postoperative bladder or bowel problems, constipation, and advice regarding toilet training.

Working in partnership

Nurses for people with intellectual disabilities will often have an in-depth knowledge of continence, with many undergoing further training in this area. It is important, however, to work in partnership with the continence advisor and build solid working relationships to ensure the person with intellectual disabilities is able to benefit from the wide range of knowledge, skills, and services available within the primary care.

Continence

Acquiring continence is a complex process; we are all born without bladder and bowel control and need to learn the necessary control and the socially acceptable places to go.

To achieve continence, we need to:
• Recognize the need to urinate or defecate;
• Identify the right place to go;
• Be able to reach the place;
• Hold on until the place can be reached;
• Pass urine or faeces once there.

Incontinence is a major problem for some people with intellectual disabilities and, while manageable when the child is small, becomes a major difficulty for parents as the person grows. It can also result in a lot of embarrassment and become a restriction on opportunities for inclusive family social events due to the risk of incontinence and challenges in finding suitable changing facilities, in particular for adults and for the disposal of incontinence products.

Promoting continence

It is important that incontinence is not accepted as inevitable just because the person has intellectual disabilities. It is clear that becoming continent will be difficult for many people, but it is important that every person is supported, using the usual 'toilet training' techniques where possible.

Communication

It is important to think about the language you use when talking to people and/or their carers about their continence problems. Remember this can be embarrassing and people may not use or know the correct terms; ask people what terms they use, and try to use these, if appropriate, when talking about their problems.

Aids, adaptations, and equipment

- The continence advisor will have a wide knowledge of the range of aids and equipment that are available from specialist companies and will be able to advise people on the most appropriate type to help to effectively manage their problem. These are often available for trial from the local services to aid independent living.
- All-in-one continence products are available for children and adults with a learning disability and can be accessed following an assessment from either a HV/continence advisor or a learning disability nurse.
- Specialist seating or toileting aids—these are available following an assessment from an OT.

Further reading

ERIC (The Children's Bowel and Bladder Charity) ℗ www.eric.org.uk (accessed 30 October 2017).
NHS England (2015). *Excellence in Continence Care: Practical Guidance for Commissioners, Providers, Health and Social Care Staff and Information for the Public*. NHS England: Reading. ℗ www.england. nhs.uk/commissioning/wp-content/uploads/sites/12/2015/11/EICC-guidance-final-document. pdf (accessed 30 October 2017).

Epilepsy nurse

The aim of epilepsy management is to maximize the individual's quality of life. An interdisciplinary/agency approach is essential: individual, parents, relatives, friends, and carers. Individuals who have intellectual disabilities and epilepsy should have access to the same specialist services as those in the general population, including epilepsy specialist nurses (ESNs).[43] Access to the ESN can depend on who manages the person's epilepsy from a medical perspective and the available services in the area. Not all individuals with intellectual disabilities who have epilepsy attend regional neurology services; their epilepsy may be managed within intellectual disabilities services, some of which have specialist epilepsy clinics. However, this varies across regions; others are managed in primary care.

Qualifications and skills

It is acknowledged that all registered nurses in intellectual disabilities are involved in supporting individuals to manage their epilepsy, joint working is essential between the role of both the registered nurse and the ESN services, given the potential complexities epilepsy and associated comorbidities.[44] ESNs are experienced registered nurses who have undertaken further specific post-registration training; qualifications held range from post-registration certificates to diploma, degree, or Masters in epilepsy. Research has shown that ESNs can lead to improvements in epilepsy care, illustrated by greater accessibility, time afforded to conduct a holistic assessment, provision of knowledgeable clinical interventions, and continuity of care, enabling the development of the therapeutic relationship between nurse and client/carer.[45] Increasingly, ESNs are independent and supplementary prescribers, allowing for more timely treatment changes. The ESN, depending on the service, will normally assess and review clients via epilepsy nurse-led clinics, telephone review, or home visits and/or relevant facilities with which the individual comes into contact.

Key principles in supporting people with epilepsy who have intellectual disabilities

- Person-centred approach;
- Accessibility to appropriate specialist services when required and continuity of healthcare;
- Promoting self-management;
- Advocating, educating, and communicating for, and on behalf of, individuals.

Role of the nurse for people with epilepsy

- *Clinical:*
  - *Holistic assessment*—to ensure proper diagnosis: using in-depth knowledge and communication skills to obtain accurate information from the individual, their family, and carers. May include: direct observation, requesting and/or enabling detailed recording, video-recording under the best interests pathway, explanation, and use of resources to enable investigative procedures (EEG, video telemetry);

- *On diagnosis of epilepsy*—provide accurate and appropriate information and advice to the individual and their family/carers to increase understanding of the condition, encouraging healthy lifestyle choices to improve seizure control and quality of life, e.g. advice on diet, recreation, alcohol. Use of counselling skills to support the individual and their family to assist the person to adapt to the changes this may create;
- *Enable timely and appropriate introduction and continuation of treatment regimens*—may include independent and supplementary prescribing where the ESN is a qualified prescriber, liaison with primary/secondary care and family/support services, as required. Provision of titration schedules, information about prescribed medication: possible adverse effects, available formulae relevant to needs. Promotion of adherence to treatment and self-administration: monitored dosage system, drug wallets, reminder systems, use of mobile phone/specialist apps. Review of response to treatment and possible adverse effects; accessible point of contact: telephone/email. Advice with respect to emergency medication if prescribed and agreeing relevant emergency management plans, as required, with the multidisciplinary team;
- *Support interdisciplinary/interagency services*—promote a balanced approach that reduces risk and maximizes opportunities, with consideration to consent, choice, and capacity: agreeing relevant epilepsy management plans, undertaking specific risk assessments, and agreeing risk management guidelines, in conjunction with the multidisciplinary team, e.g. need for a helmet, alarms, bathing, work opportunities, social activities. See also staff training in the following point.
- *Education*: establishing, provision, and review of epilepsy training programmes for interdisciplinary/interagency personnel, e.g. nurses—pre- and post-registration programmes, social care staff, education, and employers. Training programmes include epilepsy awareness and emergency management of seizures using rescue medication in the community.
- *Practice development*: the ESN ensures evidence-based practice in their own service but also collaborates with colleagues across intellectual disabilities nursing services to improve outcomes for individuals and their families/carers. Will include research and audit and is at local, regional, and national levels.

References

43 National Institute for Health and Care Excellence (2012, updated February 2016). *Epilepsies: Diagnosis and Management. Clinical Guideline.* www.nice.org.uk/guidance/cg137/resources/epilepsies-diagnosis-and-management-35109515407813 (accessed 30 October 2017).
44 Epilepsy Nurses Association (ESNA) (2013). *The Learning Disability Epilepsy Specialist Nurse Competency Framework.* www.esna-online.org.uk/ (accessed 30 October 2017).
45 Department of Health (2001). *Valuing People: A Strategy for People with Learning Disabilities for the 21st Century.* Department of Health: London.

Dementia nurse

Staff supporting people with dementia require specific knowledge, training, creativity, and insight. Rather than a 'medical model of care', a bio-psycho-social approach focused on the holistic needs of the person is needed,[46] offering a person-centred culture, acknowledging that people with dementia require emotional, social, psychological, and physical support, to maintain their quality of life.

With increased evidence of dementia in people with intellectual disability and unique, complex issues around screening, assessment, diagnosis, care, and end of life, advanced-level nursing posts are critical to supporting a person-centred nursing perspective that recognizes each person with dementia as unique, experiencing and responding differently to the challenges inherent in dementia (see ➔ Dementia, pp. 138–9).

McCarron[47] contends that addressing the care needs of people with intellectual disabilities and dementia requires leadership, a multidimensional approach, and the development of a strategic plan, which incorporates:

- Routine baseline screening, comprehensive diagnostic work-up, and consensus diagnosis, operationalized through a memory clinic model;
- The development of a continuum of residential options to support the changing needs of the person and their carer at different stages of dementia;
- Appropriate dementia-specific day programmes;
- Training and education for staff, family, and peers;
- Evidence-based research to guide practice and policy.

Standards for care[48] are also emerging as the basis for developing appropriate educational pathways to equip nurses to respond to this advanced role. Advanced and specialist nurses who have emerged within intellectual disabilities services are able to respond to dementia care challenges, develop the needed services with providers, and address problems highlighted nationally and internationally, including:

- Lack of screening and the tendency for late diagnosis;
- Implementing effective supportive interventions to address and minimize common behaviours, which challenge in dementia;
- Addressing and diagnosing health comorbidities in order to maximize health and well-being;
- Addressing end-of-life and palliative care needs of persons with end-stage terminal dementia, including support of peers, staff, and family members.[49]

Nurses with specialist training in intellectual disabilities and dementia have the following roles, and dementia-specific services for people with intellectual disabilities have begun to emerge.[50]

- *Clinical*—screenings, operation of memory clinics, work with interdisciplinary teams, and support of primary care teams and families in the diagnosis and management of symptoms of dementia.
- *Education and training*—direct delivery and support for training for professional carers, families, peers, and interdisciplinary team members on all aspects of dementia and dementia care, and supporting clinical sites for nursing students.

- *Advocacy*—negotiating the full range of support for persons with dementia and their families, including grief and bereavement support.
- *Audit and research*—participation and leadership in clinical audits, giving people with intellectual access to evidence-based interventions emerging from the dementia field, and contributing to the development of effective interventions.
- *Consultancy*—acting as a specialist resource on dementia care.

Nurses are in a prime position to advocate for, and coordinate, interdisciplinary approaches that maximize the capability of the person and their quality of life through a seamless person-centred model of care delivery.

References

46 Kitwood T (1997). *Dementia Reconsidered: The Person Comes First*. Open University Press: Buckingham.

47 McCarron M (2005). *A Strategic Plan on Dementia, Daughters of Charity Service*. Trinity College: Dublin (unpublished).

48 McCarron M, Reilly E (2010). *Supporting Persons with Intellectual Disabilities and Dementia: Quality Dementia Care Standards*. Daughters of Charity: Dublin.

49 Jokinen N, Janicki MP, Keller S, McCallion P, Force LT (2013). Guidelines for structuring community care and supports for people with intellectual disabilities affected by dementia. *Journal of Policy and Practice in Intellectual disabilities*. **10**: 1–24.

50 McCarron M, McCallion P, Reilly E, Mulryan N (2014). Responding to the challenges of service development to address dementia needs for people with an intellectual disability. In: K Watchman, ed. *Intellectual Disability and Dementia: Research into Practice*. Jessica Kingsley Publishers: London: pp. 241–69.

Child and adolescent services

Team around the child

Children with disabilities are children first and, as such, should have their needs met within child and adolescent services. Good practice guidance (such as the NSF[51] to the National Autistic Society 'You Need to Know' campaign[52]) suggests that children with disabilities should be seen by practitioners who have specialist training and who understand the particular needs of this client group. Practitioners are encouraged to work in partnership with parents/carers and with other professionals who know the child well and to form a team around that child to meet their needs most effectively. These may take the form of real teams, e.g. multi-agency child development teams or virtual ones, e.g. all professionals involved with a child reviewing their progress at school in the annual review.

Person-centred planning

It is important, wherever possible, to hear from the child themselves and to take a person-centred approach to planning intervention and service delivery. Depending on the child's needs, adapted methods of communication may be required to access the child's voice in these meetings (e.g. use of visuals or augmented communication devices).

Education healthcare plans

In the UK, education healthcare plans (EHCPs) (see government website)[51] are awarded to children with significant additional needs and, unlike the previous 'Statement of Special Educational Needs', an EHCP should include set goals for each child's health and social care, as well as their education. EHCPs are reviewed on an annual basis and last until the young person turns 25.

Diagnosis and sharing the news

Those working in children's services may inevitably be involved in the diagnosis of disability, from Down syndrome and autism to rare genetic conditions. Those involved in having to share this news with families can follow supportive guidance issued by charities such as Scope[53] to think about how they communicate in the most sensitive and supportive manner with parents/carers. There is also guidance for talking to young people (e.g. the National Autistic Society website[52] contains information on discussing autism with children and young people). Linking families to local support networks post-diagnosis is vital. Currently, each local authority has a 'local offer' on their website containing information on everything, from condition-specific support groups to Disability Living Allowance.

Positive behaviour plans

Many children with disabilities will present to services with challenging behaviour. NICE[54] has recently issued guidelines on the management of challenging behaviour which highlight that children's behaviour will have a communicative function. The Challenging Behaviour Foundation[55] has a wealth of downloadable resources, including information on how to produce a positive behaviour support (PBS) plan for children whose behaviour challenges the services. The PBS plan looks at what preventative strategies can be used, so that behaviour does not escalate strategies that might be used to de-escalate an evolving challenging situation of what parents/carers and professionals might do if there is a behavioural crisis. Each PBS plan will be bespoke to the child and should be seen as a 'living document' that will need to be updated and revised as a child grows. Key to the PBS approach is the acknowledgement that behaviour always has a function for the child and many preventative strategies can be put into place once that function is understood. The best evidence base for managing challenging behaviour in children still comes from the behavioural theory. As for children without disabilities, there are now targeted parenting group interventions, e.g. Riding the Rapids,[56] which aim to help parents of children with additional needs understand and manage their child's behaviour better and which also provide a supportive peer environment.

Guidelines for good practice

- Put on your disability glasses. Understanding the child's condition and being able to put yourself into their shoes can be enormously helpful in thinking about how you can adapt your clinical practice to best fit the needs of the young person. For example, it may be hard for some children with disabilities to wait for appointments in clinic or to manage busy and overstimulating clinic environments at all.
- Ask parents and carers about their child and plan with them what intervention may work best or what reasonable adjustments to service practice you can make.

Further reading

Jacobs M, Downie H, Kidd G, Fitzsimmons L, Gibbs S, Melville C (2016). Mental health services for children and adolescents with learning disabilities: a review of research on experiences of service users and providers. *British Journal of Learning Disabilities.* **44**: 225–32.

References

51 Gov.uk (for National Service Framework and EHCP advice and guidance). ℘ www.gov.uk (accessed 30 October 2017).
52 National Autistic Society. ℘ www.autism.org.uk (accessed 30 October 2017).
53 Scope. ℘ www.scope.org.uk (accessed 30 October 2017).
54 National Institute for Health and Care Excellence (for NICE guidelines on managing challenging behaviour). ℘ www.nice.org.uk/guidance (accessed 30 October 2017).
55 Challenging Behaviour Foundation. ℘ www.challengingbehaviour.org.uk (accessed 30 October 2017).
56 The Riding Rapids. ℘ www.encompasspsychology.co.uk/ridingtherapids.html (accessed 30 October 2017).

People with intellectual disabilities and forensic nursing

Forensic risk assessment and management

Context

It has been estimated that 'up to a third of people in prison have either an intellectual disability or learning difficulty which can affect their ability to read and to understand information (7% of prisoners have an IQ of less than 70 and a further 25% have an IQ between 70–79)'.[1]

The '*Transforming Care*' programme of work highlighted a number of people with intellectual disabilities within inpatient beds in a range of settings. The most recent model is described in *Building the Right Support* (2015).[2] Nurses have a key role working within forensic services, with some registered nurses in intellectual disabilities working as prison-in-reach practitioners, which will importantly focus on risk assessment management strategies in order to inform person centred care and treatment approaches. The Bradley Report (2009) examined the extent to which offenders of people with intellectual disabilities and mental health problems can be diverted from prison services, including people who:[3]

- 'Have not committed an offence but whose behaviour has brought them to the attention of the police;
- Have not committed an offence but whose illness or behaviour leads them to being detained under the Mental Health legislation;
- Require diversion from prison;
- Have committed a minor offence but their primary need is for treatment, and whom it is not in the public interest to detain;
- Have committed an offence and who will be prosecuted;
- Have committed an offence and may enter the prison population with a mental health problem;
- Develop a mental health problem in prison;
- Are considered unfit to plead.'[3]

Assessment of risk

Good forensic risk assessment and management is a particularly important aspect of care and treatment for some people with intellectual disabilities, as it will help to identify current presenting issues and the required care and management interventions. The process of assessment should aim to be a structured, supportive, and collaborative process.

While there are a number of tools which may be used, the *Best Practice in Risk Management* guide[4] has recommended that risk assessment tools should be seen as part of the overall clinical assessment process, and choosing the right tool for the job is a complex job.

The process of risk assessment should be person-centred, involving the individual concerned and significant others, should be inter-professional and interagency, and should enhance the therapeutic relationship between the nurse and client. The Criminal Justice Act (2003) put in place specific

---

* Reprinted from Department of Health (2009) Lord Bradley's review of people with mental health problems of learning disabilities in the criminal justice system under the Open Government License 3.0.

structures [Multi-Agency Public Protection Arrangements (MAPPA)] in England and Wales to provide added protection to members of the public and previous victims of crime from sexual and violent offenders. Through these structures, the NHS and other agencies work together in partnership with local criminal justice agencies and other bodies dealing with offenders.[5]

The consequences of poor risk assessment and management planning can be serious, not only for the individual, but also for others.

Scenario

Bill is 48 years of age. He lives with his parents and attends a local day service. He likes visiting shops and eating out but does not like crowds and noisy places. Bill has a history of physical attacks on young children. He arrives from home to the day centre in a highly agitated state. Staff supporting Bill had decided to go out for lunch, as this was something that Bill liked. It was half-term holiday from the local schools, and the height of lunchtime in the restaurant. The food was delayed, which resulted in Bill becoming increasingly agitated. While being escorted from the restaurant, Bill attacked a young child. Following this event, the police were called and an investigation was conducted. This highlighted that no risk assessment or management plan was conducted prior to, or during, the outing. When working with people with a forensic history, it is important to remember that risk plans are not static, and ongoing risk assessment and risk management planning are essential and take account of previous and present factors.

Conclusion

Risk assessment and management within a forensic history require systematic assessment, clear documentation, partnership working, and effective communication with all those involved with the person's care. It is imperative that consideration is also given to the different levels of security in which the nurse and client might be working, e.g. high-, medium-, and low-secure services. Inadequate or non-existent risk assessment and management can have serious consequences, not only for the person with intellectual disabilities, but also for others. There does not seem to have been the same extent of growth of numbers of registered nurses in intellectual disabilities working within this area, as we have seen in the general hospital and primary care settings, which is a point for commissioners to consider.

References

1 Prison Reform Trust (2013). *Lack of Support for People with Learning Disabilities Sets Offenders up to Fail*. ℜ www.prisonreformtrust.org.uk/PressPolicy/News/vw/1/ItemID/196 (accessed 9 March 2018).

2 Local Government Association and NHS England (2015). *Building the Right Support*. ℜ www.england.nhs.uk/wp-content/uploads/2015/10/ld-nat-imp-plan-oct15.pdf (accessed 9 March 2018).

3 Department of Health (2009). *Lord Bradley's Review of People with Mental Health Problems or Learning Disabilities in the Criminal Justice System*. Department of Health: London.

4 Department of Health (2007). *Best Practice in Risk Management*. HMSO: London.

5 HM Prison Service and National Offender Management Service (2014). *Multi-Agency Public Protection Arrangements (MAPPA)*. Ministry of Justice: London.

People who have offended in law

The term 'offender' can only rightfully be applied to a person who has been convicted of an unlawful act under the criminal law. In order to be convicted of an offence, there must be evidence 'beyond reasonable doubt' that the person did the unlawful act/s in question.

A range of factors, including intellectual disabilities, can affect decisions about whether or not a person should be subject to the normal processes of the criminal law. Within the criminal justice domain, intellectual disabilities is included under guidance relating to mentally disordered offenders.

Criminal responsibility

It is a fundamental assumption within the law that people who are prosecuted for unlawful acts will be held criminally responsible and liable to legal punishment. Factors that may negate or diminish criminal responsibility include considerations regarding the alleged unlawful act and about the person, including intellectual disabilities and other mental disorders. In practice, the application of the criminal law would not be considered appropriate for most people with more severe intellectual disabilities. A very small minority of people with intellectual disabilities will be prosecuted for more serious offences and found unfit to plead under the criminal procedure.

Considerations
- The alleged act (offence) must be **voluntary** (*actus reus*) and **intentional** (*mens rea*).
- Potential mitigating factors include mistake, accident, duress, and provocation.
- Personal factors/characteristics that may result in exemption or diminish criminal responsibility include mental disorders—intellectual disabilities, mental illness, personality disorder, and ASC.

The journey to a conviction

Pre-arrest and arrest

If an alleged criminal offence is reported to the police, they are required to investigate this. The police investigation can lead to the arrest of the person who is suspected of having committed the offence. The police have a substantial degree of discretion and must balance a range of considerations when they make decisions regarding the appropriateness of an arrest and the nature and seriousness of the alleged offence, including:
- The context of the alleged offence, including the setting in which the offence occurred and the ability and willingness of any victims to make a complaint and provide a reliable statement;
- The mental capacity of any offender—and the detail to which this may be affected by the presence of intellectual disabilities and other mental disorders.

Post-arrest

All people who have been arrested have certain rights that are laid down in the legalization, which include (for details, refer to legislation in the country for which you work):

- The right to remain silent;
- The right to see a solicitor in private at any time;
- The right to have someone told you are at the police station.

There are additional safeguards for people who are identified as being mentally vulnerable, including people with intellectual disabilities (➲ see Rights of person offending, pp. 426–7).

Prosecution

In most cases, the prosecuting authority, such as the Crown Prosecution Service (England and Wales), in consultation with the police, is responsible for deciding whether a person should be charged with a criminal offence and, if so, what the offence should be. The prosecuting authority applies a threshold test to these decisions:

- Is there is a realistic prospect of conviction?
- Is prosecution in the public interest?
- Will conviction result in a significant sentence?

Disposal

Disposal is the term that is used for the outcome of a successful prosecution. There are strict guidelines for the judiciary to follow regarding the sentencing options that are available, depending on the severity and circumstances of the offence and other factors. Sentencing options include community sentences (e.g. community supervision orders, fines, community service, etc.) and custodial (prison) sentences. In practice, community sentences are less likely to be considered for people with intellectual disabilities, unless specialist intellectual disabilities services are involved and advice and support is provided to the criminal justice agencies dealing with the case (see ➲ Working with criminal justice agencies, pp. 450–1).

Diversion

On many occasions, people with intellectual disabilities may be directed via court diversion schemes to receive care and support from health and welfare services. In practice, people who engage in offending behaviour are diverted away from the normal criminal justice process at various stages (see ➲ Rights of person offending, pp. 426–7; ➲ Admission for assessment, pp. 432–3; ➲ Admission for treatment, pp. 434–5).

Further reading

Department of Health (2015). *Mental Health Act 1983: Code of Practice*. Department of Health: London. ℜ www.gov.uk/government/uploads/system/uploads/attachment_data/file/435512/MHA_Code_of_Practice.PDF (accessed 30 October 2017).

Mental Health Commission (Republic of Ireland). *Mental Health Act (2001): Codes of Practice*. ℜ www.mhcirl.ie/for_H_Prof/codemha2001/ (accessed 30 October 2017).

People in prison

Being sent to prison is a punishment for a crime committed, but it should be noted that **all** prisoners or detainees should receive the same standards of healthcare that we all receive within society. In October 2015, there were 135 prisons within the UK, some of which are privately run and many of which are overcrowded. The purpose of prisons are to hold prisoners securely, reduce the risk of re-offending, and provide a safe and well-ordered establishment in which people are treated humanely, decently, and lawfully. In 2015 (October), there were 95 000 prisoners within the UK, and the figures have been increasing steadily each year. Prevalence of intellectual disabilities among adult offenders in the UK is between 2% and 10%. This is much higher for children who offend, of whom around 25% have an IQ of under 70. Research shows that the prevalence of people with intellectual disabilities in the prison population is higher (~7%) than in the general population (2.3%). While some of these people will cope adequately with a term of imprisonment, many will be very vulnerable, having difficulty coping, and struggle to access the range of services within the prison to meet their support, offence-related, and healthcare needs.

The NHS in all four UK countries has responsibility for prisoner health and work in partnership with the National Offender Management Services (NOMS). For people who have intellectual disabilities in a prison, they may come to prison with existing information about their care needs and support, but this may not have been identified in all cases. Good care and sensitive and appropriate support can reduce challenging behaviour and can help towards the reduction of re-offending.

About prisons

Prisons vary considerably in size and can cater for differing groups of people, such as only for sentenced prisoners, and others also accommodate prisoners on remand. Prisons are categorized in terms of security levels:

• Category A—prisoners whose escape would be considered highly dangerous to the public;
• Category B—prisoners who do not need the highest level of security, but for whom escape must be made difficult;
• Category C—prisoners who cannot be accommodated in open conditions but who are deemed not to have the ability or resources to make a determined attempt to escape;
• Category D—prisoners who are deemed safe to serve their sentence in open conditions.

Some prisons specialize in dealing with specific groups of offenders, particularly those convicted of sexual offences. These prisons are sometimes referred to as treatment prisons.

Prisoners may be allocated to any prison in a jurisdiction, according to their offence, security needs, and individual circumstances. There is no right to be located close to home. Information regarding particular vulnerabilities, such as those associated with intellectual disabilities, may be taken into account when a decision is made regarding allocation; however, this may not be possible if prison vacancies are severely limited.

Prison healthcare

Healthcare services in prison should include the same range of services available in the community, including primary health services, dental services, and specialist mental health, drug, and alcohol services. Many prisons have a healthcare wing to which prisoners can be admitted if their healthcare needs cannot be met on an outpatient basis. The prison service will also support prisoners who need treatment for physical health needs to access general hospital services.

Few prisons have specific services to meet the needs of people with intellectual disabilities who may need additional support to enable them to access the services that are available. Questions about mental health needs, self-harm, and suicide should be asked as part of the routine screening on reception into prison, in order that safeguards can be put in place by the prison service where required. People with intellectual disabilities may have difficulty providing accurate information regarding their own needs (see ➔ Risk of suicide, pp. 596–7).

Role of specialist intellectual disabilities services

The nurse in intellectual disabilities has a key role in working with health and justice services, directly or indirectly, and helping to make effective links with a variety of agencies. This group of staff offer the expertise, specialist skills, and knowledge that will ensure people get the best care and treatment commensurate with the wider general health services. Secure environments are considered to be challenging settings in which to work or to 'live'. Those receiving care in such settings can also be complex to care for. They typically experience greater health inequalities and are less likely to access health services. They are more likely to require assistance in prisons, for example, and less able to navigate the prison systems or to communicate their needs. In particular, nurses can:

• Establish links with prisons in their area and alert prisons to the presence of prisoners with intellectual disabilities;
• Raise awareness of the needs of people and provide advice on how these can be met in the prison setting, including access to healthcare services, education, and offence-related programmes, and links with other services;
• Provide information regarding specific needs and risks to inform the care of the person during remand or when serving a sentence;
• Provide information on how people with intellectual disabilities who cannot be adequately supported in the prison setting can be referred to specialist secure services, i.e. access to assessment for admission to secure hospital services;
• Maintain contact with the prison and contribute to release planning by attending pre-release meetings, providing information, and agreeing input if the person is returning to their local area on release.

Further reading

Department of Health (2011). *Positive Practice, Positive Outcomes: A Handbook for Professional Working in the Criminal Justice System Working with Offenders with a Learning Disability.* Department of Health: London.
Norman A, Walsh L (2014). *Nursing in the Criminal Justice System.* M&K Publishing: Keswick.

Rights of victims

All victims (sometimes referred to as injured parties) of crime have a range of rights. These rights apply, regardless of the status of the offender.

Police

When a crime is reported to the police, the alleged victim should be given an opportunity, when interviewed by the police, to describe all the effects on them. This will include physical and material harm and may also include any emotional and psychological effects/harm that have resulted from an alleged offence. This information may be taken into account in any subsequent court proceedings, e.g. it may have a bearing on the sentence if the offender is convicted. This information may also have a bearing on whether the court agrees to special measures if the victim is required to act as a witness (see ◯ People with intellectual disabilities as witnesses, pp. 430–1).

Domestic Violence, Crime and Victims Act (2004)

The Domestic Violence, Crime and Victims Act (2004) includes a Victim's Code regarding the services to be provided to victims of criminal conduct. Under specified circumstances, these services may also be available to others acting for the victim, i.e. where the victim has died or is unable to exercise/incapable of exercising their rights as a victim. There was an amendment in 2012 (Domestic Violence Crime and Victims (Amendment) Act) which broadens the scope of Section 5 of the Act to include situations where children and vulnerable adults have been seriously harmed, which previously only related to death.

Victims' rights

These rights will only be afforded if the local probation board is satisfied that the person requesting them has been the victim of an offender who has been detained or imprisoned for a sexual or violent offence.

The victim has the right to receive information about the offender, including:

- Information regarding plans for release/discharge;
- Whether or not they will be subject to licence conditions or supervision requirements;
- Whether or not they will be subject to conditions on their discharge;
- What the conditions/requirements of discharge are, including any restrictions specific to the victim;
- Information regarding any variations/changes made following release/discharge;
- Other information considered relevant to the victim.

The Victims' Code covers victims of offences committed by offenders who have been detained under mental health legislation, which deals with patients who are concerned with criminal proceedings or under sentence (see ◯ Admission for treatment, pp. 434–5). Victim support schemes are available throughout the UK and the Republic of Ireland to provide help to people to cope with crime. The police will routinely provide information about local schemes when a crime is reported.

Multi-Agency Public Protection arrangements (MAPPA)

MAPPA are the statutory arrangements for managing sexual and violent offenders. The police, probation, and prison services are the responsible authorities for MAPPA. Other public bodies, including the NHS and social services, have a duty to cooperate with MAPPA. Under MAPPA, the responsible authorities can disclose information about an offender and the plans for their management in the community to third parties, including victims and others who may be at risk.

Hospitals where offenders are detained have a duty to notify the owning MAPPA area when an offender is admitted to hospital and when there is a prospect of discharge/return to the community. The relevant MAPPA area will consider victim issues, including plans for the protection of any previous and potential future victims, and disclosure of information to others (including victims) (see → Management in the community, pp. 448–9).

People with intellectual disabilities as victims of crime

People with intellectual disabilities can also be vulnerable to becoming a victim of a crime such as physical assault, emotional and financial abuse, attack, exploitation, hate crime, or a sexual assault. Many such crimes go unreported, and the consequences can be devastating. The long-term effects of such crimes can lead to withdrawal, poor mental health, substance misuse, and self-harm. When this is the case, people should be afforded the same rights as anyone else who is a victim of crime. The nurse will have the skills required to tackle such issues and can be instrumental in giving support to someone who needs help with disclosing a crime and giving evidence, if necessary. People with intellectual disabilities are often vulnerable in their local communities and may be at increased risk of being the victims of crime; this may include hate crime.

Role of specialist intellectual disabilities services

Specialist intellectual disabilities services should raise awareness of the needs of people with intellectual disabilities and assist people to access, and make use of, support when they are the victims of crime. In a forensic context, staff have a role to inform offenders with intellectual disabilities about the rights of victims, including their right to information about future plans for the offender.

Further reading

Ministry of Justice (2014). *Victims of Crime: Understanding the Support You Can Expect*. Ministry of Justice: London.
Ministry of Justice (2015). *Code of Practice for Victims of Crime*. Ministry of Justice: London.
Ministry of Justice, National Offender Management Centre (2016). *MAPPA Guidance 2012*, version 4.1 (updated December 2016). Ministry of Justice: London.
Scottish Government (2016). *Multi-Agency Public Protection Arrangements (MAPPA) National Guidance*. Scottish Government: Edinburgh.

Rights of person offending

People with intellectual disabilities who come into contact with the criminal justice system because of offending behaviour have the same rights as others. Across the UK and the Republic of Ireland, all people within the health and justice system have rights under equality. Public services, including health and criminal justice services, are required to anticipate and prevent discrimination against people with disabilities; this includes intellectual disabilities.

People with intellectual disabilities may face particular problems, however, including a range of vulnerabilities, an increased potential for wrongful conviction, and limited access to the range of services available to non-disabled offenders (see ➔ People who have offended in law, pp. 420–1).

Police

Within each jurisdiction of the UK and the Republic of Ireland there is guidance on procedures for the detention, treatment, and questioning of people by the police.

Pre-arrest

When a crime is reported, police have a duty to investigate but also to have a substantial degree of discretion regarding the decision to arrest. In practice, the police may decide that a person with intellectual disabilities lacks the level of capacity to form intent and cannot be held fully accountable for their conduct, and conclude that arrest is therefore inappropriate.

Arrest

If a person with intellectual disabilities is arrested, they have the same rights as anyone else:

• The right to remain silent;
• The right to see a solicitor in private at any time;
• The right to have someone told you are at the police station;
• The right to look at the PACE Codes of Practice (UK) (see ➔ Rights to a solicitor, pp. 428–9).

Additional safeguards for 'mentally vulnerable' suspects

• Clinical assessment regarding fitness for detention and fitness for interview.
• Straightforward and clear explanation of the right to remain silent.
• Having an 'appropriate adult' present to support, advise, and assist the detained person, particularly when they are being questioned.
• Guidance/training for police for interviewing vulnerable suspects, including adaptations in normal police interviewing style.
• Request for a psychiatric assessment/assessment under the mental health legislation.

If these safeguards are not provided, where appropriate, the reliability of the investigation may be questioned, and evidence gathered from the suspect may be ruled inadmissible in court.

Detention

The rights of all suspects who are detained by the police are laid down, including time limits, level of care, and medical attention. The appropriate adult role includes ensuring these requirements are met.

Disposal—police

After the police have arrested a suspect and undertaken an initial investigation, they can decide between various possible courses of action. In practice, these decisions will often be made in consultation with the prosecuting authority in the jurisdiction. The decision made at this stage will depend on the severity and circumstances of the offence, and whether or not the suspect has admitted to the offence. If the suspect has intellectual disabilities (or another mental disorder), this may also affect the decision. People with intellectual disabilities should be afforded the same range of options as other suspects:

- *No further action or discontinuance*—due to lack of evidence or because prosecution is not deemed to be in the public interest.
- *Informal warning* issued by the police;
- *Non-judicial criminal punishment*—e.g. fixed penalty notice;
- *Civil enforcement*—e.g. application for antisocial behaviour order, sexual offences prevention order (see ➔ Management in the community, pp. 448–9);
- *Formal caution*—if the suspect admits to the offence and consents to being cautioned. It is important that the suspect understands the implications of admitting to the offence and the caution;
- *Police bail*—if it is considered safe, the suspect is released with conditions, pending further investigation;
- *Charge*—if the suspect is charged, a decision must be made regarding the need to detain the person or release him until he appears in court.

Courts

All cases in court are dealt with under strict rules governing court proceedings. The burden of responsibility for proving 'beyond reasonable doubt' that an offence has taken place rests with the prosecution, and all suspects have a right to defend themselves. The defence lawyer's role is critically important in protecting the rights of vulnerable defendants, as it provides the means by which information about the person, the need for psychiatric reports, evidence that the person is unfit to plead, and other mitigating factors are taken into consideration. During the course of proceedings, the court may seek psychiatric advice and remand an accused person to hospital for reports on his mental state.

Sentencing/disposal

Sentencing is subject to strict guidelines, and a pre-sentence report will normally be prepared by the probation service to inform decisions about sentencing. The court may sentence a person with intellectual disabilities to any sentence available for the offence for which they have been convicted, including custodial and community sentences. The court may also consider expert reports (including psychiatric reports) and make a disposal under the mental health legislation (see ➔ Admission for treatment, pp. 434–5).

Rights to a solicitor

When a person is arrested in the UK and the Republic of Ireland, they should be informed of their right to a solicitor and consult a solicitor in private at any time and to have one provided to be present when being interviewed by the police. The legal rights of mentally disordered suspects, including those with intellectual disabilities, are best ensured by the presence of a legal advisor at the police station and when the suspect is interviewed by the police.

Police responsibilities

The police custody officer is responsible for ensuring that suspects know their legal rights. All suspects should be verbally informed of their right to legal advice. The words that are used are: 'You have the right to an independent solicitor free of charge.'

Further information about the right to legal advice is normally given in writing in the form of a Notice to Detained Persons, which highlights the right to:

• Speak to a solicitor at any time, day or night, at no cost to you, when in the police station. This can be on the telephone or face-to-face in the police station. It will cost you nothing. This can only be withheld or delayed in exceptional circumstances. If you want to see a solicitor, tell the custody officer at once;
• You can speak to a 'duty solicitor' if you cannot contact your own solicitor or do not have a solicitor;
• You have the right to have a solicitor present when you are being questioned and there are limited circumstances when the police can question without a solicitor present;
• If you initially said you did not want to see a solicitor, you can change your mind and ask to speak to one;
• Under the Road Traffic legislation, you are still required to give specimens of breath, blood, and urine, if required, before you solicitor arrives.

Role of the solicitor

When a solicitor is called to attend to someone in custody, they are expected to:

• Provide advice on the relevant legal process and the range of options available;
• Support clients who are unfamiliar with these processes and circumstances. This is especially relevant when a person detained is considered to be vulnerable at that time;
• Make sure that all activities, including the interview, are undertaken in an appropriate way;
• Make clear and accurate independent records of all that happens;
• Explore the options for the person to be released from detention;
• Advise their client on their rights and obligations under the relevant codes of practice [Police and Criminal Evidence Act 1984 (PACE) in the UK].

If the person with intellectual disabilities is under 18 years old and/or has mental health problems or a learning disability, they can have someone with them at certain times.[6] They are usually a parent, a guardian, or a carer and are called an **'appropriate adult'**. If the detained person does not have someone, the police can arrange for someone to come from the appropriate adult service. The job of the appropriate adult is to ensure that the police respects the person's rights.

Role of the nurse for people with intellectual disabilities

Suspects with intellectual disabilities can be at greater risk when they are accused of offences if they do not understand and exercise their right to legal advice. Intellectual disabilities nurses in forensic and criminal justice liaison roles can assist the police to support suspects with intellectual disabilities through the period of detention and interviews by the police by:

• Explaining the information contained in the Notice to Detained Persons in straightforward and clear language;
• Ensuring that suspects with intellectual disabilities know that they are entitled to have a solicitor to support them and give them legal advice;
• Encouraging people with intellectual disabilities who are suspected of an offence, arrested, and held in police custody to exercise their right to legal advice;
• Working with the police and other agencies to raise awareness of the needs and vulnerabilities of people with intellectual disabilities in the criminal justice system (see ➔ Rights of person offending, pp. 426–7; ➔ Working with criminal justice agencies, pp. 450–1).

Further reading

Cotter L (2015). Are the needs of adult offenders with mental health difficulties being met in prisons and on probation? *Irish Probation Journal.* **12**: 57–78.

Home Office (2017). *Revised Code of Practice for the Detention, Treatment and Questioning of Person by Police Officers. Police and Criminal Evidence Act 1984: Code of Practice C.* Home Office: London. ⅋ www.gov.uk/government/publications/pace-code-c-2017 (accessed 30 October 2017).

References

6 Landman R (2016). *People with Learning Disabilities in the Criminal Justice System. A Guide for Carers and Learning Disability Services.* ARC England: Chesterfield.

People with intellectual disabilities as witnesses

People with intellectual disabilities are at least as likely to witness crime as others in the general population and may be at increased risk of being victims of crime. The presence of intellectual disabilities may, however, be taken as an indication that a person is unable to provide reliable information in order to make a statement to the police and is unable to act as a witness in criminal proceedings. It may also adversely influence the questioning approach of police who may not understand the ability of a person with intellectual disabilities to give reliable evidence.[7,8] A range of provisions is available to enhance the evidence provided by vulnerable and intimidated witnesses, including people with intellectual disabilities.

Special measures

When dealing with people with intellectual disabilities, a range of 'special measures' can be used to facilitate the gathering and giving of evidence by vulnerable and intimidated witnesses.

The police

- Detailed guidance for the police regarding how to plan and conduct interviews with vulnerable and intimidated witnesses (including children).
- Video-recorded interview in the presence of a responsible adult who will ensure that the witness understands questions asked and provides reliable information.

Court proceedings

If a person with intellectual disabilities is required to act as a witness in court, their capacity to give reliable evidence may be called into question as part of the defence case. With the agreement of the court, special measures can be made available to assist a person with intellectual disabilities to participate in court proceedings as a witness:

- Screens to shield the witness from the defendant;
- Live link to enable the witness to give evidence and be cross-examined from outside the court room via a video link;
- Exclusion from the court of members of the public and the press;
- Removal of wigs and gowns by judges and barristers;
- A video-recorded interview may be admitted to the court as the witness's evidence in chief. If a video-recorded interview has been agreed to, a video-recorded cross-examination may also be admissible;
- Examination of the witness via an 'intermediary' (see ➜ Intermediaries, p. 431);
- Aids to communication—provided that the communication can be verified and understood by the court;
- Protection of the witness from cross-examination by the accused person;
- Restrictions on evidence and questions about the witness's sexual behaviour.

Intermediaries

All witnesses who are considered vulnerable can get help from an intermediary.[9] Intermediaries come from a range of professional backgrounds and are specially trained for the role. Vulnerable witnesses are matched to a suitably skilled intermediary on the basis of individual need. The role of the intermediary is to help witnesses at each stage of the criminal justice process to understand questions and to communicate on behalf of the witness where required.

Witness support schemes

Witness support schemes are not able to advise on specific cases but do provide emotional and social support for vulnerable witnesses at all stages of the criminal justice process, including police interview, and prior to and during court proceedings/trial.

Roles for specialists in intellectual disabilities

- Witnesses who are known to have intellectual disabilities are generally interviewed by police officers, with additional training in the case of alleged sexual offences, but less often in the case of non-sexual offences—specialists in intellectual disabilities should raise awareness of the need for appropriately trained officers to interview people with intellectual disabilities when non-sexual offences are reported.
- It is rare for the police and prosecuting authority to consult specialists/experts in intellectual disabilities about witnesses' disabilities or their implications—specialist services for people with intellectual disabilities should raise awareness of available expertise and engage with criminal justice agencies to provide expert advice on the effects of intellectual disabilities for those who are victims or witnesses.
- The availability of special measures to adult witnesses with intellectual disabilities is still limited—specialists in intellectual disabilities, particularly those in criminal justice liaison roles, should raise awareness/advocate for the wider use of special measures where these could assist intellectual disabilities witnesses to give evidence.
- Many witnesses with intellectual disabilities would benefit from specialist support and preparation prior to appearing in court, but it is not always clear which agency is responsible for providing this—specialists in intellectual disabilities should raise awareness of their services and work jointly with witness support schemes to facilitate access to preparation and support for intellectual disabilities witnesses who are required to attend court.

Further reading

Beckene T, Forrester Jones R, Murphy GH (2017). Experiences of going to court: witness with intellectual disabilities and their carers. *Journal of Applied Research in Intellectual Disabilities.* 2017 Mar 31. doi: 10.1111/jar.12334. [Epub ahead of print].

References

7 Antaki C, Richardson E, Stokoe E, Willott S (2015). Can people with intellectual disability resist implications of fault when police question their allegations of sexual assault and rape? *Intellectual and Developmental Disabilities.* 53: 346–57.

8 Brown D, Lewis C, Stephnes E, Lamb M (2017). Interviewers' approaches to questioning vulnerable child witnesses: the influences of developmental level versus intellectual disability status. *Law and Criminological Psychology.* 22: 332–49.

9 Hepner I, Woodward M, Stewart J (2015). Giving the vulnerable a voice in the criminal justice system: the use of intermediaries with individuals with intellectual disability. *Psychiatry, Psychology And Law.* 22: 453–64.

Admission for assessment

Many nurses for people with intellectual disabilities in forensic roles work in inpatient services; these may be open units or units ranging from low to medium, or even high security. Often nurses may also not work in forensic settings but find themselves nursing patients who have offended and are admitted into admissions units. Admission into hospital may be voluntary or involuntary for assessment. Involuntary admission of people for assessment is governed by the mental health legislation in each jurisdiction, including the Mental Health Act 1983 (England and Wales, amended in 2007), the Mental Health (Northern Ireland) Order 1986, the Mental Health Act 2001 (Republic of Ireland), and the Mental Health (Scotland) Act 2015. Readers should refer to their own specific legislation for section numbers and details of the provision.

Involuntary admission

Involuntary admission to hospital can take place only if a person is suffering from a mental disorder within the meaning of the mental health legislation and detention in hospital is necessary for their own health and safety and/or the protection of other people. Mental disorder means any disorder or disability of the mind. A person with intellectual disability cannot be considered to be suffering from a mental disorder within the meaning of the mental health legislation, unless their disability is associated with abnormally aggressive or seriously irresponsible conduct.

The mental health legislation also provides civil arrangements for compulsory admission to hospital and guardianship. It also provides arrangements for patients who are concerned with criminal proceedings or under sentence to be detained in hospital for assessment and/or treatment of the mental disorder.

Assessment or treatment

It can be unclear whether a person who needs to be detained should be admitted for assessment or treatment (see Table 11.1). People who are admitted for assessment will often need and receive treatment, and people who are admitted for treatment will often need to be assessed as part of the treatment process. The core focus of assessment for most people with intellectual disabilities will be to gain an understanding of problematic and offending behaviour, and any association between their intellectual disabilities and behaviour that could result in harm to self and/or others.

Indications for assessment

- The person has never previously been admitted to hospital and/or has not been in regular contact with specialist services.
- The diagnosis/cause of the person's problems is unclear. Previously established treatment/interventions require reformulation, including assessment of the potential for informal treatment.
- The presenting needs/condition of the person are judged to have changed since an earlier involuntary admission.

Table 11.1 The Mental Health Act 1983: admission for assessment

Section no.	Purpose	Duration	Requirements
Part II: Compulsory admission to hospital and guardianship			
Section 2	Admission for assessment	Up to 28 days	Evidence of mental disorder/cannot be assessed without detention
Section 4	Admission for assessment in an emergency	Up to 72h	Urgent necessity with a view to admission for assessment under S.2
Section 5(2)	Doctor holding power	Up to 72h	Patient already receiving treatment for mental disorder as in-patient—with a view to admission for assessment under S.2
Section 5(4)	Nurses holding power	Up to 6h	Evidence of immediate risk of harm—need to secure attendance of responsible/approved clinician
Section 135	Warrant for the police to search for, and remove, a patient to place of safety for a mental health assessment	Up to 72h	Evidence to suggest mental disorder and need for a mental health assessment
Section 136	Police power to remove a person from a public place to a place of safety for a mental health assessment	Up to 72h	Evidence to suggest mental disorder and need for a mental health assessment
Part III: Patients concerned in criminal proceedings or under sentence			
Section 35	Remand to hospital for report on mental condition of the accused	Up to three periods of 28 days—not to exceed 12 weeks in total	Evidence to suggest that an accused person who is to be remanded awaiting trial or sentence is suffering from mental disorder that requires assessment in hospital

Further reading

Department of Health (2015). *Revised Mental Health Act Code of Practice.* Department of Health: London.
Mental Health Commission (2009). *Code of Practice on Admission, Transfer and Discharge to and from an Approved Centre.* Mental Health Commission: Dublin.
Scottish Government. *Code of Practice.* www.gov.scot/Topics/Health/Services/Mental-Health/Law/Code-of-Practice (accessed 15 March 2018).

Admission for treatment

Often nurses may also not work in forensic settings but find themselves nursing patients who have offended and are admitted into admissions units. Many nurses for people with intellectual disabilities in forensic roles work in inpatient services; these may be open units or units ranging from low to medium, or even high security. The involuntary admission of people for treatment is governed by the mental health legislation in each jurisdiction, including: Mental Health Act 1983 (see Table 11.2) (England and Wales, amended 2007), the Mental Health (Northern Ireland) Order 1986, the Mental Health Act 2001 (Republic of Ireland), and the Mental Health (Scotland) Act 2015. Readers should refer to their own specific legislation for section numbers and details of the provision.

Involuntary admission to hospital can take place only if a person is suffering from mental disorder within the meaning of the mental health legislation and detention in hospital is necessary for their own health and safety and/or the protection of other people. People admitted into hospital for treatment can be admitted on a voluntary, or more often involuntary, basis through use of mental health legislation. If detained as a result of court proceedings, they may also have a restriction order that is implemented by the Ministry of Justice/Department of Justice (Northern Ireland) and equivalent bodies in other jurisdictions. People may be admitted because there has been an allegation of offending that is under criminal investigation or evidence that their behaviour is placing them at risk of committing a criminal offence.

Treatment

Treatment should be focused on the 'offending risk' that resulted in their need for admission to hospital. Treatment for forensic patients is based on the recovery/rehabilitation model. Treatment plans may include psychological formulation, behavioural interventions, offence-specific treatment (e.g. sex offender treatment programmes), treatment for an underlying mental illness, social skills programmes, substance misuse/addiction programmes, and cognitive skills programmes (e.g. dialectical behaviour therapy). Treatment should be specific to the individual criminogenic need and result in risk assessment and management strategies that balance the person's ability to manage their own risk with the need for any external management strategies to maintain a non-offending lifestyle. Some people who are admitted involuntarily for treatment will also require treatment for an existing mental illness.

Appropriate treatment test

The availability of appropriate treatment is a requirement of detention to hospital for treatment of a mental disorder. Treatment must be appropriate, taking into account the nature and degree of the person's mental disorder and all the other circumstances of the person's case. The Revised Code of Practice provides extensive guidance regarding this test.

Table 11.2 The Mental Health Act 1983: admission for treatment

Section no.	Purpose	Duration	Requirements
Part II: Compulsory admission to hospital and guardianship			
Section 3	Admission for treatment	Two periods of 6 months and then renewable annually	Suffering from mental disorder which needs treatment in hospital and cannot be treated without detention
Part III: Patients concerned in criminal proceedings or under sentence			
Section 36	Remand of accused person to hospital for treatment	Up to three periods of 28 days—not to exceed 12 weeks in total	Evidence an accused person who is to be remanded awaiting trial or sentence is suffering from mental disorder which requires treatment in hospital
Section 37— with or without restriction order (S.41)	Hospital order—power of courts to order hospital admission for treatment May include Ministry of Justice restrictions in discharge (S.41 Mental Health Act)	Two periods of 6 months and then renewable annually	Conviction for an imprisonment offence— requires treatment in hospital for mental disorder. Hospital order replaces sentence
Section 38	Interim hospital order	Period of 28 days renewable by the court for a total period not exceeding 1 year	Conviction for an imprisonment offence. Requires period of treatment in hospital to allow assessment regarding appropriateness of S.37
Section 47—with or without restriction order (S.49)	Transfer to hospital of a person serving a prison sentence May include Ministry of Justice restrictions in discharge (S.49 Mental Health Act)	S.49 restriction order expires	Person serving a sentence of imprisonment requires treatment for mental disorder in hospital

Data sourced from the Department of Health (2015) Revised Mental Health Act Code of Practice. London: DoH, Mental Health Commission.

Further reading

Department of Health (2015). Revised Mental Health Act Code of Practice. Department of Health: London.

Mental Health Commission (2009). Code of Practice on Admission, Transfer and Discharge to and from an Approved Centre. Mental Health Commission: Dublin.

Scottish Government. Codes of Practice. www.gov.scot/Topics/Health/Services/Mental-Health/Law/Code-of-Practice (accessed 15 March 2018).

Emergency holding powers

If considered necessary for a person already in hospital to undergo an assessment and they wish to leave hospital, it is possible under mental health legislation across the UK and the Republic of Ireland to prevent this person from leaving hospital by the use of 'emergency holding powers'. These are for use in an emergency only, and the need to use these can often be averted by discussions with the person and highlighting concern for them and the need for an assessment to be undertaken. Use of these emergency holding powers should be through careful monitoring in services to ensure they are being used appropriately and what alternative strategies could be put in place to reduce their use.

The use of emergency holding powers of people for treatment is governed by the mental health legislation in each jurisdiction, including the Mental Health Act 1983 (England and Wales, amended 2007), the Mental Health (Northern Ireland) Order 1986, the Mental Health Act 2001 (Republic of Ireland), and the Mental Health Act (Scotland) Act 2015. The detention of people for assessment and treatment of a mental disorder in England and Wales is governed by the Mental Health Act 1983 (revised 2007). Sections 5(4) and 5(2) of the Mental Health Act 1983 make provision for patients who are already in hospital informally to be detained for a short period in order for a Mental Health Act (MHA) assessment to be undertaken. In Northern Ireland, the detention of people for assessment and treatment of a mental disorder is governed by the Mental Health Order 1986. Part II of this order can be used by a registered nurse to detain a patient who already resides in hospital if they meet the grounds for detention (if they are a danger to themselves or others); the patient must be assessed by a medical officer within 6 hours of the form being completed.

Use of Section 5(2)

The provisions under Section 5(2) can be used by a doctor or an approved clinician to detain a patient who is already in hospital informally for treatment of a mental disorder for up to 72 hours.

Indications for use

- The doctor or approved clinician in charge of the treatment of the patient (or their nominated deputy) has concluded that an application for admission under the MHA should be made.
- Detention of the patient under Section 5(2) is necessary in order for an application for admission to be made.

Considerations and safeguards

- Section 5(2) can be invoked only by the doctor or approved clinician (or their nominated deputy) in charge of the treatment of the patient's mental disorder.
- Detention commences from the moment the doctor or approved clinician's report has been delivered to the hospital managers.
- Section 5(2) can be used only for people who are already being treated for a mental disorder as inpatients and cannot be used for anyone attending hospital as an outpatient.

- When Section 5(2) is invoked, hospital staff may use the minimum reasonable force to prevent the patient from leaving the hospital (see ➔ Use of restraint, pp. 444–5).

Other settings

Emergency holding powers can be used only in hospital settings, including NHS hospitals and registered independent hospitals. For predictable emergencies and crisis situations in other settings, contingency plans can be agreed as part of a community care package. If a person is prevented from leaving, this may constitute restraint. Any use of restraint may have to be justified under common law doctrine of necessity, which provides general power to take the steps that are reasonably necessary and proportionate to protect others from immediate risk of significant harm. If it is considered necessary to regularly prevent a person from leaving, consideration should be given regarding the need for a legal framework.

Guardianship Section 7 and Section 37 of MHA 1983—this is a framework for working with a patient in a community setting where this cannot be provided without compulsory powers. This may include a condition of residence to which the person can be returned, if required.

Deprivation of liberty safeguards of MHA 2005—an application for deprivation of liberty can be made for a person who lacks capacity, if this is necessary and justifiable in their best interests and there is no less restrictive alternative. This protects staff who are responsible for the person's care and safety and provides legal safeguards to the person whose liberty is curtailed (see ➔ Use of restraint, pp. 444–5).

Other agencies—police/criminal justice system

The police have a range of powers to detain people where this is necessary to protect against harm and/or in order to investigate alleged crimes:

- Powers to remove a person suspected of being mentally disordered to a place of safety under Sections 135 and 136 of the Mental Health Act 1983;
- Powers to arrest and detain people suspected of committing an unlawful act (see ➔ People who have offended in law, pp. 420–1);
- Powers to restrain a person to protect life and property;
- Conditions of residence as part of bail arrangements and community (probation) orders.

Further reading

Department of Health (2008). *The Mental Capacity Act 2005 Deprivation of Liberty Safeguards Addendum to the Mental Capacity Act Code of Practice*. Department of Health: London.

Department of Health (2015). *Revised Mental Health Act Code of Practice*. Department of Health: London.

Guidelines and Audit Implementation Network (2011). *Guidelines on the Use of the Mental Health (Northern Ireland) Order 1986*. Regulation and Quality Improvement Authority: Belfast. ℗ rqia.org.uk/RQIA/files/4e/4ee9ff634-be47-4398-afc9-906a20ff3198.pdf (accessed 15 March 2018).

Mental Health Commission (2009). *Code of Practice on Admission, Transfer and Discharge to and from an Approved Centre*. Mental Health Commission: Dublin.

Scottish Government. *Codes of Practice*. ℗ www.gov.scot/Topics/Health/Services/Mental-Health/Law/Code-of-Practice (accessed 15 March 2018).

Nurse's holding power

If it is considered necessary for a person already in hospital to undergo an assessment and they wish to leave hospital, it is possible under mental health legislation across the UK and the Republic of Ireland to prevent this person from leaving hospital by the use of 'emergency holding powers'. These are for use in an emergency only, and the need to use these can often be averted by discussions with the person and highlighting concern for them and the need for an assessment to be undertaken. Use of these emergency holding powers should be through careful monitoring in services to ensure they are being used appropriately and what alternative strategies could be put in place to reduce their use.

A nurse in the UK can detain a voluntary patient for 6 hours, and in the Republic of Ireland, it can be for up to 24 hours. The use of emergency holding powers of people for treatment is governed by the mental health legislation in each jurisdiction, including the Mental Health Act 1983 (England and Wales, amended 2007—Section 5.1), the Mental Health (Northern Ireland) Order 1986 (Section 5.4), the Mental Health Act 2001 (Republic of Ireland—Section 23), and the Mental Health Act 2015 (Scotland—Section 229).

These provisions can be used by a registered nurse (mental health or intellectual disabilities) to detain a patient who is already in hospital for treatment of a mental disorder for up to 6 hours (24 hours in the Republic of Ireland). Once these powers have been invoked, the patient must be assessed within the required time period by a doctor or an approved clinician who has the power to use further emergency holding powers or arrange involuntary admission for assessment and treatment (see ➔ Emergency holding powers, pp. 436–7).

Indications for use
- Immediate necessity to prevent the patient from leaving the hospital for the sake of their own safety and/or the protection of others.
- Not practicable to secure the attendance of a practitioner who uses alternative holding powers or to arrange involuntary admission to hospital (see ➔ Emergency holding powers, pp. 436–7).

Considerations and safeguards
- A nurse cannot be instructed by anyone else to use these powers to detain a patient.
- In reaching a decision to use these powers, the nurse should fully assess the circumstances and presenting needs of the patient, including:
  - How soon arrangements can be made for the patient to be assessed by a doctor or an approved clinician;
  - Whether the patient can be persuaded to remain until they can be assessed by a doctor or an approved clinician;
  - The harm that might occur if the patient leaves hospital before they can be assessed by a doctor or an approved clinician.

- The registered nurse who is responsible for invoking the emergency holding powers must record the decision, the reasons for it, and the time it was invoked in the patient's records. This record must then be sent to hospital managers.
- When these powers are invoked, hospital staff may use the minimum reasonable force/restrictions to prevent the patient from leaving the hospital (see ➲ Use of restraint, pp. 444–5).
- If a doctor or an approved clinician has not attended within the required time frame, the patient must be released from detention.

Further reading

Department of Health (2008). *The Mental Capacity Act 2005 Deprivation of Liberty Safeguards Addendum to the Mental Capacity Act Code of Practice.* Department of Health: London.

Department of Health (2015). *Revised Mental Health Act Code of Practice.* Department of Health: London.

Guidelines and Audit Implementation Network (2011). *Guidelines on the Use of the Mental Health (Northern Ireland) Order 1986.* Regulation and Quality Improvement Authority: Belfast. ℘ rqia.org.uk/RQIA/files/4e/4ee9f634-be47-4398-afc9-906a20ff3198.pdf (accessed 15 March 2018).

Mental Health Commission (2009). *Code of Practice on Admission, Transfer and Discharge to and from an Approved Centre.* Mental Health Commission: Dublin.

Scottish Government. *Codes of Practice.* ℘ www.gov.scot/Topics/Health/Services/Mental-Health/Law/Code-of-Practice (accessed 15 March 2018).

Mental Health Review Tribunal

Across the four countries of the UK, and the Republic of Ireland, arrangements for Mental Health Review Tribunals (MHRTs) are in place on the basis of mental health legislation. The Tribunal's function is 'to provide mental health patients with a safeguard against unjustified detention in hospital or control under guardianship by means of a review of their cases from both the medical and non-medical points of view'.[10-14]

Purpose

- An independent judicial body for detained patients to appeal against detention.
- To review the cases of detained and conditionally discharged patients.
- To review the cases of patients subject to Community Treatment Orders and Guardianship Orders.

Mental Health Review Tribunal rules

MHRTs must be arranged and conducted in accordance with rules laid down in mental health legislation in each jurisdiction.

Applying for a Mental Health Review Tribunal

Applications must be made in writing. Hospital managers have a duty to ensure that patients, and their nearest relative (unless the patient requests otherwise), are informed of their right to apply for an MHRT. Applications are made when:

- The patient is first detained in hospital for assessment or treatment, or made subject to a Guardianship Order;
- A patient is transferred from guardianship to hospital or discharged from hospital subject to a Supervised Community Treatment Order;
- When detention in hospital is renewed;
- When a Supervised Community Treatment Order is extended or revoked;
- When the patient's status under mental health legislation changes. (see ➔ Admission for assessment, pp. 432–3; ➔ Admission for treatment, pp. 434–5; ➔ Management in the community, pp. 448–9.)

Under specified circumstances when the patient has not exercised the right to apply for an MHRT, managers of the hospital must make an application on behalf of the patient.

Composition

- The MHRT must comprise at least three members, including a legal member, medical member, and a non-medical member.
- The legal member will be the chair.
- Non-legal members are required to have some relevant specialist expertise.

Powers of a Mental Health Review Tribunal

- To direct discharge of a detained patient if they are not satisfied the patient is suffering from a mental disorder (within the meaning of the mental health legislation) to a nature or degree that warrants detention in hospital.
- To direct discharge of a detained patient if detention is not justified in the interests of the health and safety of the patient and/or for the protection of others.
- To specify that a patient must be discharged on a date in the future.

Considerations

In reaching a decision about whether to direct discharge, the MHRT must consider all relevant circumstances of the case, including:

- The availability of appropriate treatment and the likelihood of treatment alleviating or preventing deterioration in the patient's condition;
- The likelihood of the patient being able to care for themselves, to be able to obtain the care they need, or to guard against serious exploitation.

Role of the nurse for people with intellectual disabilities

- Inform the patients of their rights under detention on admission and repeated at other times, if required.
- On admission for treatment, the nurse should ensure the patient is aware of his/her rights to apply for an MHRT.
- Take all possible steps to provide information about MHRTs in a form that is accessible and understandable to the patient. Use easy-read material to enhance capacity to understand, if required, and repeat this information as frequently as necessary.
- Assist patients who are physically unable to do so (e.g. unable to read or write) to apply for an MHRT. This may include making a written application on their behalf or enabling access to advocacy services.
- Inform patients of the process of automatic referral for an MHRT.
- Ensure detained patients are aware of their entitlement to free legal advice and representation.
- Assist detained patients to request the services of an appropriate legal representative.
- Offer the patient access/referral to independent advocacy.
- Provide the necessary support and assistance to enable detained patients to have contact with their legal representative.
- Support the patient through the process, and provide support on the day of the tribunal and after the outcome received.
- Contribute to the multidisciplinary team to assessments that inform reports for consideration by the MHRTs.

Further reading

Department of Health (2015). *Revised Mental Health Act Code of Practice*. Department of Health: London.

Royal College of Psychiatrists (2015). *A Guide to Mental Health Tribunals*. Royal College of Psychiatrists: London. ℘ www.rcpsych.ac.uk/healthadvice/problemsdisorders/guidementalhealthtribunals.aspx (accessed 15 March 2018).

References

10 Mental Health Review Tribunal Northern Ireland. *Courts and Tribunals*. ℘ www.courtsni.gov.uk/en-GB/Tribunals/MentalHealthReview/Pages/default.aspx (accessed 15 March 2018).
11 Mental Health Tribunal for Scotland. ℘ www.mhtscotland.gov.uk/mhts/Home/Welcome_to_the_Mental_Health_Tribunal (accessed 15 March 2018).
12 gov.uk (England). *Apply to the Mental Health Tribunal*. ℘ www.gov.uk/mental-health-tribunal (accessed 15 March 2018).
13 Mental Health Review Tribunal for Wales. ℘ www.wales.nhs.uk/sites3/page.cfm?orgid=816&pid=34216 (accessed 15 March 2018).
14 Mental Health Commission (Republic of Ireland). *Mental Health Tribunals*. ℘ www.mhcirl.ie/for_H_Prof/Mental_Health_Tribunals/ (accessed 15 March 2018).

Mental Health Act Commission

There is a body in each of the four countries in the UK and the Republic of Ireland to safeguard the interests of all people detained under mental health legislation. The Mental Health Act Commission/Mental Health Commission is empowered to review care and treatment provided to detained patients in NHS and independent hospitals and care homes. The names and structures of these organizations vary across jurisdictions, but the remit is broadly similar. This role is under the remit of the Care Quality Commission (England and Wales), the Regulation and Quality Improvement Authority (Northern Ireland), the Mental Welfare Commission (Scotland), and the Mental Health Commission (Republic of Ireland).

Broad functions of the bodies

- To review the operation of the mental health legislation in respect of patients liable to be detained.
- To visit and interview in private patients detained under the mental health legislation in health service and registered independent hospitals (including mental health nursing homes).
- Investigate complaints that fall within the remit of the body.
- To appoint medical practitioners and others to give second opinions where this is required under the mental health legislation.
- To monitor the implementation of the mental health legislation code of practice.
- To provide regular reports to the government relating to the operation of the mental health legislation.
- Inspecting the quality of services provided through reviews of clinical and social care governance arrangements and listening to, and acting on, patients' experiences.
- To regulate a wide range of services delivered by the health service bodies and by the independent sector (including intellectual disabilities and mental health services).
- To be responsible for preventing ill treatment, preventing or redressing loss or damage to patients' property/finances, and remedying any deficiency in care or treatment.
- To terminate improper detention in a hospital.
- To work collaboratively with people, local groups, and larger organizations who use your services.
- To use the best available evidence to make fair decisions.
- To act appropriately if you have any concerns about services not meeting the required standards of safety or quality.
- To provide reports on the quality of care services to assist people in making their own decisions about which services they may choose to use.

Structure and roles

These bodies comprise lay people, lawyers, doctors, nurses, social workers, psychologists, and other specialists. Commissioners work at local and area levels to keep the operation of the mental health legislation under review.

Local commissioners

- Visit detained patients.
- Examine patient records.

- Take up immediate issues on behalf of detained patients.
- Identify issues for action and decide how they can be resolved.
- Maintain supportive, but objective, relationships with local services who provide care and treatment to detained patients.

Area commissioners
- Coordinate the work of the body.
- Develop and maintain working relationships with providers, social services departments, user groups, and other relevant agencies.
- Provide annual reports to the boards of all providers who deal with detained patients.

Second-opinion doctors
When a detained patient is incapable of giving consent or refusing to consent to treatment, the responsible clinician or approved clinician has a duty to obtain a second opinion. The bodies are responsible for the appointment of second-opinion doctors for this purpose. A second opinion is required for *detained patients* who lack capacity to consent:
- When medication is continued beyond the first 3 months of treatment;
- If ECT is to be used.

Other safeguards
- Hospital managers hearings;
- Independent mental health advocates;
- MHRTs;
- PALS.

Further reading
Care Quality Commission (England). ✆ www.cqc.org.uk/content/mental-health (accessed 15 March 2018).
Department of Health (2015). *Revised Mental Health Act Code of Practice*. Department of Health: London.
Mental Health Commission (Republic of Ireland). ✆ www.mhcirl.ie (accessed 15 March 2018).
Mental Health Review Tribunal Northern Ireland. *Courts and Tribunals*. ✆ www.courtsni.gov.uk/en-GB/Tribunals/MentalHealthReview/Pages/default.aspx (accessed 15 March 2018).
Mental Health Review Tribunal for Wales. ✆ www.wales.nhs.uk/sites3/page.cfm?orgid=816&pid=34216 (accessed 15 March 2018).
Mental Welfare Commission for Scotland. ✆ www.mwcscot.org.uk (accessed 15 March 2018).

Use of restraint

People with intellectual disabilities are at an increased risk of being restrained, and while this may be acceptable practice in emergency situations, it can also result in major abuse of human rights such as those seen in Winterbourne View and Aras Attracta in recent years. It has been found that the term 'restraint' is open to much interpretation in intellectual disabilities services.[15] A key definition is 'deliberate acts on the part of other person(s) that restrict an individual's movement, liberty and/or freedom to act independently' (p.14).[16]

Types of restraint

- Mechanical restraint—physical security, including locked doors, baffle locks, keypads, fences, and use of seclusion;
- Physical restraint—one or more members of staff holding the person, moving the person, or blocking their movement;
- Technological surveillance—includes tagging, pressure pads, closed-circuit television, and door alarms;
- Chemical restraint—use of medication to restrain movement, including regular and as-required medication;
- Indirect/psychological restraint—can include telling someone that what they want to do is not allowed and depriving people of their lifestyle choices, not providing the assistance a person needs to undertake desired activities (see ➔ Behavioural interventions, pp. 316–8).[16]

When can restraint be used?

Restraint should always be considered to be a final resort when other interventions have failed or are at clear risk of failing to protect the safety of an individual or people near to them. It should be used within clearly agreed local policies and always for the ultimate benefit of the person with intellectual disabilities. It is recognized that, in some situations, restraint may be necessary such as:

- Where the patient's behaviour has the potential to cause harm or is causing harm to themselves, e.g. deliberate self-harm, attempted suicide, other dangerous actions;
- Where the patient's behaviour has the potential to cause harm or is causing harm to other people, e.g. violence;
- To prevent a person from leaving who is subject to legal orders, e.g. detained under mental health legislation.

Principles underpinning the use of restraint

Restraint should only be used as a last resort, and when used, it should ensure that:

- The person's airway, breathing, and circulation are always protected and 'face-down' restraint is avoided;
- The least restrictive option of restraint at the time should be used and pain should not be deliberately caused as a path of restraint;
- Only people detained under the mental health legislation should be secluded;
- There should be clear personalized plans to support anyone considered to be at risk of being restrained or subject to other restrictive practices;
- The planning, reviewing, and evaluating of care and support should actively involve people with intellectual disabilities, carers, and family members.

In addition, staff should also:
- Have respect for privacy and dignity;
- Use the least restrictive option available to manage risk;
- Be proportionate—using only the force necessary to respond to the risk;
- Complete assessments to identify and address the underlying reasons for violence and self-harm (see ➲ Forensic risk assessment and risk management, pp. 418–9);
- Use restraint only for as long as necessary to manage the risk of harm;
- Use only those techniques for which they are trained and competent in.

Considerations

Legal and ethical issues

All interventions that constitute restraint must be justifiable under the common law doctrine of necessity, which provides general power to take the steps that are reasonably necessary and proportionate to protect others from immediate risk of significant harm. Nurses should be aware that restraining another person without their consent may constitute a criminal offence. The need to protect staff must always be properly balanced with the duty to provide care and protection.

All nurses who are involved in the use of restraint are accountable for their own practice and must abide by current professional standards and the policy of their employing organization relating to the use of restraint

Negotiated care plans or advanced directives

Wherever possible, the views of clients/patients should be taken into account when care/management plans are developed. This can include negotiated plans where specific approaches can be agreed in advance in the event of restraint being necessary.

Safety

It must be recognized that there is always a risk of harm when restraint is used. There is clear evidence that death can occur during restraint of a highly resistant person in a face-down position. This is called positional asphyxia. Organizational policies and training should include safeguards against this risk.

Further reading

Department of Health (2014). *Positive and Proactive Care: Reducing the Need for Restrictive Interventions*. Department of Health: London.

Heyvaert S, Saenen L, Maes B, Onghena P (2014). Systematic review of restraint interventions for challenging behaviour among persons with intellectual disabilities: focus on experiences. *Journal of Applied Research in Intellectual Disabilities*. **28**: 61–80.

References

15 Regulation and Quality Improvement Authority (2014). *Awareness and Use of Restrictive Practices in Mental Health and Learning Disability Hospitals*. Regulation and Quality Improvement Authority: Belfast.

16 Department of Health (2014). *Positive and Proactive Care: Reducing the Need for Restrictive Interventions*. Department of Health: London. ℘ www.gov.uk/government/uploads/system/uploads/attachment_data/file/300293/JRA_DoH_Guidance_on_RP_web_accessible.pdf (accessed 15 March 2018).

Keeping yourself safe

Nursing at times involves working directly with people who may engage in a range of behaviours that have the potential to cause harm to others. Personal safety is an important consideration for all nurses. All registered nurses have a responsibility for their own safety. Nursing staff, along with other professional colleagues, have a professional duty of care and must always be aware that people with intellectual disabilities may behave differently when under stress or confused. Communication is a critical component of care in order to de-escalate and to explain situations and expectations. In addition, organizations that employ nurses to work with people who have the propensity to harm others have a duty to ensure that staff are appropriately trained and supported to work safely.

Types of harm

Nurses may encounter a range of potentially harmful behaviour in the course of their practice. This places them at risk of various types of harm:

- Physical injury as a result of being a victim of violence and/or as a result of involvement in the management of violent incidents or physical interventions and restraint (see ➔ Use of restraint, pp. 444–5);
- Emotional and psychological harm as a result of the demands of the role and associated with working in direct care roles with people who have significant difficulties in relationships with others;
- Risk of harm as a result of indirect actions, e.g. allegations made by patients/clients;
- Risk of sexual harm due to sexual assault and/or abusive behaviour;
- Risks associated with the nature of this area of practice, including those arising from involvement in decision-making about risk and the potential for things to go wrong.

Risk assessment and management

A thorough and objective understanding of the needs and risks of patients is a key component for safe practice.

- Take all available information into account and avoid unnecessary risks.
- Do not compromise your own safety—take time to familiarize yourself with information about the person and avoid shortcuts. Tell senior colleagues if you are concerned that you lack the necessary knowledge and understanding to keep yourself safe.
- Ensure all activities that could give rise to risk are discussed and agreed with the person's care team and others involved in the person's care and management.
- All nurses strive to develop positive therapeutic relationships with their patients; never conclude that a special relationship with the person will protect you from harm. Always balance factual information regarding previous behaviour and risks with other opinions, including impressions gained from your personal relationship with the person.
- Always abide by agreed risk management plans, regardless of whether you consider these overly cautious or restrictive.

Physical danger

Some nursing roles involve working with people who engage in violent be-haviour and pose a risk of injury or harm to others, including staff.

- Staff should receive training in the management of disturbed and violent behaviour (see ➲ Use of restraint, pp. 444–5).
- Clear policies and guidance should be in place regarding the management of violence, covering all types of interventions used to manage potentially dangerous behaviour, including restraint, observations, seclusion, and training. Always familiarize yourself with these policies, and report any issues that affect your ability to abide by them.
- Additional safeguards should be provided for staff where they are deemed necessary. These may include personal and environmental alarm systems, use of mobile phones, seclusion facilities, debriefing, and other staff support arrangements and policy on lone working.

Recording and reporting

- Always share any concerns with colleagues, and use formal reporting procedures to record and report any, and all, concerns that could affect your own safety and/or the safety of others. This may include statements and opinions expressed by patients, as well as threats and statements of intent to harm other people.
- Report all incidents, including those which could have resulted in harm (near misses) and less serious incidents that are indicative of risk.
- If you are a victim of violence, you may report this to the police. Even though the police response may be affected because the incident involves a person with intellectual disabilities, you have the same rights as any other victim (see ➲ Rights of victims, pp. 424–5).

Code of conduct

All nurses must abide by their code of conduct/ethics.[17,18] These documents include important requirements for safe practice:

- Respect people's confidentiality—you must disclose information if you believe someone may be at risk;
- Share information with colleagues and effective teamworking;
- Keep clear and accurate records;
- Maintain clear professional boundaries;
- Professional duty of candour (NMC, 2015).

In the interests of clients, patients, and registrants, registered nurses have professional indemnity insurance in the event of claims of professional negligence. The forensic process is adversarial, and nurses may experience serious conflicts between their caring and custodial/public protection roles. Role clarity is essential for safe practice, and nurses must ensure that they always work strictly within the boundaries of their role and competence.

Further reading

Norman A, Walsh L (2014). *Nursing in the Criminal Justice System*. M&K Publishing: Keswick.

References

17 Nursing and Midwifery Council (2015). *The Code: Professional Standards of Practice and Behaviour for Nurses and Midwives*. Nursing and Midwifery Council: London.
18 Nursing and Midwifery Board for Ireland (2014). *Code of Professional Conduct and Ethics*. Nursing and Midwifery Board for Ireland: Dublin.

Management in the community

For some people, a prison sentence may be the right option, but for some, community orders have been shown to be effective in both cost and quality of outcome, for both the person and society. A variety of orders can be considered from treatment programmes that should be complied with. These options need to be available and understood by the sentence, and nursing staff have a crucial role in helping to advise, guide, and support such options. For many offenders, a community disposal will be sufficient and will enable them to receive ongoing input and supervision without recourse to a custodial sentence. Offenders with intellectual disabilities should have access to the same range of community options as other offenders. This can be problematic, unless additional support is available to help the person understand what is required of them and to assist them to abide by any conditions that may be imposed to manage the risk of harm. For many offenders, a shared approach that involves joint working between the criminal justice system, specialist intellectual disabilities services, and social services will provide the most effective means of reducing re-offending and managing the risk of harm.

Options for community management

Community sentences

Community sentences are a combination of punishment and interventions to change the offender's behaviour. Community sentences can also include a condition that the offender participates in treatment and can be used to encourage an offender to deal with problems that might be contributing to their offending, i.e. drinks and drugs, mental disorder. A range of different orders have recently been replaced with a single generic community order (previously called a probation order), which can be personalized to a specific offender, with a range of possible conditions and requirements:

- Compulsory/unpaid work;
- Participation in specified activities, including offending behaviour programmes, and attendance for treatment of associated problems, e.g. mental health problems, drug or alcohol problems;
- Prohibition from certain activities;
- Curfew;
- Exclusion from specified areas;
- Residence requirement;
- Supervision by the probation service;
- Technological restrictions, including tagging.

A community sentence is not available, unless the offender is able to give an informed indication that they are willing and able to comply with the order itself and any requirements. It should not be assumed that people with intellectual disabilities cannot benefit from a community sentence. Specialist intellectual disabilities services can advise the probation service and the courts regarding the use of community sentences and advise on how offenders can be supported to understand and comply with any requirements and to benefit from the order.

Civil enforcement

These orders are intended to manage harmful behaviour in the community. The orders can be made by lower courts (in their civil capacity) or a county court. The police can apply for an order.

Antisocial behaviour orders (ASBOs)
- The police and other agencies can apply for an ASBO.
- Application must be supported by evidence of antisocial behaviour.
- Order includes specified conditions to prevent antisocial behaviour.
- Breach of the order is a criminal offence.

Sex offender prevention orders (SOPOs)
- The police can apply for a SOPO.
- Application must be supported by evidence of behaviour that is sexually risky or indicative of the risk of sexual harm.
- May include general and specific prohibitions, e.g. to remain at a specified distance from a local school, not to enter parks.
- Breach of the order is a criminal offence.

Appropriate behaviour contracts (ABCs)

An ABC is an informal agreement with the police in the form of a written contract agreed and signed at a meeting involving the individual. Potential for legal action to be taken can be stated in the contract. People with intellectual disabilities can benefit from these arrangements, but care should be taken to ensure that the person concerned has the capacity to understand what is expected of them and the consequences if they fail to abide by the requirements of the civil enforcement order. Specialist staff in intellectual disabilities can help people to understand these orders and provide advice to the police regarding appropriate requirements.

Multi-Agency Public Protection Arrangements (MAPPAs)

MAPPAs are the statutory arrangements for managing sexual and violent offenders. The police, probation, and prison services are the responsible authorities for MAPPA (see ➔ Multi-Agency Public Protection arrangements (MAPPA), p. 425). The MAPPA provides structures and mechanisms for agencies to come together to agree risk management plans, including plans for people being released from prison.

Joint working

The most effective means of community management is through joint and collaborative working between the various agencies that have a responsibility for public safety. This shared approach should provide shared decision-making about risk. Wherever possible, the responsibility for risk should also be shared with the individual concerned. Intellectual disabilities services should engage with partners in other agencies to ensure that all reasonable steps have been taken to support people in their communities.

Further reading

KeyRing. *KeyRing and the Criminal Justice System.* ✍ www.keyring.org/cjs (accessed 30 October 2017).
NHS England (2015). *Transforming Care for People with Learning Disabilities: Next Steps.* ✍ www.england.
nhs.uk/wp-content/uploads/2015/01/transform-care-nxt-stps.pdf (accessed 30 October 2017).
The Ideas Collective (2015). *Keeping out of Trouble: Alternatives to Prison or Hospital for People with
Learning Disabilities Who Get into Trouble with the Law.* ✍ ec.europa.eu/epale/sites/epale/files/
keeping-out-of-trouble.pdf (accessed 30 October 2017).

Working with criminal justice agencies

There is a great deal of guidance for professionals in the criminal justice system and staff in health and welfare organizations which focuses upon interagency and joint working with mentally disordered offenders. The need for effective collaboration is a central tenet of the code of conduct/ethics of nurses in the UK and the Republic of Ireland.[19,20] Decisions on law enforcement, diversion from the normal process of criminal law, and disposal options for people with intellectual disabilities who are alleged to have committed offences and/or who are convicted are inconsistent and, at times, seem arbitrary.

The criminal justice system

Across the UK, the NOMS has overall responsibility for correctional services and provides a bridge between custodial and community services. The criminal justice system is made of several agencies that have general responsibilities in terms of crime prevention and reduction, and specific responsibilities to address the needs and risks of offenders and alleged offenders. These agencies work closely together to fulfil their responsibilities and provide a range of custodial and community services. The main services that make up the criminal justice system are the:
• Police;
• Probation service;
• Prison service;
• Courts.

Multi-Agency Public Protections Arrangements

MAPPAs are the statutory arrangements for managing sexual and violent offenders. The police, probation, and prison services are the responsible authorities for MAPPAs. Other public bodies, including the NHS and social services, have a duty to cooperate with the MAPPAs. The MAPPA approach to collaborative working can be applied to specialist health roles that involve joint working with criminal justice agencies.

Criminal justice liaison

People with intellectual disabilities who get into trouble with the law constitute a small minority group who are not a high priority for the criminal justice system. Criminal justice agencies need specialist advice and input to adequately address the particular needs of this group and improve access to the responses, services, and interventions available to all offenders where these are appropriate and could manage and reduce the risk of offending.

Nurses for people with intellectual disabilities can provide valuable support in the form of criminal justice liaison roles:
• Supporting people with intellectual disabilities who get into trouble with the law to understand their own situations and the decisions that are made as part of the criminal justice process;
• Developing working relationships with local criminal justice agencies, including the police, the probation service, prisons, and the courts;

- Developing a knowledge base regarding the operation of the criminal justice system and identifying points at which practical help, specialist advice, input, and support could be beneficial;
- Providing advice to inform decisions about people with intellectual disabilities;
- Providing advice/information regarding other services.

Role clarity is absolutely essential when working at the interface between health services and the law:
- At all times, be aware that you may be called upon to justify/defend your opinions in a legal arena.
- Work strictly within the boundaries of your role and competence.
- Get full support from your line manager/employer for all aspects of your practice.
- Communicate and discuss the details of your involvement with your team and through clinical supervision.
- Seek advice and support from others in similar roles, including practitioners in other areas, if required.
- Undertake training that equips you for the role, including training specific to mentally disordered offenders and the law as it applies to people with mental disorder.

Joint working
The most effective means of supporting people with intellectual disabilities who have offended is through joint and collaborative working between the various agencies that have a responsibility for public safety. This shared approach should provide shared decision-making about risk. Wherever possible, the responsibility for risks should be shared with the individual concerned. Intellectual disabilities services should engage with partners in other agencies to ensure that all reasonable steps have been taken to support people in their communities.

Further reading
Kelly E, Ní Laoi M (2015). *Working with Young People Involved in the Juvenile Justice System* (across Ireland). www.youth.ie/sites/youth.ie/files/Chapter%208%20-%20working%20with%20young%20people%20involved%20in%20the%20Juvenile%20Justice%20System%20-%20all%20Ireland_0.pdf (accessed 30 October 2017).

Ministry of Justice (2016 updated December 2016). *National Offender Management Centre (2016) MAPPA Guidance 2012 version 4.1*. Ministry of Justice: London.

Norman A, Walsh L (2014). *Nursing in the Criminal Justice System*. M&K Publishing: Keswick.

Scottish Government (2016). *Multi-Agency Public Protection Arrangements (MAPPA) National Guidance*. Scottish Government: Edinburgh.

References
19 Nursing and Midwifery Council (2015). *The Code: Professional Standards of Practice and Behaviour for Nurses and Midwives*. Nursing and Midwifery Council: London.

20 Nursing and Midwifery Board for Ireland (2014). *Code of Professional Conduct and Ethics*. Nursing and Midwifery Board for Ireland: Dublin.

Lifestyles and intellectual disability nursing

Citizenship

The concept of citizenship is based on the relationship between the individual and the state. It embraces the idea of reciprocity between rights and responsibilities, between both citizen and state. If one accepts the existence of rights, there must be a corresponding acceptance of duties. Typically someone may be referred to as a 'good citizen', because they live up to their responsibilities in society. As part of the reciprocal relationship, it is believed that the state has an obligation to meet the welfare needs of all of its citizens. The principle of representation is fundamental in society. It is connected closely with the concept of citizenship which centres on this relationship between the individual and the state. It has been suggested that citizenship as a status is bestowed on those who are full members of a community.[1] Marshall[1] has described three elements of citizenship: civil, political, and social. The civil element comprises the rights which are necessary for individual freedom. These include personal liberty, freedom of speech, thought, and faith, and the right to own property and conclude valid contracts. The right to justice, a significant civil right, is the legal right to defend all of one's rights on an equal basis by means of the legal process. The political element concerns participation in the exercise of political power at local and/or national level. It may involve participation either as an elector or as a member of an elected body (local government, parliament), which is invested with political authority. The social element includes the right, to some degree, of economic welfare and security, as well as the right to share in the social heritage and to live life according to the standards prevailing in a society. Citizens require access to social resources, including health, education, and social services, in order to further their own, as well as other people's, civil and political rights. A central aim of more recent health and social policy has been to give people more say in the services they use. Health services and local authorities, which provide health and social services, are required to consult with service users and user organizations. The consumer's voice is important and particularly significant for members of vulnerable groups such as people with intellectual disabilities.

Recent years have seen developments in policy and practice in England, Wales, Northern Ireland, Scotland, and the Republic of Ireland relating to the welfare and interests of disadvantaged groups.[2] In the UK, the implementation of the Human Rights 1998 promotes egalitarian principles. Article 14 states that '*the rights and freedoms set forth in this Convention shall be secured without discrimination on any ground*' (Human Rights Act, 1998).[3] Whereas these rights had existed previously, the advantage of the Human Rights Act is that it enables challenges to be made in UK courts.

In 2001, the UK government set an agenda for people with intellectual disabilities in a White Paper *Valuing People: a New Strategy for Learning Disability for the 21st Century*.[4] The White Paper sought to promote the civil, political, and legal rights of people with intellectual disabilities, and these were expressed as four pillars; choice, rights, inclusion, and independence. Following this agenda, in the UK, individuals have noted substantial improvements in the services they access, as well as representation for their civil rights.[5] Such rights have been monumental development for people with intellectual disabilities. More recently, the government has taken forward an agenda to deinstitutionalize services by laying out the following vision for all disabled people: *'By 2025, disabled people in Britain should have full opportunities and choices to improve their quality of life and will be respected and included as equal members of society'*.[6]

In the Republic of Ireland, the term 'decongregation' is used to refer to the development of smaller and more community-based living settings.[7]

References

1 Marshall TH (1991). *Citizenship and Social Class and Other Essays*. Pluto Press: London.
2 Gilbert T, Cochrane A, Greenwell S (2005). Citizenship: locating people with learning disabilities. *International Journal of Social Welfare*. 14: 287–96.
3 *The Human Rights Act (1998)*. The Stationery Office: London.
4 Department of Health (2001). *Valuing People: A New Strategy for the 21st Century*. The Stationery Office: London.
5 Hatton C, Emerson E, Lobb C (2005). *Evaluating the Impact of Valuing People Report of Phase 1: A Review of Existing National Datasets*. Institute for Health Research: Lancaster.
6 Prime Minister's Strategy Unit (2005). *Improving the Life Chances of Disabled People: Final Report*. Cabinet Office: London.
7 Health Service Executive (2011). *Time to Move on from Congregated Settings: A Strategy for Community Inclusion*. Health Service Executive: Dublin. www.hse.ie/eng/services/list/4/disability/congregatedsettings/ (accessed 31 October 2017).

Supported living and home ownership

In 2011, Mencap[9] found that the majority of people with intellectual disabilities in England and Wales known to local authorities lived in one of four types of accommodation: family and friends (38%), registered care home (22%), supported accommodation (16%), and as tenants in accommodation provided by local authorities or housing associations (12%) and in privately rented accommodation (3%). In the UK and Ireland, there continues to be an emphasis on the role that local services should play in supporting a person's right to live independently.[9]

Supported living

Supported living might best be thought of as a range of residential alternatives for people with intellectual disabilities; however, central to all alternatives are living in one's own home and participating in one's own community—this has become known as inclusion, and with all planning centred on the individual. Supported living is a model of living that supports an individual's wish to live in the way they want, rather than fitting into existing services.[10] Supported living was developed in the USA, born from frustration of the then dominant residential alternatives for people with intellectual disabilities.

Mencap[11] described supported living as people with intellectual disabilities being supported in a house owned by either a private landlord or a housing association, and having a tenancy agreement. It is argued that supported living is a better option, compared with traditional models of care.

Supported living increases independence over time by reducing the level of support required and empowering people with opportunity to take risks and eventually to move to more independent living.[12] People with intellectual disabilities who live in supported living accommodation have better engagement with their community and satisfaction with life. Supported living promotes a person's lifestyle and social inclusion and enables development and growth. People with intellectual disabilities in supported living are given greater power of services they use, resulting in a significantly reduced need for inpatient care.[10]

Many local authorities in the UK have changed services from residential care to supported housing for people with intellectual disabilities. The change focuses on achieving wider access to welfare benefits and having a tenancy. The aim of supported living is to achieve choice, control, and community inclusion, but in the past, it has been much less of a focus.[11]

In the report on developing supported living options for people with intellectual disabilities, it was stated that:

> 'People with intellectual disabilities are one of the most socially excluded groups in society and this is primarily a result of an historical segregation of services that unintentionally deny people their own home, choice and control and a decent income; factors which ultimately deny citizenship and social inclusion'.[13]

The funding model with supported living is split between social services and health funding and the welfare benefit system. The former pays for the necessary care and support required, while the latter pays only for housing and everyday living costs.[13]

There are identified challenges to the development and provision of independent living arising from aspects such as limited housing and support services to meet the increased demands and failure by services and family members to plan for future housing and support needs.

Home ownership by people with intellectual disabilities

Home ownership for people with long-term disabilities (HOLD) is an option where someone with disabilities can own their own home, which is administered by a housing association, who is the registered social landlord.[14] In this option, an individual finds a property they want to buy, then the housing association buys the property and sells part of it to the individual; they have an option to buy more of it in the future. They rent the other part, making the housing association responsible for repairs and the condition of the property. This is a good home ownership option for people with intellectual disabilities, as it has worked well for others, and it is secure. The disadvantage is that it can become complicated, and not all landlords offer the HOLD option and obtaining a mortgage can be difficult.

Further reading

Cocks E, Thoresen S, Williamson N, Boaden R (2014). The individual supported living (ISL) manual: a planning and review instrument for individual supported living arrangements for adults with intellectual and developmental disabilities. *Journal of Intellectual Disability Research*. **58**: 614–24.

Isaacson NC, Cocks E, Netto JA (2014). Launching: the experiences of two young adults with intellectual disability and their families in transition to individual supported living. *Journal of Intellectual and Developmental Disability*. **39**: 270–81.

Transforming Care and Commissioning Steering Group (2014). *Winterbourne View – Time for Change: Transforming the Commissioning of Services for People with Learning Disabilities and/or Autism*. Transforming Care and Commissioning Steering Group: London.

References

9 Mencap (2012). *Housing for People with a Learning Disability*. Mencap: London.

10 Housing and Support Alliance (2016). *What is Supported Living?* ℘ www.housingandsupport.org. uk/what-is-supported-living-bf (accessed 31 October 2017).

11 Mencap (2017). *Supported Living Services*. ℘ www.mencap.org.uk/advice-and-support/services-you-can-count/supported-living-services (accessed 31 October 2017).

12 Wood A, Greig R (2010). *Supported Living: Making the Move Developing Supported Living Options for People with Learning Disabilities*. National Development Team for Inclusion: Bath.

13 Houlden A (2015). *Building the Right Support: A National Plan to Develop Community Services and Close Inpatient Facilities for People with a Learning Disability and/or Autism who Display Behaviour that Challenges, Including those with a Mental Health Condition*. ℘ www.england.nhs.uk/wp-content/uploads/2015/10/ld-nat-imp-plan-oct15.pdf (accessed 31 October 2017).

14 Housing and Support Alliance (2016). *Home Ownership*. ℘ www.housingandsupport.org.uk/home-ownership-bf (accessed 31 October 2017).

Village communities

Village communities have been defined as: '*[a] service operated by [an] independent organisation comprising houses clustered on one site together that share facilities*', whereas an intentional community was defined as '*services operated by [an] independent sector organisation comprising houses and some shared facilities on one or more sites based on philosophical or religious belief*'.[15]

Village communities

The origins of such communities lie in the Camphill Village movement, established by Dr Karl König in Scotland during the 1940s.

This movement is based on the educational theories of Rudolf Steiner (1861–1925), and it was from his philosophy that the idea of therapeutic communities was developed.[16]

Therapies are supported by anthroposophical ideas and homeopathic medicines, which, alongside the community experience, are designed to: '*foster the harmonious development of the whole human being – body, soul and spirit – to create a healthy balance between thinking, feeling, and with activity and to engender morality, social co-operation and responsibility*'.[17]

In such communities, residents, according to their abilities, contribute what they can to the well-being of other members. The idea is to foster mutual help and understanding in an environment that seeks to counter some of the supposed 'harmful' ways of modern life.

Non-disabled members of the community are not referred to as carers, rather as coworkers. They do not receive financial remuneration for their efforts, and the nature of the relationship between other village members is based on equality.

Intentional communities

The problem with the definition of '*village communities*' is that not all such communities can be properly described as villages, and so an alternative term '*intentional communities*' has emerged, which perhaps describes some of them more accurately. There are other types of residential community, and these include L'Arche, a federation of communities in the UK, France, Denmark, Belgium, Norway, and the USA, as well as in India, along with Cottage and Rural Enterprise and the Home Farm Trust. A recent publication by Jackson[18] provides compelling reading, broadening the range of day and residential options for people with learning disabilities. In this sense, he makes a contemporary case for intentional and supportive communities.

Further reading

Grant G, Ramcharan P, Flynn M, Richardson M (2010). *Learning Disability: A Life Cycle Approach to Valuing People*, 2nd edn. Open University Press: Milton Keynes.

Hft. ℬ www.hft.org.uk (accessed 31 October 2017).

L'Arche in the UK. ℬ www.larche.org.uk (accessed 31 October 2017).

Orchard Trust. ℬ www.orchard-trust.org.uk (accessed 31 October 2017).

References

15 Department of Health (2001). *Valuing People: A New Strategy for Learning Disability for the 21st Century. CM 5086.* The Stationery Office: London; pp. 70–5.

16 Jackson R (1999). The case for village communities for adults with learning disabilities: an exploration of the concept. *Journal of Learning Disabilities for Nursing, Health and Social Care.* 3: 110–17.

17 Fulgosi L (1990). Camphill communities. In: S Segal, ed. *The Place of Special Villages and Residential Communities.* AB Academic Publishers: Oxford; pp 39–48.

18 Jackson R (2017). *Back to Bedlam: What Kind of Future Face People with Learning Disabilities.* Centre for Welfare Reform: Sheffield. ℘ www.centreforwelfarereform.org (accessed 31 October 2017).

Residential alternatives

In most Western countries, residential care for people with intellectual disabilities has, at some point, been influenced by political, ideological, and economic factors. Given that people with intellectual disabilities have been, and still are, often misunderstood, this has sometimes resulted in inappropriate residential care being offered to them and their families. In this section, a range of residential alternatives for people with intellectual disabilities are outlined.

Hospital-type accommodation

An example of past inappropriate residential care was that of hospital-type accommodation. Contemporary care provision has seen the closure of most long-stay intellectual disabilities hospitals; however, some residential care provision, known as 'residential campuses', have remained. Generally speaking, these types of provision retain therapists and nursing and medical staff and provide a specialist focus on care. Whereas 2009 saw the closure of the last 'long-stay' hospital in England,[19] closure rates in other countries have moved at a slower pace; overall some resistance has remained towards the closure of this type of accommodation. This has resulted in some services moving into the private sector. Voids left by closure in this area have largely been redistributed to 'supported housing' schemes and independent living accommodation and residential-style accommodation.[20]

Policy

Current policy related to provision of residential alternatives for people with intellectual disabilities is dependent on local provision in each geographical location.[20] Policy remains committed towards ensuring that people with intellectual disabilities fundamentally have the right to choose where to live.[19] However, for many people with intellectual disabilities, obstacles remain in relation to this issue.[20]

Current provision

Literature has identified that people with intellectual disabilities in England typically live in the following types of residential alternatives:
- 38% with friends and/or family;
- 22% in a registered care home;
- 16% in supported accommodation;
- 12% as tenants in accommodation provided by local housing association;
- 3% in privately rented accommodation; and
- 9% in other non-specified accommodation types.[20]

In other parts of the UK and Ireland, provision of residential alternatives remains patchy. There is still much work required in the area of imagining and providing residential services in order to truly reflect the needs, aspirations, and choices of people with intellectual disabilities and their families regarding where and how they live.

Conclusion

Overall although much progress has been made in this area, there is still a long way to go to meet individual choices in this area.

Further reading

Health Service Executive (2011). *Time to Move on from Congregated Settings: A Strategy for Community Inclusion*. Health Service Executive: Dublin. ℘ www.hse.ie/eng/services/list/4/disability/congregatedsettings/ (accessed 31 October 2017).

References

19 Department of Health (2009). *Valuing People Now: A New Three-Year Strategy for People with Learning Disabilities*. Department of Health: London.
20 Mencap (2017). *Supported Living Services*. ℘ www.mencap.org.uk/advice-and-support/services-you-can-count/supported-living-services (accessed 31 October 2017).

Risk management

Definition

Whereas risk assessment and management (see ➐ Forensic risk assessment and management, p. 418) looked at the topic in the context of forensic nursing, this section looks more broadly at risk in the context of lifestyles. There are many definitions of risk management currently available, but broadly risk management in healthcare may be broken down into two aspects:[21]

- **Strategic risk management**, in which the emphasis is on doing 'the right thing'; this should be stated clearly within an organization's business plans, operational policies and procedures, and risk registers. It is important that all staff make themselves aware of their role and responsibilities in relation to an organization's risk management processes;
- **Operational risk management** where the emphasis is on ensuring that all staff are 'doing things right'. This has clear links to nurses' code of conduct, clinical competency and governance, and general management of services.[22,23] The care programme approach provides a systematic framework for managing risks in clinical settings (see ➐ Forensic risk assessment and management, p. 418). As operational risk management is an ongoing process, there is a clear need that this is linked with practitioners' ongoing development and should be linked, for all staff, to the knowledge and skills framework and clinical and management supervision processes.

Following the outcomes of the *Mazars Report* (2016),[24] all NHS organizations need to have robust systems in place to review deaths of people with intellectual disabilities who access services.

Policy

Within the NHS, organizations are mandated to have clear policies and procedures for the management of risk within organizations. There are many organizations that are relevant to healthcare delivery and risk management, including the Care Quality Commission (CQC), Regulation and Quality Improvement Authority (RQIA), Health Information and Quality Authority (HIQA), Health and Safety Executive, NICE, and NHS Litigation Authority.

All individuals are accountable for maintaining their knowledge around risk management policies and strategies within their organization and in other agencies. Nurses should know how this relates to their day-to-day practice and be able to communicate risk issues.

Person-centred approach to risk management

It is important that the nurse working with people with intellectual disabilities adheres to the organizational policy and approach to risk management; they have a responsibility to keep the person safe, while not restricting them from experiencing a full and meaningful life. Nurses should question when institutionalized or blanket approaches are used because of one individual where this has impacted on the rights of other individuals.

When supporting an individual to manage risks associated with their life-style, it is crucial to determine that the person has the capacity to make decisions specific to that particular risk. When someone makes an unwise decision, this does not imply incapacity. It is essential that, when addressing issues of capacity, nurses are fully compliant with the latest capacity legislation or policy guidance within the country they are practising.

Conclusion

It is imperative that individuals and organizations learn the lessons from these reports and implement changes in order to promote opportunities for people with intellectual disabilities to develop new opportunities, while at the same time effectively assessing and managing risks that may affect the person. It is vital that the nurse incorporates a model for learning lessons and disseminating within their practice, supervision, and organization. The nurse revalidation process provides all with an opportunity to reflect and demonstrate that they are continually improving their practice. The role and dilemma facing nurses in intellectual disabilities services are to balance the rights and choices of the people they are supporting to lead an independent life and to experience new opportunities, while not exposing people to un-necessary dangers or being too restrictive.

Further reading

Aras Attracta Swinford Review Group (2016). *Time for Action: National Priorities Arising from National Consultation*. Health Service Executive: Dublin.

References

21 NHS Litigation Authority (2007). *Pilot Risk Management Standards for Mental Health and Learning Disability Trusts*. NHS Litigation Authority: London.

22 Nursing and Midwifery Council (2015). *The Code: Professional Standards for Practice and Behaviour for Nurses and Midwives*. Nursing and Midwifery Council: London.

23 Nursing and Midwifery Board of Ireland (2014). *Code of Professional Conduct and Ethics for Registered Nurses and Registered Midwives*. Nursing and Midwifery Board of Ireland: Dublin.

24 Green B, Bruce MA, Finn P, et al. (2015). *Mazars Report: Independent Review of Deaths of People with a Learning Disability or Mental Health Problem in Contact with Southern Health NHS Foundation Trust April 2011 to 2015*. NHS England: London. ℘ www.england.nhs.uk/south/wp-content/uploads/sites/6/2015/12/mazars-rep.pdf (accessed 31 October 2017).

Productive work

Many people with intellectual disabilities want to work. They can become productive workers if given the opportunity. Indeed, it is vital that this happens. Being a worker:

- Increases their status within the family and society, and they are seen as having talents and abilities;
- Reduces their dependency on others; it takes away some of the strain of care-giving within families and services;
- Enhances their self-esteem and self-confidence; being trusted with responsibilities brings other personal gains in mental and physical well-being;
- Provides opportunities for socializing; relationships can be formed and a greater range of social supports accessed.

Opportunities for work

As Fig. 12.1 shows, there are many opportunities for people to become productive workers. These can be grouped into three strands.

Home-based work

This can start at an early age, as children and teenagers learn to care for themselves, e.g. eating, washing, and dressing. These family-based experiences can be extended into household chores such as cooking and cleaning. As their competence grows, a variety of house maintenance tasks become possible, e.g. window cleaning, painting, gardening. These skills can be used in their own homes, but this type of work can also be done for neighbours and friends on a voluntary basis. Indeed, these skills may form the basis for obtaining paid work. Families and schools are key to promoting these forms of work opportunities.

Preparation for employment

This strand provides opportunities for acquiring the generic skills required to hold down a job, e.g. time-keeping, communication, and cooperation, as well as the specific competences needed to undertake certain jobs. These skills can be acquired as part of training courses undertaken in schools and colleges, alongside work experience opportunities in realistic settings. Voluntary work also offers many opportunities to acquire and develop work-related skills, e.g. assisting in a charity shop, helping in old people's homes, or care-taking duties in a community centre. Increasingly, schools promote these options, as well as colleges and specialist employment services.

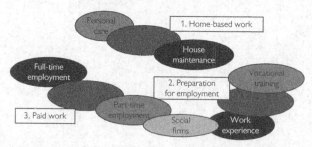

Fig. 12.1 Opportunities for productive work.

Options for paid work

Growing numbers of people with intellectual disabilities are attaining their ambition to be in paid employment. In the past, this type of work has been mainly around 'sheltered' employment, specifically for persons with disabilities. However, fears of exploitation have seen these options replaced by 'social firms', in which workers with disabilities are treated more as employees or as trainees. Part-time, paid employment with one or more employers can be especially suited to people with disabilities and avoids some of the problems around reduction in social security benefits. Nonetheless, full-time employment has been possible for some and reduces greatly their dependency on social services. Self-employment opportunities are also developing, e.g. baking specialty products. The advent of specialist employment services for people with disabilities has increased the options for paid employment.

Creating productive workers

Start young

Children can learn self-help skills from an early age and should be encouraged to take responsibility for certain tasks around the house. These skills can be further developed in the teenage years and into adulthood. However, it is never too late for people to learn.

Common expectations

Person-centred planning is the forum in which the young person, the family, schools, and support staff can identify 'work' goals across the spectrum shown in Fig. 12.1, and plan together on how they will support the person's learning. These expectations include completing work to a high standard. Shoddy performance should be discouraged.

Opportunities to work

Experience of work is vital to help young people to test out their talents and appreciate what particular jobs entail. This will also help them to acquire the discipline needed to ensure the job is completed efficiently.

Building intrinsic motivation

Work needs to be personally satisfying, and ways of making it so should be incorporated into any training strategy, e.g. by identifying their preferences and ensuring they feature in the work.

Social skills

Among the reasons for people failing in paid employment is a lack of social skills needed to work as part of a team, and acting immaturely. Hence attention needs to be paid to the wider employability skills, as well as the specific skills required by particular jobs.

Forward planning

Progress reviews will help to identify potential difficulties before they become major problems, and revised plans drawn up to overcome them. Career development plans will provide a context for any further training and help to chart job progression.

Further reading

In Control. ℘ www.in-control.org.uk (accessed 31 October 2017).
McConkey R (2011). Leisure and friendships. In: HL Atherton, DJ Crickmore, eds. *Learning Disabilities: Toward Inclusion*, 6th edn. Elsevier: Oxford; pp. 431–48.

Supported employment

Supported employment is founded on the principle of 'place and train', rather than 'train then place', which had dominated work opportunities within intellectual disabilities services in the past. The goal of supported employment is to find paid employment for the person, in line with their talents and interests. He or she is trained 'on the job' by a 'job coach' who also adjusts the working environment, if necessary, and enlists the assistance of coworkers to provide additional monitoring and support. The job coach gradually fades out but remains in contact with employers and coworkers to give further advice and support.

Specialist supported employment services have been established in many locations. In the main, these have served clients with mild and moderate disabilities, although there are examples of people with severe disabilities and challenging behaviours also benefiting. They take referrals from various sources, such as school-leavers, further education colleges, and career advisors, as well as from individuals and their families.

These services approach employers and undertake an analysis of jobs available in each setting. A profile will be completed of each jobseeker, including their present competences, interests, and past experiences. Arrangements will be made for clients to have 'work tasters' by placing them with local businesses for a defined period of time. Also further training courses may be arranged, notably those that lead to an accredited award such as a National Vocational Qualification (NVQ) Level 1.

Clients will be assisted in drawing up a curriculum vitae and coached in interview skills. When they are successful in gaining a position, a 'job coach' will be allocated who will teach the skills required for the job to the client in the workplace. The job coach will attend alongside the person until such time as the client can competently complete the work—this may extend from days to weeks. During the training phase, the salary of the new worker may be reduced to reflect the level of their productivity. However, the goal is for the client to be paid at least the national minimum wage or the going rate for that particular post.

The job coach maintains periodic contact with the client, the coworkers, and employer and is available to offer advice and support, should any difficulties arise. Regular job reviews will be undertaken, in line with the client's career development plans.

There is growing evidence for the cost benefits of these services in getting people into paid work, alongside high levels of user satisfaction. To date, only a minority of people have been able to access these services, and issues around long-term support have not been resolved. One solution is to engage a wider range of staff in seeking and supporting people in work settings, e.g. staff in supported living schemes could be allocated this function, and personal assistants paid through Direct Payments.

Six key steps in structured teaching

Set learning targets

These should be tasks of interest to the person and for which he or she has some of the necessary competences. In other words, it is not going to prove too difficult for them to learn.

Graded step

The task is broken down into discrete steps, so that the person can practise doing one step at a time. When they have accomplished one, they can move to doing two steps, then three, and so on.

Praise

Learners' achievements need to be recognized with praise. This serves the dual purpose of letting learners know they are correct, while making them more willing to persevere. Equally, any mistakes should be quickly pointed out and an example given of the correct action.

Practice

It takes practice for any new skill to be done fluently across different settings and to a consistent standard. 'Over-learning' is recommended for people with intellectual disabilities to minimize mistakes.

Realistic settings

Learning and practice are best done in the actual setting where the task is to be performed. Although some practice can be done in 'pretend' settings, the person still has to transfer their skills to the real world. People with learning disabilities can find this difficult to do.

On-the-job learning

Job coaches use structured techniques to teach people work skills. These strategies have a long history of success with people with intellectual disabilities, e.g. in teaching self-care and household skills. These techniques are based around careful observation and ongoing assessment of each person's competences in one-to-one teaching sessions. Although it may take people with intellectual disabilities longer to learn, they can achieve levels of competence on a par with non-disabled peers. Various training manuals are available to guide frontline staff in how they can implement these and other training strategies.

Social security benefits

One of the main disincentives to entering into paid employment is the impact of earnings on social security benefits paid to people with intellectual disabilities and their families. Advice should be sought from benefit specialists about the best way of structuring earnings from employment to avoid loss of entitlements.

Further reading

British Association for Supported Employment (BASE). ℘ www.base-uk.org/our-work (accessed 19 March 2018).

Lysaght R, Šiška J, Koenig O (2015). International employment statistics for people with intellectual disability: the case for common metrics. *Journal of Policy and Practice in Intellectual Disabilities*. 12: 112–19.

Networks of support and friends

Everyone needs the support of other people throughout their lives. Often this comes from family and friends, rather than formal services. For people with intellectual disabilities, it is the reverse. They rely overly on services and the staff in them. Most people with intellectual disabilities have few friends, irrespective of where they live. Many lead lonely and isolated lives, and this is often unnoticed. Of all the assessments carried out by nurses with people with intellectual disabilities, one often not fully explored is an examination of their friendships and social relationships.

The benefits of friendship are well known. It means having the company of others, times of laughter and adventure, people to give you advice and guidance, practical help, emotional support, and protection, and, above all, friends to whom you can show love and affection and who will do the same for you. Quality of life studies constantly stress the importance of friendships, and this is no less so for people with intellectual disabilities. Nurses need to promote friendships if they are to promote the health and well-being of people they support. Promoting friendships has its risks. Might they choose the wrong kind of person? Could they be taken advantage of? Will they get hurt if the friendship is not reciprocated? These risks can be managed and they are not an excuse for inaction.

Friendships are founded on three fundamentals (see also Fig. 12.2):
- Friendships cannot be made for other people; friends choose one another. At best, we can build up a network of acquaintances, out of which friendships may develop;
- Friendships usually grow out of shared interests and activities and from among people already known to the person. This is the starting point;
- Friends choose one another. You need to constantly consult and listen to the people you are trying to help. We must not impose our values and desires onto another.

In this section and in ➔ Encouraging friendships, pp. 470–1, three interlinked strategies are described for promoting friendships and building networks of support.

Expanding social networks

A social network is composed of people who interact socially. We belong to many different networks. We can make this happen for people with intellectual disabilities by getting them involved in leisure, work, and family networks. Often their closest friends will be among other people with a disability—certainly that is how many experience an intimate relationship.

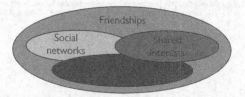

Fig. 12.2 Strategies for promoting friendships.

Creating shared interests

Discover the person's interests by talking with them and giving them opportunities to try new things. Photographs will prompt them to remember. Build their self-confidence and encourage a spirit of adventure in trying new things. There are literally hundreds of indoor and outdoor pursuits in which people can get involved.

Respecting self-determination

People are looking for, and get, different things from friendships. We need to support their informed choices. Avoid being judgemental, but equally explain the safeguards and risks that are relevant. Discretely observe the interactions if you have concerns.

Getting acquainted

There are three approaches nurses can use to help people become better acquainted with people from their local community.

Supporting community involvement

People need to be supported to be involved in community activities. Doing some form of work in social settings can provide regular contact with other people (see ➲ Productive work, pp. 464–5). This can be voluntary or part-time paid work. The volunteer bureau is a good source of information. Citizens Advice Bureaus will let you know about clubs and societies that meet locally. Support staff may be needed to support people initially in joining these groups.

Supporting friendships through invitations

We can support people with intellectual disabilities to invite their family, friends, neighbours, and workmates, and so on to their home or their centre. Celebrations are a good excuse. Make sure people spend time in activities together. Likewise they need to be supported in accepting invitations to meet other people.

Planning and recording relationships

Each person's individual plan must document the significant friendships in their lives—with photos and contact details listed—and the range of interests and activities in which they participate. All staff should receive training on the importance of social relationships in the lives of people they support. This rarely happens at present, as it is not seen as a priority. The high turnover rates among support staff makes it essential to record the valued relationships in people's lives, so that continuity of support is provided.

Further reading

Lysaght R, Šiška J, Koenig O (2015). International employment statistics for people with intellectual disability: the case for common metrics. *Journal of Policy and Practice in Intellectual Disabilities.* 12: 112–19.

Mason P, Timms K, Hayburn T, Watters C (2013). How do people described as having a learning disability make sense of friendship? *Journal of Applied Research in Intellectual Disabilities.* 26: 108–18.

McConkey R, Collins S (2010). Promoting social inclusion through building bridges and bonds. In: M Nind, J Seale, eds. *Understanding and Promoting Access for People with Learning Difficulties: Seeing the Opportunities and Challenges of Risk.* Routledge: Abingdon; pp. 127–39.

McConkey R, Dunne J, Blitz N (2009). *Shared Lives: Building Relationships and Community with People who have Intellectual Disabilities.* Sense Publishers: Rotterdam.

Tilly L (2012). Having friends – they help you when you are stuck from money, friends and making ends meet research group. *British Journal of Learning Disabilities.* 40: 128–33.

Encouraging friendships

In this section, two approaches are described that have proved somewhat successful in developing friendships. There are other ways too through which friendships can emerge, such as advocacy groups and employment opportunities, when friendships are a bonus from other intended outcomes.

Circles of support

The idea of 'circles of support' or a 'circles of friends' began in Canada as a means of supporting people to belong to their local community.[25] In essence, the concept is very simple—a group of people meet regularly to support a person who needs extra assistance to enrich their social and community life.

The circle might include family members, such as siblings, cousins, aunts, and uncles, alongside neighbours and acquaintances, coworkers of people in work settings, and members of clubs, churches, etc. who know the person. The size of the circle does not matter—a few interested people can make a start. However, paid professional workers are not usually members, although they can have a key role in facilitating the formation of the circle or acting as 'go-betweens' for the supported person.

The circle meets from time to time to explore with the person and each other the contributions they are making to each other's lives. Activity plans might develop as to how the circle supports the person in the coming weeks and months.

'In all circles of support, people are encouraged to dream'

Without a vision of what might be possible, the old routines and disappointments persist for the person with intellectual disabilities. Fulfilling their dreams[26] often involves taking risks, but: '*the circle itself is a safety-net and each time a new risk is safely negotiated greater encouragement is generated to renew the risk-taking effort*'.[26]

The idea of 'circles of support' can be taken forward in a number of ways. For example, Key Ring is a housing provider for people with intellectual disabilities; it works to build networks of mutual support among tenants living within a geographical area and, alongside this, builds networks into and among the local community.[27] Another approach is the development of day services through the development of social networks for clients by helping them make use of opportunities for education, recreation, and employment in their local communities.[28]

There is a definitive way for the type and structure of circles of support, and these are very much influenced by the local contexts and by the wishes and needs of the person with intellectual disabilities, as identified in their person-centred plan. Indeed, the richest plans often develop when a circle of support is recruited to assist in developing the person-centred plan, rather than leaving this to paid support staff.

Befrienders

People can be recruited to act as 'buddies' or 'befrienders' for a person with a disability, on either a paid or voluntary basis. They are best thought of as another form of support staff, such as a personal assistant, although a genuine, mutual friendship may develop. Often their role is to accompany the person to leisure activities they both enjoy. Unlike paid staff, they are linked with one person and their times are flexible. Variations of this idea are found in recruiting host families who are prepared to take a child or an adult into their homes for short breaks or acting as job coaches in introducing people to work settings (see ➲ Supported employment, pp. 466–7).

With the advent of individualized (direct) payments, people with intellectual disabilities or their family carers may recruit and employ their own befrienders. Befriending schemes need to be planned and implemented carefully to be successful. In particular, a lot of effort has to go into the recruitment and selection of befrienders. Similarly, payments of expenses or fees need to take account of implications for tax and social security payments. Increasingly, these schemes are provided by agencies who specialize in this form of service provision, usually voluntary organizations.

- Find out if such schemes operate in your area; the local volunteer bureau is a good starting point;
- Identify the particular ways that a befriender might support the person with intellectual disabilities. This will help you to arrive at a 'person specification' for the befriender;
- Explore a range of options for linking the person with other people, in addition to seeking a single befriender. Remember too that people with intellectual disabilities can make very good befrienders of each other;
- Service staff involved with the person should introduce themselves to the befrienders and give them their contact details. From time to time, contact them to find out how things are going, as well as doing it for the person with intellectual disabilities;
- In life, friendships come and go. The loss of a friendship is more noticeable the fewer friends one has, hence the need to develop circles of support alongside befrienders.

Further reading

Buddy Buddies. ℔ www.bestbuddies.org/ (accessed 31 October 2017).
Circles Network. ℔ www.circlesnetwork.org.uk/ (accessed 31 October 2017).
McConkey R (2010). Promoting friendships and developing social networks. In: G Grant, P Ramcharan, M Flynn, M Richardson, eds. *Learning Disability: A Life Cycle Approach*, 2nd edn. Open University Press: Maidenhead; pp. 329–42.
Carers UK. ℔ www.carersuk.org/search/shared-care-network (accessed 19 March 2018).

References

25 Neville M, Baylis L, Boldison SJ, et al. (1995). *Circles of Support: Building Inclusive Communities*. Circles Network: Rugby.
26 Neville M, McIver B (2000). Circles of support. In: B Kelly, P McGinley, eds. *Intellectual Disability: The Response of the Church*. Lisieux Hall Publications: Chorley; pp. 18–21.
27 Simons K (1998). *Living Support Networks: An Evaluation of the Services Provided by KeyRing*. Pavilion Publishing: Brighton.
28 Towell D (2000). Achieving positive change in people's lives through the national learning disabilities strategies: lessons from an American experience. *Tizard Learning Disability Review*. 5: 30–6.

Retirement

Over the last decade, there has been a continued growth in the numbers of people with intellectual disabilities living into old age. This is a reflection of improved medical, health, and social care that this population has received when compared with previous generations. However, the issues surrounding ageing within this changing population are also placing an increased demand on the mainstream older person services, intellectual disabilities services, and specialist services required to meet the needs of this population.[29,30]

Guiding principles

Do not be age-fixated!

Ageing for adults with intellectual disabilities can begin from 50 years, 40 years for those with Down syndrome. However, people with intellectual disabilities are a diverse group, and assumptions of premature ageing can impact on how service provision is planned for this population. People with certain conditions, such as Down syndrome, may present with age-related health conditions early, e.g. sensory, musculoskeletal, and early-onset dementia. Hence services designed for older persons may need to use functional entry criteria, rather than age as entry criterion. It is also important to consider that ageing for a person with intellectual disabilities can be a time of real opportunity.

Active ageing

Healthy and active ageing is a concept promoted broadly by many, including the WHO.[30] It embraces a life course approach and promotes the opportunity for people of all ages to live healthy, active, safe, and socially inclusive lifestyles.

Older people with intellectual disabilities want similar experiences to other older individuals without intellectual disabilities. They want to remain actively involved in the activities that they enjoy, as well as maintain their skills and keep learning. They want to feel empowered by having a meaningful role and keeping their independence. Feeling safe and having a sense of security are also vital, as well as having satisfying relationships and support when needed. It is important for older people with intellectual disabilities to have optimal health and fitness and living arrangements that truly meet their needs and help them maintain a level of independence.[29,34]

Barriers to ageing

It is important to address the barriers that exist for older people with intellectual disabilities and ensure that they are facilitated to access the services and opportunities that are available within their local communities.[31]

Individual

Older persons with intellectual disabilities may require additional support to access mainstream community opportunities (e.g. personal support, transport, participation). There is a responsibility on disability services, as well as mainstream community projects/programmes, to facilitate access and linkage to opportunities, as well as ongoing support, when required. Negotiating different services and collaboration between statutory and voluntary/charitable community services is vital in ensuring access for all older people with intellectual disabilities.[32]

Social networks

Largely, adults live in distinct social spaces, with support from a small group of family, peers, and paid staff. They can have little social contact/support outside their formal activities/opportunities; however, with support from peers, befrienders, and volunteers, older people with intellectual disabilities can play a valuable role within their communities.[33,34]

Stigma and discrimination

A legacy of discrimination and segregation towards people with intellectual disabilities has led to large numbers of older adults living 'in', but not 'within', their communities. To date, communities have been largely unaware of, and ill-prepared to support, the needs of this population.

References

29 Bigby C (2002). Ageing service-users with a lifelong disability: challenges for the aged care and disability sectors. *Journal of Intellectual and Developmental Disability*. 27: 231–41.

30 World Health Organization (2000). *Ageing and Intellectual Disabilities – Improving Longevity and Promoting Healthy Ageing: Summative Report*. World Health Organization: Geneva.

31 Ward C (2012). *BILD Factsheet: Older People with a Learning Disability*. British Institute of Learning Disabilities: Birmingham.

32 Stancliffe RJ, Wilson NJ, Bigby C, Balandin S, Craig D (2014). Responsiveness to self-report questions about loneliness: a comparison of mainstream and intellectual disability-specific instruments. *Journal of Intellectual Disability Research*. 58: 399–405.

33 Hogg J, Lambe L (1999). *Older People with Intellectual Disabilities: A Review of the Literature on Residential Services and Family Care Giving*. Foundation for People with Learning Disabilities: London.

34 Lawrence S (2008). Examining pre-retirement and related services offered to service users with an intellectual disability in Ireland. *Journal of Intellectual Disabilities*. 12: 239–52.

Retirement options

An active retirement is the 'third age' or 'young old' for most European citizens and can be too for older people with intellectual disabilities. Their options can include the following.

Availing of mainstream community services for older persons

In all localities, there are various activities organized for older persons, e.g. luncheon clubs, tea dances, photography clubs, and bingo. People with intellectual disabilities can, and should be, supported to join by having a staff member or volunteer to accompany them. Bigby et al. in Australia have developed a transition-to-retirement (TTR) programme, developed for employees of a large multi-site disability employment service in Sydney, Australia. By involving non-disabled older people as 'mentors', the programme promotes the concepts of participation and inclusion to effect successful partial retirement of older people with intellectual disabilities. The TTR programme consists of three main components: promoting the concept of retirement, laying the ground-work for inclusion of would-be retirees with intellectual disabilities in the community, and constructing the reality. The programme highlights the importance of supporting meaningful inclusion of people with intellectual disabilities in their communities.[39]

Retirement clubs and home-based pursuits

Groups of retired persons may wish to meet for a programme of activities designed to suit their interests and capacities. These groups could be located in a leisure or community centre, with the members taking responsibility for a programme, which can include outings and visits, as well as centre-based events. Friendship circles can invite one another to their homes for coffee mornings or afternoon tea, or to take part in organized activities such as craft circles or to sing songs. A visiting 'tutor' may be recruited to provide activities such as yoga or aromatherapy.

All-age pursuits and befrienders

In most localities, there are opportunities that include all ages of people, e.g. faith communities, spectator sports, and clubs. Older persons can be encouraged to join, and perhaps this is best done when they are younger, as this will provide continuity for them. Volunteer helpers of a similar age can be recruited to visit the person at home, to transport them to activities, and to befriend them at social events or activities.

Family placement (short breaks)

Similarly, families could be recruited to offer short breaks in their home to older persons, on either a daytime or an overnight basis. These schemes have proved particularly suitable for persons with intellectual disabilities who have taken on caring roles with their ageing parents or those with complex needs being cared for by ageing parents.

Planning for the fourth age

An active retirement gives way to a fourth age that is typified by increased dependency on others through the onset of secondary health conditions associated with impairment or long-term poor healthcare or chronic conditions. However, planning for the future (future planning) is vital in ensuring that the principles of active ageing are maintained, although it can be even more challenging to fulfil them.[35]

- A plan for the future will set out the preferred options of the person (as far as they can be ascertained) and those of their family carers regarding their living and support arrangements. The plan must be based on assessed needs of the individual with intellectual disabilities, as well as the views of family carers, while maintaining the wishes of the older person with intellectual disabilities (family-centred approach).
- Like the general population, most older people with intellectual disabilities want to continue living in their own home.[36] Any necessary housing adaptations can be planned and undertaken in advance. Where possible, the older person's voice should be considered in arranging any move/transfer to supported living/nursing/residential care.
- The availability of general healthcare services to provide additional, and perhaps specialist, support, e.g. palliative care, should be explored and referrals made as appropriate.
- Regular assessments and reviews of care needs should be undertaken to avoid delays in accessing additional support. Whenever possible, the same team of support staff should continue to provide the bulk of the care.[37]
- Support staff should be trained in advance in caring for persons at the end of life and in the procedures to be followed on the death of the person they have supported.[38]

References

35 Heller T, Miller AB, Hsieh K, et al. (2000). Later life planning: promoting knowledge of options and choice making. *Mental Retardation.* **38**: 395–406.

36 Hogg J, Lambe L (1999). *Older People with Intellectual Disabilities: A Review of the Literature on Residential Services and Family Care Giving.* Foundation for People with Learning Disabilities: London.

37 Lawrence S (2008). Examining pre-retirement and related services offered to service users with an intellectual disability in Ireland. *Journal of Intellectual Disabilities.* **12**: 239–52.

38 British Institute of Learning Disabilities (2012). *Older People with a Learning Disability.* British Institute of Learning Disabilities: Birmingham.

39 Bigby C, Wilson N, Stancliffe R, Balandin S, Craig D, Gambin N (2014). An effective program design to support older workers with intellectual disability to participate individually in community groups. *Journal of Policy and Practice in Intellectual Disabilties.* **11**: 117–27.

The law

Mental Health Act 1983

Purpose

The scope, structure, and purpose of the MHA 1983 (amended 2007) are outlined in Section 1 of the Act. It states that the Act makes provision for the compulsory detention and treatment in hospital of those with mental disorder. The MHA was amended by the MHA 2007, but it is still termed the MHA 1983. The Act comprises ten parts:

• Application of the Act;
• Compulsory admission to hospital and guardianship;
• Patients concerned with criminal proceedings or under sentence;
• Consent to treatment;
• MHRTs;
• Removal and return of patients within the UK;
• Management of property and affairs of patients;
• Miscellaneous functions of local authorities and the Secretary of State;
• Offences;
• Miscellaneous and supplementary.

Definitions

Mental disorder '*includes mental illness, arrested or incomplete development of mind, psychopathic disorder and any other disorder or disability of mind*'.[1]
The Act then offered three subcategories of mental disorder:

• 'Severe mental impairment—a state of arrested or incomplete development of mind, which includes severe impairment of intelligence and social functioning and is associated with abnormally aggressive or seriously irresponsible conduct on the part of the person concerned;
• Mental impairment—a state of arrested or incomplete development of mind (not amounting to severe impairment), which includes significant impairment of intelligence and social functioning, and is associated with abnormally aggressive or seriously irresponsible conduct on the part of the person concerned.
• Psychopathic disorder—a persistent disorder or disability of mind (whether or not including significant impairment of intelligence), which results in abnormally aggressive or seriously irresponsible conduct on the part of the person concerned.'[1]

The definitions of 'severe mental impairment' and 'mental impairment' were the ones most pertinent to the field of intellectual disabilities nursing. It should be noted that intellectual disabilities alone was not a reason for detention under the Act. These definitions became applicable under the Act when 'associated' with 'abnormally aggressive' or 'seriously irresponsible conduct'. These definitions were abolished under the MHA 2007 and replaced by a single simplified definition which is applied throughout the Act and is: '*Mental disorder means any disorder or disability of the mind; and mentally disordered shall be construed accordingly.*'[1]

---

* Text extracts in this section reproduced from Department of Health (2007) Mental Health Act 2007. London: HMSO © Crown Copyright, under the Open Government License 3.0.

This single definition means that some people who were previously excluded from the protections of the Act, such as those with acquired brain injury, could now be subject to the Act.

The Act defines learning disability as a: 'state of arrested or incomplete development of mind which includes significant impairment of intelligence and social functioning', and under the Act 'learning disability is in general regarded as a mental disorder because it is a disability of the mind'.[1] It is important to note that under the amended Act, 'a learning disability can only be considered a mental disorder if it is associated with seriously irresponsible or abnormally aggressive conduct'.[1]

This applies to all sections that relate to longer-term compulsory treatment or care for mental disorder, in particular Sections 3, 7 (guardianship), and 17A (supervised community treatment).

Mental Health Act 1983 Amended 2007—major amendments

This new Act became law in July 2007, and its main amendments came into force in October 2008. The major changes to the Act are:

- *Criteria for detention*—this includes an appropriate medical treatment test;
- *Professional roles*—a broadening of the range of practitioners [(including registered nurses in learning disability (RNLDs)] who can take on the roles currently performed by approved social workers and responsible medical officers. These new roles are those of the approved mental health practitioner and the approved clinician;
- *Nearest relative*—this gives patients the right to apply to have the nearest relative displaced if there are reasonable grounds for doing so;
- *Supervised community treatment*—allows for some people with mental disorder to receive compulsory treatment in the community;
- *MHRT*—a reduction in time before cases are referred to the tribunal;
- *Age-appropriate service*—those under 18yrs who are admitted to hospital for a mental disorder must be accommodated in suitable environments;
- *Advocacy*—a duty by a national authority to make arrangements for the provision of independent advocates;
- *ECT*—there are new safeguards for patients.

The change that applies most directly to people with intellectual disabilities relates to Section 1 of the MHA 1983.

The new Act has only one definition of mental disorder, which applies throughout the Act. The categories of severe mental impairment, mental impairment, and psychopathic disorder are abolished. The single definition is: 'Mental disorder means any disorder or disability of the mind; and mentally disordered shall be construed accordingly.'[*][1]

The MHA is law in England and Wales. In Scotland, only those parts of the Act defined in Section 146 apply, and otherwise mental disorder is under the Mental Health (Care and Treatment) (Scotland) Act 2003. In Northern Ireland, only those parts defined in Section 147 apply; the rest is under the Mental Health (Northern Ireland) Order 1986 (amendment) (Northern Ireland) Order 2004.

Further reading

Department of Health (2015). *Reference Guide to the Mental Health Act 1983.* ℘ www.gov.uk/government/uploads/system/uploads/attachment_data/file/417412/Reference_Guide.pdf (accessed 31 October 2017).

Mental Health Northern Ireland (Northern Ireland) Order 1986 (amendment) (Northern Ireland) Order 2004. ℘ www.legislation.gov.uk/nisi/1986/595 (accessed 31 October 2017).

Scottish Parliament (2003). *Mental Health (Care and Treatment) (Scotland) Act 2003.* ℘ www.legislation.gov.uk/asp/2003/13/contents (accessed 31 October 2017).

References

1   Department of Health (2007). *Mental Health Act 2007.* HMSO: London.

Compulsory admission to hospital for assessment and treatment

Compulsory admission to hospital under the MHA 1983 for assessment and treatment is largely covered by the three sections of the MHA outlined below.

Section 2—admission for assessment

This allows for a person to be detained in hospital for assessment for up to 28 days. This period should allow for an assessment to be made. If it is believed that the person needs to be detained further, it is customary to implement Section 3 for this purpose. An application can be made by the nearest relative or an approved mental health practitioner who has seen the person within the 14 days leading up to the signing of the application. Two medical recommendations are required for this Section to be used. One of these recommendations must be from an approved doctor under Section 12 of the Act.

Circumstances

An application can be made if it is felt that:
- An individual is suffering from a mental disorder of a degree that warrants detention in hospital for assessment or for assessment followed by treatment for at least a limited period;
- The individual should be detained in the interests of their own health and safety or to protect others.

This Section may be appropriate if:
- The person has not been detained before and diagnosis/prognosis are currently unclear;
- Significant time has elapsed between admissions;
- The effectiveness of compulsory treatment under the MHA is not currently known.

Section 3—admission for treatment

This Section allows for the detention of a person for treatment for a maximum period of 6 months, after which it can be renewed for a further 6 months, and then for 12 months at a time. It requires the recommendation of two doctors, one of whom must have had specialist training to undertake this role.

Circumstances
- The person is suffering from a mental disorder.
- The person has a learning disability that is associated with abnormally aggressive or seriously irresponsible conduct.
- The treatment is necessary for the health and safety or protection of others, and it cannot be provided unless s/he is detained under this Section.

Section 4—emergency admission for assessment

Provisions of this section allows emergency detainment for assessment.

Duration is for up to 72 hours. Renewal is not possible, but by means of a second medical recommendation, Section 4 can be converted into Section 2 during this period.

Circumstances

- The recommendation must indicate the urgent nature of the application, such that detention under Section 2 would result in unacceptable delay.
- The application can be made by the approved mental health practitioner or the nearest relative and be supported by one doctor who must have examined the person within the previous 24 hours.
- Section 2 requirement of obtaining a second medical representation would involve an undesirable delay.

It should be noted that Sections 5(2) and 5(4) (outlined in ➔ Emergency holding powers, pp. 484–5) are also used for compulsory detention under the Act.

Further reading

Department of Health (2015). *Mental Health Act 1983: Code of Practice.* Department of Health: London. ℀ www.gov.uk/government/uploads/system/uploads/attachment_data/file/435512/MHA_Code_of_Practice.PDF (accessed 30 October 2017).

Guidelines and Audit Implementation Network (2011). *Guidelines on the Use of the Mental Health (Northern Ireland) Order 1986.* Regulation and Quality Improvement Authority: Belfast. ℀ rqia.org.uk/RQIA/files/4e/4ee9f634-be47-4398-afc9-906a20ff3198.pdf (accessed 30 October 2017).

Mental Health Commission (Republic of Ireland) (2001). *Mental Health Act (2001) Codes of Practice.* ℀ www.mhcirl.ie/for_H_Prof/codemha2001/ (accessed 30 October 2017).

Emergency holding powers

Detention of people in mental health and intellectual disabilities services is currently governed by the MHA (England and Wales). The corresponding legislation in other jurisdictions in the UK is the Mental Health (Care and Treatment) (Scotland) Act 2003 and the Mental Health (Northern Ireland) Order 1986 (amendment) (Northern Ireland) Order 2004. In the Republic of Ireland, the relevant legislation is the MHA (2001). This chapter outlines the main provisions of Section 5(2)—Detention of an inpatient, and Section 5(4)—Nurses' holding powers.

Section 5(2)—Detention of an inpatient

This section allows for an approved doctor or approved clinician (AC) to detain an informal patient for up to 72 hours by reporting to hospital managers. Before this period of time elapses, an application can be made for Section 2 or 3 to be applied, or the individual can revert to informal status. Although this section can be used only by doctors and ACs, nurses need to be aware of it as it will affect the care and management of the client.

Section 5(4)—Nurses' holding powers

This section allows for the RNID or registered mental nurse to prevent a person from leaving an inpatient environment if it is considered to be in their best interests or that of others and that it is not practicable to secure the immediate attendance of a doctor or an AC. This holding power can last for up to 6 hours. As soon as it starts, a doctor or an AC with authority to detain the individual must be alerted, and when the doctor or AC arrives, the nurse's holding power ceases.

Clinical considerations that may lead to the nurse applying Section 5(4) include:

• The person's stated intent;
• The likelihood of suicide;
• The person's current behaviour, particularly any changes from the usual;
• The likelihood of violence;
• Any recently received news from relatives or friends;
• Any recent disturbances within the ward/hospital environment;
• The person's known unpredictability.

Legal/procedural considerations when applying Section 5(4)

Section 5(4) can only be applied to a person who is an inpatient being treated for a mental disorder. It cannot be applied to a person being treated in a general hospital for a physical illness and who becomes mentally unwell. It should be noted that because of the limited timespan during which a person can be detained under Section 5(4), there is no right of appeal.

The MHA dictates that the nurse (using form H2) must make a report to management as soon as possible after applying Section 5(4). The person detained under Section 5(4) must be informed of their rights as soon as possible after the Section has been applied. Persons detained under Section 5(4) cannot have medication administered against their will, as this Section is not governed by Part 4 of the Act (consent for treatment). Section 5(4) allows a nurse to use minimal restraint to prevent the person from leaving the hospital. The decision to use Section 5(4) is the responsibility of the nurse applying it. No one can instruct a nurse to implement this section.

Further reading

Department of Health (2015). *Mental Health Act 1983: Code of Practice*. Department of Health: London. ℰ www.gov.uk/government/uploads/system/uploads/attachment_data/file/435512/MHA_Code_of_Practice.PDF (accessed 30 October 2017).

Guidelines and Audit Implementation Network (2011). *Guidelines on the Use of the Mental Health (Northern Ireland) Order 1986*. Regulation and Quality Improvement Authority: Belfast. ℰ rqia.org.uk/RQIA/files/4e/4ee9f634-be47-4398-afc9-906a20ff3198.pdf (accessed 30 October 2017).

Mental Health Commission (Republic of Ireland) (2001). *Mental Health Act (2001) Codes of Practice*. ℰ www.mhcirl.ie/for_H_Prof/codemha2001/ (accessed 30 October 2017).

Mental Health (First Tier) Review Tribunals

In essence, a mental health tribunal is empowered by law to adjudicate about mental health treatment by conducting independent reviews of patients with a mental disorder who are detained in psychiatric hospitals or under community treatment orders and may be subject to involuntary treatment. MHRTs comprise the following members:
- A legal representative;
- A medical practitioner;
- A community/specialist member.

The Mental Health Tribunal in England is now technically known as the First Tier Tribunal (Mental Health) but, in practice, is still more usually referred to as the Mental Health Tribunal. It should be noted the First Tier Tribunal system was established in England in 2008 and other parts of the UK have different systems:
- The MHRT for Northern Ireland was developed under the Mental Health (Northern Ireland) Order 1986;
- The MHRT for Scotland was created in 2005 as part of the Mental Health (Care and Treatment) (Scotland) Act 2003;
- The MHRT for Wales is legislated within the same MHA as England, but it is run separately according to the Wales rules 2008.

Readers should pursue further reading in order to understand how the MHRTs are configured within each constituent part of the UK.

The process of appeal might vary, and this is dependent on which Section of the Act a person is being detained under. These variations pertain to issues such as when a person can appeal, who can appeal on a person's behalf, and the interim period between appeals. Readers should therefore read further to clarify the stipulations relating to specific sections; however, in broad terms, Sections 66 and 69 of the Act allow for appeals to the MHRT where an individual has been:
- Admitted for assessment under Section 2;
- Admitted for treatment under Section 3;
- Received into guardianship under Section 7;
- Made subject of a hospital order or guardianship order by the court under Section 37;
- Detained (or made subject to guardianship) for a further period under Section 20;
- Deemed to have a different form of mental disorder from that originally cited;
- Transferred from guardianship to hospital;
- Made subject to either a restriction order or a restriction direction;
- Conditionally discharged;
- Made subject to supervised discharge.

Appeals can also be made to the MHRT if the nearest relative has been:
- Barred by the responsible medical officer from discharging the individual detained in hospital;
- Replaced by the acting nearest relative as the result of a court order.

Applications

Most tribunal hearings are the result of applications made by, or on behalf of, the patient, in some cases by the nearest relative. The Act also requires hospital managers to refer to the MHRT any patient admitted under Part II of the Act who, on renewal of the Section, has not had a tribunal hearing within the previous 6 months.

The powers of the MHRT

The MHRT can discharge individuals from certain Sections of the Act. Individuals detained under Section 2 must be discharged if:

• They are not suffering from a mental disorder (as defined in Section 1 of the Act—see ➲ Mental Health Act 1983, pp. 478–9) that requires detention for assessment or if that Section cannot be justified in the best interests of the detained person or others.

The MHRT can also discharge individuals from Sections other than Section 2 if it is satisfied that:

• The person is not suffering from a mental disorder that needs detention for treatment, or if detention cannot be justified in the interests of the health and safety of the person or others, or if discharged the patient would not be a danger to themselves or others.

The role of the nurse

• To provide reports for the MHRT, if required;
• To give evidence to the MHRT, if required;
• To ensure the patient has the required information about the appeal;
• To assist in finding legal representation;
• To manage the process of appeal.

Procedures before the MHRT hearing

• Applications must be made in writing;
• Assistance should be offered and given to patients in completing the application form and in seeking legal advice;
• Patients should be informed of their rights—particularly to legal representation;
• The nearest relative should be informed of their right to attend the hearing and of their right to provide information before the hearing.

Further reading

Department of Health (2015). *Mental Health Act 1983: Code of Practice*. Department of Health: London. ♒ www.gov.uk/government/uploads/system/uploads/attachment_data/file/435512/MHA_Code_of_Practice.PDF (accessed 30 October 2017).

Guidelines and Audit Implementation Network (2011). *Guidelines on the Use of the Mental Health (Northern Ireland) Order 1986*. Regulation and Quality Improvement Authority: Belfast. ♒ rqia.org.uk/RQIA/files/4e/4ee9f634-be47-4398-afc9-906a20ff3198.pdf (accessed 30 October 2017).

Johnstone S, Miles S, Royston C (2015). *Mental Health Tribunal Handbook*. Legal Action Group: London.

Mental Health Commission (Republic of Ireland) (2001). *Mental Health Act (2001) Codes of Practice*. ♒ www.mhcirl.ie/for_H_Prof/codemha2001/ (accessed 30 October 2017).

The Equality Act 2010

The Equality Act came into force in England, Scotland, and Wales on 1 October 2010. It brought together over 116 pieces of legislation (some of which were outlined in the 1st edition of this handbook) into this single Act. The intention of this Act is to provide a legal framework to protect the rights of individuals and to promote a more equal society. The main pieces of legislation that were outlined in the 1st edition of this handbook that have been merged into, and replaced by, the Equality Act in England and Wales are:

• The Race Relations Act 1975;
• The Disability Discrimination Act 1995;
• The Employment Equality (Religion or Belief) Regulations 2003;
• The Employment Equality (Sexual Orientation) Regulations 2003;
• The Employment Equality (Age) Regulations 2006.

The Act offers explicit instruction about how organizations such as the NHS and its employees, including nurses, should operate in non-discriminatory ways in relation to nine protected characteristics:

• Age;
• Disability;
• Gender reassignment;
• Marriage and civil partnerships;
• Pregnancy and maternity;
• Race—including ethnic or national origins, colour, and nationality;
• Religion or belief (political views are excluded);
• Sex (gender);
• Sexual orientation.

Within Northern Ireland, the provision of equality legislation is covered within the Northern Ireland Order, and in particular Section 75 which includes the additional categories of dependents and political opinion.

Any of the protected characteristics can apply to people with intellectual disabilities, but it should be noted an individual is defined as being disabled under the Act if they: ' … *[have] a physical or mental impairment that has a "substantial" and "long-term" negative effect on your ability to do normal daily activities …* '[2]

Discrimination

The Act also offers explicit guidance on discrimination which is defined as '*the practice of treating individuals less fairly than other people or groups*'. The Act identifies five categories of discrimination:

• Direct—treating one individual less favourably than another because they belong to a particular protected characteristic group;
• Indirect—this can occur if rules, policies, and practices that apply to everyone disadvantage people who share a particular protected characteristic;
• Discrimination by perception—this is discrimination based on a perception that an individual or group possesses a particular protected characteristic, even when this is not the case;

- Associative discrimination—an individual cannot be discriminated against because they are associated with another person who possesses a protected characteristic;
- Third-party harassment—unwanted conduct affecting the dignity of people in the workplace that might be related to a protected characteristic.

The Equality Act is an important piece of legislation that impacts on how people with intellectual disabilities are treated. Nurses should be aware of how the Act can enable them to help support people with intellectual disabilities in non-discriminatory ways and to ensure they are treated equally. The Equality Act introduced the equality duty that applies to public authorities which are often the employers of RNIDs. The intention of the Equality Duty is to eliminate discrimination and to promote equality (see ➲ Further reading). It should be noted that, under Section 217 of the Act, with limited exceptions, the Act does not apply to Northern Ireland.

Further reading

Equality and Human Rights Commission (2014). *The Essential Guide to the Public Sector Equality Duty and Non–Devolved Public Authorities in Scotland and Wales.* ℘ www.equalityhumanrights.com/sites/default/files/psed_essential_guide_-_guidance_for_english_public_bodies.pdf (accessed 31 October 2017).

The Equality Act 2010 (Statutory Duties) (Wales) Regulations 2011. ℘ www.legislation.gov.uk/wsi/2011/1064/pdfs/wsi_20111064_mi.pdf (accessed 31 October 2017).

The Equality Commission for Northern Ireland (2010). *Section 75 of the Northern Ireland Act 1998. A Guide for Public Authorities.* Equality Commission for Northern Ireland: Belfast. ℘ www.equalityni.org/ECNI/media/ECNI/Publications/Employers%20and%20Service%20Providers/S75GuideforPublicAuthoritiesApril2010.pdf (accessed 31 October 2017).

References

2 *Equality Act 2010.* The Stationery Office: London. ℘ www.legislation.gov.uk/ukpga/2010/15/contents (accessed 31 October 2017).

Sexual Offences Act 2003

Summary

The Sexual Offences Act 2003 is an Act of Parliament that became law on 1 May 2004. It updates and makes many changes from the Sexual Offences Act of 1956 (which had been amended in 1976 and 1994). The major purpose of the Act is to govern non-consensual sexual behaviour. It is an extensive piece of legislation, and therefore readers requiring more extensive detail should consult ➔ References, p. 491. The Act is divided into a number of Sections. The Sections most relevant to people with intellectual disabilities, their carers, and nurses are Sections 30–41. For the purposes of the Act, intellectual disability falls under the umbrella term 'mental disorder'. This is the same definition used in the MHA 1983, as amended by the MHA 2007, and is 'any disorder or disability of the mind'. This definition ensures the protection of people with intellectual disabilities.

The most relevant sections
- Sections 30–33—relate to offences against people who cannot legally consent to sexual activity because of a mental disorder impeding choice.
- Sections 34–37—relate to offences against people who may or may not be able to consent to sexual activity but who are vulnerable to inducements, threats, or deceptions because of mental disorder.
- Sections 38–41—relate to specific offences committed by care workers who engage in sexual activity with a person with a mental disorder receiving care in the setting at which they work.

Role of the nurse

The role of registered nurses for people with intellectual disabilities should involve working within the provisions of the Act, monitoring for potential infringements covered by it, and acting accordingly. More information and guidance in relation to the role of registered nurses for people with intellectual disabilities and safeguarding is provided in the section ➔ Dealing with abuse, pp. 498–9. Under the Act, any sexual activity between a care worker and a person with a mental disorder is prohibited while that relationship continues. A relationship of care is one in which a person with a mental disorder (intellectual disabilities) is regularly or likely to be involved face-to-face with another person where their care needs arise from a mental disorder. This applies to both paid and voluntary people and includes:
- Doctors, nurses, advocates, cleaners, and medical receptionists;
- Care home and agency workers;
- People who provide care within the individual's home;
- People involved in face-to-face care who escort those with a mental disorder on regular outings;
- Friends or family members if they provide care, assistance, or services relating to the individual's mental disorder.

The Act covers the following areas that relate to care worker offences:
- 'Sexual activity with a person with a mental disorder—this covers all intercourse and sexual touching of any part of the body, clothed or unclothed, with the body or an object.

- Causing or inciting sexual activity—this relates to causing or persuading a person with a mental disorder to engage in any sexual activity with someone else or making them strip or masturbate. This offence applies even if the intended sexual activity does not take place.
- Sexual activity in the presence of a person with a mental disorder—it is an offence to engage in sexual activity when you know you can be seen by a person with a mental disorder who is in your care or that you intend/believe that they can see you and where you gain sexual gratification from them watching you.
- Causing a person with a mental disorder to watch a sexual act—it is an offence to intentionally cause someone with a mental disorder to watch someone else engaging in sexual activity. This includes looking at pornography, photos, and webcams and where it is for your own sexual gratification. This is not intended to prevent sex education.
- Exceptions—there are situations in which care workers' offences apply. These are where a care worker is legally married to the person with a mental disorder or it can be proved that the sexual relationship predated the relationship of care and as long as the sexual activity was lawful.'[3]

References

3 *The Sexual Offences Act 2003*. The Stationery Office: London. ℘ www.legislation.gov.uk/ukpga/ 2003/42/contents (accessed 31 October 2017).

The Care Act 2014

The Care Act 2014 builds on recent reviews and reforms, replacing numerous previous laws and policy guidance (including the NHS and Community Care Act 1990 and the Community Care Direct Payments Act 1996 and No Secrets 2000), to provide a coherent approach to adult social care in England. Part One of the Act (and its Statutory Guidance) consolidates and modernizes the framework of care and support law; it sets out new duties for local authorities and partners, and new rights for service users and carers. The Act came into force on 1 April 2015, and the main components of the Act are:

- A new emphasis on well-being (physical, mental, and emotional)—the new statutory principle of individual well-being underpins the Act and is the driving force behind care and support;
- Prevention—local authorities (and their partners in health, housing, welfare, and employment services) must now take steps to prevent, reduce, or delay the need for care and support for all local people;
- Integration—the Act includes a statutory requirement for local authorities to collaborate, cooperate, and integrate with other public authorities, e.g. health and housing. It also requires seamless transitions for young people moving to adult social care services.

'Well-being' is a broad concept. It is described as relating to the following areas, in particular:

- Personal dignity (including treatment of the individual with respect);
- Physical and mental health and emotional well-being;
- Protection from abuse and neglect (this covers safeguarding obligations, and the role of the registered nurses for people with intellectual disabilities in relation to this is outlined in the section ➋ Dealing with abuse, pp. 498–9;
- Control by the individual over their day-to-day life (including over care and support provided and the way they are provided);
- Participation in work, education, training, or recreation;
- Social and economic well-being;
- Domestic, family, and personal domains;
- Suitability of the individual's living accommodation;
- The individual's contribution to society.

Domains

- Domain 1: preventing people from dying prematurely—this domain covers how successful the NHS is in reducing the number of avoidable deaths;
- Domain 2: enhancing the quality of life for people with long-term conditions—this domain covers how successfully the NHS is in supporting people with long-term conditions to live as normal a life as possible;
- Domain 3: helping people to recover from episodes of ill health or following injury—this domain covers how people recover from ill health or injury and, wherever possible, how it can be prevented;

- Domain 4: ensuring that people have a positive experience of care—this domain looks at the importance of providing a positive experience for patients, service users, and carers;
- Domain 5: treating and caring for people in a safe environment and protecting them from avoidable harm—this domain explores patient safety and its importance in terms of quality of care to deliver better health outcomes.

The Act identifies the statutory duties of local authorities in relation to assessing people's needs and their eligibility for publicly funded care and support. The Act states that local authorities must:

- Carry out an assessments of anyone who appears to require care and support, regardless of their likely eligibility;
- Focus the assessment on the individual's needs and how they impact on their well-being, and the outcomes they want to achieve;
- Involve the individual in the assessment and, where appropriate, their carer or someone else they nominate;
- Provide access to an independent advocate to support the individual's involvement in the assessment, if required;
- Consider other things besides care services that can contribute to the desired outcomes (e.g. preventive services, community support);
- Use the new national minimum threshold to judge eligibility for care and support.

All of the local authority's duties under the Act can apply to people with intellectual disabilities and their carers; however, two duties in particular can have great significance in improving the well-being of people with intellectual disabilities and their carers:

- Following an assessment, there is a duty to produce a care and support plan and to offer a personal budget. There is a duty to review plans to make sure they continue to meet people's needs;
- The rights of carers are strengthened—local authorities must carry out an assessment of a carer's needs where they appear to have needs;

Registered nurses for people with intellectual disabilities working in Wales should be aware that the devolved Welsh government has produced the Social Services and Well-being (Wales) Act, which provides further guidance on how people in need of care can be assessed and how services can be delivered to meet their needs (see ➲ Further reading)

Further reading

Department of Health (2014). *Care and Support Statutory Guidance: Issued under the Care Act 2014.* ℘ www.gov.uk/government/uploads/system/uploads/attachment_data/file/315993/Care-Act-Guidance.pdf (accessed 31 October 2017).

Social Services and Well-being (Wales) Act 2014. ℘ www.legislation.gov.uk/anaw/2014/4/pdfs/anaw_20140004_en.pdf (accessed 31 October 2017).

Human Rights Act

The Human Rights Act 1998 is an Act of Parliament that came into force on 2 October 2000. The Act makes the European Convention of Human Rights (ECHR) (see ➔ European Convention of Human Rights, pp. 496–7) enforceable in UK courts. In effect, the Act does not create any new rights but provides ways for cases to be heard in UK courts, rather than the European Court of Human Rights. It should be noted that if cases are unsuccessful in UK courts, they can be taken to the European Court. One notable example of this was HL v UK (2004) ECHR 471 which directly led to the Bournewood ruling and the development of the MCADOLS (for further information, see ➔ Mental Capacity Act: Deprivation of Liberty Safeguards, pp. 510–11). The human rights covered under the Act are:

- 'The right to life;
- Prohibition of torture;
- Prohibition of slavery;
- The right to liberty and security;
- The right to a fair trial;
- The right not to be held guilty of a criminal offence that did not exist in law at the time at which it was committed;
- The right to privacy, family life, home, and correspondence;
- The right to freedom of thought, conscience, and religion;
- The right to freedom of expression;
- The right to freedom of assembly and association;
- The right to marry;
- The right to the protection of property;
- The right to education;
- The right to free elections;
- The right to the rights and freedoms set out above without discrimination on any grounds.'*

Not all of these rights are absolute, as some may be conditional and could be denied in certain circumstances. This is partly because a key purpose of the Act is to balance the rights of the individual against the rights of another individual and the greater public good. The Act is not designed to bring actions against private individuals. The purpose of the Act is to affect the way public authorities behave and to ensure that they attend to the human rights listed above.

It is recognized that adults with intellectual disabilities constitute a client group that is vulnerable to having their human rights compromised or denied. The government's Joint Committee on Human Rights (JCHR) has acknowledged this and, in March 2008, called for evidence to support this assertion. The JCHR commented that: *'The Committee is concerned that adults with learning disabilities in health and residential settings suffer neglect, abuse, discrimination and indifference. Although the Committee welcomes the announcement by the Department of Health of an independent inquiry into the healthcare of adults with learning disabilities, it considers that the Department of Health could do much more to promote culture change and a human rights-led approach.'*4

The views of the JCHR reflect an increasing awareness that the human rights of people with intellectual disabilities can be denied. There is an expectation that the Human Rights Act will contribute to a growing 'rights culture' within public services in relation to how people with intellectual disabilities are treated. The Equality Act (see ➡ The Equality Act, pp. 488–9), and *Valuing People*[5] (see ➡ Principles and values of social policy and their effects on intellectual disability, pp. 24–5) both supplement the Human Rights Act in supporting a rights culture.

The nurse's role

Working within a person-centred multidisciplinary and multi-agency context in relation to the Human Rights Act, the registered nurse for people with intellectual disabilities should:

- Where necessary, question care practices within organizations if it is felt that they violate human rights;
- Understand policies and procedures related to escalating and raising concerns—the *Code: Professional standards of practice and behaviour for nurses and midwives*[6] and the right to freedom of expression covered by the Human Rights Act both support the right to escalate and raise concerns ('whistleblow'). Nurses also need to be aware of and act according to the Royal College of Nursing guidance that outlines the duty of candour;[7]
- Ensure that they receive appropriate training and support.

Nurses who are concerned that the human rights of an individual with intellectual disabilities are being breached can:

- Take the individual's concerns seriously;
- Seek advice from the Citizens Advice Bureau or an advocacy group;
- Seek advice from a local authority care manager or the community team in intellectual disabilities services.

Further reading

Nursing and Midwifery Board of Ireland (2014). *Code of Professional Conduct and Ethics for Registered Nurses and Registered Midwives*. Nursing and Midwifery Board of Ireland: Dublin.

References

4 Joint Committee on Human Rights (2007). *A Life Like Any Other? Human Rights of Adults with Learning Disability*. ℘ www.publications.parliament.uk/pa/jt200708/jtselect/jtrights/40/40i.pdf (accessed 31 October 2017).

5 Department of Health (2001). *Valuing People: A New Strategy for Learning Disability in the 21st Century*. Cmnd 5086. HMSO: London.

6 Nursing and Midwifery Council (2015). *The Code: Professional Standards of Practice and Behaviour for Nurses and Midwives*. Nursing and Midwifery Council: London.

7 Royal College of Nursing (2015). *Duty of Candour*. ℘ www.rcn.org.uk/get-help/rcn-advice/duty-of-candour (accessed 31 October 2017).

European Convention on Human Rights

The ECHR was developed by the Council of Europe in 1950, with the intention of protecting human rights and fundamental freedoms. The Convention established the European Court of Human Rights, which can examine the case of any person who feels that their rights have been violated under the Convention. The ECHR forms the basis of the Human Rights Act 1998 (see ➔ Human Rights Act, pp. 494–5) which made the ECHR enforceable in UK courts. Along with other legislation such as *Valuing People*[8] and the *Equality Act*,[9] the ECHR contributes to developing the 'rights culture' within the field of intellectual disabilities. The convention covers the following rights/articles.

Articles

- The obligation to respect human rights;
- The right to life;
- The prohibition of torture;
- The prohibition of slavery;
- The right to liberty and security;
- The right to a fair trial;
- No punishment without the law;
- The right to respect for private life;
- The right to freedom of thought, conscience, and religion;
- The right to freedom of expression;
- The right to freedom of assembly and association;
- The right to marry;
- The right to effective remedy;
- The prohibition of discrimination;
- The right to property, education, and free elections.

Protocol 1

The government has concerns that the rights listed above may be denied to some people with intellectual disabilities. The JCHR has concerns in the following areas:

- Article 1—because of fundamental issues associated with humanity, dignity, equality, respect, and autonomy;
- Article 2—because of the very poor standard of medical care, which poses a risk to life;
- Article 3—because of the way some people with intellectual disabilities are treated, particularly in healthcare settings;
- Article 8—due to a variety of factors, including barriers to participating in community activities, which is covered under this article of the convention.

Nurses should examine their personal practice and the operation of the services they provide by using the human rights outlined above as a checklist.

Further reading

Joint Committee on Human Rights (2008). *A Life Like Any Other? Human Rights of Adults with Learning Disabilities: Seventh Report of Session 2007–08*. Joint Committee on Human Rights: London. ℘ www.publications.parliament.uk/pa/jt200708/jtselect/jtrights/40/40i.pdf (accessed 31 October 2017).

References

8 Department of Health (2001). *Valuing People: A New Strategy for Learning Disability in the 21st Century*. Cmnd 5086. HMSO: London.
9 *The Equality Act (2010)*. ℘ www.legislation.gov.uk/ukpga/2010/15/contents (accessed 31 October 2017).

Dealing with abuse

Abuse of people with intellectual disabilities is more often that what many people are prepared to belief, and the likelihood is that RNIDs will come across it at some point in their career and will need to deal with it. Abuse can be categorized into 'types', and these are listed in the *Care and Support Statutory Guidance* (issued under the Care Act 2014, pp. 193–4). *Care and Support Statutory Guidance* gives comprehensive guidance on how services should respond to the abuse of vulnerable people from an organizational and collaborative perspective and encourages all workers, including nurses to be vigilant to adult safeguarding concerns and to act on these concerns by raising and escalating them. Guidance documents for Scotland, Wales, Northern Ireland, and the Republic of Ireland are provided in ➔ Further reading p. 499. The duty of candour, as outlined by the Royal College of Nursing, and *The Code: Professional Standards of Practice and Behavior for Nurses and Midwives* also reinforce the necessity of raising and escalating concerns.

The Care Act stipulates that local authorities are the lead agency for coordinating protection frameworks, and it is the responsibility of the police to investigate allegations of abuse. Nurses should therefore be aware of their obligation to raise and escalate concerns and consider how they should respond in individual cases of abuse and how to act on their concerns by informing the appropriate people through the recognized channels, who will then investigate the issue and take necessary action. Although there are different types of abuse, and abuse can occur within many contexts, there are some universal principles that can be applied in all instances.

Therefore, if a nurse comes across a disclosure of abuse, they should:
- Be empathic;
- Stay calm;
- Be aware that medical evidence may be required and act accordingly to secure this, following advice and in collaboration with police services;
- Let the person know that they have done the right thing, it is not their fault, you are taking it seriously, and other people may need to know;
- Inform them that, in some circumstances, the police and the local authority may be informed without their consent;
- Record as soon as possible what has been said/occurred;
- Consider to whom to report the information;
- Make sure the person is and remains safe.

Nurses should not:
- Breach confidentiality by passing on information to anyone other than on 'a need-to-know basis' when this is necessary to protect a person or people by;
- Press the person for more detail by asking overly leading questions;
- Be judgmental or blaming; and
- It is vitally important that nurses clearly understand how to raise and escalate concerns both within and, if necessary, outside of their organization and understand their role within the interagency framework set out in *Care Support and Statutory Guidance* in relation to safeguarding procedures. Explicit guidance for nurses when raising and escalating concerns is set out in the NMC document *Raising Concerns: Guidance for Nurses and Midwives*.

Further reading

Department of Health (2014). *Care and Support Statutory Guidance: Issued under the Care Act 2014.* www.gov.uk/government/uploads/system/uploads/attachment_data/file/315993/Care-Act-Guidance.pdf (accessed 31 October 2017).

Department of Health, Social Services and Public Safety/Department of Justice (2015). *Adult Safeguarding Prevention and Protection in Partnership.* Department of Health, Social Services and Public Safety, Department of Justice: Belfast. www.health-ni.gov.uk/publications/adult-safeguarding-prevention-and-protection-partnership-key-documents (accessed 31 October 2017).

Health Service Executive (2014). *Safeguarding Vulnerable Persons at Risk of Abuse. National Policy and Procedures.* Health Service Executive: Dublin. www.hse.ie/eng/services/publications/corporate/personsatriskofabuse.pdf (accessed 31 October 2017). (This document is being updated at the time of writing; please refer to the Health Service Executive website for the most recent document.)

Nursing and Midwifery Board of Ireland (2014). *Code of Professional Conduct and Ethics for Registered Nurses and Registered Midwives.* Nursing and Midwifery Board of Ireland: Dublin.

Nursing and Midwifery Council (2015). *The Code: Professional Standards of Practice and Behaviour for Nurses and Midwives.* Nursing and Midwifery Council: London.

Nursing and Midwifery Council (2015). *Raising Concerns: Guidance for Nurses and Midwives.* Nursing and Midwifery Council: London.

The Scottish Government (2007). *The Adult Support and Protection (Scotland) Act 2007.* Scottish Government: Edinburgh. www.legislation.gov.uk/asp/2007/10/contents (accessed 31 October 2017).

The Welsh Assembly (2014). *Social Services and Well-being (Wales) Act 2014. Code of Practice and Statutory Guidance.* Cardiff: The Welsh Assembly. socialcare.wales/hub/sswbact-codes (accessed 31 October 2017).

Diversion from custody schemes

Diversion from custody is a method of redirecting people with intellectual disabilities and a mental disorder from the criminal justice system to hospital or suitable community settings where they can receive treatment appropriate to their needs. There are three principal reasons why this is necessary.

Those with intellectual disabilities and/or a mental disorder can fall through the net of support services and gravitate into the criminal justice system. The standard of care for this client group in prison is recognized as being poor. Prisons are not classified as hospitals for detention under the MHA 1983, and therefore people cannot be detained under the Act for appropriate treatment in prison.

There have been a number of policy initiatives within the past four decades, as follows:

• The Butler report 1975 which was influential in the development of medium secure units;[10]
• The Home Office circular 66/90 of 1990 which recommended diversion from custody wherever possible;[11]
• The Reed Report 1992 which recommended nationwide provision of appropriately resourced court assessment and diversion schemes, as well as other measures that support diversion;[12]
• The Bradley Report 2009 which strengthened the recommendations from the Reed Report and added other recommendations.[13]

Both the Reed and Bradley Reports have been influential. The Bradley Report offered recommendations aimed at improving the treatment of people with mental health problems or intellectual disabilities during all stages of their contact with the criminal justice system, with the intention of improving the processes relating to diversion from custody. The stages of the criminal justice system on which the Bradley Report made recommendations are:

• Early intervention, arrest, and prosecution;
• The court process;
• Prison, community sentences, and resettlement;
• Delivering change through partnership.

The MHA 1983 allows for a number of mechanisms to be used to divert people from custody. Readers should consult the MHA 1983 and associated literature in order to understand in detail how each one of the following applies in practice:

• Section 2—admission for assessment;
• Section 3—admission for treatment;
• Section 4—emergency admission for treatment;
• Section 35—remand to hospital for report on mental condition;
• Section 37—hospital and guardianship order;
• Section 37/41—restricted hospital order;
• Section 38—interim hospital order;
• Section 45A—hospital direction order;
• Section 47—removal to hospital of sentenced prisoners for treatment;

- Section 48—removal to hospital of other (remand) prisoners (for urgent treatment);
- Section 136—removal of mentally disordered persons found in public places. This is used by the police to take people to a place of safety, i.e. a mental health unit, rather than into custody.

It is important to understand that diversion from custody does not, in most instances, equate to the discontinuation of criminal proceedings.[14] Clearly, diversion from custody schemes presents the opportunity for nurses to work in a specialized role as designated diversion 'officers' or through involvement with the process as part of a broader remit.[15] Nurses working in this specialized role will need to be able to carry out thorough assessments of individual needs, including that of risk and its management, and this can be done by accessing:

- Educational history—including evidence of special educational needs;
- Level of literacy/numeracy;
- Official documents from health, social services, and criminal record information;
- Interviews with the individual and carers;
- The use of appropriate assessment tools such as the Hayes Ability Screening Index (HASI).[16]

From this, the nurse can draw up, or contribute to, pre-sentencing reports that offer options for diversion from custody. In order for this to work successfully, the nurse or team will need access to beds in specialist facilities.

References

10 Home Office and Department of Health and Social Security (1975). *Committee on Mentally Disordered Offenders.* HMSO: London.

11 Home Office (1990). *Provision of Mentally Disordered Offenders (circular 66/90).* HMSO: London.

12 Department of Health (1992). *Reed Report: Review of Mental Health and Social Services for Mentally Disordered Offenders and Others Requiring Similar Services: 1: Final Summary Report (Cm 2088).* HMSO: London.

13 Department of Health (2009). *The Bradley Report: Lord Bradley's Review of People with Mental Health Problems or Learning Disabilities in the Criminal Justice System.* Department of Health: London.

14 Nacro (2004). *Findings of the 2004 Survey of Court Diversion/Criminal Justice Mental Health Liaison Schemes for Mentally Disordered Offenders in England and Wales.* Nacro: London.

15 Birmingham L (2001). Diversion from custody. *Advances in Psychiatric Treatment.* 7: 198–207.

16 Hayes S (2000). *Hayes Ability Screening Index.* University of Sydney: Sydney.

Appropriate adult

The Police and Criminal Evidence Act (PACE) 1984[17] stipulates that all people <17yrs and those >17yrs with mental health problems and intellectual disabilities must have an appropriate adult present when they are being questioned by the police or asked to provide or sign a written statement while in police custody. The purposes of this are to assist and protect the welfare of vulnerable people who have difficulty in understanding their legal rights and may be at risk of providing unreliable and misleading information. It is the responsibility of the custody officer to identify those who require an appropriate adult and to arrange it, so that procedures relating to the detained person are conducted in the proper manner. The custody officer must inform the detained person of their rights, and this includes the circumstances in which it is deemed appropriate for an appropriate adult to be present.

An appropriate adult can be

- A parent;
- A guardian;
- Any responsible person who is at least 18yrs and is neither a police officer nor employed by the police;
- Those with experience in helping people with intellectual disabilities;
- A social worker or registered nurse for people with intellectual disabilities who is not involved with the offence as a witness, victim, or suspect, and who has not received either admissions or denials from the detained person before attendance at the police station.

Role and function of the appropriate adult

- To assist with communication between the police and the detained person;
- To advise, support, and generally assist the detained person, particularly when they are being questioned;
- To ensure that the police are acting properly and fairly;
- To observe that the police are respecting the rights of the detained person and to tell them if it is believed they are not doing so.

What the appropriate adult should avoid doing

- Acting as a passive observer;
- Discussing the alleged offence with the detained person;
- Answering questions on behalf of the detained person;
- Giving legal advice—this is the responsibility of a solicitor.

The rights of the appropriate adult

- To intervene during an interview if it is felt necessary and in the best interests of the person, in order to help them communicate with the police;
- To speak privately to the detained person at any time;
- To be informed why the detained person is being held;
- To inspect the written records (the custody record) of the person at any time;

- To see copies of the Codes of Practice that outline the powers and responsibilities of the police;
- To request a break in any interview if the person is distressed or ill, to seek legal advice, or to consult with the detained person;
- To be present during any procedure that requires the detained person to be given information or have it sought from them.

Further reading

Home Office (1984). *Police and Criminal Evidence Act*. HMSO: London.

Leggett J, Goodman W, Diani S (2007). People with learning disabilities experiences of being interviewed by the police. *British Journal of Learning Disabilities*. 35: 168–73.

National Appropriate Adult Network. ℘ www.appropriateadult.org.uk (accessed 31 October 2017).

The Representation of the People Act (RPA) 2000

The RPA 2000 amended the RPA 1983; its principal aim is to increase voter participation in elections. Historically, people with intellectual disabilities and/or a mental disorder were excluded from voting. It was a widely held assumption that these client groups were, and some still seem to think are, not eligible to vote, often because of issues relating to capacity. This is not the case, and people with intellectual disabilities have the same right to vote as anyone else (see ➲ Further reading), although the situation for those detained under the MHA 1983 requires some explanation. The RPA 1983 made voting extremely difficult for those detained under the MHA 1983, because in order to vote, a person must have been resident at a voting address for 6 months. For those detained for lengthy periods under the MHA 1983, this effectively prevented them from voting, as psychiatric hospitals were not recognized as voting addresses. In 1999, Mind submitted a case to the ECHR, claiming that this situation violated Protocol 1 of the Convention. Subsequently, Clause 4 of the RPA 2000 amended this issue and now states those patients (both voluntary and detained) who live in a mental hospital and have mental capacity can register to vote at the hospital address or another address with which they have a local connection.

Exceptions

Please note that these arrangements only apply to patients in mental hospital who are not detained offenders, and that therefore those detained on remand or the following sections (MHA 1983) are ineligible to vote:
- Section 37;
- Section 38;
- Section 44;
- Section 45A;
- Sections 46, 47, or 51(5).

RPA 2000 criteria for entitlement to register as a voter are:
- Citizenship—British, other Commonwealth, or a citizen of the Republic of Ireland;
- Age—18yrs, although if not 18yrs, you may be able to register to vote in elections following the 18th birthday;
- Residency—you must be resident in the constituency where you will vote;
- You must be on the electoral register;
- You must not be subject to any legal incapacity to vote.

The RPA 2000 does not make specific reference to intellectual disabilities. This client group is covered under the generic term 'mental disorder'. Whereas the Act does not categorically state that people with a mental disorder (or intellectual disabilities) are ineligible to vote, they can be prevented from doing so if they are deemed to lack mental capacity (see ➲ Mental Capacity Act 2005, pp. 508–9).

Arrangements for voting

The RPA 2000 stated that patients detained under the MHA 1983 can only vote via *proxy* or by *post*.[17]

Role of the registered nurse for people with intellectual disabilities

Nurses may be in a position to:
- Inform individuals of their right to vote;
- Explain the process;
- Be involved in assessment of mental capacity;
- Liaise with advocacy/legal and other services;
- Escort voluntary patients who can vote to a polling station.

Further reading

United Response, Every Vote Counts. *Learning Disabilities*. ♠ www.everyvotecounts.org.uk/ information-for-politicians/learning-disabilities/ (accessed 31 October 2017).

References

17 HM Government (2000). *Representation of the People Act*. HMSO. London.

Consent to examination, treatment, and care

Consent in relation to people with intellectual disabilities is a potentially contentious issue due to a variety of interrelated factors. People with intellectual disabilities are often perceived to lack capacity to give valid consent; they are often in unequal power relationships in which others consent on their behalf. Due to the complexities relating to consent, readers should consult the recommended reading provided at the end of this section. For the purposes of this section, consent will be divided into:

• Seeking consent—people with capacity;
• Consent when adults lack capacity;
• Compulsory treatment under the MHA 1983.

Seeking consent—people with capacity

For consent to be valid, a person must be:

• Capable of taking that particular decision (in other words 'competent');
• Acting voluntarily, and not under coercion, duress, or pressure from others;
• Provided with enough information to enable them to make a decision.

People who have given their consent to a procedure/intervention can withdraw their consent at any time. If they appear to withdraw consent during treatment, then it is good practice to stop it, unless it puts the person's life at risk. Those with capacity can refuse treatment, even if to do so is detrimental to their health and well-being. Legally, it is irrelevant whether a person signs a form to give consent or does so verbally or non-verbally. The key factor in valid consent is whether the person has capacity (see Mental Capacity Act 2005, pp. 508–9). Succinctly, for people to give valid consent for treatment, they must be able to: 'Comprehend and retain information relevant to the decision, particularly in relation to the consequences of having or not having the treatment, and use and consider this information in the decision making process'.[18]

RNIDs and others should see seeking consent and ascertaining capacity as a process that involves individual person-centred ways of explaining treatments. This can be done via augmented communication methods, using easy-to-understand language, pictorial guides, or conveying information through a close carer or family member.

Consent when adults lack capacity

Some people with intellectual disabilities lack capacity to give valid consent at specific times and for specific decisions; however, it is possible for treatment to be lawfully provided if the treatment is deemed to be in the person's best interests. Although the Act states that no one can give consent on behalf of an adult who lacks capacity to give consent, and this includes their parents, there are exceptions to this. The Court of Protection and personal welfare deputies under the MCA can make medical treatment decisions on an individual's behalf. Legally, it is the health professional responsible for the treatment who decides whether the treatment is in the person's best interests.

In practice, most decisions taken by the responsible professional will be after discussion with, and agreement from, a multidisciplinary team, carers, and family. A decision on what is in a person's best interests should not be based on medical treatment/intervention alone. Matters such as general well-being, relationships, social issues, and spiritual/religious beliefs should also be considered. When a proposed treatment is controversial, e.g. sterilization, and interested parties strongly oppose it, then the doctor responsible for the treatment can and should seek a court decision on best interests.

Compulsory treatment under the Mental Health Act 1983

The consent to treatment provisions are covered under Part IV in Sections 56–64. Some key areas are outlined below in relation to those who have capacity but refuse to consent to treatment.

Section 58 specifically applies to medication, and *Section 58(A)* to ECT. It requires consent or a second opinion and applies to detained patients. It allows for medication to be given without a second opinion for a period of 3 months after it was first given. It is mandatory that the responsible clinician or approved clinician discusses the treatment plan with the person in order to gain consent before this period elapses. If consent is not gained, then a second opinion must be sought from a CQC-appointed second-opinion appointed doctor (SOAD). If after consultation with both a nurse and another professional involved in the individual's treatment, there is agreement from the SOAD, then treatment can continue after the initial 3 months.

Section 62 allows for treatment that is immediately necessary, as long as it is not irreversible or hazardous. The treatment should be carried out under the direction of the approved clinician, and attempts should be made to seek the opinion of the SOAD, but in practice, this is not always possible.

Section 63 allows for any treatment to be given without consent that is not covered by Sections 57 (implantation of hormones) and 58. Treatment under this section can cover many things, including care, rehabilitation, and psychotherapy. Once again, this should be done under the direction of the approved clinician; however, nurses may be involved in the delivery of these treatments.

Further reading

Department of Health (2001). *Seeking Consent: Working with People with Learning Disabilities.* HMSO: London.

Department of Health, Social Services and Public Safety (2003). *Consent Guides for Healthcare Professionals.* Department of Health, Social Services and Public Safety: Belfast. ℘ www.health-ni.gov.uk/publications/consent-guides-healthcare-professionals (accessed 31 October 2017).

Health Service Executive (2013). *National Consent Policy.* Health Service Executive: Dublin. ℘ www.hse.ie/eng/services/list/3/nas/news/National_Consent_Policy.pdf (accessed 31 October 2017).

Royal College of Nursing (2017). *Principles of Consent. Guidance for nursing staff.* Royal College of Nursing: London. ℘ www.rcn.org.uk/professional-development/publications/pub-006047 (accessed 31 October 2017).

References

18 Office of the Public Guarding (2014). *Mental Capacity Act: Making Decisions. How to Make Decisions under the Mental Capacity Act 2005.* ℘ www.gov.uk/government/collections/mental-capacity-act-making-decisions (accessed 31 October 2017) (for the Mental Capacity Act, the Code of Practice, and other related documents).

Mental Capacity Act 2005

The MCA 2005 (England and Wales) is a hugely influential policy initiative that has the potential to affect many aspects of the lives of people with intellectual disabilities. One such aspect is that of consent, and you are strongly advised to read ➜ Consent to examination, treatment, and care (pp. 506–7), in conjunction with this section. The MCA 2005 received Royal Assent in April 2005; some parts of the Act became active in April 2007, but most of the Act came into force in October 2007. The main aim of the Act is to provide a statutory framework to empower and protect people (>16yrs) who may lack capacity to make some decisions for themselves—including those with intellectual disabilities. Section 1 of the Act sets out five underpinning principles, as follows:

- *A presumption of capacity*—every adult has the right to make their own decisions, and they must be assumed to have capacity to do so unless it is proved otherwise;
- *Individuals being supported to make their own decisions*—an individual must be given all practicable help before anyone treats them as not being able to make their own decisions;
- *Unwise decisions*—just because an individual makes what could be considered to be an unwise decision, they should not be treated as lacking capacity to make that decision;
- *Best interests*—an act done or a decision taken under the Act for, or on behalf of, a person who lacks capacity must be done in their best interests;
- *Least restrictive option*—anything done for, or on behalf of, a person who lacks capacity should be the least restrictive of their basic human rights and freedoms.

What the Act does

- *Assessing lack of capacity*—it sets out a single clear test for assessing whether a person lacks capacity at a particular time. The Act states that no one can be judged as lacking capacity as a result of a medical diagnosis, condition, age, appearance, or behaviour;.
- *Best interests*—the Act provides a checklist of factors that decision-makers must work through in order to decide what is in a person's best interests. Under the Act, those involved in caring for the person lacking capability have the right to be consulted in relation to best interests.
- *Acts in connection with treatment*—Section 5 of the Act gives statutory protection from liability where a person is performing an act connected to caring for the person who lacks capacity.
- *Restraint*—the Act defines restraint in relation to those who lack capacity as any restriction of liberty or movement, whether or not the person resists. Restraint is permissible if those using it reasonably believe it is necessary to the individual and that it is a proportionate response (see ➜ Use of restraint, pp. 522–3).
- *Lasting powers of attorney*—the Act allows for a person to appoint an attorney to act on their behalf, should they lose capacity in the future.

- *Court-appointed deputies*—deputies are able to take decisions on welfare, healthcare, and financial matters, as authorized by the new Court of Protection.
- *Court of Protection*—this new court has jurisdiction over the whole Act. The court can make declarations, decisions, and orders affecting those who lack capacity. It is particularly important in resolving complex and disputed dilemmas relating to consent and best interests and appoints deputies for those unable to make decisions.

The Office of the Public Guardian will be responsible for the supervision of attorneys and deputies, and liaising with other agencies such as the police and social services to respond to any concern relating to attorneys and deputies.

- *Independent Mental Capacity Advocate*—an IMCA is someone appointed by a person who lacks capacity to act and speak for themselves if they do not have anyone, such as family or friends, who can do this for them. IMCAs are involved only where decisions need to be made about serious medical matters or a change in the person's accommodation.
- *Advance decisions to refuse treatment*—the Act has created statutory rules so that people can make a decision in advance to refuse treatment, should they lack capacity in the future.
- *A criminal offence*—the Act has created a new criminal offence, which is that of ill treatment or neglect of a person who lacks capacity.
- *Research*—the Act introduces rules about research and allows for it to be carried out and involve people who lack capacity, so long as it is approved by an ethics committee.
- *Exclusions*—the Act acknowledges that some decisions cannot be made by someone on behalf of a person who lacks consent, because they are governed by other laws or are of a very personal nature. These include marriage, sexual relationships, and voting. People can also still be treated compulsorily under the MHA (see ➔ Consent to examination, treatment, and care, pp. 506–7).
- *Code of Practice*—a statutory Code of Practice that accompanies the Act provides comprehensive guidance for all those who work with, or care for, those who lack capacity. It clearly sets out, in 16 chapters, the responsibilities of all relevant parties, with specific reference to nurses. Readers are strongly advised to review the Code of Practice.

Further reading

Green M, Cowley J (2015). *A Practical Guide to the Mental Capacity Act 2005: Putting Principles of the Act into Practice*. Jessica Kingsley Publishers: London.

Office of the Public Guarding (2014). *Mental Capacity Act: Making Decisions. How to Make Decisions under the Mental Capacity Act 2005*. ℜ www.gov.uk/government/collections/mental-capacity-act-making-decisions (accessed 31 October 2017) (for the Mental Capacity Act, the Code of Practice, and other related documents).

Scottish Government (2000). *Adults with Incapacity (Scotland) Act 2000: Codes of Practice*. ℜ www.gov.scot/Topics/Justice/law/awi/010408awiwebpubs/cop (accessed 31 October 2017).

Mental Capacity Act: Deprivation of Liberty Safeguards

All the articles and rights outlined in the Human Rights Act, to some degree, influence and underpin good nursing practice; however, it is very important to note that Article 5 has resulted in some significant changes in practice relating to the capacity to consent and issues of best interests that can apply to some people with intellectual disabilities. These changes are known as the Deprivation of Liberty Safeguards (MCADOLS) which is a part of the MCA. They originated as a result of the Bournewood judgement that related to a man with intellectual disabilities and autistic spectrum condition who lacked capacity to consent to admission to a specialist unit and from which he was subsequently prevented from leaving, irrespective of having been admitted 'informally'. This was seen to be in breach of Article 5 of the ECHR which is '*the right to liberty and security*'. The Act came into force in 2009. In Scotland, the legislation that covers these issues is the Adults with Incapacity (Scotland) Act 2000. Both Northern Ireland and the Republic of Ireland have legislation in the area of capacity which has been approved and is in the process of being taken forward for implementation; all of these documents are based on similar principles. The key intention of MCADOLS is to treat a person in a care environment if it is deemed in their best interests to do so and they lack the capacity to consent to be in that care setting. MCADOLS are usually applied to people with a disorder or disability of the mind (including intellectual disabilities) associated with difficulties with capacity to consent. MCADOLS tend to be applied more often to people with intellectual disabilities and those with dementia than other client groups. They apply to people in hospitals and care homes, and NOT those sectioned under the MHA 1983. Deprivation of liberty can be:

- Physical restraint;
- Medication given against a person's will;
- Complete control over a person's care or movements for a long period;
- Making decisions on behalf of individuals;
- Deciding whether to release a person into the care of others;
- Refusing to discharge an individual;
- Restricting contact with a person's friends or family.

Authorization for the deprivation of liberty must be obtained from the local authority or NHS trust and consider the following:

- Age—over 18;
- Any mental disorder—this includes dementia;
- Mental capacity—does the person have capacity?
- Best interests;
- Eligibility—does the person meet the requirements to be detained under the MHA?
- No refusals—has there been any advance decisions? Any conflict with the lasting power of attorney?

It should be noted that the Law Commission is currently considering reforms to MCADOLS legislation and that new guidance is likely to be available in 2017.

Further reading

Department of Health, Social Services and Public Safety (2010). *Deprivation of Liberty Safeguards Interim Guidance.* ℅ www.health-ni.gov.uk/sites/default/files/publications/dhssps/revised-circular-deprivation-of-liberty-safeguards-october-2010.pdf (accessed 31 October 2017).

Ministry of Justice (2008). *Mental Capacity Act (2005): Deprivation of Liberty Safeguards – Code of Practice to Supplement to the Main Mental Capacity Act 2005 Code of Practice.* The Stationery Office: London. ℅ webarchive.nationalarchives.gov.uk/20130107105354/http:/www.dh.gov.uk/en/Publicationsandstatistics/Publications/PublicationsPolicyAndGuidance/DH_085476 (accessed 31 October 2017).

Scottish Government (2000). *Adults with Incapacity (Scotland) Act 2000: Codes of Practice.* ℅ www.gov.scot/Topics/Justice/law/awi/010408awiwebpubs/cop (accessed 31 October 2017).

Common law and duty of care

Common law is based on decisions made by judges that are derived from previous cases that have set precedents/legal principles that other judges follow. It is an ancient form of law that is grounded in jurisprudence. It is different from statute law, which is law made by Parliament. The notion of duty of care stems from common law, and some of the cases that set legal principles are important in influencing nursing practice and are outlined in this section. Duty of care can be considered to be a formalization of the implicit responsibilities held by an individual towards another individual in society. It is not a requirement that duty of care is defined by law, but it often develops through the jurisprudence of common law. In summary, there is a strong connection between common law, duty of care, and negligence.

Duty of care is a key element of ethical and professional nursing conduct, and guidance is incorporated into guidance on ethics and conduct provided by professional regulators and is updated on an ongoing basis.[19–21]

The common law that underpins duty of care comes from the 1932 case of Donoghue v Stevenson, from which the judge stated that:

'*You must take reasonable care to avoid acts or omissions which you can reasonably foresee would be likely to injure your neighbour*' (cited in Dimond 2015, p. 46).[22]

In other words, there is a duty of care if a person can see that their actions are reasonably likely to cause harm to another. In the field of nursing, this underpins the duty of care that a nurse has to the patient.

The issue of accountability is extremely important in nursing, as nurses can be called to account for their actions in a court of law. If this occurs, then the proceedings are very likely to be based on the nurse giving an account of their actions relating to a breach of their duty of care, which is often construed as negligence. Common law via the law of tort (this includes negligence) provides a framework for how care should be delivered and whether it falls short of the required standard. The common law principle that underpins decisions on the standard of practice is the Bolam Test (Bolam v Friern Hospital Management Committee 1957). The key principle of the Bolam Test is:

'*When you get a situation that involves the use of some special skill or competence, then the test as to whether there has been negligence or not is ... the standard of the ordinary skilled man exercising and professing to have that special skill.*'[23]

In other words, the standard against which a nurse is judged is that of a reasonably competent practitioner working within accepted parameters. In some instances, an expert witness may be called on to give their opinion as to whether a nurse was performing their duties to the standard of a reasonably competent practitioner. Duty of care may be owed by a number of different professionals and organizations to the same individual. The nurse who actually delivers care or performs the task in question has a primary duty of care to the individual. Where a task has been delegated by a more experienced nurse, it may be this person who has the primary duty of care.

Vicarious liability

An organization providing care and employing nurses may owe a duty of care to the individual being cared for, as will the nurses themselves, and the organization may be liable for systemic errors. An example of this would be harm caused to a person who had been physically restrained because an organization had not ensured that staff were adequately trained in control and restraint techniques.

Indemnity

It is a mandatory requirement of the NMC[19] and NMBI[21] Codes that nurses must have an indemnity arrangement which provides appropriate cover for any practice they take on as a nurse or midwife.

Withdrawing care

It is acknowledged that, in some circumstances, nurses may withdraw their duty of care. The Royal College of Nursing offers advice on when a nurse might consider withdrawing care and also provides a list of circumstances that might lead to the withdrawal of treatment.

> If you find yourself in a situation where you may have to consider withdrawing care, you should firstly consider your rationale for taking such action very carefully.
>
> The following situations may justify a refusal to treat, the withdrawal of care, or the finding of an alternative:
> - There is physical violence, or the fear of;
> - There is sexual or racial harassment;
> - There are health and safety hazards, e.g. lack of appropriate equipment;
> - The care required is outside the scope of competence or training (another practitioner should be identified who does have the necessary skills and training sought);
> - There is conscientious objection;
> - The client/patient is known to you in a personal capacity;
>   You are asked to do something unlawful/in breach of the Code.

Situations off duty

If a nurse encounters an emergency while not on duty, they do not have a legal duty to intervene. If the nurse does decide to intervene, then they take on a legal duty to act reasonably and within the parameters of their best skills and knowledge. Although the nurse does not have a legal duty to intervene, the professional regulator codes place a professional duty on nurses at all times.[19–21] In the event of an emergency outside of work, it is reasonable for a nurse to act in a proper manner, e.g. giving support and comfort without direct intervention. However, at all times, nurses must be mindful of their own safety.[20]

References

19 Nursing and Midwifery Council (2015). *The Code: Professional Standards of Practice and Behaviour for Nurses and Midwives.* Nursing and Midwifery Council: London.
20 Nursing and Midwifery Council (2017). Information for nurses and midwives on responding to unexpected incidents or emergencies. ◌ www.nmc.org.uk/news/news-and-updates/information-for-nurses-and-midwives-on-responding-to-unexpected-incidents-or-emergencies/ (accessed 31 October 2017).
21 Nursing and Midwifery Board of Ireland (2014). *Code of Professional Conduct and Ethics for Registered Nurses and Registered Midwives.* Nursing and Midwifery Board of Ireland: Dublin.
22 Dimond D (2015). *Legal Aspects of Nursing*, 7th edn. Pearson: Harlow.
23 Bolam v Friern Barnet HMC (1957) 2 All ER1184. *Advice Sheet: Duty of Care.* Nursing and Midwifery Council: London.

Safeguarding adults

Until the Care Act came into force on 1 April 2015, there had been no English legislation that specifically dealt with the safeguarding of adults who might be at risk of abuse and neglect. Prior to the Care Act 2014, in 2000, the Department of Health had provided statutory guidance within the *No Secrets: Guidance on Developing and Implementing Multiagency Policies and Procedures to Protect Vulnerable Adults from Abuse*. The guidance provided by *No Secrets* has been replaced by new legislation which is set out in Sections 42–46 and Schedule 2 The Care Act 2014. The law is designed to protect adults who:

• Have care support needs;
• Are experiencing, or are at risk of, abuse or neglect; and
• Because of their care and support needs, cannot protect themselves against actual or potential support needs.

Abuse

Abuse is a generic term that is open to wide interpretation. It can be a single act or it can be systematic repeated acts. It can occur within institutions and as a result of institutionalization. It can occur within families and in public places. It is a violation of one person's human and civil rights by another. The Act specifies that exploitation is a common theme and identifies other examples of abuse such as:

• Physical abuse;
• Sexual abuse;
• Psychological abuse;
• Financial or material abuse;
• Neglect and acts of omission;
• Organizational abuse;
• Modern slavery;
• Domestic abuse, including honour-based violence;
• Self-neglect.

The Care Act enshrines six key principles which are:

• Empowerment;
• Prevention;
• Proportionality—proportionate and least intrusive response appropriate to the risk presented;
• Protection—support and representation for those in greatest need;
• Partnerships—local solutions through services working together within their communities;
• Accountability.

The overall aims of the Act in relation to safeguarding are to:

• Prevent harm and reduce the risk of abuse and neglect;
• Address the cause of the abuse or neglect;
• Wherever possible, stop abuse and neglect;
• Raise public awareness in order that communities can be involved in safeguarding alongside professionals;
• Safeguard adults in empowering ways that support them making choices and having some control over their lives;

- Focus on improving the lives of the adults concerned;
- Provide accessible information and support about staying safe; and
- Raise concerns.

The Act emphasizes the importance of cooperation between health and social care and other public sector professionals and the importance of multi-agency approaches to safeguarding. The law requires local authorities to make enquiries if there is 'reasonable cause' to suspect an adult with care needs is, or is at risk of, being abused or neglected. Every local authority must establish 'Safeguarding Adults Boards' which include representatives from a wide range of organizations. These Boards have a duty to arrange case reviews where there has been a serious incident. It should be noted that the Care Act applies to England only. In Scotland, safeguarding legislation is set out in the Adult Support and Protection (Scotland) Act 2007. In Wales, the Social Services and Well-Being (Wales) Act 2014 is the legislation that makes specific provision for 'adults at risk'. Links to relevant documents for Northern Ireland and the Republic of Ireland are provided under ➜ Further reading.

The Act emphasizes the importance of healthcare workers, and this includes registered nurses for people with intellectual disabilities, 'being alert to possible signs of abuse and neglect and acting on their concerns'.

Readers should, in conjunction with this section, also refer to ➜ Dealing with abuse (pp. 498–9) and be aware of, and use, the guidance provided in the NMC document *Raising concerns: Guidance for Nurses and Midwives* (NMC 2015). This should be read in conjunction with Parts 16 ('act without delay if you believe that there is a risk to patient safety or public protection') and 17 ('Raise concerns immediately if you believe a person is vulnerable or at risk and needs extra support and protection') of the Code (NMC 2015).

Further reading

Department of Health (2014). *Care and Support Statutory Guidance: Issued under the Care Act 2014*. 🔗 www.gov.uk/government/uploads/system/uploads/attachment_data/file/315993/Care-Act-Guidance.pdf (accessed 31 October 2017).
Department of Health, Social Services and Public Safety/Department of Justice (2015). *Adult Safeguarding: Prevention and Protection in Partnership*. Department of Health, Social Services and Public Safety/Department of Justice: Belfast. 🔗 www.health-ni.gov.uk/publications/adult-safeguarding-prevention-and-protection-partnership-key-documents (accessed 31 October 2017).
Health Service Executive (2014). *Safeguarding Vulnerable Persons at Risk of Abuse. National Policy and Procedures*. Health Service Executive: Dublin. 🔗 www.hse.ie/eng/services/publications/corporate/personsatriskofabuse.pdf (accessed 31 October 2017) (this document is being updated at the time of writing; please refer to the Health Service Executive website for the most recent document).
Nursing and Midwifery Board of Ireland (2014). *Code of Professional Conduct and Ethics for Registered Nurses and Registered Midwives*. Nursing and Midwifery Board of Ireland: Dublin.
Nursing and Midwifery Council (2015). *The Code: Professional Standards of Practice and Behaviour for Nurses and Midwives*. Nursing and Midwifery Council: London.
Nursing and Midwifery Council (2015). *Raising Concerns: Guidance for Nurses and Midwives*. Nursing and Midwifery Council: London.
Scottish Government (2007). *The Adult Support and Protection (Scotland) Act 2007*. Scottish Government: Edinburgh. 🔗 www.legislation.gov.uk/asp/2007/10/contents (accessed 31 October 2017).
Welsh Assembly (2014). *Social Services and Well-being (Wales) Act 2014. Code of Practice and Statutory Guidance*. Welsh Assembly: Cardiff. 🔗 socialcare.wales/hub/sswbact-codes (accessed 31 October 2017).

Nurse prescribers

In the UK, the control and administration of medicine are governed by the Medicines Act 1968. Under the original Act, nurses could not prescribe medicines. This situation was altered by the Medicinal Products: Prescription by Nurses, etc. Act 1992[24] that amended Section 58 of the Medicines Act 1968 to allow some limited nurse prescribing. This Act came into force in 1994 and stipulated that nurse prescribing would be limited to registered nurses, midwives, and HVs. In 1999, the Department of Health extended the range of potential prescribers,[25] and this has enabled RNIDs to become nurse prescribers. There are three main types of nurse prescriber.

Community practitioner nurse prescribers (CPNPs)

These are prescribers who have successfully completed the NMC Community Practitioner Nurse Prescribing course (V100). The majority of nurses who do this are district nurses, public health nurses, community nurses (including community learning disability nurses), and school nurses. They are qualified to prescribe from *Nurse Prescribers Formulary for Community Practitioners* only. This formulary includes appliances, dressings, pharmacy, general sales list, and 13 prescription-only medicines.

Supplementary nurse prescribers

These nurses can prescribe any medication listed in the *British National Formulary* (*BNF*),[26] identified on a clinical management plan, and within their scope of practice. Supplementary prescribing legally allows nurses to prescribe from a wider range of medication applicable to the field of intellectual disabilities than that available within the formulary of independent nurse prescribing. Supplementary prescribing is based on clear limitations set out in the clinical management plan, which must be agreed with the individual patient, and in consultation with an independent prescriber who must be a doctor or dentist. These plans must be signed by both the nurse and doctor.

Nurse independent prescribers

These prescribers can prescribe any licensed medicine for any medical condition within their competence, including some controlled drugs. The Department of Health has laid down criteria regarding the eligibility of those wishing to become nurse prescribers.[27] In summary, they should be able to study at degree level, have 3yrs post-registration experience (the preceding one in the clinical area in which they wish to prescribe), and have the ability to assess client needs. The benefits of nurse prescribing include:[28]

- Professional flexibility;
- Recognition of the nurse's increased skills and responsibilities;
- Improved multidisciplinary working;
- Removing some barriers to patients accessing medication;
- More effective/efficient/timely healthcare;
- Improved ability to help patients and carers manage medication;
- Early intervention.

References

24 Medicinal Products: Prescription by Nurses etc. Act 1992 (commencement No 1 order 1994) Statutory Instrument 1994 No.2408 (C.48). HMSO: London.

25 Department of Health (1999). *Review of Prescribing, Supply and Administration of Medicines.* Crown Report II. HMSO: London.

26 British Medical Association, Royal Pharmaceutical Society of Great Britain. *British National Formulary.* British Medical Association, Royal Pharmaceutical Society of Great Britain: London. (Ensure you are always using the most up-to-date version.)

27 Department of Health (2006). *Patients' Access to Medicines: A Guide to Implementing Nurse and Pharmacist Independent Prescribing within the NHS in England.* HMSO: London.

28 Royal College of Nursing. *Nurse Prescribing.* www.rcn.org.uk/get-help/rcn-advice/nurse-prescribing (accessed 31 October 2017).

Physical assault

A 'zero tolerance' campaign towards assault of staff has been introduced in many health services, with the intention of minimizing the risk to staff.[29] The initiative advocated by the government covers all NHS staff and environments. The campaign documentation describes violence as:

'any incident where staff are abused, threatened or assaulted in circumstances related to their work, involving an explicit or implicit challenge to their safety'.[29]

A note of caution is necessary in relation to zero tolerance, in so far as nurses and other professionals must remain alert to the possibility that behaviour which involves threatening, abuse, or assault of staff may have another cause, e.g. head injury, confusional state, or metabolic disorder. It is essential that staff clearly assess the possible reasons for such behaviour and are not blinkered by a blind adherence to 'zero tolerance'.

Working with people with intellectual disabilities can present challenges that are, in some cases, different from other areas of nursing practice. Some people with intellectual disabilities:

- Have learnt to respond in inappropriate ways to their environment, and the consequences of this behaviour have been reinforcing for individuals;
- Display behaviour that may be viewed by some people as threatening or abusive to communicate their needs that would otherwise remain unmet;
- Show threatening or abusive behaviour that may be associated with a condition (e.g. mental illness, epilepsy);
- Show behaviour that is a response to abuse;
- May use behaviour to draw attention to something, e.g. pain.

The above is not an exhaustive list but indicates the complexity of distressed behaviours that some people with intellectual disabilities use in order to communicate their distress. Physical assault in the field of intellectual disabilities might include:

- Biting;
- Scratching;
- Nipping;
- Grabbing;
- Slapping;
- Punching;
- Poking;
- Hair pulling;
- Head butting;
- Throwing objects;
- Using weapons;
- Choking;
- Inappropriate touching.

The management of physical assault in intellectual disabilities can be outlined from the perspectives of clinical aspects and organizational responses. Nurses involved with working in direct contact with people who may physically assault need to consider clinical and management aspects. From a clinical perspective, management and limitation of physical assault can be aided by:

- Training—staff working in environments where physical assault may occur should receive mandatory training in restraint, break-away techniques, and de-escalation (see ➔ De-escalation, pp. 520–1);
- Adequate staffing levels so that clients and staff are safe from harm;
- The ability to closely observe people to identify and respond promptly to triggers that may lead to assault;
- Functional analysis—the process of gaining an understanding as to why people may become physically aggressive (record antecedents, behaviours and consequences for individual);
- Access to, and the ability to provide, clinical supervision;
- The use of self as a therapeutic tool in order to build relationships with clients;
- Good communication techniques, including augmented communication;
- The ability to work within an interdisciplinary framework;
- Knowledge of the appropriate use of medications prescribed for the person;
- Structured interventions to help clients manage their anger;
- Recording and reporting of incidents using appropriate incident reports;
- Individual client risk management.

From an organizational perspective, management and limitation of physical assault can be aided by:
- Producing and disseminating robust policies;
- Involving criminal justice/forensic services (see ➔ Chapter 11);
- Adopting strategies for risk management;
- Managing resources so that staff engaged in individual client work can operate safely, given the considerations outlined above;
- Structured post-incident support/staff counselling;
- Providing systematic collation and interpretation of trends emanating from incident reports;
- Managing the environment to ensure it is as therapeutic as possible/ commissioning of services based on best practice;
- Ensuring staff have the necessary knowledge, skills, and confidence to competently undertaken their role, including staff with a specific role in responding to threatening, abusive, or assaultive behaviour.

References

29 Department of Health (2014). *Positive and Proactive Care: Reducing the Need for Restrictive Interventions*. Department of Health: London. ℡ www.gov.uk/government/uploads/system/uploads/attachment_data/file/300293/JRA_DoH_Guidance_on_RP_web_accessible.pdf (accessed 31 October 2017).

De-escalation

Challenging behaviour, physical assault, and some self-injurious behaviours can sometimes be avoided through the use of de-escalation. For the vast majority of people, aggression and physical assault are an uncommon occurrence that usually arises due to an environmental trigger and results in some physiological changes that can make an aggressive outburst almost inevitable. This phenomenon is part of the 'assault cycle,[30] which has the following phases:

- Baseline behaviour—this is a person's usual pattern of behaviour, which, for most people, does not include violence;
- Trigger phase—something in the person's environment causes them to become increasingly agitated;
- Escalation phase—the person deviates more and more from their baseline behaviour and they become increasingly less likely to respond to any form of rational behaviour;
- Crisis phase—physical assault is likely to occur and the least effective response is to attempt to reason with the person;
- Plateau/recovery phase—a gradual reduction in agitation;
- Post-crisis or depression phase—this is when the person dips below their usual baseline behaviour and they may feel exhausted and depressed.

The assault cycle is linked to physiological changes, particularly in the trigger, escalation, and crisis phases when adrenaline is being quickly released into the body for 'flight or fight'. De-escalation is based on intervention before a person reaches the crisis phase, so that a violent incident can be avoided. Nurses need to be vigilant for any changes from baseline behaviour in the trigger and escalation stages and for any known triggers that cause a person to become violent. Experienced nurses with extensive knowledge of the people in their care will usually be able to recognize the triggers that affect individuals and behavioural changes that signify entry into the trigger phase. Such behavioural changes might include:

- Pacing;
- Hand wringing;
- Fist clenching;
- Muttering;
- Being red-faced or pale;
- Standing tall;
- Making gestures;
- Rapid breathing;
- Direct and prolonged eye contact;
- Any major change in behaviour;
- Tensing of muscles.

To avoid a violent incident, the nurse can use the following techniques.

Non-verbal

- Create a distance between self and client;
- Move towards a safer place and avoid corners;
- Consider access to exits;

- Mood matching;
- Mirroring;
- Intermittent eye contact;
- Open posture/avoid squaring up;
- Keep both hands visible;
- Display calmness;
- Avoid sudden movements.

Verbal

- Speak slowly, gently, and clearly; if more than one member of staff is involved, only one should speak and give instructions;
- Lower your voice;
- Do not argue, confront, make threats, or give ultimatums;
- Listen;
- Give clear, brief, and assertive instructions;
- Use open questions;
- Show concern/empathy;
- Do not patronize;
- Acknowledge grievances and frustrations;
- Depersonalize issues.

The above are all well-recognized de-escalation techniques and can be used with people with intellectual disabilities, particularly those with verbal speech. For some people with more profound and complex needs, de-escalation may involve identifying and altering environmental triggers such as:

- Temperature—too hot or cold;
- Noise levels;
- Overstimulation/understimulation;
- Inability to communicate a need, e.g. hunger, thirst, need to go to the toilet;
- Lights—too bright or too dim;
- Too many people;
- Too many demands being placed on the person;
- Illness/pre-existing condition;
- Change in routine (often in autism).

Further reading

Department of Health (2014). *Positive and Proactive Care: Reducing the Need for Restrictive Interventions*. Department of Health: London. ℘ www.gov.uk/government/uploads/system/uploads/attachment_data/file/300293/JRA_DoH_Guidance_on_RP_web_accessible.pdf (accessed 31 October 2017).

Lowry M, Lingard G, Neal M (2016). De-escalating anger: a new model for practice. *Nursing Times*. 112: 4–7. ℘ www.nursingtimes.net/roles/mental-health-nurses/de-escalating-anger-a-new-model-for-practice/7009471.article (accessed 31 October 2017).

References

30 RN.com. *The Assault Cycle*. ℘ https://lms.rn.com/courses/2033/page5149.html (accessed 31 October 2017).

Use of restraint

It is widely acknowledged that the use of physical restraint is an undesirable, but sometimes inescapable, practice but that it can be used as long as it is the last resort and a proportionate response, and the method is the least restrictive form of restraint. It is imperative, therefore, that nurses make sure that both staff and those who may be subject to being restrained know how and why someone may be restrained. Readers are advised to consult the Department of Health 2014 policy document *Positive and Proactive Care: Reducing the Need for Restrictive Interventions* because it offers comprehensive guidance on the use of restraint.

Restraint can take many forms
- Physical restraint—by members of staff;
- Use of mechanical devices/equipment;
- Seclusion/time out;
- Manipulation of the environment, e.g. baffle locks;
- Medication.

In summary, restraint can be a spectrum of interventions, ranging from the insidious to physical restraint. Restraint is most likely to be used for behavioural management issues that include:[31]
- Physical attacks on others;
- Self-injurious behaviour;
- Destructive behaviour;
- Refusal to participate in treatment programmes;
- Prolonged verbal abuse and threatening behaviour;
- Going missing;
- Risk of physical injury by accident;
- Prevention of harm to others;
- Severe and prolonged overactivity likely to lead to exhaustion.

Restraint can be justified if it is likely to prevent significant harm to others, and it should also be noted that it can be in the client's best interests to use restraint. Restrictive interventions can be:
- Either planned—as part of an agreed multidisciplinary treatment/care plan, which will include explicit detail on the process of restraint, risk assessment(s), the condition/vulnerability of the individual, and roles and responsibilities of staff; or
- Emergency and unplanned interventions that must still be guided by best practice principles.

Purposes of restraint
- To take immediate control of a dangerous situation;
- To contain/limit the patient's freedom for no longer than is necessary;
- To end, or reduce significantly, the danger to the patient or others.

Physical restraint is distressing for both staff and clients, and its use can lead to physical harm and psychological damage; it can be counterproductive in a therapeutic sense. Therefore, if restraint is carried out, it must be done within the parameters of defined policy, as indicated above, and, wherever possible, it must be explained to those who may be restrained how and why restraint could be used. Readers who work in areas where restraint is commonly used must receive mandatory training on control and restraint and break-away techniques. It is also the case that all preventative measures should be taken to minimize the need for restraint and that de-escalation should be attempted (see ➔ De-escalation, pp. 520–1).

Further reading

Department of Health (2014). *Positive and Proactive Care: Reducing the Need for Restrictive Interventions*. Department of Health: London. ☞ www.gov.uk/government/uploads/system/uploads/attachment_data/file/300293/JRA_DoH_Guidance_on_RP_web_accessible.pdf (accessed 31 October 2017).

Autism Act 2009

In 2008, the National Autistic Society lobbied the English government to recognize and support people with ASCs through an Act of Parliament. The Autism Act 2009 was pioneering, as it was the first disability specific law in England. It is important to note that this Act relates to England only. Other government agencies in the UK and Ireland have outlined similar aspirations in their own strategies: *Refreshed Autistic spectrum condition Strategic–Action Plan Wales*, *Scottish Strategy for Autism Outcomes Approach* in Northern Ireland, and *The Autism Strategy 2013–2020* and services in the Republic of Ireland are being shaped by the Autism Bill (2012). The English Act ensured two key items: a duty on the government to produce a strategy for adults with autism (this strategy was published in 2010) and a duty on the government to enable the production of statutory guidance for local councils and local health authorities.

Fulfilling and Rewarding 2010

The autism strategy *Fulfilling and Rewarding Lives*, published in 2010, sought to improve access to health and social care for people with autism. It was acknowledged that people with comorbidity of intellectual disabilities and an ASC were supported within specialist learning disability services and appropriate autistic services were sporadic and largely inaccessible for the majority of people with an ASC without an intellectual disability. This strategy made far-reaching recommendations, calling for:

• Autism awareness and training;
• Government-commissioned autism awareness training;
• Examples of autism awareness and training;
• Diagnosis of autism;
• Diagnostic pathways;
• Community care—linking diagnosis to individual need;
• Developing services and support;
• Personalization and transition;
• Examples of developing services and support, and employment;
• Examples of good practice in employment;
• Useful resources, and local planning and autism partnership boards;
• Examples of good practice in local planning, and useful resources for local planning.

Think Autism (Department of Health, 2014)

In 2014, the Department of Health reviewed the first autism strategy and produced a Think Autism strategy. There were three key proposals in this second autism strategy; these are in addition to existing duties of the 2010 strategy and were expected to make an impact to the lives, services, and support for adults with autism. These proposals were:

• The establishment of Autism Aware Communities and Think Autism community awareness projects;
• Autism Innovation Fund—funding for projects to promote innovation in services;
• Better data collection and joined-up advice and information services.

To demonstrate commitment, the UK (English) government invested £4.5 million towards the Autism Innovation Fund and Autism Aware Community Programme. There were many innovations, including short films about people's lives. In addition, the Think Autism strategy reinforced expectations of the government set out in the 2010 strategy. This included local authorities reporting on data about people with autism, GPs making autism a priority for training and awareness, and autism awareness training made available to all general healthcare professionals and disability employment advisers in job centres.

Progress report

In 2016, the Department of Health England published a progress report, following baseline assessments carried out in 2011 and a follow-up assessment in 2013. All progress across the Autism Act and its subsequent strategies were measured under areas listed in the previous section. Increased awareness of autism was identified within the report as being a direct result of health and social care professionals being trained, many on a mandatory basis. Additionally, e-learning training packages for staff and managers improved understanding of autism. Also reported was the establishment of better pathways to diagnosis, with less bureaucracy in establishing a diagnosis and receiving appropriate services. Less successful was the implementation of strategies to encourage employers to recruit and retain people with autism within their workforce. Additionally, far greater awareness across services was still thought necessary around sensory impairments and sensory processing disorder. In summary, the Department of Health and the National Autistic Society have made significant improvements across services and within society in general.

Further reading

See Department of Health Strategy publications for your country

Research and intellectual disability nursing

Introduction

This chapter examines research and intellectual disability nursing. Nursing is relatively new to the world of research. Although nurses have used research findings for many years, it is only in recent decades that they have been required to undertake research or to study it systematically during pre- and post-registration nursing education. In the 1990s, British nursing education moved from hospital-based schools of nursing to universities, and this brought a requirement that all nurses engage with research. This primarily has taken the form of nurses ensuring that their practice is evidence-based, but for a smaller group, it has led to the direction of, and participation as researchers in, research projects.

This chapter is an introduction to some of the key concepts in nursing research that are most relevant to intellectual disability nursing. The major methodologies of quantitative and qualitative research are outlined, to help in identifying and evaluating their use in practice. Some of the stages of the research process are outlined, so that you will know what to look for when reading research or what to start with if you want to pursue your own research ideas. Finally, the chapter examines some of the issues that are important to intellectual disability nursing research. These include ethical issues that are fundamental to all research, as well as working with people with intellectual disabilities, carers, and children.

Definitions of terms

Readers who are not familiar with research may find some of the terms difficult. Most are like a lot of nursing terms that are simply shorthand to mean things that would take a great deal of time to explain every time that they are used. Some of the terms used in this chapter will be explained in the context that they are used, but this section defines some of the main ones that are used.

- *Research* is the systematic approach to discovering or developing knowledge.
- *Participatory research* is research that involves its participants as an integral part of its method.
- *Methodology* is the intellectual framework that is used in a research project.
- *Research methods* are the techniques that are used within the methodological framework.

The two primary methodologies are quantitative and qualitative research.

- *Quantitative research* uses experimental methods. Research is particularly concerned with reliability, generalization, control of variables, testing hypotheses, and statistical association between variables, and is often large-scale in nature.
- *Qualitative research* uses naturalistic methods and examines the social world or 'lived experience' of people. Research is less concerned with reliability and generalization, and is descriptive in style and small-scale in nature, and engages directly with participants.

Further reading

Flood S, Bennet D, Melsome M, Northway R (2013). Becoming a researcher. *British Journal of Learning Disabilities*. **41**: 288–95.

Northway R, Hurley K, O'Connor C, et al. (2014). Deciding what to research: an overview of a participatory workshop. *British Journal of Learning Disabilities*. **42**: 323–7.

Tilly L, Money F; Making Ends Meet Research Group (2015). Being researchers for the first time: reflections on the development of an inclusive research group. *British Journal of Learning Disabilities*. **43**: 121–7.

Defining areas for research

An area for research must be clear, achievable, and manageable within the available resources. This section will concentrate on how to bring clarity to areas of research.

Most researchers start with a broad question or a vague area of enquiry. Readers can probably think of their own examples, and they may be similar to the following:

- Why do people with intellectual disabilities have poorer health than the rest of the population?
- How can people be encouraged to adopt healthy lifestyles?
- How can a nurse be sure that they are adopting the correct interventions for someone whose behaviour disturbs others?

The first step in defining an area for research is to think carefully about your idea(s) and to discuss this with colleagues. A literature review is then required to find out what has already been written (see ➡ Undertaking a literature review, p. 530). The literature review will unearth research that has already been carried out and may provide answers to your question. It is more likely going to lead to a refinement of the area of research.

However, sometimes it is found that the literature related to your question is sparse. This may require you to re-examine the original broad area for your research; it will possibly need to be broken down to more discrete questions to ensure that it is clear and that you are clear about the parameters.

As an illustration, the first question, from the examples above, is now going to be broken down.

Why do people with intellectual disabilities have poorer health than the rest of the population?

There are several elements to this broad question that have to be broken down. For the sake of simplicity, this will be done through a series of questions.

What is meant by 'people with intellectual disabilities' in this context?
The researcher needs to be very clear about the remit of their enquiry. Is the definition going to include all people with intellectual disabilities? Is there a difference between the health of people with profound and complex disabilities and those with less complex needs? It may be that this is what the research is really trying to tease out. Perhaps the comparison will be with people with intellectual disabilities and the general population, in which case both will still need to be defined. This is often referred to as inclusion and exclusion criteria.

What is the evidence for the underlying assumption that people with intellectual disabilities have poorer health?
There is a clear assumption behind the broad research question, and the researcher needs to be quite clear that there is a body of evidence to demonstrate that this assumption is correct. It may be demonstrated adequately within the literature, but even so, the researcher needs to be sure that it is right for the question being asked. If it is not in the literature, then can it be

demonstrated through statistics or observation, or is it simply a 'gut' feeling? If the evidence is not clear, then the area for research will have to be significantly refined to: 'Do people with intellectual disabilities have poorer health than the rest of the population?'

What is meant by health?

Health is a very difficult concept to define, although there are some generally accepted measures that help to clarify the health status of groups. Morbidity and mortality figures tend to be used to draw broad lessons. Morbidity refers to the incidence of a particular disease; mortality refers to a measure of the number of deaths due to a particular disease/cause. You may be more interested in positive states of health, in which case evidence based on a method such as quality of life surveys may be more useful. Other issues to consider are whether your interest is in the health status from an individual point of view or whether there needs to be an attempt to introduce objective measures.

What is the general population?

There are figures published for illness rates in the general population, and these are nationally defined. Reference to these will help in making broad comparisons, but the research will still need to be very clear about the nature of the comparisons to be made and between which groups.

In this example, a broad research question has been turned into several smaller questions that need to be addressed in order to define the area for research. It may be that one of the narrower questions becomes one that develops into the final research question for a specific research project.

Whatever is decided, the research area needs to be achievable. This will require you to consider:

- Can the question be answered?
- Is enough known about the background to the topic?
- Is enough known about all the elements of the research question?

The research area to be studied needs to be made manageable within the available resources of the research team. It is of little use having an achievable project that can be managed only by a much larger research team, unless you can successfully bid for the resources.

Undertaking a literature review

At its simplest, a literature review is a systematic summary of what is already known about a subject.

A literature review involves two main stages:
- A literature search;
- Making sense of the findings of the research.

Literature search

First of all, you need to know what you are looking for. There is an enormous amount of literature published about some subjects and very little about others, and it is important to start with a clear idea of what you want to find out. Most literature searches are now conducted through electronic databases, and while this has made searching literature much more accessible, the amount of material retrieved can be overwhelming. If you are lucky, you may have a library in the organization where you work, and if so, you are well advised to use the services of a librarian or an information specialist to help you. If not, you can undertake a simple search for material using an Internet-based search engine such as Google Scholar. However, please be aware that searches using popular search engines throw up a large number of references, and it is not always easy to discriminate between different forms of material. It is important to use your critical skills in assessing the important from the unimportant material.

Some simple tests to use are:
- Has the article been subject to peer review?
- Does the article say how it came to the findings?
- Is the article a piece of journalism or opinion-based?
- Is the article written by a professional?
- Has the author written anything else?
- Is the author's work referenced by others?

These questions can help you to assess whether an article is useful for your literature review and whether the information is reliable. Of course, you may find that your search reveals that there have already been reviews written about the subject in which you are interested; such reviews will be your first port of call, although there may be more recent material in print and you will have to find this.

You will need to establish criteria for inclusion in your literature search. Most search engines will help you with this. Typically you may wish to restrict your search to a particular time period and to a particular language. The search engine will do this for you if you set the parameters to the search that you think is necessary. You may also wish to restrict your search to particular types of research, such as large-scale studies or smaller in-depth research using only a few subjects. It is usual to refine search criteria as you find out the amount of material with which you are dealing.

Making sense of the findings of the research

Once you have completed your initial search, you will need to make sense of the material. In an ideal world, you will have unearthed enough material to tell you what you need to know without being overwhelmed. However, you may find that you need to further refine your criteria in order to be able to make use of the material. You can do this by narrowing the dates or by restricting your criteria to primary research papers or possibly to a narrower subject. Whatever you decide will involve a critical analysis of the material that you have found.

When you have done this and have satisfied yourself about the quality of the research that you have found, you will need to arrange it in a way that makes sense to you and to others. This will become the literature review itself. It is usually helpful to develop a table or some other means of grouping the research by categories such as:

- Method used;
- Number of subjects;
- Key findings;
- Limitations.

The use of a structured approach, such as Preferred Reporting Items for Systematic Reviews and Meta-Analyses (PRISMA), provides a framework for reviewing published articles and enables comparison with previous literatures reviews that have used this approach.

Once you have done this, it is time to write up your review. Your table or list of themes may be sufficient for what you need. If you wish to publish your literature review, however, or put it into a report, you will need to include an account of how you conducted your review, as well as the main findings. Key questions to ask about the papers that you have considered are:

- Are there any trends?
- Are there any gaps in the literature?
- Does the literature lead to new research questions?

Further reading

Parahoo K (2014). *Nursing Research: Principles, Process and Issues*, 3rd edn. Palgrave Macmillan: London.
Preferred Reporting Items for Systematic Reviews and Meta-Analyses (PRISMA). ℘ www.prisma-statement.org (accessed 31 October 2017).

Qualitative approaches

Qualitative research is subjectivist and encompasses research designs and methods such as:

• Grounded theory;
• Phenomenology;
• Phenomenography;
• Ethnography;
• Ethnomethodology;
• Documentary analysis;
• Action research;
• Case studies;
• Narrative analysis-based approaches.

Qualitative approaches are anti-methodological, idiographic, hermeneutic, and inductive, in which the research seeks to explore and describe, and usually interpret subjective information provided by participants.

The underlying assumption of qualitative approaches is the need to examine the whole in order to understand phenomena within multiple temporal and spatial realities.

Qualitative study designs are useful in areas where there is little known about the phenomenon under investigation. Qualitative research aims to contextualize information; provide meaning, purpose, and insight into human behaviour, perceptions, experiences, emotions, and social processes; apply findings to individual cases; and explore sources of hypotheses.[1] Given the absence of an overarching framework and the diversity of designs and methods that may be used within qualitative approaches, together with approaches to data analysis and interpretation, it will be necessary to refer to authoritative textbooks such as those in ➔ Further reading, p. 533.

Sampling

All sampling within qualitative projects is non-probability or non-random, and deliberate and purposive. In seeking to generate a sample, the focus is on identifying sources of data that are relevant to the phenomena under investigation. Therefore, approaches such as convenience, snowball, quota, or theoretical sampling may be used. The sample size within a qualitative study will be smaller than quantitative projects, with an emphasis on the flexibility and depth and richness of data obtained, rather than the quantity or ability to represent an overall population. Many qualitative studies have samples of <20 participants, and some have used single-case study designs.

Data collection

Qualitative data may include words, songs, poetry, and still or moving images, and will depend on the research aim of the specific project. Often a combination of approaches is used to collect data, including:

• Semi-structured interviews;
• Unstructured interviews;
• Diary entries;
• Focus groups;
• Observations (participant, non-participation, video-recorded);
• Questionnaires (largely for biographical information).

Depending on the design, data may be collected on one occasion, but in many projects, data are collected on more than one occasion to provide opportunities for data saturation or take account of temporal changes.

Data analysis

The framework for data analysis will be determined largely by the specific research design used within the project. A number of analysis frameworks exist, with differing approaches such as grounded theory analysis, interpretative phenomenological analysis, and qualitative content analysis. These approaches have a different number of steps and different titles of steps, but they are similar overall in so far as moving from initial thoughts about key points, to identifying emergent themes and sub-themes. The detail of individual analysis frameworks, and the need for robustness and clear audit trails in qualitative data analysis is discussed fully in the following sections.

Further reading

Creswell JW (2014). *A Concise Introduction to Mixed Methods Research*. Sage: Thousand Oaks.
Denzin NK, Lincoln YS, eds. (2017). *The Sage Handbook of Qualitative Research*, 5th edn. Sage: London.

References

1 Guba EG, Lincoln YS (2004). Competing paradigms in qualitative research: theories and issues. In: SN Hesse-Biber, P Leavy, eds. *Approaches to Qualitative Research: A Reader on Theory and Practice*. Oxford University Press: Oxford; pp. 17–38.

Quantitative approaches

The central tenets of quantitative research approaches are that truth is singular and fixed, and that research has to be objective, reliable, valid, generalizable, and reductive/deductive. Quantitative research is positivist and there are four main types:
- Descriptive;
- Correlational;
- Causal–comparative/quasi-experimental;
- Experimental.

Quantitative research designs include:
- Randomized controlled trials (RCTs);
- Surveys;[2]
- Cohort studies.

Quantitative research adopts deductive approaches to generating knowledge that includes observable relationship(s) between independent and dependent variables. An independent variable is something that can be manipulated to bring about a predicted effect (hypothesis). This can be accounted for by a change to an independent variable. This is often referred to as a cause-and-effect relationship.

In quantitative research, further work conducted in a different setting under the same conditions should result in this cause-and-effect relationship being replicated. This is important because this implies an ability to generalize findings. Research in this genre attempts to emulate the natural sciences and is concerned with the generation and testing of knowledge, and thereby the construction of theory. The most important characteristics of quantitative research are clarity, replicability, reliability, and validity.

Understanding quantitative research requires time, patience, and a detailed knowledge of the study design, sampling methods, and sample calculations, descriptive and inferential analysis methods and statistics, statistical interpretations, and the significance of any findings; and for this reason, the reader is strongly advised to refer to authoritative textbooks such as those shown in ➔ Further reading, p. 535.

Sampling

The approach to sampling needs to be logical and consistent with the overall study design and the research question(s).

Probability

Probability refers to a range of sampling approaches used by the researcher to select a random sample of sources of data or participants from the population being studied, e.g. simple random sampling, systematic random sampling, and stratified random sampling.

Non-probability

Non-probability refers to a range of sampling approaches used by the researcher to select a non-random sample of participants from the population being studied, and these may include:
- Proportional and non-proportional quota sampling;
- Judgemental or purposive sampling;
- Expert sampling;
- Snowball sampling.

Data collection methods
- Questionnaires;
- Structured interviews;
- Observation;
- Scales;
- Physiological measurement.

Data analysis
There are predominantly two types of statistics: descriptive and inferential. Broadly, in quantitative research, statistical analysis is a three-step process, focusing on:
- Summarizing and reducing data;
- Descriptive-level analysis;
- Relationship analysis.[2]

The extent and type of analysis are dependent on the research design and variables sample (level of measurement—nominal, ordinal, interval, or ratio). The data can be analysed either through descriptive or inferential statistics using a computer software such as SPSS.

Descriptive statistics
Measure of central tendency—mean, median, and mode; also used are frequency distribution, standard deviation, and range.

Inferential statistics
Inferential statistics are used to describe and make inferences about a population. A wide range of inferential statistical analyses are possible, but the following types are commonly used, and they are relatively easy to interpret:
- One-sample test of difference/one-sample hypothesis test;
- Confidence interval;
- Contingency tables and chi-square statistics;
- *t*-test or analysis of variance (ANOVA);
- Pearson correlation;
- Bi-variate regression;
- Multi-variate regression.

Further reading
Creswell JW (2014). *A Concise Introduction to Mixed Methods Research*. Sage: Thousand Oaks.
Denzin NK, Lincoln YS, eds. (2017). *The Sage Handbook of Qualitative Research*, 5th edn. Sage: London.
Parahoo K (2014). *Nursing Research: Principles, Process and Issues*, 3rd edn. Palgrave Macmillan: London.

References
2 Punch K (2003). *Survey Research: The Basics*. Sage: London.

Ethical issues in research

All research with human participants or information relating to real people should meet the following ethical values.

- Beneficence (to do good);
- Non-maleficence (not to cause harm);
- Autonomy (to treat people with respect and provide them with the kinds of information they need to make informed decisions);
- Justice (to try and ensure that, through the research, some justice is served).

Seeking permission

All research projects have ethical aspects that need careful consideration in relation to aspects such as informed consent, specifically regarding the purpose and potential negative consequences of participation, confidentiality, anonymity, security of data, and the use of findings. Researchers should clarify local research governance requirements and must ensure that all necessary approval has been obtained before any recruitment to, or data collection within, a research project commences.

Given the personal, and often sensitive, nature of the information collected when research involves people with intellectual disabilities, care must be taken in developing and undertaking research in an ethically defensible manner.[3] In order to involve people with learning or intellectual disabilities in research, it is good practice to ensure that ethical approval is obtained from an established ethical committee, e.g. in a university, local authority, or healthcare organization. Within the NHS, for example, the Health Research Authority (HRA), set up in 2011, approves research projects through research ethics committees (RECs), and these exist across England, Scotland, Wales, and Northern Ireland. Local RECs are also in place across the Republic of Ireland and normally aligned to Health Service Executive structures/areas.

In nearly all cases that involve people with learning or intellectual disabilities, this will require the researcher to demonstrate how they will ensure that they have obtained informed consent, as well as giving due consideration to capacity to consent; this is usually achieved through the development of 'accessible' information sheets about the research, along with 'accessible' consent forms.[4] These are usually in the form of straightforward information sheets that use simple language and are frequently supported with pictures from picture databases such as Change.[5]

Further reading

Comstock G (2013). *Research Ethics: A Philosophical Guide to the Responsible Conduct of Research*. Cambridge University Press: Cambridge.
NHS Health Research Authority (HRA). www.hra.nhs.uk/ (accessed 31 October 2017).
Pittaway E, Bartolomei L, Hugman R (2010). 'Stop stealing our stories': the ethics of research with vulnerable groups. *Journal of Human Rights Practice*. 2: 229–51.
The Research Ethics Guidebook. www.ethicsguidebook.ac.uk/ (accessed 31 October 2017).
Zaner RM (2015). *A Critical Examination of Ethics in Health Care and Biomedical Research: Voices and Visions*. Springer: London.

References

3 Department of Health (2001). *Seeking Consent: Working with People with Learning Disabilities.* Department of Health: London.
4 Department of Health (2010). *Making Written Information Easier to Understand for People with Learning Disabilities: Guidance for People who Commission or Produce Easy Read Information – Revised Edition.* Department of Health: London. ℳ www.gov.uk/government/uploads/system/uploads/attachment_data/file/215923/dh_121927.pdf (accessed 31 October 2017).
5 Change. ℳ www.changepeople.co.uk/ (accessed 31 October 2017).

Involving people with intellectual disabilities in the research process

It is now increasingly recognized that people with intellectual disabilities can actively contribute to, and enhance, the development, planning, and conducting of research as co-researchers, and there is an increasing expectation upon researchers to provide opportunities and support for this to happen.[6] There is a requirement by many major research funders for researchers seeking funding to demonstrate 'public patient involvement' (PPI) in their research. Even when it is not a requirement of the researcher funder, it will often be expected by RECs as good practice.

Public involvement in research is defined as 'research being carried out 'with' or 'by' members of the public, rather than 'to', 'about', or 'for' them' (Hayes et al., 2012, p. 6).[7] The above requirements are a major shift from the historical position of people having research 'done to them', in which they were the subjects of the researcher the studied, the analysed, but never the participant.[8] Today contemporary researchers are charged with the responsibility of making their research accessible and inclusive to people with intellectual disabilities.

Kinds of involvement

Since the development of the concepts of participatory research leading to emancipatory research within the general disability field, a 'natural progression has been to incorporate these principles into research with people with intellectual disabilities'.[8] Within the context of researchers in services for people with intellectual disabilities, this means the direct involvement of people with intellectual disabilities in activities such as:
• 'Joint grant holders or co-applicants on a research project;
• Identifying research priorities;
• As members of a project advisory or steering group;
• Commenting on, and developing, patient information leaflets or other research materials;
• Undertaking interviews with research participants;
• User and/or carer researchers carrying out the research'.[7]

A review of the literature specific to 'inclusive' research[9] with people with intellectual disabilities identified three main ways of doing inclusive research:
• 'Where people with an intellectual disability give advice about what to do;
• Where people with an intellectual disability lead and control research;
• Where people with and without intellectual disability work together as a group with different jobs based on their different interests and skills'.[9]

Planning for, and supporting, the involvement of people with intellectual disabilities in research

A review of the literature highlighted a number of potential ethical (e.g. obtaining informed consent and assessing capacity) and practical challenges (e.g. recruitment, data collection, analytic strategy, researcher interpretation) that need to be considered in planning inclusive research.

All of these challenges can be addressed with careful planning, opportunities for discussion, and preparation of people with their involvement in inclusive research. This preparation should be undertaken as a research team with all people involved and sharing their thoughts and ideas in a supportive discussion. It is important that information about the role of all researchers is prepared in a format that makes it accessible to all researchers and clearly states the roles and responsibilities of all researchers involved. Opportunities to discuss what involvement in research projects could mean for people, how support will be available, and how questions are explored and answered are important in building confidence and ability among people with intellectual disabilities involved in research. As with all novice researchers, there is a need for effectively paced mentorship and support, as new knowledge and skills are developed to maximize the contribution people can make to research projects.

Further reading

Journal of Applied Research in Intellectual Disabilities (2014). Volume 27, Issue 1. New Directions in Inclusive Research. ℘ onlinelibrary.wiley.com/doi/10.1111/jar.2014.27.issue-1/issuetoc (accessed 31 October 2017).

References

6 Bigby C, Frawley P, Ramcharan P (2014). Conceptualizing inclusive research with people with intellectual disabilities. *Journal of Applied Research in Intellectual Disabilities*. **27**: 3–12.

7 Hayes H, Buckland S, Tarpey M (2012). *Briefing Notes for Researchers: Public Involvement in NHS, Public Health and Social Care Research*. National Institute for Health Research/Involve: Eastleigh. ℘ www.involve.nihr.ac.uk (accessed 31 October 2017).

8 Northway R (2000). The relevance of participatory research in developing nursing's research and practice. *Nurse Researcher*. **7**: 40–52.

9 O'Brien P, McConkey R, Garcia-Iriarte E (2014). Identifying the key concerns of Irish persons with intellectual disability. *Journal of Applied Research in Intellectual Disabilities*. **27**: 65–75.

Mixed methods

Traditionally, research has been viewed as fitting into either a quantitative 'positivistic' or a qualitative 'interpretative' paradigm. While both approaches have important contributions to research projects and have been used in most previous studies within intellectual disability, they are only able to provide a partial view of what may be complex situations. At times, these two paradigms have been portrayed as completely separate, and not compatible to being used together. However, as the value of using mixed methods approaches has been more widely recognized, that view has been regularly challenged and is now largely rejected. There is now a growing awareness of the potential contribution of a mixed methods design.[10]

Rationale for using mixed methods design

When planning research, nurses need to consider in detail the research question(s) being asked and, in light of that, the various approaches that may be used to 'answer' the research question(s). A mixed methods design recognizes that, in real-life experiences, there is no 'single real world', but rather a number of perceived 'real worlds', and the challenge is to gain an understanding of these worlds and their interconnectedness from differing, yet complementary, perspectives.

With the increased recognition of the complexity of most human experiences and the limitations of other more traditional research designs, the use of a mixed methods design provides an opportunity to gain broader insights into the wider experience and identify the potential connections and influences that may exist, which will not be illuminated by using purely quantitative and qualitative approaches.

The use of a mixed methods approach provides the opportunity to:
• Enhance validity of research findings through providing corroboration of these across different research methods (triangulation);
• Illustrate, clarify, and amplify the meaning of constructs or relationships;
• Gain a further understanding of the complexity of issues which can be taken forward through exploring the inconsistencies across differing research perspectives (development);
• Enhance theoretical insights, hypothesis generation, and instrument development through providing alternative views and perspectives of the area under investigation.

Sampling, data collection, and data analysis

When using a mixed methods design, the procedures for sampling, data collection, and data analysis will be guided by whether that aspect of the study is qualitative or quantitative in nature. However, four key decisions are:
• Which approach (quantitative or qualitative) has priority in the overall mixed methods design?
• How will the quantitative and qualitative aspects of the overall study be sequenced?
• How will the qualitative and quantitative aspects of the study fit together? Will the overall design keep these as separate components of the study, or will each preceding phase directly influence what comes after it within a more integrated approach?

- How will data analysis be undertaken? As with sequencing of data collection, will data analysis be dealt with in separate components (combined only in the final discussion) or presented as an integrated process?

Some notes of caution

As with all research designs, the selection of the design and methods must be linked to research questions, and not selected on the basis of which approach the researcher prefers or whether it is a 'new fad'. Likewise the use of a mixed methods design must be justified in light of the research question(s) being asked. Care must be taken to select approaches that are consistent with the aspect of the project to be addressed, and not to breach the logic of each individual component of the research design, in order that they could be defensibly applied, or else the resultant research design will be best described as 'mixed-up methods'. It is also important to recognize that the collection of some 'qualitative' data in response to open-ended questions in a questionnaire is not a mixed methods study; it is still a quantitative study with some open-text answers. These are often analysed through content analysis, and this does not provide a separate stream of data.

Mixed methods designs are also more complex than single quantitative or qualitative designs. Nurses considering using them should remember that although the outcome may be more comprehensive, mixed methods studies can take longer to complete, may have additional costs involved for time and equipment, and require an understanding (in researcher or supervisor) of both quantitative and qualitative paradigms and how these may be blended together.

Given the diversity of designs and methods that may be used within mixed methods approaches, together with approaches to analysis and interpretation, to build on the overview provided in this section, it will be necessary to refer to authoritative textbooks such as those shown in ➔ Further reading.

Further reading

Plano Clark VL, Ivankova NV (2015). *Mixed Methods Research. A Guide to the Field*. Sage: Thousand Oaks.

Tashakkori A, Teddlie C (2010). *The Handbook of Mixed Methods in Social and Behavioral Research*, 2nd edn. Sage: Thousands Oaks.

References

10 Creswell JW (2014). *A Concise Introduction to Mixed Methods Research*. Sage: Thousand Oaks.

Audit

An audit has similarities to research. Both need to be carried out in systematic ways and aim to find things out. They also have to have regard for ethical principles. The fundamental difference is that research is defined by the aim of creating new knowledge. Audit can be defined by the aim of measuring existing service provision. Informal audit, like research, should be part of the work of every nurse because it helps answer the question about how the individual's and the organization's practice is affecting care.

Clinical audit has been defined as follows:

'Clinical audit is a quality improvement cycle that involves measurement of the effectiveness of healthcare against agreed and proven standards for high quality and taking action to bring practice in line with these standards so as to improve the quality of care and health outcomes.'[11]

An audit uses research methods and research findings to investigate existing practice and usually makes comparisons with practice elsewhere or with specific benchmarks. In other words, is the organization doing what it should be doing, says it is doing, or aspires to do?

A clinical audit is closely associated with improving patient care. NICE makes this clear in its guidelines, which include the following questions as part of a clinical audit cycle:[11]

- What are we trying to achieve?
- Are we achieving it?
- Why are we not achieving it?
- Doing something to make things better?
- Have we made things better?
- Back to point 1. What are we trying to achieve?

Audits do not normally need formal ethical approval but should still follow ethical guidelines, e.g. data should be confidential and users of services should not be coerced in any way into taking part in an audit. It has been suggested that some research studies may have been changed into audits in order to avoid complex ethical scrutiny.[12]

Many organizations have audit teams, and it is important to consult them prior to undertaking audits within your organization. They will likely have clear guidelines to be followed. NICE suggests that an audit needs to be properly supported both financially and with appropriate time. It should be part of the organization's work, and it should involve people who use the service, who may have different priorities than the professionals.[12]

In the absence of organizational guidelines, the following need to be taken into account:

- What is the aim of the audit (what are you trying to find out)?
- Is the issue important enough for an audit?
- Is the issue an organizational priority?
- Are there any benchmarks to be measured against?
- How can the information that you need be obtained?
- Is it going to be possible to change things following the audit?
- How is the audit to be carried out?
- Are there sufficient resources for the audit?

Methods that can be used for an audit are very similar to those used in research projects. Some typical methods are:

- Reviewing case notes;
- Analysis of complaints;
- Analysis of critical incident reports;
- Direct observations of care settings or waiting areas;
- Satisfaction surveys;
- Review of admission and discharge statistics;
- Workload analysis.

Quite apart from research and audit, there is the process of 'service development'. This approach does not fit neatly into either 'research' or 'audit', but generally service development does adopt systematic approaches. These might include collection and analysis of previous literature, taking baseline measurements, and comparing these with post-service changes. Therefore, such approaches often attempt to describe/measure the impact of a particular service development, e.g. changes to the well-being of a person with intellectual disabilities or improvements in organizational effectiveness.

Further reading

Healthcare Quality Improvement Partnership (2016). *Best Practice in Clinical Audit.* ℛ www.hqip.org. uk/resources/best-practice-in-clinical-audit-hqip-guide/ (accessed 31 October 2017).

References

11 Burgess R, ed. (2011). *New Principles of Best Practice in Clinical Audit.* Radcliffe: London.
12 Paxton R, Whitty P, Zaatar A, Fairbairn A, Lothian J (2006). Research, audit and quality improvement. *International Journal of Health Care Quality Assurance.* **19**: 105–11.

Evidence-based care

All health and social care should be based on the best available evidence. Arguably, most recipients of care, given the chance to express an opinion, would expect, or at least hope, that this was so. However, nurses will sometimes struggle to cite the evidence behind some of their practice. This problem is not specific to nurses; many professionals, when put 'on the spot', will find it difficult to cite the evidence behind some of their decisions. It will be reassuring to know that to be an evidence-based practitioner does not require us to be able to make reference to a peer-reviewed article every time we make a decision about our practice. However, nor does it mean justifying decisions for practice by arguing that 'we've always done it this way' or 'this is the way I was taught' or 'it's commonsense'.

Melnyk[13] and colleagues suggest that, despite the benefits of evidence-based care, it is not practised consistently across the world. Among the reasons for this is that many clinicians misunderstand evidence-based care and assume that it takes too much time. They also suggest that there is a lack of organizational support and poor educational preparation for nurses. This supports anecdotal evidence that evidence-based practice in nursing is frequently seen as the use of a range of evidence to support clinical decision-making and that such evidence is not restricted to published research findings.

All nurses need to be able to use research. Northway[14] suggests that the evidence generated through research improves standards and the quality of care and that nurses should therefore have skills relating to research awareness, critical appraisal, reflection, and decision-making.

There are a variety of ways in which evidence-based care can be fostered. Some of them are dependent on the organization that employs the nurses, but there is also a responsibility for individual nurses to ensure that they are up-to-date with practice. There is now a wealth of information available, and it is probably more of a task to sift through the material than to find it in the first place. The following are ways in which nurses can keep up-to-date and help ensure that they are adopting evidence-based practice:

• Regularly reading journals relevant to the specific area of practice;
• Maintaining links with electronic discussion networks;
• Searching library databases (the NHS Library is ideal for this—𝄞 www. evidence.nhs.uk;
• Discussing research with colleagues;
• Participating in a journal club.

Whereas nurses should be able to evaluate research critically for themselves, it is important to remember that papers published in peer-reviewed journals have already been through critical review and are likely to be more reliable than other publications or Internet resources. Many researchers would go much further than this and suggest that there is a clear hierarchy of evidence. The following types of evidence are acceptable:[15]

• 'Experimental (randomized clinical trials, meta-analyses, and analytic studies);
• Non-experimental (quasi-experimental, observational);
• Expert opinion (consensus, based on published literature and consensus process, commissioned reports);
• Historical or experiential'.[15]

Further reading

Aveyard H, Sharp P (2013). *A Beginner's Guide to Evidence-based Practice in Health and Social Care*. McGraw Hill Education: New York, NY.
National Institute for Health and Care Excellence. ℘ www.nice.org.uk (accessed 31 October 2017).

References

13 Melnyk BM, Gallagher-Ford L, Long LE, Fineout-Overholt E (2014). The establishment of evidence-based practice competencies for practicing registered nurses and advanced practice nurses in real-world clinical settings: proficiencies to improve healthcare quality, reliability, patient outcomes, and costs. *Worldviews on Evidence-Based Nursing*. 11: 5–15.
14 Northway R (2009). Researching learning disability nursing. In: M Juke, ed. *Learning Disability Nursing Practice: Origins, Perspectives and Practice*. Quay Books: London.
15 Tranmer JE, Squires S, Brazil K, et al. (1998). *Factors that Influence Evidence-based Decision Making. National Forum on Health. Canadian Health Action: Building on the legacy*. Volume 5. Making Decisions: Evidence and Information. Multimondes: Quebec.

National occupational standards and professional requirements

Nursing and Midwifery Council

(🔗 www.nmc.org.uk)

Origins of the NMC

The NMC was established as a response to the Nursing and Midwifery Order 2001 by Westminster legislation in 2002. The NMC replaced the UK Central Council for Nursing, Midwifery, and Health Visiting (UKCC). It consists of over 600 000 nurses and midwives.

Purpose of the NMC

The NMC regulates nurses and midwives in England, Wales, Scotland, and Northern Ireland and maintains a register of nurses and midwives allowed to practice in the UK. The NMC has a key role in the protection of members of the public who use/receive nursing services. They develop and publish standards relating to education, conduct, and performance. These published standards are used as the benchmarks against which to assess the practice of a nurse and what constitutes high-quality nursing care. The NMC requires nurses and midwives to keep their skills and knowledge up-to-date and uphold professional standards and established processes of investigating and taking action in relation to any allegations above the practice of registered nurses, midwives, and HVs.

Key responsibilities of the NMC

- Maintaining a register of nurses and midwives permitted to practise in the UK;
- Setting entry criteria to the register;
- Overseeing standards to quality-assure professional education and training;
- Ensuring nurses and midwives maintain and develop their skills and knowledge;
- Ensuring nurses and midwives uphold professional standards;
- Carrying out investigations on nurses and midwives who fall short of agreed standards of practice through misconduct, lack of competence, or being unfit to practice. Following due process, a number of sanctions may be applied, including removal of the nurse from the NMC Register, preventing them from practising as a nurse or midwife in the UK;
- Addressing public complaints and concerns;
- Advising on, and implementing, social policy.

NMC publications

The NMC supports nurses in their professional practice by providing a wide range of essential and helpful resources, including the following.

Standards—🔗 www.nmc.org.uk/standards/
- The code for nurses and midwives;
- Standards of proficiency for nurse prescribers;
- Standards of competence for registered nurses.

Guidance—⏣ www.nmc.org.uk/standards/guidance/

Guidance documentation are also provided, and these should be read alongside the relevant standards. Such guidance includes:
- Raising concerns: guidance for nurses and midwives;
- Social media guidance;
- The professional duty of candour.

The nurse is responsible for keeping abreast of such policy developments as they evolve over time.

Maintaining or restoring your registration

The NMC maintains a live register of all nurses eligible to practise legally in the UK. It is the responsibility of the registered nurse to maintain their professional registration with the NMC. Details of the requirements are outlined in the section ➋ Maintaining ongoing professional registration, p. 555. Further details are also available from the following microsites:
- Maintaining registration—⏣ www.nmc.org.uk/registration/staying-on-the-register/
- Restoring registration—⏣ www.nmc.org.uk/registration/returning-to-the-register/

It is essential that the NMC has up-to-date contact details for registrants in case they need to provide them with any important updates or contact them for any reason such as fitness to practice.

Fitness to practise

(⏣ www.nmc.org.uk/concerns-nurses-midwives/what-we-do/what-is-fitness-to-practise/)

The NMC defines fitness to practise as the nurse having ' ... the skills, knowledge, good health and good character to do their job safely and effectively' (NMC 2016).

Nurses are required to adhere to *The Code: Professional Standards of Practice and Behaviour for Nurses and Midwives* (⏣ www.nmc.org.uk/standards/code/). The NMC is required by law to investigate all allegations made against individual nurses. Allegations can include:
- Misconduct;
- Lack of competence;
- Not having the required proficiency of English;
- Behaviour of a criminal nature;
- Serious ill health—whether physical, mental, or psychological, etc.

Following initial investigation, the nurse may be asked to appear before a public hearing and, if found guilty, they may receive a sanction, or have conditions placed on their practice, or be removed from the register permanently or for a set period of time. See the microsite ⏣ www.nmc.org.uk/concerns-nurses-midwives/. Details of charges, hearings, and outcomes are published. Examples of real cases may be found at ⏣ www.nmc.org.uk/concerns-nurses-midwives/hearings/hearings-sanctions/.

Students of nursing also have a duty to report concerns they may have about a nurse's fitness to practise.

Support available from the NMC

The NMC provides an online registration confirmation service for the public, especially employers. Free publications are also available to keep practitioners, students, and the general public informed about the Council's work.

NMC address

Nursing and Midwifery Council, 23 Portland Place, London, UK. W1B 1PZ.

Finally

The standards and guidance from the NMC develop over time. It is the nurse's responsibility to regularly check their website to keep abreast of current developments with regard to policy and practice. It is important to ensure that the NMC always has up-to-date contact details for nurses and, through this, the NMC can send nurses any necessary information.

Further reading

Nursing and Midwifery Council UK. ℜ www.nmc.org.uk (accessed 31 October 2017).

Nursing and Midwifery Council (2015). *The Code: Professional Standards of Practice and Behaviour for Nurses and Midwives.* Nursing and Midwifery Council: London.

Nursing and Midwifery Council (2015). *Raising Concerns: Guidance for Nurses and Midwives.* Nursing and Midwifery Council: London.

Nursing and Midwifery Board of Ireland

Origins

Bord Altranais agus Cnáimhseachais na hÉireann (the Nursing and Midwifery Board of Ireland) (NMBI) is a statutory body established under the Nurses and Midwives Act 2011 and replaced by An Bord Altranais (The Nursing Board). Currently, over 65 000 nurses and midwives who practise in Ireland are registered.

Objectives

The NMBI has two statutory objectives:
• To safeguard the general public; and
• To ensure the professionalism of nursing and midwifery practices.

Duties

The NMBI establishes and oversees the implementation of standards to ensure quality in education, registration, and professional conduct of nurses and midwives in the Republic of Ireland.

To ensure quality health and social care to clients, their families, and carers, this is achieved by:
• Maintaining a live register;
• Instructing nurses and midwives on how to maintain and enhance competences within their scope of intellectual disability nursing practice;
• Accrediting and reviewing educational programmes at pre-registration and post-registration levels;
• Establishing and ensuring standards of practice through a code of professional conduct and ethics and through fitness to practise processes;
• Addressing public complaints and concerns;
• Advising on, and implementing, social policy.

NMBI publications

(⌘ www.nmbi.ie/Standards-Guidance)

The NMBI support nurses in professional decision-making and quality practice through the development of standards and guidelines such as:
• Code of professional conduct and ethics;
• Scope of practice;
• Medication management;
• Nurses' use of social media;
• Recording clinical practice;
• Ethical conduct in research.

The NMBI also offers a help centre where nurses may find answers to frequently asked questions regarding the above documents. The microsite is ⌘ www.nmbi.ie/Help-Centre. The nurse is responsible for keeping abreast of such policy developments as they evolve over time. Nurses may also raise with the NMBI issues that arise in practice on which they require further clarification or guidance.

Maintaining or restoring your registration

The NMBI maintains a live register of all nurses eligible to practise legally in Ireland. It is the responsibility of the registered nurse to maintain their professional registration with the NMBI. Details of the requirements are

outlined in the section ➲ Maintaining ongoing professional registration, p. 555. Further details are also available from the following microsites:
- Maintaining registration—🖰 www.nmbi.ie/Registration;
- Restoring your registration—🖰 www.nmbi.ie/Complaints/Application-To-Restore-Registration.

It is essential that the NMBI has up-to-date contact details for registrants, as they may need to provide them with any important updates or contact them for any reason such as fitness to practise.

Fitness to practise

The NMBI is legally obliged to consider written complaints against nurses through its fitness to practise processes. If a complaint is made regarding nurses' practice, it may relate to limited knowledge, poor or unfair practice, poor health, or criminal behaviour.

Following initial investagation and the hearing of a complaint, if the Fitness to Practice Committee finds against a nurse, then a sanction is imposed on the individual. Sanctions may include an advice or admonishment, or a censure, in writing, a fine not exceeding €2000, conditions in which the nurse can continue to practise, and the suspension or removal from the register. Certain sanctions, such as removing the nurse from the register, must be approved by the High Court. The details of charges, hearings, and outcomes are published. Examples of real cases may be found at 🖰 www.nmbi.ie/Complaints/Findings-Decisions.

Students of nursing also have a duty to report concerns they may have about a nurse's fitness to practise. Further information regarding grounds for complaining, the complaints process, and sanctions are available at the microsite 🖰 www.nmbi.ie/Complaints/Findings-Decisions.

Support available from the NMBI

The NMBI provides an online registration confirmation service for the public, especially employers, and a free and confidential advice service for nurses and midwives. Free publications are also available to keep practitioners, students and, the general public informed about the Board's work.

NMBI address

Nursing and Midwifery Board of Ireland, Bord Altranais agus Cnáimhseachais na hÉireann, 18-20 Carysfort Avenue, Blackrock, Co Dublin.

Finally

The standards and guidance provided by the NMBI develop over time. It is the nurse's responsibility to regularly check the website of the NMBI to keep abreast of current developments in policy and practice. It is important to ensure that the NMBI always has up-to-date contact details for nurses and, through this, they can send nurses any necessary information.

Further reading

Nursing and Midwifery Board of Ireland. 🖰 www.nmbi.ie/Home (accessed 31 October 2017).
Nursing and Midwifery Board of Ireland (2014). *Code of Professional Conduct and Ethics for Registered Nurses and Registered Midwives*. Nursing and Midwifery Board of Ireland: Dublin.

Obtaining initial professional registration

To work as a nurse in the UK (Great Britain and Northern Ireland) or the Republic of Ireland, you must first register with the relevant statutory nursing registration body for that country. It is illegal to work as a nurse in these countries if you are not on their 'live register'. If someone wishes to work as a registered nurse in England, Scotland, Wales, or Northern Ireland, they must first register with the NMC. If they want to work as a nurse in the Republic of Ireland, then they must first register with the NMBI.

After they have successfully completed their approved nursing education programme, the higher education institution or university will forward students' successful competency details to the nursing body in the state in which they trained, e.g. the NMC or NMBI. They will also need to ascertain whether potential registrants are in good health and of good character. If these are acceptable, the NMC or NMBI will then forward an application form to the student to fill out, along with details of the registration fee which will need to be paid.

Nursing competences

Competency refers to an individual's ability, in terms of their values, knowledge, and skills, to be able to complete something in an efficient or successful manner to a defined standard. Nursing competences are set and regulated by the NMC in the UK and the NMBI in the Republic of Ireland. Such competences, as well as requirements and standards to ensure patient quality and safety, develop over time and it is the responsibility of the registered nurse to be up-to-date with, and achieve, these at all times. Nurses can do this by regularly visiting their respective registration authority's website, reading their correspondence and newsletters, and keeping up-to-date with nursing news and developments in the professional press.

Further reading

Nursing and Midwifery Board of Ireland. ℳ www.nmbi.ie/Home (accessed 31 October 2017).
Nursing and Midwifery Council. ℳ www.nmc.org.uk (accessed 31 October 2017).

Maintaining ongoing professional registration

In the Republic of Ireland

To continue practising as an RNID in the Republic of Ireland, individuals must:
* Be on the NMBI intellectual disability nursing division of the 'active' register;
* Pay the NMBI annual retention fee;
* Comply with any fitness to practise requirements, restrictions, or conditions attached to their registration.

In the UK

Since April 2016, nurses are required to go through the NMC's 'revalidation' once every 3yrs if they wish to continue practising. 'Revalidation' is a process whereby each nurse demonstrates, through evidence, that they continue to be fit to practise and therefore should be allowed to remain on the NMC register.

The nurse is required to provide evidence for:
* *Annual fee*—the nurse is required to pay the sum for that year;
* *Practice hours*—the nurse has practised a minimum of 450 hours over the previous 3yrs since their last registration or when they joined the register;
* *Continuing professional development* (CPD)—the nurse has completed 35 hours of CPD applicable to their scope of practice as a nurse since their last registration or when they joined the register;
* *Practice-related feedback*—the nurse is required to have gained five pieces of practice-related feedback since their last registration or when they joined the register;
* *Written reflective accounts*—the nurse is required to have five written reflective accounts since their last registration or when they joined the register; these must be documented on an approved form;
* *Reflective discussion*—the nurse is required to have had a reflective discussion with another nurse on the NMC active register about the content of their five written reflective accounts on their CPD and/or practice-related feedback and/or an event or experience in their practice and how it is linked to the NMC Code;
* *Health and character*—the nurse is required to declare if they are of good health and character, and to report any criminal offence convictions or formal caution;
* *Professional indemnity arrangement*—the nurse is required to have an indemnity arrangement when practising;
* *Confirmation*—the nurse is required to verify declarations made in their application by demonstrating to an appropriate confirmer that they have complied with the revalidation requirements.

The NMC has a revalidation microsite, and this contains additional details and templates of the forms to be completed as part of the portfolio.

Further reading

Nursing and Midwifery Board of Ireland. ℛ www.nmbi.ie/Home (accessed 31 October 2017).
Nursing and Midwifery Council Revalidation microsite. ℛ revalidation.nmc.org.uk (accessed 31 October 2017).

Career development within services for people with intellectual disabilities

When you are registered as a learning/intellectual disabilities nurse, there are many career opportunities available within health and social care. As well as working within intellectual disabilities-specific services, you can work for children's, mental health, hospice, and general health services as staff nurses, managers, consultants, eductaionalists, and liaison nurses.

Developing your career

Continuing to advance your career can assist you in attaining professional goals and achieving greater care satisfaction. Steps to consider are to:
• Develop a career plan for the next 5, 10, or 20 years. Review goals annually and amend your plan as required. Aim high;
• Identify and document the steps needed for you to achieve your career goal(s), e.g. training/education to attend to enhance your knowledge base, new job and/or clinical experiences to develop your nursing competency and proficiency. Develop a structured plan to achieve these steps;
• Pursue each step in your plan. Evaluate each step regularly;
• Seek career and/or clinical opportunities such as advanced positions, or take on further responsibilities within your existing role.

Examples of roles in which registered nurses practise

Staff nurse

Staff nurses may facilitate the holistic care of people with an intellectual disability in a wide range of health and social care settings, including residential, day-care, independent living, and family settings. Nurses work across the lifespan supporting children, young adults, and older people in residential and community services. Some clients may have multiple and complex disabilities; others may require support to live independently and achieve their own lifestyle goals. The nurse draws on their professional knowledge and skills to meet health and social care in meaningful ways for the client.

Clinical nurse manager

The nurse manager is responsible for the day-to-day management of nursing teams and services which provide care. They lead the development of policy, services, and clinical pathways.

Nurse teacher

Nurse educators play a pivotal role in shaping the future generation of nurses, as well as supporting registered nurses to maintain their competency and develop their areas of specialism. Educationalists work in universities, third-level institutions, and services. University websites are a useful starting point for exploring what courses are currently available.

Nurse researcher

There are opportunities for nurses to advance the profession's knowledge and understanding of intellectual disabilities through carrying out primary research.

UK clinical nurse specialists

Clinical nurse specialists are registered professionals with a master's degree or higher. They demonstrate high levels of clinical excellence in research and evidence-based practice specific to their scope of nursing competency. They are the central clinician of quality person and family-centred care to people with a learning disability.

UK nurse consultant

The nurse consultant's primary role is to ensure better quality clinical outcomes for people with an intellectual disability; 50% of their time is spent directly facilitating people with an intellectual disability to live the life they wish to live. Responsibilities include:

- Developing their own clinical practice;
- Being research-active;
- Actively developing and providing education, training, and continuous development to other nurses;
- Linking nursing and medicine at strategic, leadership, and managerial levels;
- Developing guidelines and protocols in practice.

Irish clinical nurse specialist

Clinical nurse specialists' clinical competencies are at a higher level to those of a staff nurse and include expertise in patient/client advocacy, education and training, audit and research, and consultancy at inter- and intra-disciplinary and multi-agency levels.

The clinical nurse specialist has in-depth clinical experience and competencies. Clinical nurse specialists carry out their roles and responsibilities safely and effectively, have evidence of CPD, and have successfully completed a recognized post-registration qualification in their specialist practice area (Begley et al., 2010; pp. xxiv–xxv).[1]

Irish advanced nurse practitioner (ANP)

Advanced intellectual disabilities nursing practice is performed by 'autonomous, experienced practitioners who are competent, accountable and responsible for their own practice' (Begley et al., 2010; p. xxii).[1]

ANP core concepts

Autonomy in clinical practice, expert practice, professional and clinical leadership, and research.

ANP competencies

ANPs demonstrate proven competencies at a high level of clinical practice under six domains (NMBI, 2015; pp. 6–14):

- Professional values and conduct of the registered ANP;
- Clinical decision-making;
- Knowledge and cognitive competencies;
- Communication and interpersonal competencies;
- Management and team competencies;
- Leadership potential and professional scholarship.

ANP must
- Be an RNID;
- Work in an accredited ANP post;
- Use high levels of knowledge and skills in their scope of clinical practice;
- Hold a postgraduate qualification at master's degree or higher level, with a substantial clinical assessment module, in an area specific to their area of nursing practice;
- Have a minimum of 7yrs post-registration experience;
- Have substantive hours at supervised advanced practice level;
- Demonstrate a high level of leadership and management;
- Provide evidence of CPD.

Postgraduate courses

Universities and other third-level educational institutions offer a wide range of postgraduate certificates, diplomas, master degrees, and doctorates to qualified intellectual disability/learning disability nurses to enhance their practice and advance their careers. Examples include ℘ nursing-midwifery. tcd.ie.

Further reading

Norton C, Sigsworth J, Heywood S, Oke S. (2012) An investigation into the activities of the clinical nurse specialist. *Nursing Standard.* 26: 42–50.

Nursing and Midwifery Board of Ireland (2015). *Scope of Nursing and Midwifery Practice Framework.* Nursing and Midwifery Board of Ireland: Dublin.

Nursing and Midwifery Board of Ireland (2017). *Advanced Practice (Nursing) Standards and Requirements.* Nursing and Midwifery Board of Ireland: Dublin. ℘ www.nmbi.ie/NMBI/media/ NMBI/Advanced-Practice-Nursing-Standards-and-Requirements-2017.pdf?ext=.pdf (accessed 31 October 2017).

References

1 Begley C, Murphy K, Higgins A, et al. (2010). *Evaluation of Clinical Nurse and Midwife Specialist and Advanced Nurse and Midwife Practitioner Roles in Ireland (SCAPE): Final Report.* National Council for the Professional Development of Nursing and Midwifery: Dublin.

Nursing and Midwifery Board of Ireland (2015). *Scope of Nursing and Midwifery Practice Framework.* Nursing and Midwifery Board of Ireland: Dublin; pp. 6–14.

Chapter 16

Independent regulators of care quality

Care Quality Commission: England

The Care Quality Commission (CQC) is the independent regulator for health and social care in England.[1,2] The CQC publishes standards for services and undertakes inspections of hospitals, care homes, dentists, and GP surgeries. The role of the CQC is to ensure that services provided to the public are safe and of a high quality. In order to achieve this, they undertake inspection visits to services and publish standards against which to monitor, inspect, and regulate services. The outcomes of the monitoring visits, including the ratings provided to services, are published on their website for anyone who wishes to read them. This can be an important consideration for an individual or their family members when considering which services to use. The CQC identifies what good, as well as outstanding, care should look like. Through their inspection visits, they can seek to make sure that services meet or exceed the required standards of service.

The CQC carries out its role in a number of ways that include:

• 'Making sure services meet fundamental standards of quality and safety;
• Registering care service providers that are able to demonstrate they meet standards;
• Monitoring, inspecting, and regulating care services to ensure they continue to meet the standards;
• Protecting the rights of vulnerable people, including those whose rights are restricted under the MHA;
• Listening to, and acting on, experiences of people using services;
• Involving people who use services;
• Working in partnership with other organizations and local groups;
• Challenging providers with poor performance;
• Making fair and authoritative judgements supported by the best information and evidence;
• Taking action if services fail to meet standards;
• Carrying out in-depth reviews to look at care across systems;
• Reporting on quality of care, including ratings to help people choose services'.[*1]

Following an inspection visit and a review of the evidence from documentation and observations, each service will be given a ranking.

There are four levels of rating:

• **Outstanding**—the service is performing exceptionally well;
• **Good**—the service is performing well and meets the CQC's expectations;
• **Requires improvement**—the service is not performing as well as it should and the CQC has told the service how it should improve;
• **Inadequate**—the service is performing badly and the CQC has taken action against the person or organization that runs it.[1]

If a service is identified as now meeting the required standards of care, further actions are taken to ensure services are monitored more frequently until the services have improved to meet the necessary recommendations put in place by the CQC. For further information on this, refer to the CQC's guide to special measures. Also of importance to note is that any NHS Trust that the CQC places in 'special measures' must publish their monthly action reports on NHS Choices.

References

1 Care Quality Commission. *Who We Are*. ℜ www.nhs.uk/NHSEngland/thenhs/healthregulators/Pages/carequalitycommission.aspx (accessed 31 October 2017).
2 Care Quality Commission. *About Us: What we do and how we do it*. ℜ www.cqc.org.uk/sites/default/files/documents/20131108%206657_CQC_Aboutus_A5_Web%20version.pdf (accessed 31 October 2017).

Care regulation in Scotland

Scotland has two national bodies responsible for the regulation of care services: *NHS Health Improvement Scotland* and *The Care Inspectorate*. Both organizations came into being in April 2011, forming a single body for healthcare services and another for social work and social care services, following the *Crerar Review* in 2007 and *The Public Services Reform (Scotland) Act 2010*.[3,4]

NHS Health Improvement Scotland

NHS Health Improvement Scotland is the national health improvement organization that is part of the Scottish NHS, replacing *NHS Quality Improvement Scotland*. One of the main priorities of the organization is to implement the Scottish Government's *Healthcare Quality Strategy* across NHS Scotland.[5] The organization comprises six units with specific roles related to improving the quality and standard of patient care in Scotland.

• Healthcare Environment Inspectorate (HEI);
• Scottish Health Technologies Group (SHTG);
• Scottish Health Council (SHC);
• Scottish Intercollegiate Guidelines Network (SIGN);
• Scottish Medicines Consortium (SMC);
• Scottish Patient Safety Programme (SPSP).

The *HEI* undertakes safety and cleanliness inspections of healthcare services across NHS Boards in Scotland to ensure standards of care are met and maintained and improvements made.[6] The *SHTG* provides advice and guidance about the clinical and cost-effectiveness of existing and new technologies that can impact on the care of patients in Scotland, e.g. through the publication of *Health Technology Assessment* reports such as antimicrobial wound dressings.[7] The advice supports planning and decision-making in NHS Boards.

The *SHC* undertakes activities to ensure that NHS Scotland involves people in decisions about their health services by focusing on how NHS Boards include patients and involve the public in decisions about their health services. The role of *SIGN* is to improve the quality of healthcare for patients in Scotland by developing evidence-based clinical practice guidelines. All the guidelines are developed by multidisciplinary working groups, with representation from patient and carer groups and professions across Scotland. Over 130 have been published, focusing on, for example, breast cancer, schizophrenia, hepatitis C, and epilepsy.[8-11] All guidelines can be downloaded, free of charge, from the NHS Health Improvement Scotland website (℘ www.healthcareimprovementscotland.org).

The *SMC* reviews and analyses information produced by the manufacturers of medicines to identify their benefits to patients and ensure value for money to the NHS in Scotland and they are adopted efficiently into clinical practice.[12] The SMC comprises pharmacists, senior clinicians, and health economists, as well as representatives from NHS Boards across Scotland, the pharmaceutical industry, and patient groups.

NHS Health Improvement Scotland has developed inspection methodologies to undertake scrutiny and service reviews to ensure hospitals are clean and safe and the needs of older people are met in acute care.[13] The organization also reviews and regulates independent healthcare providers, based on national care standards.[14–17] Supporting the improvement in the quality of care in the NHS in Scotland is the *SPSP*. The SPSP is a Scottish national initiative that delivers the NHS Scotland *Healthcare Quality Strategy* to improve the safety of healthcare and minimize avoidable harm. The SPSP work programme focuses on acute hospital care to minimize the risk of healthcare-associated infections and improve the care of older people in acute hospitals, maternity and children, primary care, mental healthcare, and medicines.

The Care Inspectorate

Following the *Crerar Review* in 2007 and *The Public Services Reform (Scotland) Act 2010*, the Care Inspectorate was established in April 2011 as a single regulatory body for social work and social care services. The Care Inspectorate regulates a wide range of organizations that provide care services, including local authorities, private care providers, charities, and voluntary organizations.

Some 15 000 care services are regulated by the Care Inspectorate. In delivering their regulatory and scrutiny functions, the Care Inspectorate aims to ensure that vulnerable people are safe and have a national scrutiny programme which focuses on four specific areas: (i) the care and support provided to the users of services; (ii) the management and leadership provided by care services; (iii) the quality of staffing provided within care services; and (iv) the care environment. The Care Inspectorate has also produced service self-assessments that are completed by care services as part of the scrutiny process.[18–20] A series of national care standards have been developed and published to enable scrutiny of regulated care services—*Services for children and young people, Services for adults, Services for everybody*, and *Independent healthcare services*.[21–23] The national care standards inform the scrutiny process, following which services are awarded grades from 1 to 6. Reports based on the service review are published online and are available to the public, so that users of services and their carers know the standards provided and can make informed choices about which service to select to provide their care and support (⌨ www. careinspectorate.com). Another function of the Care Inspectorate is to undertake investigations of complaints made by users and their carers about regulated care services.[24]

References

3 Scottish Government (2007). *The Crerar Review: The Report of the Independent Review of Regulation, Audit, Inspection and Complaints Handling of Public Services in Scotland.* The Stationery Office: Edinburgh.

4 *Public Services Reform (Scotland) Act 2010.* The Stationery Office: Edinburgh.

5 Scottish Government (2010). *The Healthcare Quality Strategy for NHS Scotland.* The Stationery Office: Edinburgh.

6 NHS Health Improvement Scotland (2014). *Ensuring Your Hospital is Clean and Safe.* NHS Health Improvement Scotland: Edinburgh.

7 NHS Health Improvement Scotland (2015). *Antimicrobial Wound Dressings (AWDs) for Chronic Wounds: Health Technology Assessment Report 13.* NHS Health Improvement Scotland: Edinburgh.

8 NHS Health Improvement Scotland (2013). *SIGN 134: Treatment of Primary Breast Cancer.* NHS Health Improvement Scotland: Edinburgh.

9 NHS Health Improvement Scotland (2013). *SIGN 131: Management of Schizophrenia.* NHS Health Improvement Scotland: Edinburgh.

10 NHS Health Improvement Scotland (2013). *SIGN 133: Management of Hepatitis C.* NHS Health Improvement Scotland: Edinburgh.

11 NHS Health Improvement Scotland (2015). *SIGN 143: Diagnosis and Management of Epilepsy in Adults.* NHS Health Improvement Scotland: Edinburgh.

12 NHS Health Improvement Scotland (2015). *A Guide to the Scottish Medicines Consortium.* NHS Health Improvement Scotland: Edinburgh.

13 NHS Health Improvement Scotland (2015). *Independent Healthcare Regulation: Inspection Methodology.* NHS Health Improvement Scotland: Edinburgh.

14 Scottish Executive (2005). *National Care Standards: Independent Specialist Clinics.* The Stationery Office: Edinburgh.

15 Scottish Executive (2005). *National Care Standards: Independent Hospitals.* The Stationery Office: Edinburgh.

16 Scottish Executive (2005). *National Care Standards: Hospice Care.* The Stationery Office: Edinburgh.

17 Scottish Executive (2006). *National Care Standards: Dental Services.* The Stationery Office: Edinburgh.

18 Care Inspectorate (2015). *Self-Assessment: Care Homes for Learning Disabilities.* The Care Inspectorate: Dundee.

19 Care Inspectorate (2015). *Self-Assessment: Care Homes of Older People.* The Care Inspectorate: Dundee.

20 Care Inspectorate (2015). *Self-Assessment: Care Homes for Mental Health Problems.* The Care Inspectorate: Dundee.

21 Care Inspectorate (2005). *National Care Standards: Care Homes for People with Learning Disabilities.* The Care Inspectorate: Dundee.

22 Care Inspectorate (2009). *National Care Standards: Housing Support Services.* The Care Inspectorate: Dundee.

23 Care Inspectorate (2009). *National Care Standards: Care at Home.* The Care Inspectorate: Dundee.

24 Care Inspectorate (2015). *Unhappy About a Care Service? Find out what you can do.* The Care Inspectorate: Dundee.

Care Inspectorate Wales

Introduction

Care Inspectorate Wales (CIW) regulates and inspects care and social services in Wales and aims to make sure that these services are safe and provide good care. The four strategic priorities of the CIW for 2017–20 are:

- 'To consistently deliver a high quality services;
- To be highly skilled, capable and responsive;
- To be an expert voice to influence and drive improvement;
- To effectively implement legislation.' (p. 6).[25]

The CIW work closely with Healthcare Inspectorate Wales (HIW) (⅁ hiw. org.uk/) which has a similar stated purpose related to healthcare provisions in Wales.

Remit of the CIW

The remit of the CIW covers the registration and inspection of the following: 'adult services including care homes, adult placement schemes and domiciliary care agencies, children's services including care homes, fostering and adoption services, boarding schools, residential special schools and further education colleges and childcare and play services including child minders, crèches, nurseries, out of school clubs and play schemes' (p. 4).[25]

The CIW also reviews social services departments in Wales and undertake national reviews to monitor the overall performance of services.

Inspections may occur at any time, including evenings and weekends, with the majority of CIW inspections unannounced. The inspections are designed to examine how well services meet the national standards for services set in Wales (⅁ careinspectorate.wales/providingacareservice/ our-inspections/?lang=en). Only fostering, adoption, childminders, and open play facilities have any advance notice of an inspection visit, which is required in order to ensure availability of service providers.

The CIW states that, during an inspection, staff will gather information through a range of approaches, designed to provide a clear picture of services. Inspectors will be involved in talking and listening to people using the services, their relatives, and staff members. They will also seek to speak to service managers and professionals visiting the services. Inspectors may also use a Short Observational Framework for Inspection (SOFI) observing people, as well as reading relevant documentation, including policies and records. Inspectors may also use questionnaires to gather information from people using the services, their relatives, and professionals.

An inspection report is completed with 28 days and sent to the service. If all requirements are met, no further action is required. In the event that all requirements and conditions are not met, the CIW will issue a non-compliance notice that will set out the regulations not being achieved, the evidence of this, and the actions required within a clear timescale, after which a check on compliance will be made.

If a service becomes a concern, the CIW has options in relation to enforcement action, which include formal meetings with service providers, sharing concerns with other relevant agencies, and taking urgent action, including, if necessary, suspending a service, cancelling registration, and/or seeking prosecution.

Changes to legislation

Implementation of the Regulation and Inspection of Social Care (Wales) Act 2016 which was passed on 18 January 2016 will lead to changes in the regulation and inspection of social care services in Wales. These changes are designed to result in more robust protection for people using the services and lead to improvements in the processes of regulation. The changes arising from this legislation in relation to regulation and inspection will be fully implemented by April 2019, and updated information and useful learning resources can be found at ℘ www.ccwales.org.uk/regulations and ℘ careinspectorate.wales/about/changes-to-legislation-and-policy/regulation-and-inspection-social-care-bill/?skip=1&lang=en.

CIW resources

The CISSW (former name for CIW) and the HIW undertook a national inspection of care and support for people with intellectual disabilities in Wales and produced an overall report, as well as individual service reports, in June 2016. Overall, a series of 13 recommendations were identified under three key areas, namely: providing effective care and support, understanding need, and leading in partnership with people (℘ careinspectorate.wales/docs/cssiw/report/160628overviewen.pdf). Both the CIW and HIW websites provide additional up-to-date and useful resources for staff working in services for people with intellectual disabilities.

References

25 Care Inspectorate Wales (2018). *Strategic Plan 2017–2020*. Care Inspectorate Wales: Merthyr Tydfil.

Regulation and Quality Improvement Authority: Northern Ireland

Introduction

The Regulation and Quality Improvement Authority (RQIA) was, in April 2005, under the framework of the Health and Personal Social Services (Quality, Improvement, and Regulation) (Northern Ireland) Order (2003). The RQIA is responsible for monitoring and inspecting the availability and quality of health and social care services and encouraging improvements in the quality of these services through its programme of inspection, investigation, and review.

Public confidence in health and social care services in Northern Ireland is assured through independent, proportionate, and responsible regulation. Through its activities, the RQIA makes an independent assessment of a wide range of health and social care services, to determine if the care being delivered is safe, effective, and compassionate. It also considers whether these services are well led and meet the required standards.

Remit of the RQIA

The RQIA manages the registration and inspection of regulated health and social care services, which include care homes for adults and children, agencies providing domiciliary care workers and nurses, day-care services, and a wide range of independent healthcare services such as independent hospitals and private dental treatment. The majority of the RQIA's inspections are unannounced, examining how, and to what degree, services achieve the regulations and service-specific standards of care, as well as the management of their estates, medicines, and safeguarding service users' finances. Inspections are conducted by the RQIA's team of experienced nurses, social workers, pharmacists, estates, and finance officers.

The RQIA's approach to inspection is underpinned by the five principles[26] of effective regulation which require them to be 'transparent, accountable, proportionate, consistent, and targeted'.[26]

The RQIA also inspects general hospitals, examining the quality of care and leadership within specific wards or clinical areas. This is in addition to an ongoing programme of infection prevention/hygiene inspections at a range of health and social care facilities, including hospitals. The RQIA's inspection reports highlight both good practice and areas of concern. This allows the RQIA to drive improvements for all those using these hospital facilities and services. It also inspects services providing radiological procedures, including X-rays and radiotherapy, to protect service users from inappropriate or unnecessary exposure to ionizing radiation. It is responsible for the oversight of health and social care in places of detention, including Northern Ireland's prisons, children's secure accommodation, and facilities for people with mental ill health or intellectual disabilities.

The RQIA collaborates with health and social care organizations throughout Northern Ireland in order to encourage the delivery of high-quality services through an ongoing, planned programme of governance, service, and thematic reviews.

Since 2015, the Guidelines and Audit Implementation Network (GAIN) joined the RQIA. The GAIN's role is to promote leadership in safety and quality in health and social care. Services can apply for funding for audit projects that seek to improve outcomes for patients, clients, and carers through the development, implementation, and audit of regional guidelines. In 2010, the GAIN published guidelines on caring for people with learning disability in general hospitals.[27] The implementation of these guidelines was reviewed by RQIA in 2014.[28]

Services for people with intellectual disabilities

Within Northern Ireland, the RQIA also has the responsibility to review services provided to people with intellectual disabilities and people with mental illness who are subject to the Mental Health (Northern Ireland) Order 1986. This Order was amended in 2009 to give the RQIA responsibility for 'preventing ill treatment, remedying any deficiency in care or treatment, terminating improper detention in a hospital or guardianship, and preventing or redressing loss or damage to a patient's property'.[26] During inspections, RQIA inspectors speak to people with intellectual disabilities about their experiences of receiving care, and people using the services should be made aware of their right to speak to RQIA inspectors during a visit.

In addition, the RQIA monitors detention forms completed to detain a person in hospital, the appointment of Part II doctors who have the authority to recommend that a person is compulsorily admitted to hospital for assessment, and the appointment of SOADs who have the authority to provide a second opinion in relation to Part IV of the Mental Health (Northern Ireland) Order 1986.

RQIA resources

The RQIA provides a wide range of very useful resources on its website ✆ www.rqia.org.uk, which are relevant to nursing staff providing care and support for people with intellectual disabilities. These include guidance of the public and for service providers, information on legislation and standards, and all its inspection and review reports.

References

26 Better Regulation Task Force (2003). *Principles of Good Regulation*. Better Regulation Task Force: London.

27 Guidelines and Audit Implementation Network (2010). *Guidelines on Caring for People with a Learning Disability in General Hospitals*. Guidelines and Audit Implementation Network: Belfast. (This document is being reviewed at the time of writing and may become 'Best Practice Statements on Caring for People with a Learning Disability in General Hospitals' (2018); ensure you check the RQIA website for the latest version of the document.)

28 Regulation and Quality Improvement Authority (2014). *Review of the Implementation of Guidelines and Audit Implementation Network (2010): Guidelines on Caring for People with a Learning Disability in General Hospitals*. Regulation and Quality Improvement Authority: Belfast.

Health Information and Quality Improvement Authority: Republic of Ireland

Introduction

In the Republic of Ireland, the safety, quality, and accountability of health and social care provision is overseen by the Health Information and Quality Authority (HIQA). Since 2007, this statutory, publicly funded agency has undertaken roles and responsibilities as legally required by the Health Act 2007, the Children Act 2001, and the Child Care Act 1991. RNIDs have a professional responsibility to, and are accountable for, maintaining the highest quality of care at all times (NMBI 2014).

Remit of the HIQA

The HIQA follows agreed national care standards which aim to enhance patient safety and the quality of services they receive:

- Developing and promoting standards of safe, quality, and accountable health and social care;
- Monitoring compliance of services to national standards through periodic inspects of designated centres;
- Monitoring healthcare safety and quality;
- Monitoring children's services;
- Addressing complaints or concerns from the public;
- Evaluating the clinical effectiveness of new health technology;
- Establishes security standards for the collection and dissemination of health data.

The HIQA is responsible for driving the standards of health and social care in services for children, older people, and people with a disability, including intellectual disabilities. The HIQA ensures the registration and inspection of all public, private, and voluntary health and social care services. Their duty is to inspect and re-register such providers every 3yrs. Services are permitted to function only if they have been first registered and approved by the HIQA. Inspection visits are a mixture of announced or unannounced visits and may occur at any time of the day or night.

Inspections undertaken by the HIQA are carried out by trained individuals from a wide range of health and social care professions. Such inspections focus on the rights of people receiving services, safeguarding people from abuse, person-centred care and support, effectiveness of care, leadership, governance, and management, how resources are used, workforce responsiveness, and the storage and use of information.

HIQA resources

The HIQA provides nurses with a wide range of free resources to better support people with an intellectual disability. Such resources are available at ℰ www.hiqa.ie. Available information includes guidance to the general public and health and social care professionals such as nurses and organizations providing care; standards such as those for residential care settings (HIQA 2009, 2012, and 2013); guidance on national policy and legislation; and inspection reviews undertaken to date. All inspection reports and enforcement information are available in the public domain and can be sourced by the nurse from the microsite ℘ www.hiqa.ie/social-care/find-a-centre/inspection-reports.

HIQA addresses
- Head office: Unit 1301, City Gate, Mahon, Cork, T12 Y2XT;
- Dublin regional office: George's Court, George's Lane, Dublin 7, D07 E98Y.

Finally
The standards and guidance from the HIQA develop over time. It is the nurse's responsibility to regularly check their website to keep abreast of current developments with regard to policy and practice.

Further reading
Children Act (2001). The Stationary Office: Dublin.
Child Care Act (1991). The Stationary Office: Dublin.
Health Act (2007). The Stationary Office: Dublin.
Health Information and Quality Authority (2009). *National Quality Standards for Residential Care Settings for Older People in Ireland*. Health Information and Quality Authority: Cork.
Health Information and Quality Authority (2012). *National Standards for Safer Better Healthcare*. Health Information and Quality Authority: Cork.
Health Information and Quality Authority (2013). *National Standards for Residential Services for Children and Adults with Disabilities*. Health Information and Quality Authority: Cork.
Nursing and Midwifery Board of Ireland (2014). *Code of Professional Conduct and Ethics for Registered Nurses and Registered Midwives*. Nursing and Midwifery Board of Ireland: Dublin.
Health Information and Quality Authority. ℘ www.hiqa.ie (accessed 31 October 2017).

Chapter 17

Practice resources

Healthcare resources

Recognized for many years is that generally people with intellectual disabilities have poorer physical and mental health than does the general population. The most common causes of death continues to be respiratory and circulatory disease, and this includes heart disease. People with intellectual disabilities are also more likely to have epilepsy and mental health and sensory problems, and a growing number will have diabetes. They can also have trouble with equity of access and equity of health outcomes when using general healthcare services. This section notes some useful resources to help develop an understanding of issues related to healthcare and people with intellectual disabilities.

Confidential Inquiry into Premature deaths of People with Learning Disabilities (CIPOLD)

This major report, funded by the Department of Health, explored the deaths of 247 people with intellectual disabilities occurring during 2013–14. They compared these to the deaths of people who did not have intellectual disabilities. This inquiry has provided a useful review of the literature and made a number of important recommendations to improve the health and access to general healthcare services for people with intellectual disabilities. For more information, follow the link below:

🔗 www.bris.ac.uk/cipold/confidential-inquiry/ (accessed 31 October 2017).

Improving Health and Lives Learning Disabilities Observatory (IHaL)

The IHaL organizationally is located in Public Health England. It maintains data and monitors and undertakes reviews on the health of people with intellectual disabilities and their experience of using healthcare services in England. It undertakes numerous projects and has a website that provides a vast amount of information that includes data on people with intellectual disabilities. It collates data at local authority level in England, as well as provides examples of reasonable adjustments such as hospital passports that are available to share with others. For more information, follow the link below:

🔗 www.improvinghealthandlives.org.uk/ (accessed 31 October 2017).

Scottish Learning Disabilities Observatory (SLDO)—learning disabilities and autism information portal

The SLDO's new website presents information to support health improvement for people with learning disabilities and autism. This was set up with funding from the Scottish Government to better understand health and address health inequalities. Based in the Institute of Health and Wellbeing at the University of Glasgow, its portal brings together detailed data of age profiles and health status, along with where these populations live by local authority and health board area. For more information, follow the link below:

🔗 www.sldo.ac.uk/ (accessed 31 October 2017).

UK Health and Learning Disability Network

This is a national/international network of people with an interest in the health of people with intellectual disabilities. Members include people with learning disabilities, including nurses, doctors, allied health professionals and other therapists, commissioners, and educationalists. The Network produces an informative, regular email newsletter called *Health Stones*. It has a focus on problem-solving, information sharing, and networking. For more information, follow the link below:

℘ www.mentalhealth.org.uk/learning-disabilities   (accessed   20 March 2018).

Easyhealth

Easyhealth is a website that is a one-stop shop to locate 'accessible' health information for people with intellectual disabilities and is regularly updated. Easyhealth makes its own information and hosts other useful accessible information in the form of leaflets, videos, and links to other useful organizations. For more information, follow the link below:

℘ www.easyhealth.org.uk/ (accessed 31 October 2017).

Understanding Intellectual Disability and Health

This website provides some very useful resources for medical, nursing, and other healthcare students. It is also useful for everyone working in healthcare who encounter people with intellectual disabilities. It was developed in association with St George's Hospital, Beyond Words, Hertfordshire NHS Foundation Trust, As One, and the University of Hertfordshire. For more information, follow the link below:

℘ www.intellectualdisability.info/ (accessed 31 October 2017).

Learning Disability Health toolkit by Turning Point

This document written by nurses in intellectual disabilities is aimed at informing parents and supporters of people with intellectual disabilities some of what they will need to know to allow them on a day-to-day basis to improve and maintain their health. For more information, follow the link below:

℘ www.turning-point.co.uk/learning-disability/resources.aspx (accessed 31 October 2017).

SeeAbility

This charity aims to enrich the lives of people with sight loss and multiple disabilities across the UK. They provide a range of services, including literature and easy-read factsheets and films about eye care for people with learning disabilities. For more information, follow the link below:

℘ www.seeability.org/ (accessed 31 October 2017).

National Hearing and Learning Disabilities Special Interest Group (HaLD SIG)

The HaLD SIG is a network of professionals with a dual interest in people with intellectual disabilities as well as hearing loss. It aims to raise awareness of the high prevalence of hearing loss in this group of people and improve clinical practice of those working with this group, as well as increase the evidence base and knowledge around hearing loss and intellectual disabilities by undertaking projects, setting up working groups, and contributing to research and publications. For more information, follow the link below:

℘ www.hald.org.uk (accessed 31 October 2017).

Behaviour management resources

For more information, as well as downloadable resources from the groups in this section, follow the links provided.

Challenging Behaviour Foundation (CBF)

Established in 1997, this national charity seeks to support and provide information about people with severe intellectual disabilities whose behaviour challenges services. It provides information relating to challenging behaviour, as well as links for family members. It also provides events for family members in order that they can learn about supporting those with behaviours that are thought of as challenging. It is also able to advocate for family members. It is able to give support to family members and professionals through a peer support network. The CBF has produced a wide range of resources concerning challenging behaviour that includes:

- Information sheets;
- Information packs;
- DVDs.

Their resources are free of charge to family carers. For more information, follow the link below:

℗ www.challengingbehaviour.org.uk/ (accessed 31 October 2017).

Autism Speaks

Founded in 2005, Autism Speaks as become an international organization seeking to learn more about people with autism and the best ways to support them. It is able to provide research funding both to understand the causes as well as explore the nature of autism. It also has an important advocacy role that is related to supporting people with autism and their families. It has produced a toolkit in relation to challenging behaviours, which is a useful resource for staff as well as family members supporting people with autism. For more information, follow the link below:

℗ www.autismspeaks.org/ (accessed 31 October 2017).

Autism Education Trust (AET)

The AET focuses on ensuring children and young people with autism receive high-quality education to support them. It produces a wide range of educational materials and undertakes research into effective practice for educating and supporting children and young people with autism. The AET has produced a number of resources to help manage challenging behaviour. For more information, follow the link below:

℗ www.autismeducationtrust.org.uk/Global/News/Resources%20to%20help%20manage%20challenging%20behaviour.aspx (accessed 31 October 2017).

Crisis Prevention

This excellent resource provides the top ten positive behaviour supports. These supports are presented in the format of an online resource. For more information, follow the link below:

🖄   www.crisisprevention.com/Blog/September-2010/Top-10-Positive-Behavior-Support-Online-Resources (accessed 31 October 2017).

NHS Education for Scotland

This resource provides an interactive online learning resource on positive behaviour support. For more information, follow the link below:

🖄   www.nes.scot.nhs.uk/media/570730/pbs_interactive_final_nov_12.pdf (accessed 31 October 2017).

Special Education Support Service

This website has created a Behaviour Resource Bank, which contains a range of online resources regarding strategies for managing behaviour. For more information, follow the link below:

🖄 www.sess.ie/behaviour-resource-bank (accessed 31 October 2017).

Children and young people resources

For more information, as well as downloadable resources from the groups in this section, follow the links provided.

Mencap

Mencap is a national charity in England that acts as a collective advocacy and a service provider organization, which seeks to improve the lives of people with intellectual disabilities. They have an enormous range of resources; for the purposes of this section, supportive material about young people is presented. Notwithstanding it is worth searching Mencap's website for a rich source of resources. For more information, follow the link below:

🔗 www.mencap.org.uk/advice-and-support/children-and-young-people (accessed 31 October 2017).

Similar resources are available in other jurisdictions of the UK and the Republic of Ireland. For more information, follow the links below:

🔗 www.enable.org.uk/Pages/Enable_Home.aspx (accessed 31 October 2017);

🔗 wales.mencap.org.uk/?gclid=CO3fz7vR6tUCFQcQ0wodZoEJIQ&q=mencap-cymru (accessed 31 October 2017);

🔗 www.mencap.org.uk (accessed 22 March 2018);

🔗 www.enableireland.ie/donate?gclid=EAIalQobChMI04iS4NHq1QIVy7vtCh2DDw-SEAAYASAAEgLqjfD_BwE (accessed 31 October 2017).

'Paving the Way'

This is a collaborative project between the CBF and the Council for Disabled Children. It focuses on understanding the causative factors of challenging behaviours and the importance of early interventions. For more information, follow the link below:

🔗 pavingtheway.works/ (accessed 31 October 2017).

National Institute for Health and Care Excellence (NICE)

This national centre produces guidelines across a wide range of topics. A recent document is the guideline *Challenging Behaviour and Intellectual Disabilities: Prevention and Interventions for People with Intellectual Disabilities whose Behaviour Challenges*, that was published in May 2015. This report highlights the importance of early identification, assessment, and intervention and provides comprehensive outlines of how care should be delivered. For more information, follow the link below:

🔗 www.nice.org.uk/guidance/ng11 (accessed 31 October 2017).

Contact a Family

This is a national charity with local networks to support families of children with disabilities. They have a network of local workers who provide information, advice, and support to family members of children with disabilities. They have a key role in advocating for the rights of children with disabilities and their families to be valued and included in society. They have a wide range of useful and applied resources on their website that will be of interest to healthcare professionals. For more information, follow the link below:

℘ contact.org.uk (accessed 31 October 2017).

NHS Choices

This site offers guidance and resources on health matters and choices. The section of the website shown here contains details on accessible toys, play, and learning. It proposes tips, related articles, and external links. For more information, follow the link below:

℘ www.nhs.uk/Conditions/social-care-and-support-guide/Pages/accessi ble-toys-play-learning.aspx (accessed 31 October 2017).

Intensive Interaction

The homepage of the Institute provides access to a wide range of information concerning the best ways to support younger people who are still developing communication abilities. The available resources include information that is also highly relevant to working with, and supporting, people with severe or profound intellectual disabilities and multisensory impairments. For more information, follow the links below:

℘ www.intensiveinteraction.org/ (accessed 31 October 2017);

℘ thepsychologist.bps.org.uk/volume-22/edition-9/introducing-intensive-interaction (accessed 31 October 2017).

AboutLearningDisabilities

This site offers extensive information and advice on learning disabilities. It has a number of information categories, including types of disabilities, disability rights and values, education, and employment. For more information, follow the link below;

℘ www.aboutlearningdisabilities.co.uk/ (accessed 31 October 2017).

BOND Consortium

This consortium is led by young minds and has developed a resource entitled *Children and Young People with Learning Disabilities – Understanding their Mental Health*. This resource provides information about understanding the mental well-being and mental health problems faced by children and young people with intellectual disabilities. It provides practical information and resources aimed to help people with intellectual disabilities. For more information, follow the link below:

℘ hsm.manchester.gov.uk/kb5/manchester/directory/service.page?id=j GJoXgHrPqs (accessed 31 October 2017).

Centre Forum

This group has published a report in 2016 entitled *State of the Nation Children and Young People*. This highlighted the challenges that young people face in gaining access to effective mental health services. For more information, follow the link below:

℘ centreforum.org/publications/children-young-peoples-mental-health-state-nation/ (accessed 31 October 2017).

The National Elf Service

This website shares information across a number of areas of health and client groups, including in relation to services and working with people with intellectual disabilities. It is aimed at supporting professionals and making research findings more easily accessible, as well as building networks among professionals working with people who have intellectual disabilities. For more information, follow the link below:

℘ www.nationalelfservice.net (accessed 31 October 2017).

Adults and older people

For more information, as well as downloadable resources from the groups in this section, follow the links provided.

Scottish Learning Disabilities Observatory (SLDO)— learning disabilities and autism information portal

The SLDO's website presents information to support health improvement for people with learning disabilities and autism. It was established with funding from the Scottish Government in order to understand health and address health inequalities in people with intellectual disabilities. The observatory is based at the Institute of Health and Wellbeing at the University of Glasgow. The portal brings together a range of detailed data that include age profiles, health status, and where these populations live by local authority as well as health board. For more information, follow the link below:

℘ www.sldo.ac.uk/ (accessed 31 October 2017).

Understanding the lives and needs of older people— BILD's Ageing Well Project

This was a collaborative project between the British Institute of Learning Disabilities, the Alzheimer's Society, and Our Way Self Advocacy. It focuses on the experiences of older people with intellectual disabilities and their family carers. They have a range of useful resources that include a toolkit as well as videos. For more information, follow the link below:

℘ www.bild.org.uk/ageingwell (accessed 31 October 2017).

The Foundation for People with Learning Disabilities

This charity, part of the wider Mental Health Foundation, concentrates on raising awareness of, and about, people with intellectual disabilities. It seeks to support integration and inclusion in communities of people with intellectual disabilities. They provide links to many useful resources concerning health, mental health, dementia, older people, and future planning. For more information, follow the link below:

℘ files.eric.ed.gov/fulltext/ED542387.pdf (accessed 31 October 2017).

Intellectual Disability Supplement—the Irish Longitudinal Study on Ageing (IDS-TILDA)

This research programme is being undertaken in the Republic of Ireland. The programme includes many elements and seeks to explore the lived experiences of people with intellectual disabilities over the age of 40, and then compare findings to the experiences of older people from the general population. This project is underpinned by the values of *'inclusion, choice, empowerment, person-centredness, and the promotion of people with intellectual disability'*. Through the work of this programme of research, it is seeking to influence practice and thus make a contribution to the quality of the lives of those with intellectual disabilities living in Ireland. For more information, follow the link below:

℘ www.idstilda.tcd.ie (accessed 31 October 2017).

Guidance and resources on Alzheimer's dementia for carers of people with Down syndrome

Dementia is common among older people with intellectual disabilities, particularly those with Down syndrome. Importantly, it is more common among people with intellectual disabilities or members of the general population of the same age. For more information, follow the links below:

📖 www.intellectualdisability.info/mental-health/alzheimers-dementia-what-you-need-to-know-what-you-need-to-do (accessed 31 October 2017);

📖 www.scie.org.uk/dementia/living-with-dementia/learning-disabilities/ (accessed 31 October 2017);

📖 www.bild.org.uk/resources/ageingwell/dementia/ (accessed 31 October 2017);

📖 www.rcpsych.ac.uk/usefulresources/publications/collegereports/cr/cr196.aspx (accessed 31 October 2017).

National and international networks

Much is to be learnt from exchanging ideas with colleagues in other countries concerning services, legislation, and best practice relating to the support of people with intellectual disabilities. Therefore, when seeking to develop your knowledge, it is important to consider what is happening in not only your own country, but also internationally. This section has not listed the numerous 'condition-specific' organizations; these are well known and easy to locate. However, some of the broader national and international organizations that provide useful information and resources aimed at improving the lives of people with intellectual disabilities are. For more information, follow the links provided.

Developmental Disabilities Nurses Association (DDNA)

This membership association, based in the USA, is for nurses who provide care and support to people with intellectual and developmental disabilities (IDD). Any student or registered nurse can apply for membership. As an organization, it seeks to build networks among professionals working with people with IDD. For more information, follow the link below:

🔗 ddna.org (accessed 31 October 2017).

Foundation for People with Learning Disabilities (FFPWLD)

This is a charitable organization and part of the wider Mental Health Foundation. The FFPWLD concentrates on raising awareness of, and about, people with learning disabilities. It seeks to support their integration and inclusion in communities. Its work focuses primarily on employment and education; families, friends, and community; rights and equality; health and well-being; getting the rights support; and changing service delivery. It hosts a number of useful publications and resources. For more information, follow the link below:

🔗 www.mentalhealth.org.uk/learning-disabilities/our-work (accessed 31 October 2017).

British Institute of Learning Disabilities (BILD)

This membership organization, established in 1971, focuses on the rights of people with disabilities. It is a national organization that seeks to assist in transforming policy into practice. It works with a range of groups, e.g. central government departments, local authorities, national health trusts, along with service providers and other relevant organizations. Ultimately, it seeks to improve the quality of the lives of people with intellectual disabilities. The official journal of BILD is *British Journal of Learning Disabilities*. For more information, follow the links below:

🔗 www.bild.org.uk/ (accessed 31 October 2017);

🔗 onlinelibrary.wiley.com/journal/10.1111/(ISSN)1468-3156 (accessed 31 October 2017).

International Association for the Scientific Study of Intellectual and Developmental Disabilities (IASSIDD)

The IASSIDD was established in 1964 and is now acknowledged as a global network of like-minded people who work with, and/or research a range of issues that affect the lives of, people with IDD. It is a membership organization and holds numerous international conferences that seek to improve services for people with IDD. The *Journal of Intellectual Disability Research* (*JIDR*) and the *Journal of Policy and Practice in Intellectual Disabilities* (*JPID*) are both journals of the association. For more information, follow the link below:

℘ www.iassidd.org/ (accessed 31 October 2017).

Inclusion Europe and Inclusion International

Inclusion Europe and Inclusion International are both linked organizations that focus on campaigning for, as well as achieve equal rights for, people with intellectual disabilities. Both these organizations run a wide range of programmes, as well as produce reports and documents. Additionally, they hold an annual conference. For more information, follow the links below:

℘ www.inclusion-europe.eu (accessed 31 October 2017).

℘ inclusion-international.org (accessed 31 October 2017).

LDNurse.com

This website hosts a wide range of informative references and information on legislation, as well as links and blogs aimed at nurses for people with intellectual disabilities. It serves as a one-stop shop for nurses looking for further information. For more information, follow the link below:

℘ learningdisabilitynurse.com/ (accessed 31 October 2017).

The National Elf Service

This website shares interesting information spanning a range of areas concerning health and client groups, and this includes services and working with people with intellectual disabilities. It is aimed at supporting professionals and making research findings more easily accessible, as well as building networks among professionals who work with people with intellectual disabilities. For more information, follow the link below:

℘ www.nationalelfservice.net (accessed 31 October 2017).

Positive Choices

This network is for undergraduate students of intellectual disability nursing, which is seen as a positive choice (hence its name). The network meets annually at a conference hosted by a different university each year from across the five nations, which, in turn, volunteer to support and host the event. Each year, the conference is free to all undergraduate nursing students, who are supported by academic staff and clinicians from learning disabilities services, employers, and most importantly by people with intellectual disabilities. For more information, follow the links below:

🕮 positive-choices.com/ld-nursing/ (accessed 31 October 2017).

They also host a Facebook page:

🕮 www.facebook.com/groups/11271315956/ (accessed 31 October 2017).

Together 4 Change

Together 4 Change makes use of online communities that seek to support the development of services, as well as provide resources to support the health of people with social and health needs, and this includes people with intellectual disabilities. One of their key online communities is the Choice Forum. This forum addresses issues that impact on the lives of people with intellectual disabilities in the UK; however, its reach is international. It was established in 2000, in response to research demonstrating that those working with people with intellectual disabilities were isolated and could benefit from receiving support in helping them assist people with intellectual disabilities achieve more choice in their lives. The Forum runs in partnership with the Foundation for People with Learning Disabilities. For more information, follow the link below:

🕮 www.together4change.org/ (accessed 31 October 2017).

@WeLDNurses

This Twitter account connects learning disabilities nurses through regular Twitter chats by using the hashtag #WeLDNs.

Chapter 18

Emergencies

Emergency management of a person in a seizure

Status epilepticus

The majority of epileptic seizures are self-limiting, lasting >5 minutes. Status epilepticus is defined as a single, prolonged seizure or recurrent seizures without regaining consciousness in between seizures, lasting 30 minutes or more. Convulsive status epilepticus occurs in 3% of people with epilepsy; this is more often triggered by, e.g. infection and metabolic disturbance; it may result in brain injury and death. Non-convulsive status epilepticus is rare and can be difficult to diagnose; the person may present with an abnormal mental state, changes in behaviour, or cognition with diminished responsiveness.

The longer a seizure continues, the greater the risk; therefore, in practice, a seizure lasting >5 minutes or recurrent seizures warrant intervention. Emergency medication is normally recommended only if the person has a history of prolonged or recurrent seizures.[1] When emergency medication is prescribed, a balanced approach is needed to avoid overuse. Guidelines should be available as to when to administer, and this must be specific to each individual.

Emergency medication prescribed in the non-acute setting

The benzodiazepine midazolam is recommended as first-line treatment for prolonged or recurrent seizures in the community.[1] Rectal diazepam may be prescribed in particular circumstances. Midazolam is administered into the buccal cavity of the mouth (or base of the nasal passage), passes across the thin mucosal lining, is absorbed directly into the bloodstream, and travels directly to the brain, avoiding first-pass metabolism in the liver. It reduces brain excitability by strengthening brain inhibitory systems. Most seizures are stopped within minutes. Side effects of benzodiazepines include sedation, hypotension, and rarely cardiorespiratory depression and respiratory arrest. It is advised to contact emergency services on first use, if not under medical supervision. Families should be reassured this is a precaution and does not necessarily result in hospital admission. A second dose may be prescribed, depending on previous response to drug, age, weight, and other relevant factors. A third dose is infrequently prescribed in any 24-hour period. Oral benzodiazepines clobazam/diazepam may be prescribed to prevent cluster seizures when the individual regains consciousness between seizures and the seizure history identifies a pattern.

Emergency management plan

If emergency medication is prescribed, an emergency management plan is required, agreed by the prescriber, the individual where capacity allows, the parent/guardian, the nurse, or carers. Registered nurses who delegate the administration of emergency medication should follow local policy on delegation of clinical care to non-registered carers. A recording system is needed to include the time of administration of medication to seizure stopping, to enable review of effectiveness and for the treatment plan to be adjusted if necessary. This must be reviewed at least yearly and after first use.

Emergency management plan should detail

- Description of seizure type for which medication is prescribed;
- Indications for the use of emergency medication, e.g. after certain time and/or number of seizures;
- Initial dose of emergency medication;
- Usual response to treatment if known;
- If and when a second dose can be given (for same episode or further episode after specific time);
- Who can administer the medication—care staff to sign;
- When emergency assistance should be sought;
- Consent—prior consent by individual should be obtained if possible;
- Who to inform.

Follow agreed local procedures for administration of the prescribed drug. Ensure dignity and privacy, explaining all actions to the individual who may regain consciousness at any time. In some circumstances, it may not be appropriate to administer emergency medication; in such situations, emergency services must be sought in the first instance. Consider safe carriage of the medication. Risk assessment for carrying on transport may be required.

Emergency management of seizures—acute care

Emergency services should be contacted if:

- A person has a first seizure;
- The person is known to have epilepsy and has a prolonged seizure or recurrent seizures for >5 minutes and is not prescribed emergency medication;
- After administration of the first dose of emergency medication, fully prescribed emergency medication fails to work in 5 minutes;
- A person sustains an injury that requires urgent medical assessment;
- It is believed the person requires urgent medical assessment

If relevant, provide the paramedics with information regarding medications administered, prescribed AEDs, and seizure history. Management of early status in the acute clinical setting involves: securing the airway, oxygen, assessing cardiorespiratory function, establishing intravenous (IV) access, and AED treatment in accordance with local protocols and national guidelines.[1]

References

1 National Institute for Health and Care Excellence (2016). *Epilepsies: Diagnosis and Management*. Clinical guideline [cG137]. ℗ www.nice.org.uk/guidance/cg137 (accessed 31 October 2017).

Self-harm

Self-harm is a term defined as 'any act of self-poisoning or self-injury carried out by an individual irrespective of motivation'.[2] People with intellectual disabilities also engage in this type of behaviour, although the term self-injury is usually used (see ➔ Self-injury, pp. 592–3).[2]

There is a danger that people who engage in self-harming behaviour may incur censure and rejection from those around them when it is deemed a deliberate act. In supporting people who have self-harmed, the focus should also be placed on the care, support, and development of the individual. The nursing process (assessment, planning, implementation, and evaluation) can be used to organize care for individuals who engage in self-harm. Understanding the motivation for self-harm is crucial to helping a person, although it can be very difficult to determine whether the act was intentional or not in people with intellectual disabilities. Nursing assessment and care should be structured and holistic. While it is important to gain insights into the possible motivations for self-harm, this should not be the sole focus, and care should be taken to avoid negative assumptions being made about motivations, as it is not helpful.

Some reasons why people may self-harm

- Low self-esteem;
- Feelings of isolation;
- Feeling stressed;
- Past or current abuse;
- Being bullied;
- Suffered a bereavement;
- Problems with sexuality;
- Experiencing social rejection;
- A desire to end one's life;
- Severe mental illness, i.e. command hallucinations during a psychotic episode.

It can be very difficult to understand why people should want to self-harm. For some, it may provide a sense of release from emotional pain or may act as a type of coping mechanism. It may be a way of communicating to others the distress that the individual is feeling. Self-harm is often carried out in private and on parts of the body that are usually covered with clothing. As such, it can be difficult to tell if someone is self-harming, but other signs might be that the person becomes withdrawn and irritable, and is lacking energy, covering up, and not taking part in certain activities, e.g. swimming. People with intellectual disabilities may not conform to the usual pattern of self-harming and will often self-harm quite openly and injure parts of their body that are not usually covered up by clothing such as the face.

Some specific expressions of self-harming behaviour

- Swallowing poisonous substances or objects;
- Burning or scalding;
- Cutting.

Practitioners need to **listen** to the messages that clients try to communicate when they self-harm—you can listen with all your senses, particularly your eyes and ears. Remember it can be very distressing for other clients, and you should offer reassurance to those in the immediate environment.

Important considerations when nursing an individual who engages in self-harming behaviour

The individual should be

- Treated with respect and dignity;
- Treated for their injuries;
- Consulted and included in all decisions;
- Given privacy during consultation and treatment;
- Shown understanding with their coping mechanism;
- Assessed for further risk;
- Assumed to have mental capacity unless there is evidence of doubt.

They should not be

- Discriminated against;
- Forced to disclose why they self-harmed;
- Automatically considered a dangerous person;
- Punished for self-harming.

Interventions

Interventions would be similar to those for self-injury (see ➡ Self-injury, pp. 592–3).

Further reading

Dicks K, Gleeson K, Johnstone L, Weston C (2011). Staff beliefs about why people with learning disabilities self-harm: a Q-methodology study. *British Journal of Learning Disabilities.* **39**: 233–42.

Jones V, Davies R, Jenkins R (2004). Self-harm by people with learning difficulties: something to be expected or investigated. *Disability and Society.* **19**: 487–500.

Lovell A (2007). Learning disability against itself: the self-injury/self-harm conundrum. *British Journal of Learning Disabilities.* **36**: 109–21.

References

2 National Institute for Health and Care Excellence (2011). *Self-harm in over 8s: Long-term Management.* Clinical guideline [CG133]. ℞ www.nice.org.uk/guidance/cg133 (accessed 31 October 2017).

Self-injury

The term self-injurious behaviour is commonly used in services for people with intellectual disabilities to describe self-harming behaviour particularly motivated by biological factors. It may also be a learnt behaviour reinforced by responses of others, or biological responses to pain in the body. It may also be worth considering the idea that people deliberately injure themselves. For instance, if the risks of pica (eating inedible material) or poison are not known, then it would not be self-injury. However, in mental healthcare, the preferred term is self-harm, although both terms mean that the individual has injured or harmed themselves in some way (see ➔ Self-harm, pp. 590–1). Individuals who self-injure should be treated with the same respect, dignity, and privacy as other clients, regardless of whether the act of self-injury was intentional or not.

Biological causes of self-injury in people with intellectual disabilities

- Genetic syndromes such as Cornelia de Lange, Lesch–Nyhan, fragile X, and Prader–Willi;
- Neurochemical defects such as a low level of dopamine.

Remember that just because an individual has a particular syndrome does not mean that they will automatically engage in self-injurious behaviour. There is evidence that interventions such as those that relieve pain or treat gastric reflux may reduce the incidence of self-injurious behaviour. Individuals are also susceptible to the same external triggers as the general population such as:

- Impoverished environments;
- Abuse;
- Lack of activities;
- Frustration.

People with ASC may also engage in self-injurious behaviours due to:

- Having a low pain threshold;
- Obsessive and compulsive behaviours;
- Self-stimulatory behaviours;
- Inquisitiveness—experimenting to see what will happen.

Again they are also susceptible to the same external triggers as the general population. Some common types of self-injurious behaviours displayed by some individuals with intellectual disabilities include:

- Head banging and face slapping;
- Biting, pinching, and scratching;
- Eye poking and hair pulling;
- Repeated vomiting;
- Consuming inedible foods (pica), e.g. cigarettes, faeces, paper, etc.

Interventions

Short-term interventions

In an emergency, assess the severity of self-injury and respond accordingly. (When dealing with a serious incident of self-injury, e.g. poisoning, breathing difficulties, head injury, or loss of blood, you need to act quickly to prevent loss of life.) Full emergency procedures should be initiated, if appropriate—medical help, phone ambulance, accident and emergency unit, and providing emergency services with full information of the incident and client history (e.g. exact injuries, method used, timescales, complicating factors such as alcohol, methods used to respond, and their effectiveness). It is also important to remember to provide psychological support throughout the event.

Longer-term interventions
- Chemotherapeutic, e.g. medication such as naltrexone and/or fluoxetine, although medication is being used less frequently;
- Behavioural, e.g. PBS;
- Humanistic, e.g. gentle teaching;
- Cognitive, e.g. CBT, counselling.

The same principles apply as with self-harm (see ➲ Self-harm, pp. 590–1) in that the individual who self-injures has the right to be treated with the same respect and care as other clients.

Further reading

Heslop P (2011). Supporting people with learning disabilities who self-injure. *Tizard Learning Disability Review*. 16: 5–15.

Heslop P, Macauley F (2009). *Hidden Pain? Self-injury and People with Learning Disabilities*. Bristol Crisis Service for Women: Bristol. ஃ www.bristol.ac.uk/media-library/sites/sps/migrated/documents/hiddenpainrep.pdf (accessed 31 October 2017).

National Autistic Society. *Self -injurious Behaviour*. ஃ www.autism.org.uk/about/behaviour/challenging-behaviour/self-injury.aspx (accessed 31 October 2017).

Tantam D, Huband N (2009). *Understanding Repeated Self-injury*. Palgrave/Macmillan: Basingstoke.

Missing person

Missing people with intellectual disabilities are regarded as emergency situations. A detailed understanding of individual needs and past behaviour is necessary. Plans and patterns of this type of behaviour that they may undertake when missing or places they may go to can to often can be predicted from previous incidents of going missing. When a person with intellectual disabilities does not return to their place of residence or does not arrive for a planned activity somewhere else, staff and family members involved will understandably be anxious. It may also be that, in some instances, there are concerns that they may be at risk from others or themselves. In some circumstances, when a person goes missing, i.e. in supported living situations, the response will be the same as would be available for any other missing person, and this should be reported to the police immediately. When a person who was in secure care goes missing, this should also be reported to the police immediately, as there may be a perceived risk to others. In such situations, those responsible for the person's care may have specific authority to take action to locate and return them.

Terms and definitions

When an individual goes missing, care should be taken to include a description of the circumstances when recording and reporting the incident. Incident reports are an important source of information for current and future risk assessment, and they inform decisions about people's care and management. The term missing is used when people absent themselves and their whereabouts are unknown in everyday life, whether it is from home, college, work, etc. For those detained or under the provisions of the mental health legislation, specific terminology to describe missing persons is used, and how a missing person is defined in this context is often subject to their legal status, e.g. detained under the MHA. The Department of Health has issued the following definitions:[3]

- 'Escape: a detained patient escapes from a unit/hospital if he or she unlawfully gains liberty by breaching the secure perimeter that is the outside wall, fence, reception, or declared boundary of that unit;
- Attempted escape: a failed or prevented attempt by a patient to breach the secure perimeter that in the nature of the incident demonstrated intent to escape;
- Abscond: a patient unlawfully gains liberty during escorted leave of absence outside of the perimeter of the originating unit/hospital by getting away from the supervision of staff;
- Failure to return: a patient fails to return from authorised unescorted leave'.*[3]

Risk assessment for people with intellectual disabilities

Escape or absconding is often viewed as high-risk behaviour because of the potential of what might occur when the person is absent. Where this is the case, a thorough assessment specific to this area of risk should be

---

* Text extracted from DoH (2009) *Absent without Leave* © Crown Copyright under the Open Government License v3.0.

undertaken using as many sources of information as possible. All information should be checked for factual accuracy. The best indicators for future risk will come from information about previous incidents. Areas for particular attention include:

- Circumstances when risk has occurred in the past, including setting conditions, antecedents, and specific triggers;
- Likely destinations and likely contacts from previous incidents;
- Evidence regarding planning/preparation;
- Person's vulnerability/ability to manage independently;
- Evidence regarding potential risks to others;
- Evidence regarding the likelihood of safe return without intervention (see ➔ Risk management, pp. 462–3).

Risk management

Individual assessment information should be used to inform plans to address risk. Ensure that plans are developed and agreed jointly between those who are responsible for the person's care and reflect the assessed level of risk and the personal circumstances of the person, i.e. living situation, legal framework, abilities, and personal rights. These should recognize that the likelihood, immediacy, frequency, and consequences of the risk may be subject to change and be regularly reviewed and amended, as required, to address changes in identified risk and personal circumstances, including vulnerabilities. A balanced approach, including preventative strategies, plans for managed risk-taking, and emergency management strategies, should be taken.

Within services for people with intellectual disabilities, there is a duty when making decisions relating to risk of absconding that relates both to any anticipated behaviour that may occur and its potential impact on others. Often decision-making or reviews regarding leave can be disproportionate to the actual risk and can serve to keep order within the system. For positive risk-taking around leave, there are structured frameworks available such as the leave/absconding risk assessment (LARA),[4] which allows an objective and structured approach to interdisciplinary decision-making.

Further reading

Association of Chief Police Officers (2014). *Missing from Care: A Multi-agency Approach to Protecting Vulnerable Adults. A National Framework for Police and Care Providers.* ℗ library.college.police.uk/docs/APPREF/Protecting-Vulnerable-Missing-Adults-Framework-FINAL.pdf (accessed 31 October 2017).

Bartholomew D, Duffy D, Figgins N (2009). *Strategies to Reduce Missing Patients: A Practical Workbook.* National Mental Health Development Unit: London. ℗ www.scribd.com/document/36352199/A-Strategy-to-Reduce-Missing-Patients-a-Practical-Workbook (accessed 31 October 2017).

References

3 Department of Health (2009). *Absent Without Leave: Definitions of Escape and Abscond.* Department of Health: London.
4 Hearn D, Ndegwa D, Norman P, Hammond N, Chaplin E (2012). Developing the leave/abscond risk assessment (LARA) from the absconding literature: an aide to risk management in secure services. *Advances in Mental Health and Intellectual Disabilities.* 6: 280–90.

Risk of suicide

Prevalence

Suicide is the tenth leading cause of death in the world and one of the top three among those aged between 15 and 44yrs. With almost one million cases of suicide reported each year, there has been a 60% increase recorded in the last 50 years (WHO).[5] Added to this, the rates for attempted suicide have been estimated to be between 8–25 times higher, compared to suicide deaths.[6] The proportion of ♂ suicides is much greater, when compared to the ♀ rate (78% versus 22%).[6,7] There have been very few studies to investigate suicide in people with intellectual disabilities. A study in Finland followed up a nationwide sample of 2677 people with intellectual disabilities over a 35-yr period;[9] during this period, only ten suicides occurred. This is much lower than the national suicide rates in England and lower still in relation to the rates in Finland where the study was undertaken.

Risk

There are no indications in the literature to suggest any significant differences between the factors that are indicative of risk of suicide in the general population and risk among people with intellectual disabilities. The clearest single indicator for risk of suicide is the wish to die. In clinical practice, this is often referred to as suicidal intent or suicidal ideation. Factors that are statistically linked with an increased risk of suicide are:

- Being ♂ of <35yrs;
- Being in a lower socio-economic group, poor social conditions or social isolation, unemployment, alcohol and drug misuse;
- Mental illness, in particular depression and schizophrenia;
- Deliberate self-harm in the previous year;
- Imprisonment, increased for those in prison for the first time;
- Loss such as family breakdown;
- Bullying;
- Family history/previous unsuccessful attempts.

There is currently no specific suicide assessment tool for people with intellectual disabilities widely used in practice. In clinical practice, the CPA, which incorporates a general assessment of risk to self and others, is the most common framework for assessing risk. Where the CPA is not used, a policy regarding general risk assessment should be in place. The Beck's Suicidal Intention Scale is an example of a measure that can be used following an attempted suicide to focus specifically on future suicide risk.

Risk management

- All people who engage in deliberate self-harm should be asked, as far as possible, to explain in their own words why they have harmed themselves in order to assess for risk of suicide.
- A thorough assessment should be undertaken to identify underlying causes for suicidal thoughts and behaviour.
- Underlying health conditions should be treated where possible.

- Appropriate support should be provided to assist the person to address circumstances and situational factors that contribute to suicidal thoughts and behaviour.
- Plans may include access to listening or support services on a 24-hour basis. This may include general mental health services, emergency services, and helplines (e.g. the Samaritans; Lifeline—Northern Ireland).
- External management of risk may be required to prevent serious harm or death, including: admission to hospital for a period of assessment/ treatment; close observations/supervision during periods of increased risk; preventative environmental adaptations, i.e. removal of ligature points; and limited access to means of attempting suicide.

Previously, it was thought that intellectual disabilities acted as a buffer against suicide. Attitudes such as this have hampered scientific inquiry, as there are no valid estimates of suicide rates among people with intellectual disabilities. There needs to be more attention to the assessment and prediction of suicide risk and agreeing on best practices in preventing suicide. Previous reviews have found that the majority of suicide risk factors identified for people with intellectual disabilities are common to the general population, although individuals with intellectual disabilities may use more passive methods to attempt or complete suicide.[9] Reduced cognitive ability may mean that individuals may be less likely to make elaborate plans or, in some cases, to execute the act of suicide using certain more complex methods. A lack of planning may increase the risk, as behaviour may be more difficult to predict. Given the high ratio of attempted suicides, all attempts and those of self-harm need to be fully investigated, as it is the case that suicide attempts can be missed or mistaken for self-harm by clinicians. For individuals more at risk of mental illness, the launch of the UK's first suicide prevention tool for people with intellectual disabilities from Grassroots suicide prevention in 2014 is a start in addressing the lack of suicide assessment measures for people with intellectual disabilities as a gap in current clinical provision.

References

5 World Health Organization (2011). *Suicide Prevention*. World Health Organization: Geneva.
6 Moscicki EK (2001). Epidemiology of completed and attempted suicide: toward a framework for prevention. *Clinical Neuroscience Research*. 1: 310–23.
7 Office for National Statistics (2015). *Suicides in the United Kingdom, 2013 Registrations*.
8 Patja K (2004). Suicide cases in a population based cohort of persons with intellectual disability in a 35 year follow-up. *Mental Health Aspects of Developmental Disabilities*. 7: 117–23.
9 Mollison E, Chaplin E, Underwood L, McCarthy J (2014). A review of risk factors associated with suicide in adults with intellectual disability. *Advances in Mental Health and Intellectual Disabilities*. 8: 302–8.

Allergies

An allergy is an immune response caused by an abnormally high sensitivity to a normally harmless substance (or allergen). A true allergy is sensitization of the human immune system to a specific allergen, mediated by immuno-globulin E (IgE). The body produces antibodies against these allergens, with subsequent exposure leading to severe reactions. There is overreaction of the body's defence mechanism to something that is usually harmless; common reactions include sneezing, watery eyes, coughing, itchy rashes, and swelling of the lips and tongue. More severe reactions result in lowering of blood pressure, difficulty in breathing, and anaphylactic shock. Many 'allergic' reactions are not true allergies. Some food 'allergies' are due to direct effects of substances within the food on the body in predisposed individuals. Heat, sun, and cold allergies are similar, in that the body has not produced antibodies against heat/cold, but instead the individual is predisposed to respond by releasing histamine from cells in the skin, producing urticaria. An *allergen* is any substance that the body mistakenly perceives as a threat that triggers an allergic reaction.

Some of the most common allergies

- Pollen and moulds (often found indoors where humidity is high and can easily become airborne), dust mites, insect stings or bites, peanuts and tree nuts, penicillin, latex, cosmetics, e.g. make-up, creams, lotions, sprays, perfumes, powders, deodorants, bath oils, and bubble baths.

Some precautions in trying to prevent an allergic reaction

- Keep a record of known allergens for an individual and try to avoid where possible.
- Check food labels for allergy-causing ingredients.
- If the person is affected by hayfever, then monitor the pollen report.
- Consider immunotherapy for desensitization to a known allergy—under medical supervision.

Signs and symptoms of an allergic reaction

- An allergic reaction typically triggers initial symptoms in the area of contact, i.e. nose, throat, lungs, eyes, skin, stomach.
- Initial symptoms may include wheezing and/or coughing, a runny nose, sneezing, itchiness, hives, redness of the skin, rash, nausea, diarrhoea, stomach cramps, itchy eyes, swelling, puffiness, or red eyes.
- These may rapidly progress to more severe symptoms such as swelling of the face, lips, tongue, or throat, shortness of breath, tightness of the chest, or chest pain, for which emergency treatment is required.

Action in the event of an allergic reaction

- Assess the severity of the allergic reaction and ask the person and/or carers whether the person is known to suffer from an allergy.
- Identify if the person has been prescribed medication for allergic reactions and encourage them to take it, if available.
- Seek medical advice, should any signs or symptoms be detected or persist after taking prescribed medication for an allergic reaction.

- Provide reassurance, support, and information to a person with intellectual disabilities.
- Depending on the severity of the symptoms, i.e. difficulty in breathing, severe rash, altered consciousness, or history of severe reaction symptoms, contact emergency services or attend the local accident and emergency department, providing all relevant information.

Types of medications that can be used in the management of allergies

- Antihistamines;
- Decongestants;
- Corticosteroids and non-steroidal anti-inflammatory drugs;
- Bronchodilators.

Anaphylactic shock

This is an **extreme and severe allergic reaction** that affects the whole body. It may develop within minutes of contact with a trigger factor and is **potentially fatal**. Triggers may be:

- Insect sting;
- Ingestion of a particular food substance, e.g. shellfish or peanut;
- Airborne or contact with particular materials, e.g. latex;
- A specific drug.

Signs and symptoms of anaphylactic shock

- Anxiety, widespread red/blotchy skin, swelling of the tongue and throat, puffiness around eyes, difficulty in breathing that may result in gasping for air, abdominal pain, signs of shock, unconsciousness.
- Note that not all of these symptoms may be present.

Action in the event of anaphylactic shock

- Dial 999/emergency number and describe the person's symptoms.
- Aid breathing and minimize shock.
- Provide reassurance and support.
- Help the person to take any necessary medication they may be carrying.
- If person is conscious, help to sit up to help with breathing.
- If person becomes unconscious, check breathing and seek to maintain an open airway. If necessary, give rescue breaths and chest compressions, as per local policy.
- Treat any symptoms of shock until help arrives.

Further reading

National Institute for Health and Care Excellence. *Anaphylaxis: Assessment and Referral after Emergency Treatment Overview.* ℛ pathways.nice.org.uk/pathways/anaphylaxis (accessed 31 October 2017).
Resuscitation Council (UK). ℛ www.resus.org.uk (accessed 31 October 2017).

Adverse reactions to medications

Definition

An adverse drug reaction (ADR) is an untoward, unintended, or harmful reaction experienced by an individual, which is suspected to be related to a medication having been taken. This reaction may be physical and/or psychological in nature. It is estimated that 10 000 serious drug reactions and 1200 deaths are caused by prescribed medicines each year, and that they currently account for 6–7% of hospital admissions in the UK.

The simplest classification of ADRs is type A and type B.

Type A (most common)
- Predictable from the pharmacology of the drug;
- Are dose-related (occurring at a dose that is too high for an individual) and reactions are usually slow in onset;
- Increased risk in the elderly and neonates;
- Usually a reduction in dose will suffice; however, a severe reaction requires the drug to be stopped.

Type B
- Reactions are not predictable from the drug pharmacology;
- Susceptibility to this type of reaction is individualistic;
- Usually rapid in onset and are often allergic.

Reactions involve anaphylaxis (see ➔ Allergies, pp. 598–9) and usually requires the causative drug to be stopped.

Reducing the risk

- Is there clear indication for the need of the medication? If so, try and establish the dose range that allows effective control of the disease/illness.
- Review the information available on possible ADRs of the drug, and identify if there are any risks of drug interactions, i.e. polypharmacy.
- Establish patient susceptibility, e.g. pharmacokinetic issues, and any predisposing factors such as allergies and any previous ADRs.
- Consult the prescriber on any contraindications identified.

Monitoring ADRs

- Introduce a systematic approach to patient surveillance and maintain ongoing monitoring.
- Identify and use an appropriate scale for identifying adverse reactions, e.g. DAI-10, LUNSERS, UKU Side-effects Scale, Quality of Life Scale.
- Education and training for persons with intellectual disabilities and/or their carers to recognize ADRs.

Considerations

- ADRs have the potential to impact on the person's physical, psychological, and social well-being, resulting in impaired quality of life.
- Be aware that a black triangle next to a drug in the *BNF* indicates that it is either new, under intensive surveillance, or an old drug marketed in a new combination or formulation.
- Act in accordance with the NMC's standards for medicines management.

Responding to a medication error

- Respond rapidly to any actual or suspected medication error.
- Provide first-aid treatment as required.
- Immediate contact to be made with the GP/prescriber/emergency department/hospital medical staff for advice as to recommended actions.
- Keep the person with intellectual disabilities informed and reassured.
- Keep others involved in the person's care informed.
- Document the incident in the person's nursing notes, and complete all other relevant paperwork, as required by local policies and procedures.
- Increase monitoring for potential side effects.

Professional and legal requirements

This requires that medicine is given to the right person, at the right time, in the correct form, using the correct dose, via the correct route,[11] at the correct time.[12] Nurses are accountable for their actions/omissions and therefore need to be aware of their professional responsibility with regard to drug administration. Therefore, nurses need to be aware of the Medicines Act 1968 and the Misuse of Drugs Act 1971, as failure to abide by these could lead to criminal prosecution and professional conduct hearings by the NMC, as well as disciplinary action by the employer.

Final thought

Any nurse is potentially at risk of making a medication error. It is important that whether you are the contributor or an observer, you report the incident as soon as possible to minimize patient harm and to ensure appropriate advice and response.

References

10 National Coordinating Council for Medication Error Reporting and Prevention (2005). *NCC MERP: The First Ten Years —Defining the Problem and Developing Solutions*. National Coordinating Council for Medication Error Reporting and Prevention: New York, NY.

11 Nursing and Midwifery Council (2010). *Standards for Medicine Management*. ℘ www.nmc.org.uk/globalassets/sitedocuments/standards/nmc-standards-for-medicines-management.pdf (accessed 31 October 2017). (These standards are being revised at the time of writing; ensure you check the NMC website for the most recent version of these guidelines.)

12 An Bord Altranais (2007). *Guidance to Nurses and Midwives on Medication Management*. ℘ www.nmbi.ie/Standards-Guidance/Medicines-Management (accessed 31 October 2017). (These are under review at the time of this publication; please check the website for the latest document.)

Needlestick/sharps injuries

A needlestick/sharps injury is a puncture to the skin or a percutaneous injury. Nurses are at risk of exposure to infections, such as HIV and hepatitis B and C, within their practice due to blood-borne pathogens. Approximately 16% of accidents to NHS staff are caused by needlestick/sharps injuries, and there are ~40 000 reported incidents a year in the UK.[13]

Causes of needlestick/sharps injuries

- Incorrect use of equipment;
- Failure to dispose of used needles properly in puncture-resistant sharps containers;
- Non-use of safety needles;
- Recapping of needles;
- Accidental—resulting from an unexpected movement by the patient.

Reducing the risk of needlestick/sharps injury in practice

- Be aware of, and familiar with, the local needlestick/sharps injury policy which should cover:
  - Education and training;
  - Safe working practices;
  - Safe disposal of devices;
  - Use of safety needles;
  - Procedures in the event of a needlestick injury;
  - Monitoring and evaluation;
  - Procedures for reporting needlestick injuries.
- Undertake any necessary risk assessments, including environment and predictability of patient response.
- Avoid distractions while undertaking the intervention.
- Access training to refresh knowledge and skills in the correct use and disposal of sharps and in respect of infection control.
- Where available, use sharps with built-in safety features, rather than conventional needles.
- Never re-sheathe a needle.
- Promptly dispose of contaminated sharps immediately in sharps collection boxes, and ensure these are not full prior to undertaking a procedure.
- Use appropriate personal protective equipment, i.e. gloves.
- Remain up-to-date with hepatitis B immunization status.

Actions in the event of a personal needlestick/sharps injury

- *Do not suck the injury site.*
- Bleed it.
- Wash it. Decontaminate the wound by rinsing with soap and large amounts of warm water; do not scrub it.
- Dress it with an appropriate dressing.
- Inform your line manager.
- Immediately contact the relevant occupational health department for advice and support regarding appropriate medical investigations/actions.

- Outside of usual office hours, immediate attendance at the nearest minor injury unit or A&E department.
- If you are aware of a significant risk of transmission of an infectious disease, then immediate attendance at the nearest A&E department.
- Complete the relevant accident and/or incident form, as per local policy and procedure.

Actions in the event of witnessing a needlestick/sharps injury

- Provide immediate assistance and support in respect of first aid.
- *Do not suck.*
- Ensure the person contacts the occupational health department and attends the minor injury unit or A&E department, as appropriate.
- Ensure that an accident and/or incident form is completed.
- Provide support for any distress.

Further reading

Health and Safety Executive. *Sharps Injuries.* ℘ www.hse.gov.uk/healthservices/needlesticks/ (accessed 31 October 2017).

References

13 Royal College of Nursing (2013). *Sharps Safety: RCN Guidance to Support the Implementation of the Health and Safety (Sharp Instruments in Healthcare Regulations) 2013.* Royal College of Nursing: London.

Unsafe standards of care

There is continual emphasis in healthcare to improve the quality of care provided and thus to eliminate poor practice, particularly unsafe standards of care. This is achieved through standard settings at different levels, which should be continually monitored. A number of initiatives and strategies have been put in place to do this, e.g. clinical governance, benchmarking, integrated care pathways, care standards, and NSFs. These approaches set safe standards of care, which staff should follow; this is particularly important in the field of intellectual disabilities where clients may have little concept of what safety means.

Unfortunately, due to a variety of reasons, e.g. poor management, lack of competence and training, poorly developed and implemented care plans, and lack of resources, standards may fall short of what is considered safe practice. Areas in intellectual disability nursing that have been known to have had concerns raised regarding unsafe standards of care include:

• Use of restraint;
• Administration of medication;
• Manual handling of clients with profound and multiple learning disabilities;
• Feeding;
• Poor communication;
• Bathing and personal care;
• Developing independent living skills (road safety, cooking, gardening activities, etc.).

(Many of the reasons highlighted above have been identified in abuse inquiries such as those undertaken in Cornwall, and Sutton and Merton Trusts.)[14,15]

As a registered nurse, your first consideration in all activities must be the people in your care, who you should treat as individuals and whose dignity you should respect. Both the NMC (2015) and NMBI (2014) nursing codes of professional conduct indicate that you must raise concerns whenever you come across situations that put patients or public safety at risk.[16,17] Safety must never be compromised, and there is no middle ground with safety. A practice standard is either safe or unsafe; it cannot be just a little bit or moderately safe. Therefore, you should never knowingly engage in practice once it has been deemed to be unsafe. Practice should also always be based on the best available evidence.

As a registered nurse, you are personally accountable for your actions and omissions in practice and you must keep your skills and knowledge up-to-date. You should know the limits of your competence, and you should strive to take part in appropriate training that develops your competence and performance in practice. Safety is everyone's concern and should be promoted as a positive and essential activity. In caring for people with intellectual disabilities, some activities carry inherent risks, which, when properly managed, can help enormously in the development of the client. However, every risk has to be properly assessed, using a risk assessment approach.

A risk assessment should:
- Identify what is unsafe;
- Identify who is likely to be harmed and how;
- Evaluate the risks and put an action plan together;
- Record the steps taken;
- Review the actions taken and revise if necessary.

If you cannot remedy the unsafe standard of care, then you must:
- Act quickly to protect all those likely to be harmed (client, carers, colleagues, and visitors);
- In an emergency, provide care in or outside the work setting, as long as you do not put yourself or others at further risk;
- Follow set procedures for reporting risks and harm (policies, guidelines, health and safety procedures);
- Report concerns regarding the environment of care to an appropriate person and put it in writing;
- Offer reassurance to those in the immediate environment.

Further reading

Health and Safety Executive. ℻ www.hse.gov.uk (accessed 31 October 2017).
Nursing and Midwifery Board of Ireland. ℻ www.nmbi.ie/Home (accessed 31 October 2017).
Nursing and Midwifery Council. ℻ www.nmc-uk.org (accessed 31 October 2017).
NHS England. *Patient Safety*. ℻ www.nrls.npsa.nhs.uk/ (accessed 31 October 2017).
Verita (2015). *Independent Review into Issues that may have Contributed to the Preventable Death of Connor Sparrowhawk*. Verita: London. ℻ www.england.nhs.uk/wp-content/uploads/2015/10/indpndnt-rev-connor-sparrowhawk.pdf (accessed 31 October 2017).

References

14 Commission for Healthcare Audit and Inspection (2006). *Joint Investigation into the Provision of Services for People with Learning Disabilities at Cornwall Partnership NHS Trust*. Commission for Healthcare Audit and Inspection: London.
15 Commission for Healthcare Audit and Inspection (2007). *Investigation into the Service for People with Learning Disabilities Provided by Sutton and Merton Primary Care Trust*. Commission for Healthcare Audit and Inspection: London.
16 Nursing and Midwifery Council (2015). *The Code: Professional Standards of Practice and Behaviour for Nurses and Midwives*. Nursing and Midwifery Council: London.
17 Nursing and Midwifery Board of Ireland (2014). *Code of Professional Conduct and Ethics for Registered Nurses and Registered Midwives*. Nursing and Midwifery Board of Ireland: Dublin.

Recording and reporting

Good record-keeping is an essential component of effective and safe nursing practice. It helps to protect the welfare of clients, identifies risks, promotes high standards, and aids communication. It should also provide a pen picture of the assessment, planning, and delivery of individualized care. Increasingly, records are now being shared with other members of the healthcare team to produce one single comprehensive record of the client's healthcare journey.

There is no single form for recording every incident, although most organizations have standardized forms for various events.

Key features to observe when completing a record

You must

- Do it as soon as possible after the incident has occurred;
- Accurately date and legibly sign the record;
- Be clear, accurate, and concise;
- Follow a methodical and logical sequence;
- Sign, date, and time all entries;
- Ensure it is readable when copied;
- Record in terms that the client can understand;
- Identify risks/problems and actions taken to rectify such areas;
- Provide evidence of assessment, care planning, decision-making, care delivery, effectiveness of treatment, and sharing of information;
- Ensure that if you make an entry in an electronic record, it is clearly identifiable.

You must not

- Make alterations without a record of change;
- Use abbreviations, jargon, or meaningless phrases;
- Make offensive or subjective statements.

If it is appropriate, every effort should be made to involve the person with intellectual disabilities and/or carer in the completion of the record; therefore, it should be written in an understandable format. Increasingly, clients are also being encouraged to look after their own records.

Important points to remember

- Records should be held securely and confidentially.
- When delegating responsibility for completing records, you should ensure that the person is competent to do so (registered nurses remain accountable for doing this).
- In law, the view tends to be that '*if it is not recorded, it has not been done*'.
- Record events on appropriate forms or documents, and avoid making notes on scraps of paper.
- In community settings, you need to be particularly careful when sharing and transporting records. They should be kept securely, and you should ensure that only authorized personnel have access to them.

- There may be occasions where it would be appropriate to share information, e.g. emergencies, safeguarding, national security, and crime prevention. If in any doubt, you must take advice before sharing information with others.
- The loss or damage of records should be reported immediately to the appropriate person.

Access to records

The 1998 Data Protection Act gives clients the right to access their own health records (paper or computer-based records). In some exceptional circumstances, it may not be in the client's best interests for them to view the record made about them. If you make such a decision to withhold information, then a record needs to be made of the reasons for doing so.

The NMC no longer issues specific guidance documentation on record-keeping, as it is now covered in the professional code (NMC 2015).

Further reading

Important and up-to-date information for registered nurses on record-keeping can be obtained from the Nursing and Midwifery Council (NMC) website at ℬ www.nmc-uk.org (accessed 31 October 2017) and from the Nursing and Midwifery Board of Ireland website at ℬ www.nmbi.ie/Home (accessed 31 October 2017).

Barnes J, Jenkins R (2015). Record keeping and documentation. In: C Delves-Yates, ed. *Essentials of Nursing Practice*. Sage: London; pp 251–63.

Nursing and Midwifery Board of Ireland (2014). *Code of Professional Conduct and Ethics for Registered Nurses and Registered Midwives*. Nursing and Midwifery Board of Ireland: Dublin.

Nursing and Midwifery Council (2015). *The Code: Professional Standards of Practice and Behaviour for Nurses and Midwives*. Nursing and Midwifery Council: London.

Complaints

A complaint can be made by anyone, e.g. a service user, advocate, carer, or person affected or likely to be affected in some way by the actions/decisions of an individual or organization. The complainant is usually unhappy about the level of service provided, and they want an answer to their concerns. All organizations should have a complaints procedure for you to follow, and many have complaints personnel who deal with such matters.

There are generally two types of complaints—informal and formal.

Informal complaints

Most complaints are informal and made verbally in person or over the telephone, and can be dealt with on the spot without the need to formalize proceedings. Often an explanation of why things may have gone wrong, and an apology if they did, is all that is needed to satisfy the complainant. Every effort should be made to resolve the complaint at this stage; help may be required from your line manager. If the complaint cannot be resolved at this stage, then you should ask the complainant to put it in writing as soon as possible.

Formal complaints

Formal complaints are made in writing or by electronic means such as by email or text. The complainant needs to write down the exact nature of what they are complaining about. They should be advised that they also need to put down how they would like their complaint to be satisfactorily resolved.

Health professionals, such as doctors, nurses, and midwives, now have a professional duty of candour. This requires such professionals to inform the patient or client when something has gone wrong, to apologize for it happening, and then to put things right. Any short- or long-term ill effects must be fully explained to the patient, family, carer, or advocate.[18] The NMC (2015) professional code states clearly that nurses should respond professionally to any complaints made against them and to use such complaints as an opportunity to reflect on their practice.[19]

General principles when dealing with complaints

You must
- Maintain confidentiality;
- Be polite and courteous;
- Listen carefully to what is being said;
- Act promptly;
- Remain neutral;
- Be fair and open-minded;
- Give a constructive and honest response;
- Cooperate with internal and external investigations.

You must not
- Be angry or annoyed;
- Ignore the complaint in the hope it will go away;
- Make personal judgements about the complainant;
- Make promises that you or the organization cannot keep;
- Treat people detrimentally because they have complained.

Remember that dealing with complaints effectively often leads to improvements in practice. Many of the past and recent inquiries into abuses of people with intellectual disabilities highlighted that complaints were made but were not acted upon or dismissed.[20-22] It was also highlighted that very little information was made available on how to complain or produced in an easy-to-read and accessible format for people using services and their carers and relatives.

People with intellectual disabilities must be supported to make complaints. For example, they may need the support of family and friends or may require the services of an independent advocate. It is important that their complaint should be treated sensitively and without prejudice. It can be very stressful to speak out about aspects of care, particularly against the people providing such care. It should be viewed as good practice to develop client-assertive skills in this area within a culture that promotes client empowerment. A major barrier faced by people with intellectual disabilities is the dismissive attitude of others towards them. All complaints need to be acted on, and the actions taken need to be reported back to the complainant within a specified timescale.

- If an individual wishes to complain about an aspect of the NHS, then they can access information from the NHS website at ℘ www.nhs.uk/choiceintheNHS/Rightsandpledges/complaints/Pages/NHScomplaints.aspx and from the Independent Health Complaints advocacy service at ℘ www.seap.org.uk/services/nhs-complaints-advocacy/
- Members of the public have the right to complain about the fitness to practise of any registered nurse and can do so by contacting the NMC and NMBI or the national care regulator (see ➔ Chapter 16).

References

18 Nursing and Midwifery Council and General Medical Council (2015). *Openness and Honesty when Things Go Wrong: The Professional Duty of Candour.* ℘ www.gmc-uk.org/DoC_guidance_englsih.pdf_61618688.pdf (accessed 31 October 2017).
19 Nursing and Midwifery Council (2015). *The Code: Professional Standards of Practice and Behaviour for Nurses and Midwives.* Nursing and Midwifery Council: London.
20 Committee of Inquiry (1969). *Report of the Committee of Inquiry into Allegations of Ill-treatment of Patients and Other Irregularities at the Ely Hospital, Cardiff.* Cmd 3975. HMSO: London.
21 Commission for Healthcare Audit and Inspection (2006). *Joint Investigation into the Provision of Services for People with Learning Disabilities at Cornwall Partnership NHS Trust.* Commission for Healthcare Audit and Inspection: London.
22 Commission for Healthcare Audit and Inspection (2007). *Investigation into the Service for People with Learning Disabilities Provided by Sutton and Merton Primary Care Trust.* Commission for Healthcare Audit and Inspection: London.

Index